An Atlas of
OPERATIVE LAPAROSCOPY AND HYSTEROSCOPY

THE ENCYCLOPEDIA OF VISUAL MEDICINE SERIES

An Atlas of
OPERATIVE LAPAROSCOPY AND HYSTEROSCOPY

Second Edition

J. Donnez and M. Nisolle

Catholic University of Louvain
Brussels, Belgium

With a foreword by
Alan H. DeCherney
UCLA School of Medicine
Los Angeles, CA, USA

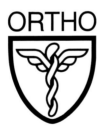

The Parthenon Publishing Group
International Publishers in Medicine, Science & Technology

NEW YORK   LONDON

Published in the USA by

The Parthenon Publishing Group Inc.

One Blue Hill Plaza

PO Box 1564

Pearl River

New York 10965

USA

Published in the UK and Europe by

The Parthenon Publishing Group Limited

Casterton Hall

Carnforth

Lancs LA6 2LA

UK

Library of Congress Cataloging-in-Publication Data

Data available on request

British Library Cataloguing in Publication Data

Data available on request

ISBN 1-84214-089-2

First published in 1994

This edition published 2001

Composition by The Parthenon Publishing Group Limited

Color reproduction by Graphic Reproductions, UK

Printed and bound by Butler & Tanner Ltd., Frome and London, UK

Contents

Part 5: Complications

Section II: Operative hysteroscopy

Members of the Department of Gynaecology

in front of

St. Luc's University Hospital (Catholic University of Louvain)

Brussels, Belgium

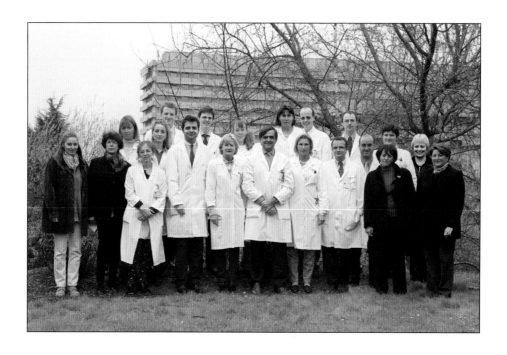

"There is no life without pressure ..."

Brussels, 31 March 2001

List of principal contributors

W. Abdul-Nour
Department of Gynecology
Catholic University of Louvain
Cliniques Universitaires St. Luc
Avenue Hippocrate 10
B-1200 Brussels
Belgium

M. Berlière
Department of Gynecology
Catholic University of Louvain
Cliniques Universitaires St. Luc
Avenue Hippocrate 10
B-1200 Brussels
Belgium

M.A. Bruhat
Gynécologie Obstétrique Reproduction Humaine
Polyclinique Hôtel Dieu
13 Bd. Charles de Gaulle
F-63003 Clermont-Ferrand Cedex
France

M. Canis
Gynécologie Obstétrique Reproduction Humaine
Polyclinique Hôtel Dieu
13 Bd. Charles de Gaulle
F-63003 Clermont-Ferrand Cedex
France

F. Casanas-Roux
Department of Gynecology
Catholic University of Louvain
Cliniques Universitaires St. Luc
Avenue Hippocrate 10
B-1200 Brussels
Belgium

C. Chapron
Gynécologie Obstétrique Reproduction Humaine
Polyclinique Hôtel Dieu
13 Bd. Charles de Gaulle
F-63003 Clermont-Ferrand Cedex
France

F. Chantraine
Department of Gynecology
Catholic University of Louvain
Cliniques Universitaires St. Luc
Avenue Hippocrate 10
B-1200 Brussels
Belgium

D. Dargent
Gynécologie Obstétrique
Hôpital Edouard Herriot
Place d'Arsonval
F-69437 Lyon
France

A.H. DeCherney
Department of Obstetrics and Gynecology
UCLA School of Medicine
10833 Le Conte Avenue 27-112 CHS
Los Angeles
California 90095-1740
USA

O. De Hertogh
Department of Gynecology
Catholic University of Louvain
Cliniques Universitaires St. Luc
Avenue Hippocrate 10
B-1200 Brussels
Belgium

J. Dequesne
Chemin des Croix-Rouges 16
CH-1007 Lausanne
Switzerland

J. Donnez
Department of Gynecology
Catholic University of Louvain
Cliniques Universitaires St. Luc
Avenue Hippocrate 10
B-1200 Brussels
Belgium

O. Donnez
Department of Gynecology
Catholic University of Louvain
Cliniques Universitaires St. Luc
Avenue Hippocrate 10
B-1200 Brussels
Belgium

J.B. Dubuisson
Service de Gynécologie et Obstétrique
Groupe Hospitalier Cochin
Pavillon Baudelocque123 Bd de Port Royal
F-75079 Paris Cedex 14
France

C. Hubinont
Department of Obstetrics
Catholic University of Louvain
Cliniques Universitaires St. Luc
Avenue Hippocrate 10
B-1200 Brussels
Belgium

P. Jadoul
Department of Gynecology
Catholic University of Louvain
Cliniques Universitaires St. Luc
Avenue Hippocrate 10
B-1200 Brussels
Belgium

C.H. Koh
2315 N Lake Dr Ste. 501
Milwaukee
Wisconsin 53211–4516
USA

G. Mage
Gynécologie Obstétrique Reproduction Humaine
Polyclinique Hôtel Dieu
13 Bd. Charles de Gaulle
F-63003 Clermont-Ferrand Cedex
France

A. Münschke
Department of Gynecology
Catholic University of Louvain
Cliniques Universitaires St. Luc
Avenue Hippocrate 10
B-1200 Brussels
Belgium

M. Nisolle
Department of Gynecology
Catholic University of Louvain
Cliniques Universitaires St. Luc
Avenue Hippocrate 10
B-1200 Brussels
Belgium

C. Pirard
Department of Gynecology
Catholic University of Louvain
Cliniques Universitaires St. Luc
Avenue Hippocrate 10
B-1200 Brussels
Belgium

S. Ploteau
Department of Gynecology
Catholic University of Louvain
Cliniques Universitaires St. Luc
Avenue Hippocrate 10
B-1200 Brussels
Belgium

R. Polet
Department of Gynecology
Catholic University of Louvain
Cliniques Universitaires St. Luc
Avenue Hippocrate 10
B-1200 Brussels
Belgium

J.L. Pouly
Gynécologie Obstétrique Reproduction Humaine
Polyclinique Hôtel Dieu
13 Bd. Charles de Gaulle
F-63003 Clermont-Ferrand Cedex
France

J.P. Qu
Department of Gynecology
Catholic University of Louvain
Cliniques Universitaires St. Luc
Avenue Hippocrate 10
B-1200 Brussels
Belgium

R. Rabinovitz
ESC Sharplan Medical Systems
Atidim Science Based
Industrial Park
Neve Sharett
PO Box 13135
61131 Tel Aviv
Israel

H. Reich
245 N Memorial Hwy
Shavertown
Pennsylvania 18708
USA

M. Smets
Department of Gynecology
Catholic University of Louvain
Cliniques Universitaires St. Luc
Avenue Hippocrate 10
B-1200 Brussels
Belgium

M.F. Spada
Department of Gynecology
Catholic University of Louvain
Cliniques Universitaires St. Luc
Avenue Hippocrate 10
B-1200 Brussels
Belgium

J. Squifflet
Department of Gynecology
Catholic University of Louvain
Cliniques Universitaires St. Luc
Avenue Hippocrate 10
B-1200 Brussels
Belgium

B.J. van Herendael
Dienst Gynecology and Obstetrics
ACZA Campus Stuivenberg
Lange Beeldekensstraat 267
B-2060 Antwerpen
Belgium

G.A. Vilos
Department of Obstetrics and Gynecology
St. Joseph's Health Care
268 Grosvenor Street
London
Ontario
Canada

A. Watrelot
Centre de Recherche et d'Etude de la Sterille-CRES
85 Cours Albert Thomas
F- 69003 Lyon
France

A. Wattiez
Gynécologie Obstétrique Reproduction Humaine
Polyclinique Hôtel Dieu
13 Bd. Charles de Gaulle
F-63003 Clermont-Ferrand Cedex
France

C. Wyns
Department of Gynecology
Catholic University of Louvain
Cliniques Universitaires St. Luc
Avenue Hippocrate 10
B-1200 Brussels
Belgium

Foreword

The second edition of *An Atlas of Operative Laparoscopy and Hysteroscopy* by Jacques Donnez and Michelle Nisolle shows a number of significant changes; the text is 20% longer and therefore has been totally rewritten and contains over 850 superb full-color illustrations. The first edition was written in 1994, and it is obvious that many advances have been made in regards to operative laparoscopy and hysteroscopy. Thus, this new text is a timely and a long-awaited addition to the literature.

Technology continues to advance and many chapters have been added, evaluating and instructing on these new technologies, including, for example, robotics and fertiloscopy. Established techniques continue to change and improve, including laparoscopic tubal anatomosis, endometrial ablation and ovarian surgery, to cite just a few.

A burgeoning field in gynecologic surgery is pelvic reconstructive surgery and its cousin, geriatric gynecology. Professors Donnez and Nisolle address this field fully and introduce a number of endoscopic procedures in order to correct these conditions. As the female population ages, this becomes more important and it foretells the disappearance of many procedures that were carried out utilizing older techniques and being replaced by minimally invasive surgery; this is a quiet revolution that is occurring in our field. The urogynecological area is covered, not only as an atlas and a how-to-do-the-surgery book, but also includes information on the pathogenesis, pathophysiology and epidemiology.

In the decade of the 1980s, endoscopic surgery was introduced on a large scale in gynecology. This was followed in the 1990s with perfection of these techniques and some innovation, but, as we move into the 21st century, it is apparent that a revolution has occurred and that gynecologic surgery will be minimally invasive surgery. There are few texts that so adequately provide in-depth information as this one does, helping to prepare us for the future.

Classic textbooks are needed in the field and this is one.

To repeat the success of any endeavour needs the writer to have courage to put forth their own ideas; some may be challenged, some may be controversial, some may be proven to be wrong over time, but, nevertheless, it is imperative that the author be creative and stimulating. There are a number of excellent examples of this on these pages including 'The concept of retroperitoneal adenomyotic disease is born' and 'Douglasectomy – torus excision – uterine suspension'.

Stimulating chapters are written in regard to the treatment of carcinoma with minimally invasive techniques; how this will play out over time is difficult to tell. Obviously, this is a very conservative area; if one allows one's imagination to be unbridled, it would appear that most gynecologic oncologic procedures will be replaced with these techniques in time. These are addressed in an extremely thoughtful manner.

Throughout the book, there is editorial consistency; this makes it easy to read and represents extensive work on the part of the editors. Basic principles are illustrated such as laser physics and operational aspects of instrumentation. Key is the fact that Professors Donnez and Nisolle address complications. The field of gynecologic endoscopic surgery has been remiss in not reporting complications; there are a number of reasons why complications must be reported, including allowing others to recognize and possibly avoid these complications by learning through the mistakes of others.

The contributors represent an international panel of experts with a great deal of experience and wisdom.

The future of gynecologic surgery will definitely be in the realm of minimally invasive endoscopic surgery. It is important for everyone to be knowledgeable on this important ever-improving field. Professors Donnez and Nisolle have provided us with a beautiful, informative and thorough text which is many things – an atlas, a textbook of gynecology, and a surgical manual.

The second edition confirms that this is truly a classic.

Alan H. DeCherney, MD
Professor and Chair
Department of Obstetrics and Gynecology
UCLA School of Medicine
Los Angeles, CA, USA

Laser physics and laser instrumentation

R. Sinai, J. Raif and R. Rabinovitz

INTRODUCTION

The utilization of the laser in advanced modern surgery owes its wide dissemination to the fact that lasers commonly used in industrial, military, commercial or scientific applications interact with biological tissue in such a way that localized and precisely controlled alterations of the cellular structure are effected irreversibly.

In the hands of the skilled surgeon, the laser becomes an instrument capable of inducing desired therapeutic effects, far beyond the scope of conventional surgical tools, such as cold knives or electrocautery probes. The laser enables the surgeon to utilize a variety of operational modalities for the treatment of diseased tissue. Precise incisions can be performed, lesions extending over large areas can be vaporized, and voluminous lesions can be debulked and destroyed by ablation or necrotization. Very often, it is possible to target the therapeutic energy selectively at cells characterized by a well-defined property (e.g. color), implementing the selectivity of the interaction process between the laser and the tissue.

Laser energy can be delivered to tissue in a variety of ways: by contact or from a distance, in conjunction with an operative microscope, through an endoscope, or with the aid of freehand tools.

Finally, laser treatments provide significant advantages, unmatched by competitive techniques; in the majority of cases the operation is largely hemostatic. Thus, the surgeon enjoys the convenience of a dry and clear field, even when operating in an environment of high vascularity. Moreover, contamination of adjacent areas is considerably reduced because of the sealing of blood and lymph vessels. The extent of injury to surrounding tissue is, to a high degree, controllable. Consequently, the risk of postoperative pain, complications or irreversible damage is diminished considerably. In some cases, the recurrence rate of the disease also appears to be reduced. The laser enables the surgeon to reach anatomical structures whose size or location renders them inaccessible to any other known surgical instrument.

The reasons for this impressive procedural variety and wealth of benefits lie in the particular properties of the laser as a special source of energy. In order to achieve the best clinical use with this surgical tool, it is necessary to understand what a laser is, how it operates, and how the parameters that govern its operation can be controlled by the surgeon.

WHAT IS A LASER?

Light as a wave phenomenon

The laser is merely a beam of ordinary light radiation. Visible light, which is a day-to-day experience in our natural environment, represents only one facet of a much broader physical phenomenon known as electromagnetic radiation.

Classical physics regards electromagnetic radiation as a wave phenomenon, much like the waves generated by throwing a stone into a pond or the audible sound waves emitted by a tuning fork (Figure 1). A wave-type phenomenon is manifested by periodic vibrations of physical quantities, such as the height of the pond surface, the air pressure or the electromagnetic field. These undergo a cyclical change in magnitude – the cycle repeating itself, in principle, over an indefinite period of time. In the case of the pond, the surface at each specific location is displaced and elevated above its rest value to a certain maximum displacement – the crest of the wave. Subsequently, the pond surface sags under gravity and a trough is created at the same location, below the same rest value. The downward displacement is equal to the displacement of the crest. The cycle repeats itself, and were it not for the dissipative forces which ultimately return the pond to the rest position, the oscillation would continue *ad infinitum*. Moreover, as a result of the temporal oscillations occurring at one particular location, adjacent areas are also set in motion and the wave propagates over the pond surface,

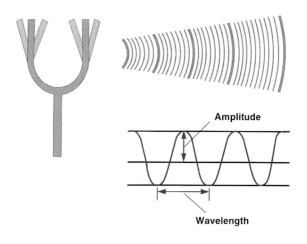

Figure 1 Sound wave generated by a tuning fork

away from the origin of disturbance, creating a sequence of crests and troughs which propagate as spatial oscillations.

A similar phenomenon occurs in the case of sound waves: the crests and troughs of the pond waves are substituted by alternate compressions and rarifications of the gas (air) through which the sound propagates.

The quantity that vibrates in the case of electromagnetic waves is an electrical field (always paired with a concurrent magnetic field to which it is related by a well-defined mathematical relation).

Four basic parameters describe the wave phenomenon:

(1) The magnitude of the displacement represents the intensity of the wave and is a direct outcome of the energy invested in its generation (the impact of the stone on the surface of the pond). This is the *amplitude* (A) of the wave (Figure 1).

(2) The *wavelength* (λ) is the distance between two successive crests or troughs (Figure 1). The unit of measurement is:

$$1 \text{ nm} = \frac{1 \text{ mm}}{1\,000\,000} \quad \text{or} \quad 1\ \mu\text{m} = \frac{1 \text{ mm}}{1000}$$

(Obviously, $1\ \mu\text{m} = 1000$ nm)

(3) The *speed* of propagation (*c*) is measured in cm/s.

(4) The *frequency* (*f*) is measured in Hertz (cycles/s) and represents the number of vibrations per second, occurring at a given spatial location. In the case of sound waves, the frequency translates into the pitch of the sound.

Wavelength (λ), speed of propagation (*c*) and frequency (*f*) are related by:

$$\lambda f = c$$

In the case of electromagnetic waves, the speed of propagation in the void is a universal constant, namely the speed of light:

$$c = 300\,000 \text{ km/s}$$

Consequently, the higher the frequency, the shorter the wavelength.

The electromagnetic spectrum

Electromagnetic radiation of different wavelengths is manifested in diverse physical phenomena:

(1) The wavelength of ordinary radio waves ranges from approximately 1000 m (AM radio waves, hundreds of kHz in frequency) to 1 m (FM radio waves, hundreds of MHz in frequency).

(2) Radar occupies the range of cm waves (frequency in GHz) in the electromagnetic spectrum.

(3) Microwaves, or mm waves used in consumer products, feature frequencies up to 100 GHz.

(4) Infrared light covers the range of wavelengths from 100 μm (very far infrared) to 0.7 μm (near infrared).

(5) Visible light occupies a very narrow region of the entire spectrum of electromagnetic radiation, from 500 nm to 700 nm. The light is visible because the rods and cones located in the human retina can detect it. These are not sensitive to wavelengths outside this range, which remain invisible to the human eye.

(6) Wavelengths shorter than visible light belong to the ultraviolet range: 100–500 nm. Beyond that region of the spectrum, we find X-rays, whose wavelength is as low as 0.1 nm, and nuclear gamma rays of much shorter wavelengths.

The concept of color originates from the interaction of the human retina with the visible region of the electromagnetic spectrum. The sense of color is determined exclusively by the wavelength of the light. The color 'red' lies at one end of the visual spectrum (long wavelength), while 'blue' lies at the opposite end (short wavelength). The white daylight generated by the sun is a mixture of several basic colors and, as such, it is *polychromatic*. It can be dispersed into the basic rainbow colors by a prism (Figure 2). Other sources emit light of a precise individual wavelength. Such radiation sources are called *monochromatic*.

The atomic theory of light

Light is a form of energy generated, emitted or absorbed by atoms or molecules. To emit energy, the atom or molecule must be aroused to an excited energy level above its ground state (in which there is no excess energy to be discharged). Atoms, like human beings, cannot sustain excitement for long periods of time. Consequently, they have a natural tendency to rid themselves of the surplus energy, subsequently emitted in the form of particles or light wave packets called photons. The wavelength of the

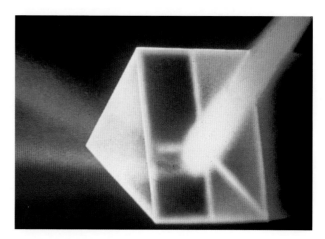

Figure 2 Dispersion of white light by a prism

emitted photon is related to the energy surplus according to:

$$\lambda = \frac{hc}{E}$$

where h is a universal constant called Planck's constant, E is the energy surplus, c is the speed of light and λ is the wavelength.

Each elementary atom or particular molecule possesses distinct and precisely determined excited energy levels. Consequently, different elements will emit photons of different energies, i.e. photons of different wavelengths. All these primary radiations are, therefore, monochromatic. The fact that sunlight is polychromatic indicates that the incandescent matter of which the sun is composed is a mixture of different elements (atoms).

Atoms can be excited by different mechanisms: they can be heated – a fact which on the atomic scale translates into intensification of their state of agitation, leading to an increase in mutual interatomic collisions; they can be excited by electrical discharge – which on the atomic scale means that they are bombarded by fast-moving charged particles; or they can be illuminated by electromagnetic radiation of a characteristic wavelength – which on the atomic scale means that they absorb photons of selective wavelength.

Atoms decay from their excited to ground state levels in two different ways (Figure 3): spontaneous and stimulated emission. The normal mechanism is spontaneous emission. At the completion of a known and calculable period of time – the lifetime of the excited level – the atom returns to its ground state, by emitting a characteristic photon of light.

In the early 1920s, Albert Einstein postulated, and proved, the existence of another mechanism – stimulated emission. An excited atom emits its characteristic photon instantaneously, even before the complete lifetime elapses, if it encounters on its journey a stimulating photon identi-

cal to, and of the same wavelength as, the one that it would have spontaneously emitted, should the lifetime have already elapsed.

Stimulated emission conforms to the following two laws:

(1) The stimulated photon travels in the same direction as its stimulator;

(2) The wave packet incorporated in the stimulated photon synchronizes itself to the wave packet of the stimulator. In other words, the two photons align their crests and troughs to act simultaneously, re-inforcing rather than cancelling one another (which is the case when crests of one wave packet align to the troughs of the other). Photons with aligned crests and troughs are called *coherent*. The end result of stimulated emission is thus a pair of photons which are coherent and travel in tandem in the same direction. Stimulated emission constitutes the basis for the invention of the laser, effected some 30 years after Einstein's discovery.

Basic principle of laser operation

To illustrate the mechanism of laser light generation, imagine a perfectly straight tube or rod, housing a very large quantity of identical atoms or molecules. At each end of the tube, reflecting mirrors are attached: the mirror at one end is totally reflective; at the other end (the output port of the laser tube), the mirror is only partially reflective (90% of the light is reflected back into the tube, while 10% is transmitted through the mirror and exits).

Imagine also that the atoms are excited to an elevated energy level by an external source (such as an illumination device or an electrical discharge). The exact instant of excitation varies from atom to atom and is governed by the rules of chance. This also applies to the spontaneous emission of photons at the end of the lifetime of each atom, which occurs at different points in time, randomly distributed. The emitted photons travel in various directions within the tube. Those hitting the tube walls are absorbed and vanish from the scene. On the other hand, a freshly emitted photon travelling in a direction parallel to the tube axis enjoys the probability of encountering another atom and, thereby, stimulating the emission of an additional photon, coherent with the stimulator and travelling in the same direction – namely, along the longitudinal axis of the tube. The two photons continue their journey, again enjoying the probability of giving rise, by a similar process, to two additional photons – all coherent with one another and all travelling along the same axis. The progression continues on and on, and eight, 16, 32, etc. photons are generated, all travelling in the same direction. This is clearly an *amplification* process that creates a very large flux of light photons.

To enhance the amplification factor further, photons that hit the totally reflective mirror, which is perpen-

Spontaneous Emission

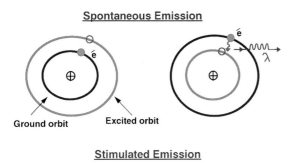

Ground orbit   Excited orbit

Stimulated Emission

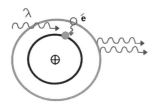

Figure 3 Photon emission modalities

dicular to the tube axis, are reflected back into the tube, and they continue to travel along the same axis in the opposite direction. Every such photon will initiate a similar chain reaction, yielding a stream of coherent photons. Even when the partially reflective mirror is hit, 90% of the photons will be returned to the tube and will continue to contribute to the amplification sequence. The remaining 10% exit at the output port, constituting the source of laser radiation (Figure 4). They represent, in absolute terms, a very intense photon beam produced by the amplification chain.

The above description of the lasing process explains the acronym 'laser': Light Amplification by Stimulated Emission of Radiation. From the above description, we also learn what are the unique properties of laser radiation that differentiate it from ordinary light:

(1)   It is monochromatic because it is generated by a collection of identical atoms, all emitting photons of the same wavelength;

(2)   It is coherent by virtue of the stimulated emission which creates coherent photons;

(3)   The laser beam, being parallel to the longitudinal axis of the tube, features a very low angular divergence. (The divergence is never nil because, in practical terms, there is always some slight misalignment of the mirrors, as they cannot be positioned precisely perpendicular to the axis.)

The clinical implications of the first and last properties are far-reaching. Monochromaticity, and its consequences in surgery, will be discussed in the next section. The low angular divergence of the laser beam enables the surgeon to take full advantage of the capabilities of classical optical systems, and to focus the laser beam precisely on the target area. The laws of physical optics imply that the size of the beam spot on the focal plane of an optical lens system is proportional to the angular divergence of the incoming beam. No matter how perfect the lens system, a largely divergent incoming beam will result in a poorly focused output beam (large spot size). Conversely, a non-divergent or minimally divergent incoming beam, such as the laser, will converge at the focal plane of a high-quality optical system, into a very small spot size (Figure 5). The flux of the photons contained in the beam is the same in both instances. Consequently, in the case of the laser beam, the same flux of photons hits a target which is much smaller. Thus, the energy deposited per unit area is much higher than in the case of ordinary divergent light, and so is the effect on tissue. The laser beam, which in itself is an intense source of energy, is further down-focused to a minuscule spot size to strongly interact with the tissue. Two results are achieved: the target area is finely pinpointed by a very precise beam, and the effect on tissue is very intense.

LASER–TISSUE INTERACTION

Physical effects of the laser on tissue

The laser effect on a tissue sample is one of transmission, reflection, scattering or absorption (Figure 6). The effect on tissue achieved by any laser commonly used in therapeutic medicine is a consequence of its absorption therein. In particular, the energy deposited by most of the commonly used lasers is transformed into heat, thereby obtaining a thermal effect on the tissue.

The types of lasers used in therapeutic medicine are confined to the visible, ultraviolet and infrared regions of the spectrum. Figure 7 presents a list of these lasers with their respective wavelengths.

Excimer lasers (a short form of excited dimers, which are short-lived unstable halogen molecules) emit light in the ultraviolet range (very short wavelength). Their absorption by the tissue leads to photochemical disintegration of large protein molecules, shaving away microstructures from the treated area. For this reason, excimers are

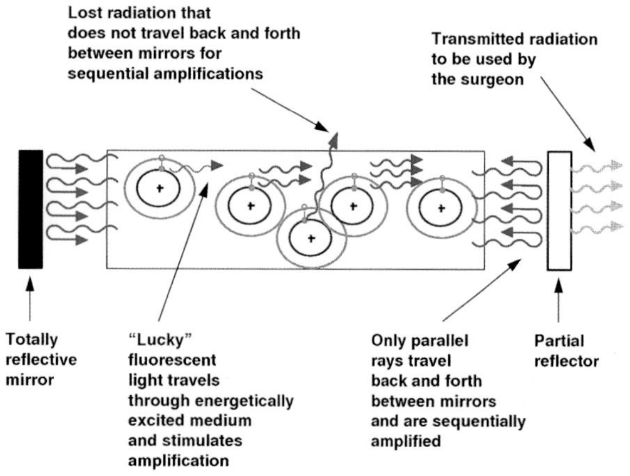

Figure 4 Operating principle of the laser

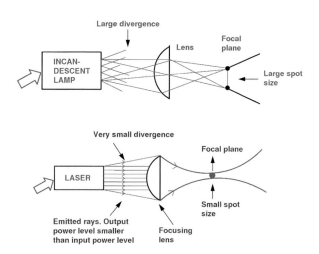

Figure 5 Spot size versus angular divergence of the beam

used in cornea refractive surgery for the treatment of myopia (photokeratomy).

Argon green lasers are used in ophthalmology for treating retinopathies related to vascular disorders of the retina bed. The monochromatic green light is selectively absorbed by the blood oxyhemoglobin, resulting in coagulation of the blood and sealing of the blood vessel.

Yellow dye and copper vapor lasers, also selectively absorbed by oxyhemoglobin, are used in dermatology and cosmetic surgery to treat vascular diseases of the skin, such as port wine stains, telangiectasias and superficial hemangiomas.

The green dye laser is used in urological lithotripsy to pulverize ureteral stones (by a photoacoustic effect). The stones strongly absorb a green light of a very defined wavelength: 508 nm.

The green dye and copper vapor lasers are also strongly absorbed by the skin melanin. Consequently, they are used for treating pigmented lesions, such as café-au-lait or age spots.

Red light is selectively absorbed by the blue and black ink used to infiltrate the skin in the production of tattoos. Certain red-colored lasers, such as alexandrite or ruby, are employed for the removal of these otherwise indelible markings.

The infrared lasers constitute the primary subject of this book. They are widely recognized by the medical community as part of the armamentarium of modern surgery. We will, therefore, elaborate further on their interaction with biological tissue.

Figure 8 illustrates the relative absorption of light in water as a function of wavelength. Because water is a major component of the cellular structure, its interaction with the laser is predominant. The CO_2 laser features a wavelength of 10.6 µm in the far infrared range. It is strongly absorbed by water, as indicated in Figure 8. CO_2 laser radiation is readily absorbed by the first few cellular layers of tissue, constituting the first 100 µm. Consequently, this is a laser used for superficial treatments.

The neodymium : yttrium–aluminum–garnet (Nd : YAG) laser features a wavelength of 1.06 µm (near infrared). Water is completely transparent to this type of radiation. Consequently, the Nd : YAG laser is ideal for the treatment of lesions located in liquid-filled cavities, such as the bladder and the uterus (filled with a distension liquid). The Nd : YAG laser is, however, strongly scattered by the tissue. Penetrating beams are scattered and folded at multiple sites, increasing the effective path length of the beam through the tissue. Nd : YAG laser light, which is absorbed to some degree by the proteins within the tissue bed, deposits energy each time absorption takes place. The end result is the creation of a deep and laterally extended ball of affected tissue, 3–5 mm in diameter (Figures 1–8 and 10).

Contact fibers allow a more controlled incisional effect with Nd : YAG lasers, with only about 1 mm of surrounding thermal necrosis.

More recently, high-power diode lasers have become available, emitting wavelengths of either 810 or 980 nm. Tissue interaction at these wavelengths resembles the interaction of the Nd : YAG laser; therefore, these diode

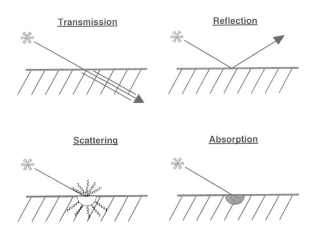

Figure 6 Laser–tissue interaction

NAME	COLOR	WAVELENGTH
Excimers	Ultraviolet	200–400 nm
Argon	Blue	400 nm
	Green	515 nm
532 Yag	Green	532 nm
Krypton	Green	531 nm
	Yellow	566 nm
Dye laser	Yellow Green	577 nm
	Red	630 nm
Helium neon	Red	630 nm
Gold vapor	Red	630 nm
Krypton	Red	647 nm
Ruby	Deep red	694 nm
Diode	Infrared	810–980 nm
Nd : YAG	Infrared	1064 nm
	Infrared	1318 nm
CO_2	Infrared	10600 nm

Figure 7 Lasers used in therapeutic medicine

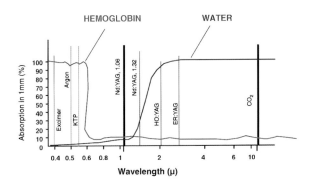

Figure 8 Absorption of laser radiation

lasers are replacing the Nd : YAG lasers in certain medical applications.

The Ho (holmium) : YAG and Er (erbium) : YAG lasers are lasers of the mid-infrared range, whose wavelength is approximately 2 μm. Both are pulsed, which means that the intense stream of photons is delivered during an extremely brief interval. These pulses are instantaneous and, therefore, very powerful, generating a shock-wave in the tissue. They are both absorbed by water, creating vapor microbubbles. The rapid expansion of the bubbles, and their subsequent micro-explosion, create the above-mentioned shock-wave effect. Er : YAG radiation is also strongly absorbed by hydroxyapatite, which has prompted its experimental use in bone surgery or in hard-tissue dental operations.

Thermal effects on tissue

Heat deposited in tissue elevates its temperature. Figure 9 summarizes how the tissue is affected, both visually and biologically, by the increase in its temperature. As long as the temperature does not reach 60°C, there is no visual change in the appearance of the tissue. Up to 45°C, the changes that occur are all reversible. Beyond that temper-

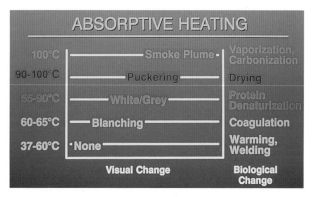

Figure 9 Thermal effects on tissue

ature, some of the cellular enzymes are destroyed and the functional operation of the cell is impaired. Between 60 and 65°C, capillary blood vessels shrink and the tissue undergoes extensive coagulation, showing distinct blanching.

It is noteworthy that the coagulation process induced by the CO_2 laser is rather different from that effected by the Nd : YAG laser. The shrinkage of the capillary vessel caused by the CO_2 laser is a result of vaporization of the water contained in the walls of the blood vessel. If, however, the CO_2 laser beam hits a vessel, it is readily absorbed by the blood liquid at its exit from the initially desiccated wall. Thus, it will never have the chance to hit the opposite wall, leaving the vessel open and, thereby, causing extensive bleeding. Hence, it is important to remember that the sharply focused beams of CO_2 lasers are inadequate for the treatment of highly vascular tissue. Conversely, Nd : YAG lasers are unhindered by the presence of the liquid medium; consequently, they can very effectively accomplish the complete coagulation of the bulk of the tissue. Nd : YAG lasers are excellent coagulators.

Temperatures between 65 and 90°C completely denature the proteins. The tissue turns a whitish color, indicative of dead cells, which subsequently slough off.

At 100°C, vaporization of the cellular water occurs. The high vapor pressure (generated by the rapid expansion of the cellular content that undergoes transformation from liquid to vapor) pushes against the cell membrane, which eventually ruptures, vigorously expelling the resulting fragments in an outgoing plume. The end effect of the entire process is the local removal of tissue matter (Figure 11).

If temperatures are raised much above boiling point, carbonization ultimately occurs.

Energy, power and power density

The rise in temperature of the tissue matter depends primarily on the amount of energy deposited on the target

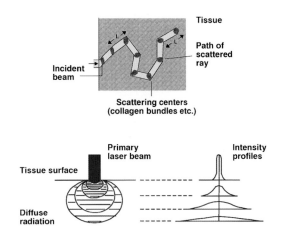

Figure 10 Scattering and penetration of Nd : YAG laser radiation

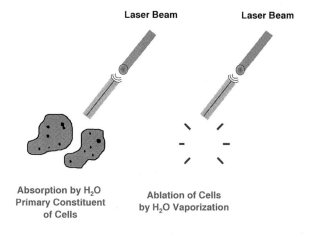

Figure 11 Laser ablation of cells by vaporization

site, as well as on the capability of the tissue to rid itself of heat by dissipating it to surrounding areas. If a large quantity of energy is deposited in the tissue before it can dissipate the heat, a rise in temperature will occur.

Energy, power and power density are the physical parameters that determine the eventual rise in temperature. Energy is measured in joules. Power is the amount of energy delivered per second and is measured in Watts (joules/s). The thermal effect of the laser is local. Thus, the physical quantity which governs the thermal response of the tissue is the amount of power delivered to a unit of area; this quantity is called *power density* and is measured in W/cm^2.

The higher the power density, the more rapid the temperature rise on and around the area where the laser beam impinges upon the tissue. In order to obtain the desired surgical effect, both power and power density can be adjusted easily. All commercial laser systems enable the user to vary the power on tissue in a continuous manner. At constant output powers, power density can be varied with the aid of optical devices, which either bring the laser beam into focus on the target site, or defocus it intentionally (Figure 12).

The shape of the cross-section of the beam in most commercial systems is approximately circular. The diameter of the beam can be decreased or increased by the respective focusing/defocusing method. Reducing the diameter of the beam spot by a factor of two represents a reduction of the spot area by a factor of four, and consequently, a four-fold increase in the power density (Figure 13).

The optical system through which the CO_2 laser beam is delivered incorporates specially designed lenses. This system is responsible for bringing the beam into focus on the tissue at the operative site. For a given optical system at a given power, the maximum power density is obtained when the beam is completely focused.

If the surgical circumstances require lower power densities (see below), the surgeon can achieve this by defocusing the beam, i.e. by increasing the diameter of the spot size and, consequently, increasing its area. Defocusing is normally effected by manually retracting the optical

system from its focused position, or by employing a focusing/defocusing device.

High power densities are required when fine incisions must be performed. Traction is applied to the tissue on both sides of the desired incision and a focused beam is aimed at the required location. The depth of the incision is a function of the power delivered and of the dwell time of the laser on each and every point of the incision. The longer the dwell time, the larger the volume of tissue removed by the laser and, therefore, the deeper the cut. But the dwell time is inversely proportional to the speed of movement of the cutting tool. In short, the depth of the incision increases with the power of the beam and decreases with the speed of movement (Figure 14).

Vaporization may be performed with a defocused beam and high power. However, in this mode, tissue ablation is not well controlled and is accompanied by excessive carbonization and deeper thermal necrosis. A significantly more effective CO_2 laser vaporization technique is based on rapid scanning of a focused beam over the area to be vaporized. This Flashscan™ technology allows extremely uniform, char-free, layer-by-layer vaporization with minimal residual thermal necrosis.

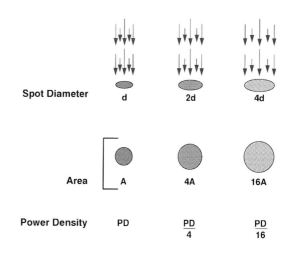

Figure 13 Diameter and area of the spot versus power density

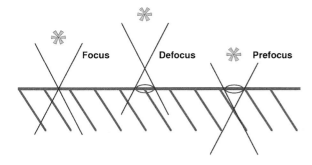

Figure 12 Focusing/defocusing the laser beam on tissue

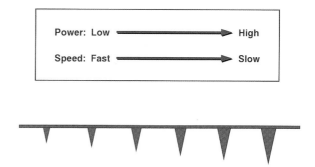

Figure 14 Depth of incision

Finally, in order to coagulate a bleeding point or an oozing area, the surgeon should defocus the laser beam, use low power and gently 'brush' the affected area.

LASER INSTRUMENTATION

CO_2 laser systems and accessories

The CO_2 laser beam is generated by a sealed gas-filled tube. The lasing gas is CO_2 and it is mixed with other types of gases which are required for different technological reasons. The excitation of the CO_2 molecules is effected by an electrical discharge.

One of the limitations of the CO_2 laser beam is that it cannot propagate very effectively through flexible fibers. Consequently, the delivery system ordinarily used in commercial products consists of a lightweight articulated arm, composed of straight, hollow, segmental tubes with reflective mirrors mounted at the joints. Hence, the CO_2 laser beam propagates in straight lines and bounces off each consecutive joint, eventually reaching the target tissue through an optical device attached to the end joint.

As the CO_2 laser is invisible to the human eye, each laser system is equipped with a red helium–neon (He–Ne) laser tube, the direction of propagation of which is coincident with the infrared beam. The red He–Ne beam enables the surgeon to aim at the target area and simulate visually on the tissue, the position and the extent of the therapeutic beam.

Manufacturers offer CO_2 laser units featuring different maximum powers from 15 to 150 W. CO_2 laser systems are composed of:

(1) A laser tube;

(2) A power supply which provides the necessary electrical energy to excite the lasing gas;

(3) A closed-circuit water-cooling system which removes excess heat from the tube and its surroundings;

(4) A control system based on a microcomputer;

(5) An articulated-arm delivery system; and

(6) A He–Ne laser tube.

Figures 15 and 16 show, respectively, a schematic diagram and a photograph of a state-of-the-art CO_2 laser system.

Accessories for CO_2 laser units are offered in different categories:

(1) Handpieces: attached to the end joint of the articulated arm and manipulated by the surgeon during the procedure (Figure 17). Usually, handpieces come in different focal lengths.

(2) Micromanipulators: devices coupled to the laser unit and mounted on the objective of an operative microscope/colposcope (Figure 18). The optical lens

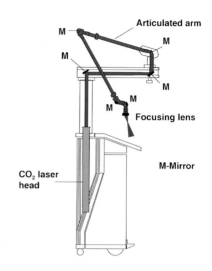

Figure 15 Schematic structure of a CO_2 laser

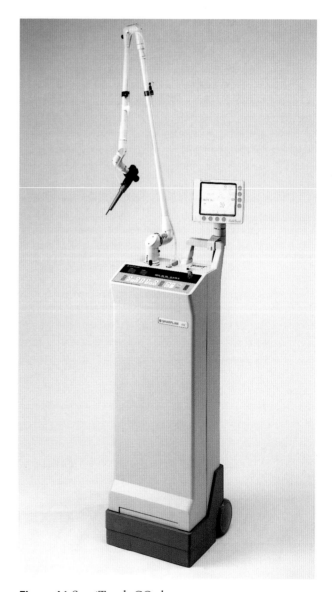

Figure 16 SurgiTouch CO_2 laser system

system enables both the red He–Ne beam and the infrared CO_2 beam to be focused at the desired distance. The surgeon observes the tissue through the objective of the microscope and steers the laser beam directly at the target tissue with the aid of a joystick that controls the gimballing of a reflective mirror.

(3) Rigid endoscopes: devices which incorporate operating channels through which the laser beam travels, as well as coupling devices which constitute the optical interface between the articulated arm of the CO_2 laser and the endoscope. A wide variety of endoscopes are available: laparoscopes (Figure 19), bronchoscopes, laryngoscopes, rectoscopes and anoscopes.

(4) CO_2 laser waveguides: rigid metallic or ceramic tubes through which the CO_2 laser beam propagates (Figure 20). They are either inserted through the operating channel of a laparoscope, or are supplied for freehand surgery to allow access to sites which

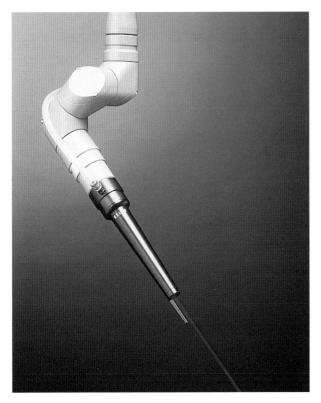

Figure 17 Focusing handpiece

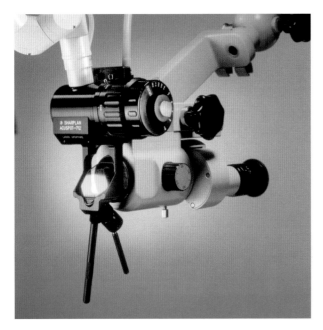

Figure 18 Acuspot micromanipulator mounted on an operative microscope

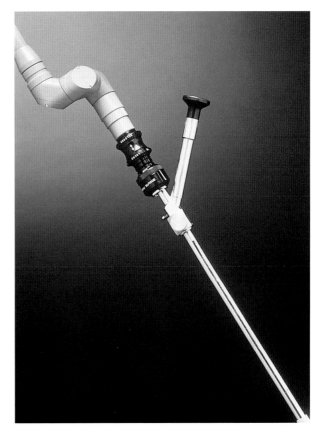

Figure 19 Laser laparoscope with laser coupler

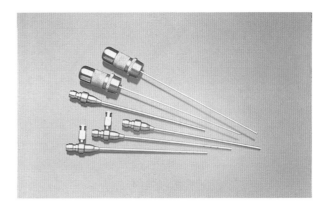

Figure 20 CO_2 laser waveguide set

are difficult to reach (such as nasal cavities when performing turbinectomies). The distal end of the rigid waveguide is brought into close proximity to the tissue and the laser beam is fired.

(5) Flexible CO_2 fibers (FiberLase™): offered by Sharplan, they are a particular type of hollow, flexible waveguide (Figure 21). Flexible fibers are used to enhance the maneuverability of the delivery device, to distance the body of the laser unit from the sterile field and to provide access to anatomical sites which are difficult to reach.

The latest generation of CO_2 lasers employs the SurgiTough Flashscan technology which significantly improves the laser's tissue vaporization capabilities. This technology, introduced by Sharplan, allows uniform, char-free, layer-by-layer tissue vaporization control with minimal residual thermal necrosis. Tissue layers as thin as 100 microns may be removed with extreme precision and excellent visual control.

Nd : YAG laser systems and accessories

The Nd : YAG laser uses a solid-state rod (garnet) in which the neodymium atoms play the active lasing role. The exciting energy is supplied by a flashlight lamp which illuminates the rod. Both are housed in a container called the resonator. The shape of the resonator is ellipsoidal and its inner surface is coated with a highly reflective material. The lamp and the rod are placed at the two focal points of the ellipsoid. The light emitted by the lamp is reflected by the internal coating of the resonator and it is collected, almost in its entirety, by the rod positioned at the opposite focal point (Figure 22).

In contrast to the CO_2 laser, Nd : YAG laser beams propagate well through commercially available glass fibers, very much like visible light. The propagation is effected by a chain of internal reflections occurring at the boundaries of the glass fiber. Hence, the delivery devices used in Nd : YAG lasers are a variety of fibers (see below) equipped with a connector that attaches to the output port of the laser system.

Manufacturers offer Nd : YAG laser units featuring different maximum powers, from 40 to 100 W. Nd : YAG laser systems are composed of:

(1) A laser head or resonator;

(2) A power supply, which furnishes the flashlight lamp with the necessary electrical energy;

(3) A closed-circuit water-cooling system, further chilled by a radiator which removes excess heat from the resonator;

(4) A control system, based on a microcomputer;

(5) A He–Ne laser tube; and

(6) An output port optical assembly to which the external glass fiber is attached.

Figures 23 and 24 show, respectively, a schematic diagram and a photograph of a state-of-the-art Nd : YAG laser system. The accessories offered with Nd : YAG systems are almost exclusively fibers. They fall into two categories:

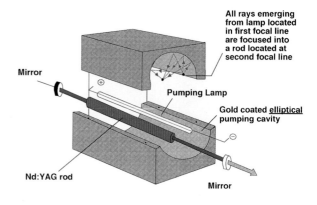

Figure 22 Internal structure of a Nd : YAG laser resonator

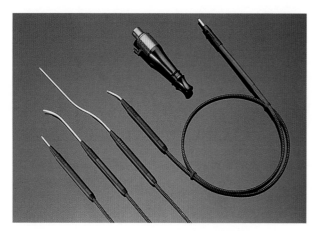

Figure 21 FlexiLase™–CO_2 laser flexible fiber set

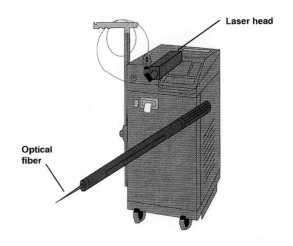

Figure 23 Schematic structure of a Nd : YAG laser

(1) Non-contact fibers, whose distal end is flat and highly polished. They operate at a short distance from the tissue, in order to create deep coagulation (Figure 25). A well-known example of their use is the treatment of superficial bladder tumors, where the fibers are inserted through a cystoscope. Non-contact fibers have no incision capability. These fibers are usually reusable. However, after a limited number of surgical procedures, they must be re-polished with the aid of a special polishing kit.

(2) Contact fibers, featuring a sharpened sculpted conical tip. The laser radiation is concentrated at the very narrow tip and the fiber functions like a hot knife, capable of performing fine incisions when in contact with the tissue (Figure 26). Moreover, the tapered fiber prevents the rays from progressing forwards, while enabling their exit through the sides of the tip. The end result is that the forward penetration is reduced, much as in the case of the CO_2 laser. The side radiation, on the other hand, produces

a hemostatic effect on the lateral surfaces of the wedge created by the incision. Contact fibers are used in a variety of configurations for freehand (Figure 27) and endoscopic applications. They feature different tip shapes (conical, hemispherical) and different diameters (400, 600, 800 and 1000 μm). They are offered as disposable, single-use, sterilized fibers.

Recently, new types of fibers have been introduced onto the market. These fibers possess a polished distal face which is inclined with respect to the fiber axis. This angle enables the fiber to emit the laser beam at right angles to its long axis. Employed transurethrally, these fibers are used to treat benign prostatic hypertrophy by coagulating the adenoma. Another type of fiber, emanating lateral diffusive radiation from an elongated segment located at its distal end, is used for the interstitial laserthermia of benign and malignant lesions.

Diode laser systems and accessories

Diode lasers include semi-conductor material as the active medium. They include either AIGaAs, which emits at a nominal wavelength of 810 nm, or InGaAs which emits at a nominal wavelength of 980 nm, as their active medium.

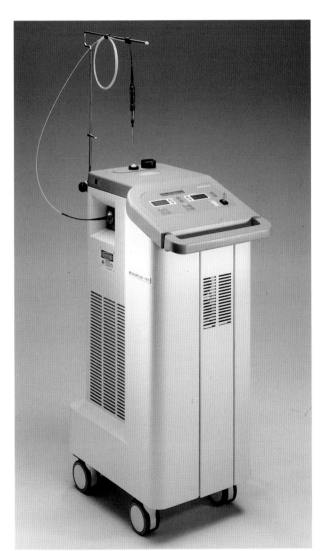

Figure 24 Nd : YAG laser system

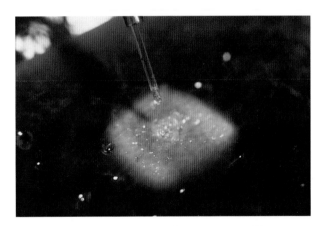

Figure 25 Coagulation effect of a non-contact fiber

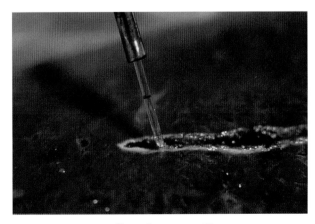

Figure 26 Cutting effect of a contact fiber

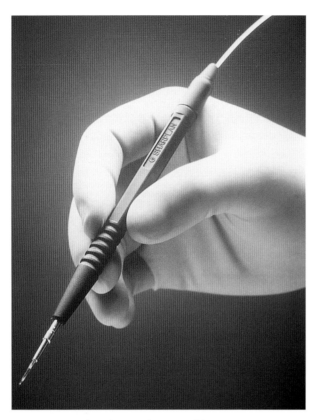

Figure 27 Freehand conical contact fiber

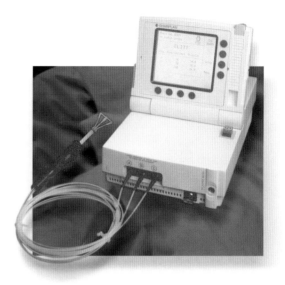

Figure 28 GyneLase™ diode laser system

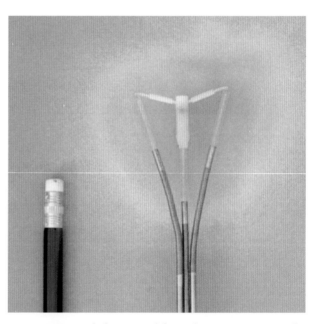

Figure 29 Laser light emitted from the GyneLase™ applicator. The disposable handset consists of three optical-light diffusers designed to conform to the shape of the uterus

These wavelengths can be changed slightly by adding aluminum or indium, respectively.

Tissue interaction at these wavelengths resembles the interaction of the Nd : YAG laser, with slightly smaller depth of penetration into tissue. The fiber optic delivery system is also similar to that of the Nd : YAG laser. The size of the diode lasers is much smaller than Nd : YAG lasers, they can be tabletop or wall-mounted units. Diode lasers are very reliable – the diode chip can last for 10 000–25 000 hours of use, and they are nearly maintenance-free. Therefore, diode lasers are replacing the Nd : YAG lasers in certain medical applications.

The GyneLase™ diode laser system offered by Sharplan is a compact tabletop system of 21 W, with 830-nm wavelength and a disposable applicator (Figure 28). The system is a second-generation, global endometrial ablation system. It simultaneously emits a laser beam through three separate parallel channels. Each channel delivers equal laser power, directing the laser beam to the target through an optical fiber and a disposable applicator.

The applicator (Figure 29) includes three optical light diffusers that are designed to transmit laser light in all directions to destroy the endometrial tissue employing Endometrial Laser Intrauterine Thermo-Therapy (ELITT™). The side diffuser arms can be manipulated individually by the operator to conform to the shape of the uterine cavity. Unlike other global endometrial ablation techniques, ELITT does not require direct contact with the endometrium to induce coagulation. The laser beam is

diffused inside the uterine cavity In all directions it, therefore, reaches the entire uterine cavity, including such inaccessible areas as the cornua. The 830-nm wavelength laser beam penetrates the uterine wall to a necessary depth and is absorbed by the hemoglobin. The absorbed light is then transformed to heat; it warms the endometrium and causes coagulation. The inherent light-scattering inside the endometrium positively contributes to the uniformity of the light distribution and resultant coagulation.

The endocervical canal is dilated to 7 mm, and the light diffuser's applicator is inserted into the uterus. The opera-

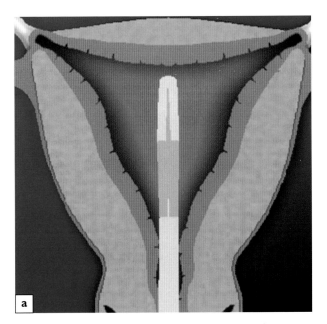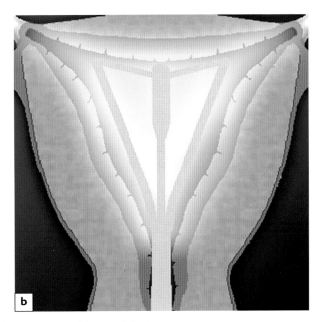

Figure 30 Simulation showing the ELITT procedure. (a) Handset insertion; (b) use of the laser

tor advances the distal end of the applicator (Figure 30a) to the fundus and adjusts the side diffusers, forming a butterfly-wing contour that conforms to the shape of the intrauterine cavity. The laser is then activated for a 7-min pre-programmed cycle (Figure 30b) that automatically terminates at the end of the cycle. The 830-nm diode laser is preset for 7 min, delivering the following pre-programmed laser intensities: 20 W during the first 90 seconds, 18 W during the next 90 seconds, and 16 W during the final 240 seconds, yielding a total energy of 7020 J at an average power density of less than 1 W/cm^2 per diffuser. No user setting or applicator maneuvering is required. The extended wings are then refolded and the applicator is removed from the uterus.

Instrumentation and operational instructions

J. Donnez and M. Nisolle

ENDOSCOPIC INSTRUMENTS

Telescopes

Telescopes used in laparoscopy are available with different viewing directions, either with or without an instrument channel. The various telescopes and their application range are briefly described below (Figure 1).

(1) 0° straightforward telescope: this telescope has the greatest application range, because it facilitates orientation and conveys an impression of the area inspected. The direction of view corresponds to the natural approach and the usual perspective. The 0° telescope is generally preferred in gynecological interventions;

(2) 30° forward-oblique telescope: this can be rotated to enlarge the field of vision. Use of the 30° telescope can be advantageous during dissection in the Douglas pouch;

(3) 45° telescope.

Telescopes without instrument channels are used in the majority of cases in gynecology, as they give a better overview and offer better image resolution.

However, in some cases, it may be more reasonable to use telescopes with an integrated instrument channel (telescope with parallel eyepiece, see Figure 1, top). These telescopes are generally 0° straightforward telescopes. The diameter of the instrument channel is 5–7 mm; thus, a correspondingly large instrument can be inserted. Additional devices can also be connected to this laparo-

scope, such as a CO_2 laser. The best example of this is for laparoscopic sterilization; tissue fragments or biopsy specimens can also be extracted through the telescope trocar with the aid of a grasping forceps, which is introduced through the telescope's instrument channel.

A disadvantage of using telescopes with instrument channels is the deterioration in the image quality. This is due to the lower light intensity that can be picked up by the video camera, when compared with telescopes that do not have an instrument channel.

A Verres optical needle with insufflation can be used in some difficult cases (Figure 2a and b) or in order to perform 'mini-laparoscopy'.

Trocars

Small passage-ways through incisions in the abdominal wall are created with the aid of trocars. The use of disposable trocars is clearly in decline in the era of cost reduction. In general, trocars with different diameters are used in surgical endoscopy. The standard sizes (Figure 3) are 5.5, 11, 12, 15 and 22 mm.

Spherical and flap valves make it possible to change operating instruments quickly, as the change can be carried out without activating the valve mechanism. *Trumpet valves* are mostly found in telescope trocars. The telescope is protected from contamination by tissue and blood particles during insertion by pressing the trumpet valve. *Sharp, pyramidal trocar tips*, on the other hand, can be positioned relatively easily. The sharp edges can sometimes damage smaller blood vessels and other organs.

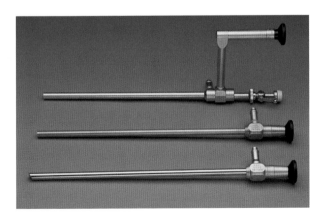

Figure 1 Telescopes used in gynecology. From top to bottom: telescope with instrument channel, 30° and 0° telescopes (Karl Storz)

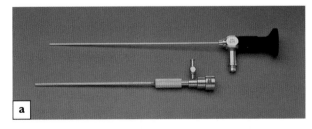
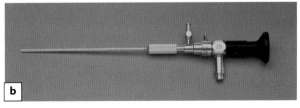

Figure 2 (a) and (b) Optical Verres needles

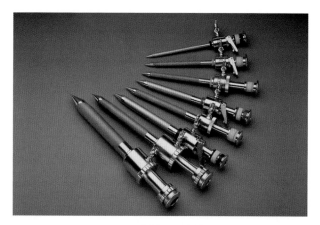

Figure 3 Trocars are available in different sizes and with various valve mechanisms (Karl Storz)

There are great differences between trocar tips (Figure 4a and b). By using spherical blunt trocar tips, the blood vessels are pushed aside and protected to a large degree. Sometimes, however, greater pressure has to be exerted during insertion. Since the skin incision for the auxiliary puncture is carried out under transillumination and the puncture itself is in full view, the choice of the trocar tip here can be regarded as being of secondary importance. Better protection to prevent the trocar slipping out of the intraperitoneal space is provided by sheaths with screw threading (Figure 5a). However, these cause increased trauma, both of the abdominal wall and of the peritoneum. Trocar reducers facilitate the surgery (Figure 5b).

INDIVIDUAL INSTRUMENTS

Grasping forceps

Atraumatic dissecting and grasping forceps (Figures 6 and 7) are particularly suitable for grasping and the liberation of hollow organs. The claws are fashioned so that trauma to the tissue should not occur.

Atraumatic grasping forceps (multi-serrated) are designed for atraumatic and precise tissue grasping, such as of ligaments during diagnosis. Grasping forceps (2 × 4 teeth) are used to grasp and liberate solid organs. Sturdy grasping forceps are indispensable in surgical endoscopy; in the case of endoscopic cyst extirpation, for example, they can help to fix the ovary capsule properly and remove the cystic bag.

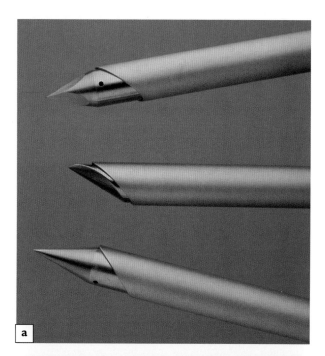

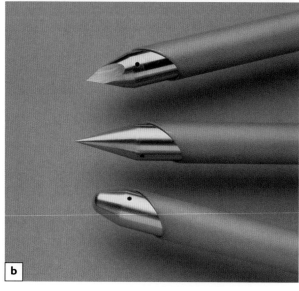

Figure 4 (a) and (b) Various trocar tips (Karl Storz)

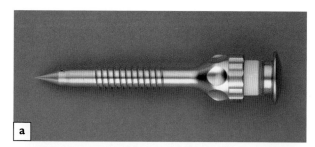

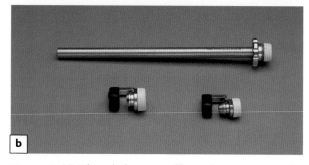

Figure 5 (a) Threaded trocar offers a better grip in the abdominal wall (Karl Storz); (b) various trocar reducers (Karl Storz)

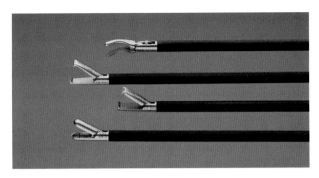

Figure 6 Grasping forceps. From top to bottom: Kelly grasping forceps (atraumatic), Manhes grasping forceps (atraumatic), Manhes grasping forceps (traumatic), biopsy forceps (traumatic) (Karl Storz)

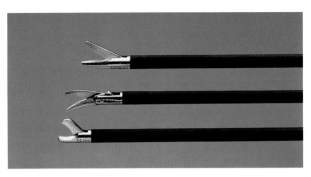

Figure 8 Laparoscopic scissors. From top to bottom: straight scissors, curved scissors and hook scissors (Karl Storz)

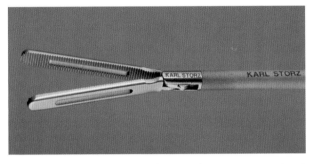

Figure 7 Intestinal grasping forceps, diameter 5 mm (Karl Storz)

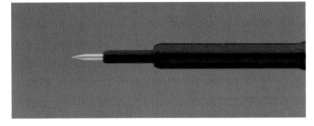

Figure 9 Monopolar high-frequency needle (Karl Storz): the tip of the needle can be retracted into the sheath

Dissecting and grasping forceps (claw forceps) are particularly designed for grasping solid structures (e.g. myomas). These forceps are used where trauma of the tissue does not have to be particularly considered.

Scissors

Hook scissors (Figure 8) are particularly suitable for transecting ligature fibers and for tissue transection. Delicate dissection can be carried out with straight scissors. Curved scissors, in general, have the same features as straight scissors. In some cases, they are easier to dissect with, because the curvature changes the viewing angle.

Coagulation instruments

The tip of a monopolar high-frequency needle (Figure 9) can be retracted into the sheath. Various bipolar forceps (Figures 10 and 11) can be introduced through a 5-mm trocar.

Additional instruments

Other 5-mm instruments are needed for laparoscopic surgery, for example, probes (atraumatic) (Figure 12, top), a needle for cyst puncture, and an irrigation-suction probe.

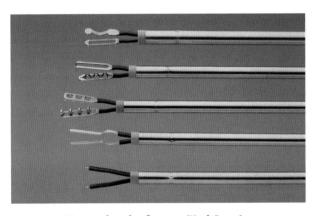

Figure 10 Various bipolar forceps (Karl Storz)

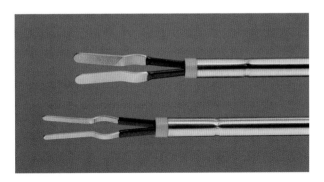

Figure 11 3-mm wide bipolar forceps (Karl Storz)

Biopsy forceps

Biopsy forceps (Figure 13) are used during diagnostic laparoscopy in cases of malignant diseases (ovarian cancer: before chemotherapy or during second-look laparoscopy) and in cases of benign disease such as endometriosis.

Needle holder

Figure 14 shows the 5-mm needle holder and the 3-mm needle holder.

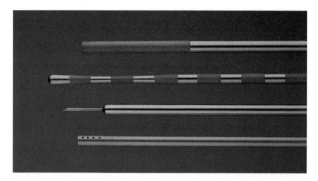

Figure 12 Additional instruments. From top to bottom: blunt puncture probe, atraumatic probe, needle for puncture, irrigation suction probe (Karl Storz)

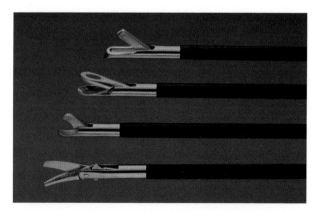

Figure 13 Biopsy forceps and scissors (Karl Storz)

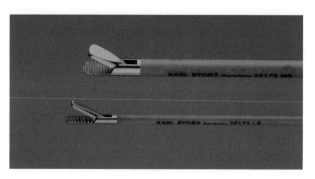

Figure 14 5-mm and 3-mm needle holder (Karl Storz)

Myoma holder

Figure 15 shows the 5-mm and 10-mm myoma holders.

Atraumatic forceps

Atraumatic forceps (Figure 16a and b) are used for prehension of the Fallopian tube or the ureter.

Intestinal probe

The intestinal probe (Figure 17) is used to push back the intestines in order to achieve a good view.

MORCELLATORS

In the past, laparoscopic surgeons were faced with the difficult problem of extraction of tissue and were often obliged to perform a suprapubic mini-laparotomy or a transvaginal extraction. The first substantial improvement was the development of the manual morcellator

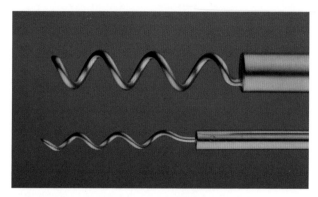

Figure 15 5-mm and 10-mm myoma holders

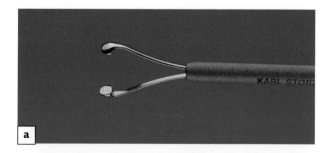

a

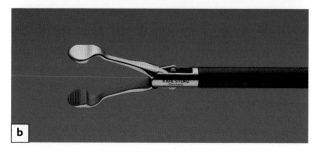

b

Figure 16 (a) and (b) Atraumatic forceps

(Semm–Wisap). Much force and time were necessary, depending on the consistency of the tissue.

In collaboration with Storz, R. Steiner developed the electromechanical morcellator (Figure 18) consisting of a motor-driven cutting tube. The speed can be selected in three stages. It is possible, with the aid of this morcellator, to extract even large amounts of tissue from the abdomen, using the size 11 trocar, in a short period of time. With 15-mm and 20-mm trocars (Figure 19), large quantities of

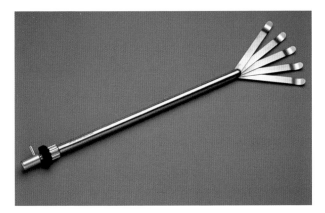

Figure 17 Intestinal probe

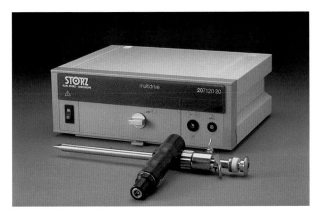

Figure 18 Electromechanical morcellator (R. Steiner, Storz)

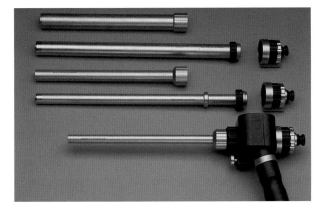

Figure 19 11-mm, 15-mm, 20-mm trocars for tissue morcellator (Karl Storz)

tissue can be extracted in this way within a few minutes. Because of the good cutting quality of the rotating morcellator, the tissue structure is minimally damaged. It also enables a reliable histological examination to be carried out.

CO₂ GAS INSUFFLATOR

A pneumoperitoneum must be created so that the organs and tissues are separated from each other and rendered accessible. Conventional gas insufflators are sufficient for a purely diagnostic laparoscopy. However, in surgical laparoscopies performed today, compensation for considerable volume losses must be made in a relatively short period of time, e.g. due to frequent suction of irrigation solutions using high-performance irrigation/aspiration units. High-flow CO_2 insufflators (Figure 20) are a basic prerequisite for surgical laparoscopy, as they offer the only option to reduce operating time to a minimum. Electronically controlled insufflators have become the preferred choice in this respect.

The insufflator's display, which the surgeon should always be able to see, gives continuous information on the following data:

(1)   The patient's intra-abdominal pressure (actual value). The pre-selected maximum intra-abdominal pressure should never exceed a value of 15 mmHg!

(2)   Flow rate: the required set value for the patient's intra-abdominal pressure must be pre-selected. The maximum flow rate (set value) must be pre-set;

(3)   Total CO_2 insufflated volume;

(4)   Gas reserve.

Some of the state-of-the-art insufflators (Figure 20) are equipped with an integrated preheating element which keeps the insufflated gas at body temperature, in order to prevent the patient from cooling down. In order to avoid the disadvantages of CO_2 insufflation, gas-less laparoscopy could be an alternative.

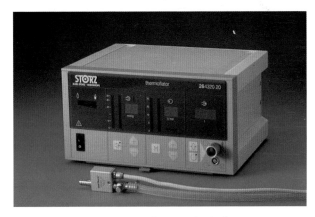

Figure 20 Thermo-insufflator (high-flow CO_2 gas insufflator) (Karl Storz)

IRRIGATION/SUCTION UNITS

Within the framework of diagnostic and surgical laparoscopy, it is often necessary to drain fluids and irrigate wound surfaces until they are clean and can be viewed adequately. Sometimes, effective irrigation can also be used for adhesiolysis (hydrodissection). Suction is performed either with an additional suction pump or by means of a central vacuum supply system. It is important that these solutions are used at body temperature.

In summary, the equipment for an operating theater for endoscopic surgery (laparoscopy) should comprise (Figure 21):

(1)   Gas insufflator;

(2)   Light source;

(3)   Video camera unit (Figure 22);

(4)   Suction irrigation device;

(5)   Monitor and documentation system (video recorder, printer or photodigitalizer for digital image storage).

THE OPERATING LAPAROSCOPE

Laser endoscopy has already been widely used in otolaryngology and gastroenterology and it is currently being investigated for clinical use in orthopedics, urology and gyne-cology. Prototype instruments for CO_2 laser laparoscopy appeared independently on three continents (developed by Bruhat and colleagues, Tadir and co-workers, Daniell and Brown, and Kelly and Roberts). The initial prototype proved to be inadequate because of loss of CO_2, accumulation of intraperitoneal smoke, and an inability to keep the beam focused in the center of the channel. Fortunately, with the development of new laparoscopic instrumentation for CO_2 laser use, the majority of technical problems have been overcome. Instruments have been developed and tested in order to ensure safe, easy, accurate and effective procedures.

The operative laparoscope for laser laparoscopy is an instrument which is 11 mm in diameter with a 7.3-mm operative channel. To use the CO_2 laser through the laparoscope, the operator simply swings the articulated arm of the laser over the operative field and attaches the BeamAlign™ coupler to the operative channel of the laparoscope (Figure 23) or to a special second-puncture laser delivery tube.

The laser coupler assembly (Figure 24) consists of the following:

(1)   Direct coupler housing. This contains a mechanical alignment mechanism which must be pre-adjusted for the specific operating laparoscope used. Once adjusted, alignment remains for multiple uses with the same laparoscope.

(2)   Interchangeable lens housing:

(a)   200-mm working distance lens housing to match beam focal length to nominal length of standard second-puncture tube, giving spot size diameter of 0.64 mm; laser beam may also be defocused;

(b)   300-mm working distance lens housing to match beam length to nominal length of single-puncture tube (and optional 300-mm second-puncture tube), giving spot size diameter of 0.70 mm; laser beam may also be defocused;

(c)   Each lens housing has a groove around it for convenient attachment of the sterile drape.

(3)   Laser arm attachment.

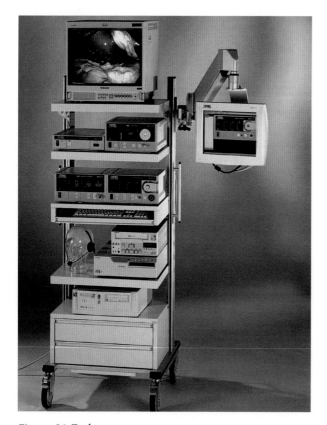

Figure 21 Endocart set-up

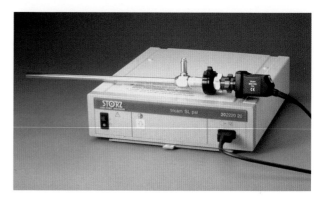

Figure 22 Endoscopic camera unit (Karl Storz)

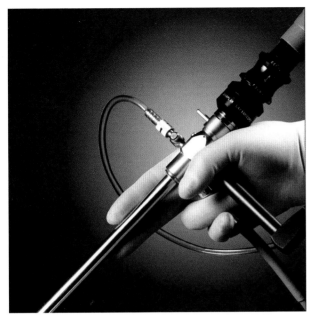

Figure 23 The single-puncture operative laparoscope for laser laparoscopy. The direct coupler containing the focusing lens is attached to the operative channel of the laparoscope

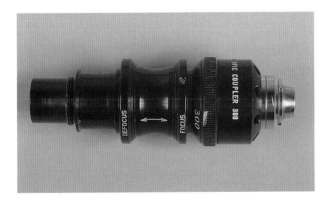

Figure 24 Laser 'direct' coupler (Sharplan, ESC)

SURGITOUCH

The Flashscanner is a miniature optomechanical scanner compatible with any Sharplan microprocessor-controlled laser (Figure 25). It consists of two almost, but not exactly, parallel folding mirrors. Optical reflections of the CO_2 laser optical beam from the mirrors cause the beam to deviate from its original direction by an angle θ (Figure 26). The mirrors constantly rotate at slightly different angular velocities, thereby rapidly varying with time between zero and a maximal value, θ_{max}. By attaching the laparoscope focusing coupler of focal length F to the Flashscan, the CO_2 laser generates a focal spot which rapidly and homogeneously scans and covers a round area of diameter $2F\tan\theta_{max}$ at the distal end of the laparoscope. For a single-puncture laparoscope ($F = 300$ mm), θ_{max} was selected to provide a round treatment area of 2.5 mm

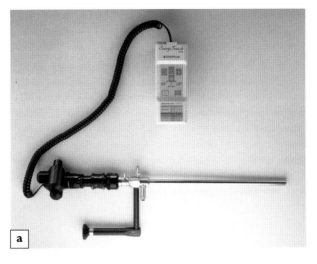

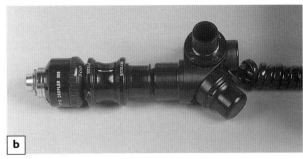

Figure 25 (a) SurgiTouch optomechanical scanner consisting of two almost, but not exactly, parallel microprocessor controlled mirrors; (b) Flashscanner connected to the direct coupler (Sharplan, ESC)

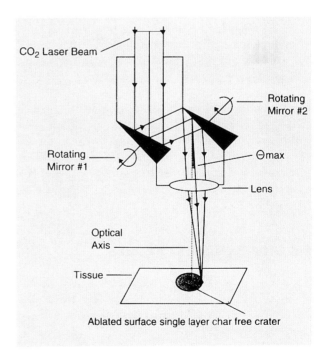

Figure 26 Optical reflections of the beam from the two mirrors cause it to be deflected from its original direction by $\theta°$

diameter. The rapid movement of the beam over the tissue ensures a short duration of exposure on individual sites within the area and very shallow ablation.

Since therapeutic CO_2 medical lasers typically generate a focused beam smaller than 0.9 mm in diameter at the laparoscope working distance, the use of the SurgiTouch with a laser power level of 30 W will generate an optical power density of greater than 50 W/mm² on tissue. This is considerably higher than the threshold for vaporization of tissue without residual carbon charring (the threshold for char-free tissue ablation is about 30 W/mm²). The time required for the SurgiTouch to homogeneously cover a 2.5-mm round area is about 100 ms. During this time, the 30-W operating laser will deliver 3000 mJ to the tissue. Since the typical energy required to completely ablate tissue is about 3000 mJ/mm³, keeping the laparoscope precisely on a single site for 0.1 s will generate a clean char-free crater of 0.2 mm in depth.

SMOKE EVACUATION

To allow a flow of fresh CO_2 down the beam channel, the CO_2 insufflation tubing is attached to this operative channel; the flow of CO_2 from the insufflator displaces smoke, which can reduce the power of the beam from the laser channel, and prevents fogging of the mirror and lens in the black coupler.

To evacuate smoke, a Verres needle can be inserted suprapubically under direct vision and transillumination, directing it towards the target site and connecting it to the smoke evacuation system. Auxiliary kits are available for synchronizing smoke evacuation with laser emission, providing automatic smoke evacuation from the target site. With the automatic smoke evacuation kit installed, smoke evacuation begins with actual laser emission and remains active for 3 s after the laser emission ceases.

If smoke disturbs the viewing field, the smoke evacuation flow can be increased, taking care not to cause a collapse of the pneumoperitoneum. The equilibrium state will be reached when the insufflation system is able to provide the amount of gas that the smoke evacuation port is releasing. If the smoke evacuation kit is installed, the expulsion of gas (smoke) can be regulated using a sterile infusion drip kit.

SECOND-PUNCTURE PROBES

The present second-puncture probe which permits the use of the CO_2 laser with the laparoscope is a double-ring probe that is 8 mm in external diameter with 5.6-mm operating channel. The second-puncture laparoscope is based on two tubes. The inner tube contains the operating channel and the insufflation port as well as the locking device for securing it to the outer tube. Two distinct outer tubes are provided: open-end and hook-tipped (Figure 27).

The outer tube includes a smoke evacuation port with stopcock. This assembly provides the user with a double-lumen second-puncture laparoscope that is easily disassembled for cleaning purposes. The hook-tipped outer tube is recommended for use in clinical situations that require a backstop to protect healthy tissue beyond the treatment site. The probe attaches to the same laser coupler assembly that is used with the operative laparoscope. A 200-mm working-distance lens is then used.

WAVE GUIDES

Rigid stainless-steel CO_2 laser waveguide probes (Figure 28) are also available. The probe is attached to the articulated arm of a CO_2 laser system. Optical transmission through these probes is not affected by manipulating the articulated arm. A conventionally used helium–neon (He–Ne) aiming beam is transmitted coaxially through the probe. The short focal length (focal place: > 0.4 mm < 2 cm from the probe top) yields a beam that defocuses within a short distance beyond the focal plane. This is expressed by a sharp drop in power density and may serve as an optical backstop.

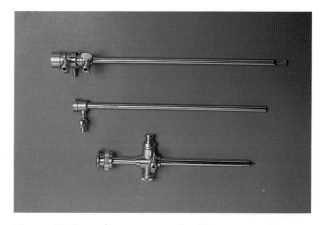

Figure 27 Second-puncture probe. From top to bottom: hook-tipped, open end, trocar

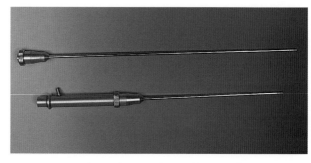

Figure 28 Rigid stainless-steel CO_2 laser probes

ACCESSORIES

Third-puncture probes are shown in Figure 29. The following operating instruments were developed in our department in collaboration with the Storz Company:

(1) Atraumatic probe;

(2) Hook for fimbrioplasty;

(3) Probe with backstop for use in vaporizing adhesions near the blood vessels;

(4) Smoke suction and rinsing tube;

(5) Double-channel probe for rinsing the pelvis and for suction.

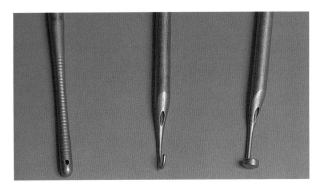

Figure 29 Third-puncture probes: left, atraumatic probe; center, hook for fimbrioplasty; right, probe with backstop. An inner channel is used for rinsing the operating field (Karl Storz)

3

Robotics in endoscopy

R. Polet, M. Nisolle and J. Donnez

Laparoscopic surgery has benefited greatly from the technological developments of the last 20 years. Paradoxically, as patient comfort has increased with minimally invasive surgical procedures, the surgical comfort of the operator has decreased due to the particular working conditions of endoscopic surgery. This problem was not addressed while the range of indications for laparoscopic surgery was being explored.

Today, the use of cameras, self-regulated insufflators, new light sources, new trocar designs and new multifunctional instruments demonstrates the ongoing and highly desirable trend towards increasing the comfort of the laparoscopic surgeon. As the array of what can be done in laparoscopic surgery and what should not be done has become clearer, it is time to think about improving surgical comfort.

ERGONOMICS IN SURGERY

Ergonomics is the scientific study of people at work with the aim of improving accuracy, productivity, training, satisfaction and safety. Its relevance to surgery seems obvious, although it has been applied less often to surgery in a formal way than to other forms of work. Ergonomics in surgery aims to increase the surgeon's comfort in his environment: this attainment of comfort comes through the surgical instrumentation and the workspace (physical ergonomics), cognitive ergonomics (how humans handle information) and organizational ('macro')ergonomics (how actors in the operative room work together).

Assistance is part of the instrumentation and poses two ergonomic issues: the loss of autonomy of the operator and the dependence on a variable human parameter, subject to skill, fatigue and availability variations.

ASSISTANCE IN LAPAROSCOPIC SURGERY

One of the constraints of laparoscopic surgery is the need to work with an assistant, experienced if possible. The assistant manages the operative visual field and helps to hold the instruments. He is actually the eye of the operating surgeon. Problems of co-operation naturally arise between the two, limiting concentration and restricting the eye–hand co-ordination of the surgeon. If the quality of assistance is not what was expected, surgery is less comfortable. In fact, the quality of the assistant goes hand in hand with the quality of the surgery.

Because of the narrowness of the endoscope, the view obtained through the laparoscope and transmitted to the video screen only represents part of the surgical field; the loss of the global view of the operative field creates some difficulty in space orientation for the surgeon. To center the operative field, the telescope must be moved along the tissue of interest. Initially, the telescope was manipulated by the surgeon himself. By doing this, the surgeon sacrifices one hand to the visual control of his operation. Manipulation of the laparoscopic instruments (laparoscopic scissors, forceps, cautery, suction–irrigation cannulas), visually controlled through the telescope, is carried out with only one functional hand. This means that the surgeon operates endoscopically with one hand only, the other instruments being delegated to an assistant, whose quality and level of interest may be very variable.

An alternative that emerged to counter this flaw was to assign manipulation of the laparoscope to an assistant; in such a situation, the surgeon gains more fluency and speed in his surgery, recovering the control of two hands working together. Unfortunately, the management of his optical field is dependent on the qualities of the assistant, whose capacity for anticipation is not always optimal; not uncommonly, the assistant is unaware of what the next step of the operation will be. As a solution, the surgeon often operates with a colleague but, considering the loss of time and money spent on surgical assistance, this solution is not optimal.

The ideal solution, therefore, is to restore to the surgeon *personal control of his own two hands and eyes without intermediates*.

Scope holding: the Lapman Project

In 1995, we launched a project to design a laparoscope-holding system able to answer, in real time, to the surgeon's commands. Static laparoscope holders do exist but are associated with a serious flaw: the impossibility of moving the endoscope without putting down one of the two operative instruments held by the surgeon. The static laparoscope holder gives the most stable image on the video screen but is unable to follow dynamically, in real time, the changes in the operative field required by the surgeon. The idea of a dynamic laparoscope holder able to displace the endoscope along the three axes under the command of an ergonomic control unit was conceived. This laparoscope manipulator was developed in collaboration with the firm Medsys (Gembloux, Belgium).

Table I Classification of laparoscopic artificial assistance devices

---

A. Laparoscope holders: hold the laparoscope only

(1)   Static: the surgeon moves the laparoscope holder manually

Examples: static holders

           Kronner

           Passist

           Siska

(2)   Dynamic: the surgeon moves the laparoscope holder by voice, finger, or head control

Examples: Aesop (Computer Motion): voice

           ImagTrack (Olympus): finger

           Lapman (Medsys): finger

           Endosista (Armstrong): head

           FIPS

B. Laparoscope holders and instrument manipulators

Zeus (Computer Motion)

Da Vinci (Intuitive)

Together with development of the manipulator, an ergonomic external control unit was developed. The question was to find which neuromuscular function could be used to achieve command of six degrees of freedom, corresponding to displacement in three dimensions. A foot pedal requires eye control and can be uncomfortable in the long run, as noted by Mettler and colleagues[1]. Besides, the foot is often already used to control coagulation. Voice interface is attractive but limited by two drawbacks: the answer to the order takes longer, slowing down the operation when the surgeon needs to move frequently, and the impossibility of moving obliquely. The fingers of the left hand were finally chosen because they belong to the surgically minor hand, whose function in dissection is limited to traction, retraction and irrigation, relatively trivial tasks in comparison with their potential.

General description

The Lapman (Figures 1 and 2) is inexpensive technology, based on electromechanical control of brakes regulating the displacement of a series of articulated arms constructed to cover the three dimensions of space. The assistant, of low bulk and mobile on motorized wheels, comprises a rolling base and a sterile autoclavable shaft, which comes connected to the scope through an easy-release system. The assistant displaces the shaft in the three dimensions, translating the displacement of the laparoscope connected to it. A laser pointer indicates the geometric center of the assistant.

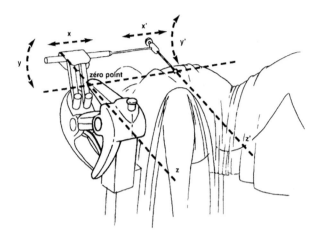

Figure 1 Lapman: principle

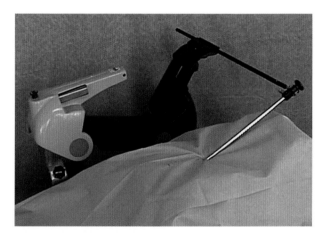

Figure 2 Lapman: external view

The human–machine interface – the hand control (Figure 3) – is a small, embedded electronic circuit, that has been moulded on the palm of the author to raise the thenar eminence towards the fingers in their natural flexed position. Six knobs corresponding to the six directions are distributed on the pad, which can be disposed along two schemes according to personal preference: three rows of two buttons, occupying the last three fingers, or two rows of three buttons, occupying the last two fingers. The unit attaches to the index finger under a sterile glove. Pressing a button leads to a radiofrequency emission that is recognized by the equipment's receiver. Pressing several buttons at once according to a dedicated scheme enables set-up actions to be realized during the calibration phase, such as switching on the laser pointer, backward/forward, upward/downward movements of the whole device or putting the arm in the neutral position. This pad is autoclavable and the batteries allow 1 h of uninterrupted activation. The set-up phase on the right side of the patient is rapid; approximation of the scope holder on the umbilicus requires a 2-min laser calibration.

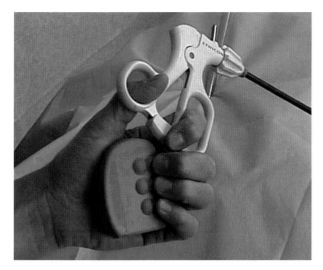

Figure 3 Lapman: hand control (comes under the glove)

As there is a learning curve to become familiar with the position of the buttons on the pad, software was developed allowing navigation in a three-dimensional pelvic environment using a palm-pad joystick connected to the serial port of the surgeon's office personal computer; it is then possible to train effectively out of theater.

Advantages

This laparoscopic manipulator has several advantages. It provides the surgeon with a steady image and gives an immediate response to the surgeon's command, positively influencing the fluency of the operation. Steadiness is obviously useful for suturing and helps in orientation. Besides restoring autonomy of vision, it allows work in conditions of reduced personnel; solo surgery for straightforward cases is carried out in very comfortable conditions, the only function for the circulating nurse being manipulation of the uterus from below. Compared to other laparoscopic assistance systems, the Lapman is not cumbersome, is easy to move on its rolling base and, for these reasons, could surely be labelled 'nurse-friendly'. The electromechanical technology is simple and robust; it is also by far the cheapest of all the engine-driven laparoscope holders ever produced. The polyvalence of the Lapman must be underlined as it allows one to perform abdominal surgery by rotating the Lapman cranially and permits operation from either side of the patient; several cholecystectomies have been performed so far with remarkable ease.

In common with all laparoscope holders, the dynamic scope holders do not cope well with the necessity of frequent moving on the target (as the movements are sequential, not oblique). These situations are encountered in extensive adhesiolysis cases, large structures (e.g. large uteri, ovarian cysts) and in operations covering two remote fields (laparoscopic promontofixation). At present, not all procedures should be tried using automated laparoscope

holders. However, compared to other modalities, the Lapman has the essential characteristic of responding instantaneously to the surgeon's command and is important on two levels: first, it will probably behave better in operative fields with a frequently moving scope; and second, it is safer as the release of the knob stops the move instantaneously. So far, nearly all laparoscopic procedures in 50 operations have been performed.

Indications in gynecological surgery

Considering the present version of the hand control, we would suggest that the Lapman is indicated in reduced personnel conditions for straightforward uncomplicated cases of laparoscopic surgery, which include, in gynecology, all adnexal surgery and small- to medium-size uterus surgery (myomectomy, laparoscopic subtotal hysterectomy (LASH), laparoscopic hysterectomy (LH)) and, in digestive surgery, gallbladder and hiatal surgery. Future developments of the hand control, by increasing the ergonomic design, will enable the surgeon to operate on more complex pathologies in restricted personnel conditions and will probably also elicit profound satisfaction in reoperating bimanually with his own visual operative field control.

Other laparoscope holders

Passive laparoscope holders

Several laparoscope holders are available on the market today. They attach to the side rail of the operative table. Their use essentially depends on the resistance to movement they can provide and the facility to change position comfortably. These holders can also be used to hold instruments. The TISKA endoarm[2,3] has been widely investigated and gives surgeons a great deal of satisfaction. Also worthy of note is the Kronner telescopic arm laparoscope holder (Figure 4); pressing an electronic control attached to the camera releases the joints for quick position changes. The position is held by gas pressure available in the operating room.

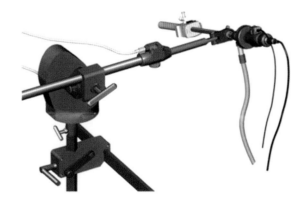

Figure 4 Kronner laparoscope holder

Passive laparoscope holders offer steady images and substitution with human assistance when needed.

Active laparoscope holders

To move in the operative field, passive laparoscope holders need to be moved by the surgeon's hand; this interrupts his concentration and limits eye–hand co-ordination. Besides providing steadiness and a substitution for human assistance, these devices have been developed to offer simultaneous vision and instrument control, as is the case in classic surgery.

The machines differ in technology, some being much more expensive than others, and in the interface used for command. Ideal characteristics should take into account cost, robustness, cumbersomeness, set-up time, user-friendliness of the control unit and response time.

Aesop 3000 (Computer Motion). Aesop (Figure 5) has come up with several control units: foot, hand and voice. Comparative studies tend to consider voice as being better than the other options[1,3-5]. Aesop 3000 is a voice-controlled surgical robot imitating the form and function of the human arm. By orally introducing simple spoken commands, the robotic arm moves the scope in the three dimensions of space. The response is almost instantaneous. Speech-recognition technology requires the surgeon to accustom the system to his voice. Each order must be specifically introduced, for the machine not to become confused with the background theater noise. The displacement in space is the sum of simple displacements and obliquity is not achieved. This model was inspired by robotic technology, which makes it the most expensive in its category, although cost-effectiveness has been demonstrated[6].

Endosista 2 (Armstrong). This system (Figure 6) holds a conventional laparoscope and camera and moves them in

sympathy with the surgeon's head, which it tracks using a headband pointer; thus, a glance at the right-hand side of the monitor causes the camera to pan in that direction. The robot only moves if the surgeon presses a footswitch, allowing different head movements at other times[4].

FIPS. The FIPS (Figure 7)[3,7] is a remote-controlled arm capable of moving a rigid endoscope with about 4° of freedom, while maintaining an invariant point of constrained motion coincident with the the trocar puncture site through the abdominal wall. The system is driven by means of a speaker-independent voice control or a finger-ring joystick clipped onto the instrument shaft close to the handle. When the joystick is used, the motion of the endoscope is controlled by the finger tip of the operating surgeon, which is inserted into the small ring of the controller in such a way as to make the motion of the fingertip correspond directly to the motion of the tip of the endoscope.

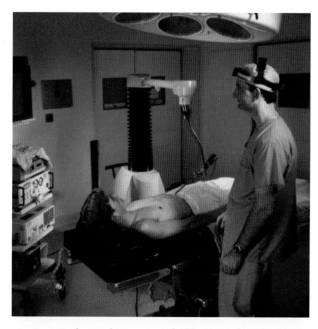

Figure 6 Endosista laparoscope holder (interface: head tilt)

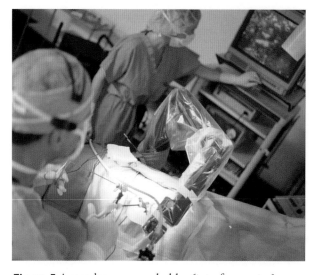

Figure 5 Aesop laparoscope holder (interface: voice)

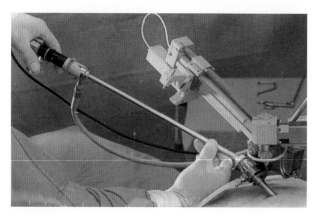

Figure 7 FIPS laparoscope holder (interface: voice or finger)

ImagTrack (Olympus). A 13-mm integrated camera/laparoscope with 80° visual field is inserted intraumbilically (Figure 8)[8,9]. Inside this immobile field (the laparoscope stands still), a mobile CCD chip is displaced in the x–y axis, under voice or fingertip control through a unit attached to the handle of the left instrument. In/out is obtained by a zooming effect. This system has already proven its feasibility in plain laparoscopic surgery. Advantages are the rapid manipulation of the lens displacement. The inability to approach organs physically could result in a reduced sense of depth perception. The integrated aspect of the camera/scope makes multi-use of the camera for other forms of surgical endoscopy impossible.

Other. There has been a very active interest in this field and other systems have been conceived, some that are still under development. Self-guided robotic control (SGRCCS)[10] is based on color tracking. The tip of one instrument is marked with a special color and the camera is programmed to follow this unnatural dye, moving the laparoscope holder so that the color always stays in the operative field. Blood does not significantly interfere. The inconvenience is that this instrument must always be in the field.

Instrument manipulation

Associated with the automated scope holder, there has been extensive development in the robotic enhancement of instrument manipulation itself. The instruments are supported by robotic arms and no longer by the human hand; the surgeon operates from a console at a distance from the patient, in the same or another room, in the same hospital or even from one in another country, through Internet connections.

The concept at the heart of this development is somewhat different: it answers the need of making some fine movements even more precise, essentially microsuturing, and not the concept of solo surgery, as the set-up and the change of instruments require the presence of an assistant at the side of the patient anyway.

Two companies have produced very proficient systems. In the Zeus (Computer Motion) (Figure 9), the surgeon is seated at an ergonomic workstation where he manipulates handles designed to resemble conventional surgical instruments. The surgeon's hand movements are translated and scaled into precise micromovements at the operating site. The Da Vinci (intuitive) surgical system (Figure 10) consists of a surgeon's console, a patient side-cart, a camera arm and proprietary instruments. At the console, the surgeon is seated viewing a three-dimensional image (two three-chip cameras, one for each eye) of the surgical field, with the instrument controls at the tip of his fingers; the wrists are naturally positioned relative to the eyes.

Technology developed in this field is far more sophisticated and (very) costly, monopolizes space, requires regular maintenance and special training of the operating room staff. However, the performance is outstanding in terms of quality and ease; these machines enhance the dexterity of the surgeon by reducing the camera moves, eliminating the tremor of the surgeon and scaling the motion. Distal articulation on the distal shaft of the instruments recreates the wrist function inside the abdomen,

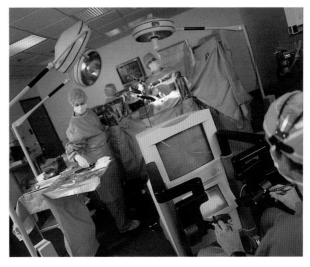

Figure 9 Zeus robot

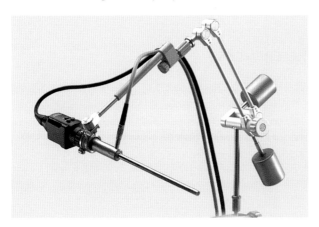

Figure 8 ImagTrack laparoscope holder (interface: finger)

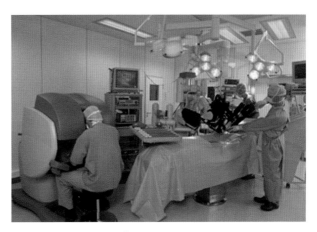

Figure 10 Da Vinci robot

adding a dimension not available with the 'chopstick' instruments used generally in laparoscopic surgery. This definitely helps in suturing small diameter structures, i.e. (re)anastomoses, vessels, tubes, ureters.

Although it is of formidable quality, the proportion of laparoscopic surgery requiring such suturing proficiency is minor. In gynecology, tubal reanastomosis appears to be the only reasonable indication[11,12], but so far this indication probably does not warrant the cost–benefit ratio. The future of these expensive devices is probably in endoscopic cardiac surgery, and, to a lesser extent, urology, gastro-intestinal tract surgery and basically all intracavitary surgery requiring microsuturing.

Fully integrated operating room

Several companies are integrating the management of the operative laparoscopic surgery theater suite into a fully surgeon-controlled environment. Insufflation, light source, coagulation, camera control, image capture, operative protocol edition, theater lighting, and internet and tele-phone consulting are centralized at the surgeon's command through PC technology controlled by voice or by a sterile-draped tactile touchscreen. Surgical robotic companies are busy integrating their robot products into this type of technology, maximizing the concept of surgi-cal ergonomy. It seems intuitively reasonable to think that our future theater suites will look very much like this!

The concept of solo surgery (Figure 11)

The development of surgeon-controlled laparoscope holders has an interesting implication: it allows the surgeon to operate in restricted personnel conditions for straightforward uncomplicated procedures. Adnexal surgery of moderate size (5–6 cm) and subtotal hysterec-tomy cases of (sub)normal size are ideally suited to laparo-scopic solo surgery, because the organ target is mobile and the amount of scope manipulation is somewhat limited. In the event of reduced personnel resources, these artificial arms render these procedures possible; solo-surgery sessions can therefore be performed in emergency cases (bleeding ectopic pregnancy, acute adnexal pathology) or planned on an elective basis, grouping, for example, trans-hysteroscopic resections and simple laparoscopic surgery cases. Table 2 lists the procedures which may be performed under these conditions.

There is no doubt that working conditions in laparo-scopic surgery will evolve in the future towards better comfort. It is hard to keep thinking that straightforward basic laparoscopic cases will always need two operators; staff shortages should not be an obstacle to the perfor-mance of endoscopic surgery. In this respect, the future developments in the field of artificial assistance need to be followed with great interest.

Table 2 Indications for the Lapman in laparoscopic solo surgery

Adnexal surgery (ovariectomy, adnexectomy, salpingo-tomy, salpingectomy, ectopic pregnancy, ovarian cystectomy)

Small- to mid-size laparoscopic hysterectomy (LH, LASH)

Myomectomy (subserosal)

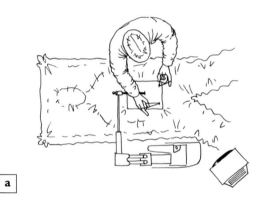

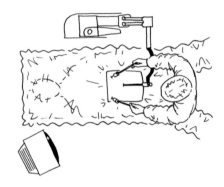

Figure 11 Solo surgery with the Lapman (a) in gynecology, (b) in abdominal surgery

REFERENCES

1. Mettler L, Ibrahim M, Jonat W. One year of experi-ence working with the aid of a robotic assistant (the voice-controlled optic holder AESOP) in gynaeco-logical surgery. *Hum Reprod* 1998;13:2748–50
2. Shurr MO, Arezzo A, Neisius B, *et al.* Trocar and instrument positioning system TISKA. An assist device for endoscopic solo surgery. *Surg Endosc* 1999;13:528–31
3. Arezzo A, Ulmer F, Weiss O, *et al.* Experimental trial on solo surgery for minimally invasive therapy.

Comparison of different systems in a phantom model. *Surg Endosc* 2000;14:955–9

4. Yavuz Y, Ystgaard B, Skogvoll E, *et al.* A comparative experimental study evaluating the performance of surgical robots aesop and endosista. *Surg Laparosc Endosc Percutan Tech* 2000;10:163–7

5. Mettler L. Robotics versus human golden fingers in gynaecological endoscopy. In Ben-Rafael Z, Shoham Z, eds. *Proceedings of The First World Congress on Controversies in Obstetrics, Gynecology and Infertility,* Prague, Czech Republic. Monduzzi Editore, 1999:152

6. Dunlap KD, Wanzer L. Is the robotic arm a cost-effective surgical tool? *AORN J* 1998;68:265–72

7. Buess GF, Arezzo A, Schurr MO, *et al.* A new remote-controlled endoscope positioning system for endoscopic solo surgery. The FIPS endoarm. *Surg Endosc* 2000;14:395–9

8. Niebuhr H, Born O. Image Tracking system. A new technique for safe and cost-saving laparoscopic operation. *Chirug* 2000;71:580–4

9. Kimura T, Umehara Y, Matsumoto S. Laparoscopic cholecystectomy performed by a single surgeon using a visual field tracking camera: early experience. *Surg Endosc* 2000;14:825–9

10. Omote K, Feussner H, Ungeheuer A, *et al.* Self-guided robotic camera control for laparoscopic surgery compared with human camera control. *Am J Surg* 1999;177:321–4

11. Falcone T, Goldberg JM, Margossian H, *et al.* Robotic-assisted laparoscopic microsurgical tubal anastomosis. *Fertil Steril* 2000;73:1040–2

12. Degueldre M, Vandromme J, Thi Huong P, *et al.* Robotically assisted laparoscopic microsurgical tubal reanastomosis: a feasibility study. *Fertil Steril* 2000;74:1020

Anatomy in relation to gynecological endoscopy

4

S. Ploteau and J. Donnez

In gynecology, as in other surgical fields, an excellent knowledge of human anatomy is necessary. Surgical progress makes this even more pertinent; laparoscopy requires, more than ever, a thorough knowledge of all the relationships between anatomic structures. If one injures the ureter, uterine artery or large vessels or if intraperitoneal bleeding occurs, it is necessary to be able to react quickly and to convert to open surgery. Experienced surgeons possess the required skills, but younger practitioners with less extensive anatomic knowledge could experience serious difficulties.

Laparoscopy reveals the undeniable aspect of anatomy as a tool of work. Without perfect knowledge of the different structures encountered during dissection, and particularly those which one would prefer not to encounter because of the dangers they evoke, laparoscopy can become hazardous due to the surgeon's lack of awareness.

We are not about to go over all the anatomic data concerning the pelvis; this information can be found in all the anatomic textbooks and, in any case, it is well known. What is required is the ability to identify, without hesitation, all the structures grasped or isolated during dissection. We will simply call back to mind some anatomic notions to ensure a safe pelvic approach during laparoscopy, and present some anatomic points which highlight potential dangers and require particular attention during surgery. In this chapter, we will describe the different steps of gynecological laparoscopy and some recent surgical techniques such as TVT (tension-free vaginal tape) and the anatomic basis of pelvic or perineal pain. For each stage of surgery, we will explain the dangerous elements which should inspire only one instinct in the surgeon: vigilance. In practice, we will describe certain strategic notions which should be perfectly understood before beginning laparoscopy, whatever the pathology: pelvic wall anatomy, pelvic cellular tissue, ureteral and broad ligament relationships.

INSUFFLATION AND PRIMARY TROCAR INSERTION

Pneumoperitoneal needle placement should be performed with rigor because it is responsible for 90% of vascular and visceral injuries. It is advisable to use a blunt needle with a perforated mandrel, mounted on a spring, to avoid any unwelcome surprises. After making the cutaneous incision, the abdominal wall is raised, particularly in thin patients, to distance the large vessels (except in cases of previous surgery in this area). For the same reason, needle placement should be perpendicular to the stretched abdominal wall, which corresponds to an angle of 45° from the horizontal.

The pneumoperitoneal needle penetrates the abdominal cavity, crossing several successive layers (Figure 1). At the umbilicus, the aponeurosis is stuck to the peritoneum and is therefore pierced in one go. Further down, on the subumbilical linea alba, the peritoneum is not stuck to the aponeurosis and one can feel the two successive jolts as the needle pierces the aponeurosis and the peritoneum. Tactile identification of these jolts is essential in order not to place the needle between the peritoneum and the aponeurosis and so induce an awkward extra pneumoperitoneum, and also so as not to advance the needle through the viscera or a vessel, when the peritoneum has already been crossed.

At this stage, there are many potential hazards and the surgeon must remain extremely vigilant at all times. During their abdominal passage, trocars can injure numerous structures. Concerning the insufflation needle, it is very important to be aware of the position of the umbilicus because of the risk of major visceral and vascular injury. The umbilicus most often projects towards the L4 (in 67% of cases), that is to say, at the level of the most anterior point of the lumbar lordosis. In fact, the umbilicus is situated opposite the aortic bifurcation in 80% of cases, to within 2 cm. The most dangerous situation is observed in thin patients when the umbilicus is perpendicular to the aortic bifurcation or, in 50% of cases, perpendicular to the left common iliac vein which crosses the promontory near the midline.

In dorsal decubitus, with flexed legs, the stretched aorta tends to move away from the abdominal wall because of sagging of the lumbar lordosis. With age, as well as in obese patients, the umbilicus tends to descend and its relation to the aorta is altered.

The insufflation needle may injure the following organs: large vessels that are even more vulnerable as they are against bone structures, the omentum, the small intestine, the transverse colon, the sigmoid and, more rarely, the left side of the liver and the stomach. For this reason, insufflation and needle insertion should be performed only after assurance that the patient's stomach and bladder are empty.

In case of doubt concerning the presence of adhesions, especially if there is a median subumbilical scar, it is recommended that insufflation be performed in the left hypochondrium area, two fingers' breadth from the costal

1 At the level of the umbilicus

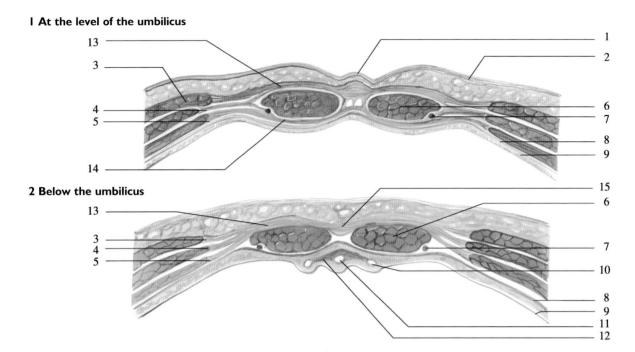

2 Below the umbilicus

1 Umbilicus	6 Rectus abdominis muscle
2 Skin	7 Epigastric artery
3 Aponeurosis of external abdominal oblique muscle	8 Transversalis fascia
4 Aponeurosis of internal abdominal oblique muscle	9 Peritoneum
5 Aponeurosis of transversus abdominis muscle	10 Medial umbilical ligament

11 Urachus (Median umbilical ligament)
12 Umbilical prevesical fascia
13 Anterior layer of rectus sheath
14 Posterior layer of rectus sheath
15 Linea alba

Figure 1 Transverse section of the abdominal wall

border, to avoid a large spleen on the lateral side of the rectus abdominis muscle. This is an area of little depression where adhesions are uncommon.

When insufflation has started, one must be vigilant at all times so as to be immediately alerted if a needle is not in the right position. With the pneumoperitoneum established, the subumbilical trocar can be carefully introduced.

ANCILLARY TROCAR PLACEMENT

Ancillary trocar placement requires the Trendelenburg position. This position forces back the bowel, increases pelvic venous circulation, thereby reducing the consequent risk of venous thrombosis, and improves blood flow. We cannot place the patient in this position before insufflation because it may lead to some modifications in the position of the needle, with the consequent risk of vascular injury. During abdominal passage, these trocars may injure two principal structures: the bladder, if it is not empty or if it is attracted to the umbilicus by an anterior scar, and the inferior epigastric vessels. These vessels are situated in the preperitoneal space (between the peritoneum and the transversalis fascia). They originate from the external iliac artery near the deep inguinal ring and go up medially towards the lateral side of the rectus abdominis muscle; they then rejoin this muscle 5 cm above the pubis. When

one of these arteries is injured, it can induce significant bleeding, but the multiplicity of anastomoses in the abdominal wall and the wealth of blood supply mean it can be sacrificed and ligated, if necessary. On the inside of these epigastric vessels is the median umbilical ligament, a vestige of the urachus, stretched between the umbilicus and the vesical apex, and the medial umbilical ligaments, obliterated umbilical arteries, which extend to the umbilicus.

Before ancillary trocar placement, it is important to identify the inferior epigastric vessels along the abdominal wall behind the rectus abdominis muscle. In thin patients, they are usually transparently visible under the peritoneum. However, locating them can be more difficult if there is thick adipose tissue. The distance between the epigastric vessels and the midline is 5–6 cm, located 5 cm above the symphysis pubis; the mean distance between the medial umbilical ligaments and the inferior epigastric vessels is 2 cm. However, humans are not made symmetrically and these distances are significantly greater on the right side than on the left. There is no significant correlation between weight and any measured distance. However, a high body mass index affects the visibility of the inferior epigastric vessels, medial umbilical ligament and ureter on the left. Once the abdominal wall is pierced, the surgeon must take care not to injure the pelvic structures, particularly vascular and visceral structures.

During laparoscopic surgery, two golden rules that must be applied in order to avoid injury to the intraperitoneal and retroperitoneal structures are knowledge of their normal anatomic localization and their visibility and appearance on the video-monitor. Compared with the laparotomic view, certain anatomic structures in the abdominal and pelvic cavity may look different during laparoscopic procedures because of the effect of pneumoperitoneal pressure, Trendelenburg positioning and the use of an intrauterine manipulator. However, magnification should enhance visualization of these structures, allowing finer dissection.

PELVIC ANATOMY IN LAPAROSCOPY

Broad ligament or operative peritoneum

When one penetrates the peritoneal cavity, one encounters the digestive viscera which are moved upwards. One is then opposite the pelvic viscera, covered with peritoneum, which define, from front to back, the *retropubic space* (of Retzius) behind the pubis symphysis, in front of the vesical wall, known for the venous plexus which is situated there; the transverse vesical fold on the vesical corpus, the vesico-uterine pouch situated between the bladder and the uterine isthmus, with its opening leading to the vesico-uterine septum. This septum is bordered below by an intimate connection between the ureters and the vagina. The *recto-uterine pouch* described by Douglas is bordered by the rectum and its fascia behind, the vagina and the uterus in front, and laterally by recto-uterine folds which extend backwards towards the pararectal fossae. Its opening leads to the *rectovaginal septum*, which is limited by the joining of the two *uterosacral ligaments* behind the cervix. The *retrorectal* space is situated between the rectal and the retrorectal fascia.

The *broad ligament* is situated laterally, a double-layer formation extending from the uterus to the lateral walls of the pelvis. Perfect knowledge of its anatomy is essential to perform adnexal and fertility surgery. It extends like a sheet across clothes lines which represent the different subperitoneal elements. Each broad ligament consists of three peritoneal mesos, the funicular meso, the mesosalpinx and the meso-ovarium, which extends with the mesometrium, below and medially.

The *funicular meso*, raised by the round ligament of the uterus, extends from the uterine horn to the deep inguinal ring. Its removal allows one to approach the *paravesical fossae* whose superior opening is situated between the umbilical artery on the inside and the iliac vascular pedicle on the outside. It is a wide and deep space; its floor consists of the elevator ani muscle and its caudal part of the iliopubic branch and Cooper's ligament. It is crossed by the obturator pedicle which emerges from the interiliac space.

The obturator nerve is the most superficial element of the pedicle and converges towards the obturator foramen. It can be recognized by its pearly white color at the level of the lateral pelvic concavity. One sometimes observes, against the superior branch of the pubis, accessory obturator vessels, branches of the inferior epigastric vessels. This paravesical space contains the obturator lymph nodes and the external iliac nodes and is therefore affected by lymphadenectomy. The potential danger at this level is from the inferior hypogastric vessels and the sometimes present accessory obturator vein, which emerges from the obturator pedicle near the foramen and ends on the inferior side of the external iliac vein, 1 or 2 cm from the femoral foramen.

The *mesosalpinx*, triangular when spread out, is bordered by the Fallopian tube above and the infundibulopelvic ligament on the outside. It contains vascular archways (infratubal, infra-ovarian and tubal branches of ovarian vessels) and the infratubal nervous plexus.

The lateral limit of the mesosalpinx is the *tubo-ovarian ligament*, partially followed by Richard's fimbrial fringe, whose role it is to loosely connect the fimbria with the ovary. It is essential that the mesosalpinx and tubo-ovarian ligament are free for good ovular capture and subsequent fertilization.

The *meso-ovarium* contains the ovarian vessels and nerves.

The *preovarian fossa* is bordered in front by the funicular fold and the mesosalpinx behind. It forms a triangle whose relief is marked by the external iliac vessels laterally and the uterine horns inside. It covers the obturator fossa and faces the appendix on the right side, and the sigmoid on the left.

The *tubo-ovarian recessus* is between the mesosalpinx and the meso-ovarium. The *ovarian fossa* is between the meso-ovarium in front, the iliac vessels on the outside, and the discrete fold of the *ureter* behind. Under its peritoneum is the obturator pedicle. Just behind, the uterine vessels are covered by the dorsal side of the broad ligament, advancing into the parametrium with the ureter.

Lateral to the ovary is the *infundibulopelvic ligament*, which contains the ovarian vessels. It crosses the external iliac vessels 2 cm in front of the ureter. It ends on the tubal extremity of the ovary. On the inside of the ovary is the *proper ovarian ligament* which emerges from the uterine horn behind and below the uterine tube, and goes to the uterine side of the ovary. The *mesometrium* extends behind, as far as the uterosacral ligaments.

The two *pararectal fossae*, whose superior opening is narrow in the sacro-iliac sinus, are not generally affected by gynecological laparoscopy. They are bordered in front by the paracervix, inside by the rectum and the uterosacral folds, with the piriformis muscle outside, the levator ani muscle below and the lateral rectal ligament behind. They are covered with peritoneum under which is the ureter.

35

They extend forwards by the paravesical space, passing under the paracervix. Access is difficult because of the presence of internal iliac and rectal vessels.

Laterally, still under the peritoneum, are the *iliac vessels*. The most accessible structure is the *external iliac artery* which continues the bifurcation of the common iliac artery. If the internal iliac artery is dissected at this level, one inevitably arrives at the anterior branches and some of its visceral branches. Situated more deeply on the inside of the artery is the *external iliac vein*. More laterally, the pelvic wall consists of the *internal obturator muscle* and its fascia.

Pelvic cellular tissue

A knowledge of pelvic cellular tissue is essential for the surgeon who operates on the pelvis. This tissue has two forms: slack zones, which can be easily dissected, and dense zones (fascia and visceral ligaments), which must be cut for dissection.

The *slack zones* are full of areolar tissue, relatively easy to dissect (retropubic space, paravesical fossae, pararectal fossae, retrorectal space, vesicovaginal septum, rectovaginal septum). The *pelvic fascia* is a dense conjunctive lamina covering the pelvic wall (parietal pelvic fascia), and forms the adventitia of the viscera (visceral fascia). The pelvic parietal fascia (or urogenital diaphragm) is not greatly affected by laparoscopy. It is, first of all, a conjunctive lamina which constitutes an effective support for the pelvic viscera because of the continuity between the parietal and visceral pelvic fascia.

The visceral pelvic fascia covers the visceral non-peritonealized surface. The thickness of this fascia is variable and it is impaired particularly on the midline in case of prolapse. Only the vaginal fascia is a thick conjunctive layer reinforced by a strong elastic network. All this fascia exchanges fibers which makes anatomic relationships much tighter and dissection more precarious. This generates risks of visceral injury, especially at the level where the connections between the viscera and the urogenital diaphragm are dynamic (at the point where each viscus passes through the pelvic fascia, between the vagina and the vesical cervix, between the vagina and the rectum).

The *visceral ligaments* are made up of densifications of pelvic cellular tissue whose visceral insertion intermingles with the perivisceral fascia. They are very resistant structures that require ligature and section for visceral mobilization. Pelvic cellular tissue looks like the stitches of a mesh, with traction on a point of this mesh provoking a reduction of the stitches and mesh densification. The greater the traction, the more pronounced the densification near the point of traction, in other words, near the viscera. These visceral ligaments are divided into two groups: the lateral ligaments go with the internal iliac artery branches and the sagittal ligaments convey the inferior hypogastric plexus branches.

There are three lateral ligaments: rectal, genital and vesical. The *genital ligament* is the strongest and constitutes the strongest means of suspension of the uterus. It comprises three continuous parts: the *parametrium*, the *paracervix* and the *paravagina*. They present, near their visceral attachments, a densification of conjunctive tissue, very rich in elastic fibers and smooth muscle fibers. The parametrium situated just above the ureter contains the uterine artery, veins and lymphatics. The sometimes present latero-ureteral cervicovaginal arteries can give the parametrium an anterior extension which is near the vesico-uteral ligament and even merged with it. The paracervix, situated under the ureter, contains the vaginal arteries, the voluminous venous plexus, and the uterovaginal lymph nodes. Contrary to the parametrium, the paracervix is frequently affected by cervical cancers. The genital ligament is also called the *cardinal ligament*.

The *vesical ligament* is located around the anterior vesical arteries, branches of the umbilical artery, and is attached to the anterior side of the paracervix. The *rectal ligament* is located around the middle rectal vessels. It is thick and disposed almost transversally on each side of the rectum. It separates the retrorectal area from the pararectal area.

The sagittal ligaments consist of the uterosacral, vesico-uterine and tubovesical ligaments. The *uterosacral ligaments* are attached to the posterolateral side of the cervix and the vaginal fornix, and run alongside the lateral sides of the rectum to be finally lost, like a broad fan, on the inside of the sacral foramen from S2 to S4. They contain few vessels, but notably the inferior hypogastric plexus nerves described by Lee and Frankenhauser. A little transverse relief joins the points of uterine origin: the *torus uterinus*. On the whole, the content of these ligaments is principally made up of nerves; vessels are few and often their surgical section does not cause bleeding or necessitate hemostasis. Moreover, the wealth of nervous elements in these ligaments is expressed by their sensitivity. Their section can soothe pain provoked by static uterine defects. They are always extremely resistant and are even very elastic. Their resistance is due to both the nervous elements and the framework of pelvic fascia.

The *vesicouterine ligaments* extend from the isthmus and the cervix to the meatus uretrae area. They are situated around the arterial and venous cervicovaginal branches and extend in front of the parametrium. In front of them, the *pubovesical ligaments* extend from the posterior side of the pubis symphysis to the vesical cervix. All these structures form the *tendinous arch of the pelvic fascia* (the genitopelvic-rectosacral arch).

The parametrium and the paracervix have an extremely important functional role in the support of the uterus and vaginal fornix. These ligaments and fascias share numerous fibers which make their individualization very difficult and their borders imprecise. A typical example is the pericervical and perivaginal fascia which turn into the uterosacral ligaments and the two paracervices, and which share fibers with the parietal pelvic fascia. This explains why removal of the cervix does not provoke prolapse because the vaginal vault is supported by the fascia.

Vascular relationships

Pelvic visceral vascularization derives from the iliac vessels but also from the abdominal vessels for the adnexa and the rectum. We will only briefly recall these elements and describe in more detail the strategic points which can be risk factors during laparoscopy. It is vital to know the dangerous anatomic areas, and carefully identify the important structures before proceeding with dissection.

Arterial relationships

The principal vascular relationship which is encountered when introducing the optic is represented by the external iliac vessels which continue outside the viscera against the lateral pelvic wall. Pelvic visceral vascularization is essentially assured by the internal iliac arteries, the ovarian arteries, and the superior rectal arteries.

The *internal iliac artery* divides into the principal visceral pelvic arteries. To see it during laparoscopy, it is necessary to push the infundibulopelvic ligament upwards. It is not necessary to cut it, as it serves as a screen against bowel inrush. It is classically divided into two branches at the level of the greater sciatic foramen. The anterior branch separates into essentially visceral branches. The

umbilical artery continues in front along the superior part of the vesical inferolateral side. It constitutes a surgical landmark which leads to the origin of the uterine artery. It then leads to the superior vesical arteries. The *uterine artery* has three segments (Figure 2):

(1) The parietal segment descends forwards from its origin against the pelvic wall as far as the ischiatic spine. It is accompanied by the umbilical and obturator arteries in front and the ureter inside;

(2) The parametrial segment: the artery branches transversally inside, under the parametrium, and crosses the ureter in front. Around this point of crossing, there are some important venous plexus and lymph vessels;

(3) The mesometrial segment is very sinuous, running alongside the lateral side of the uterus in the mesometrium. It is accompanied by the uterine venous plexus, lymphatic vessels and the sometimes present parauterine lymph nodes. The uterine artery leads to several collateral branches, including vesicovaginal branches, the cervicovaginal artery after the ureteral crossing, the sinuous cervical artery, the corporeal artery and the round ligament artery.

The *vaginal arteries* run behind the uterine artery. The *obturator artery* proceeds forwards, towards the obturator foramen. It is situated against the internal obturator muscle fascia and is bordered by the obturator nerve above

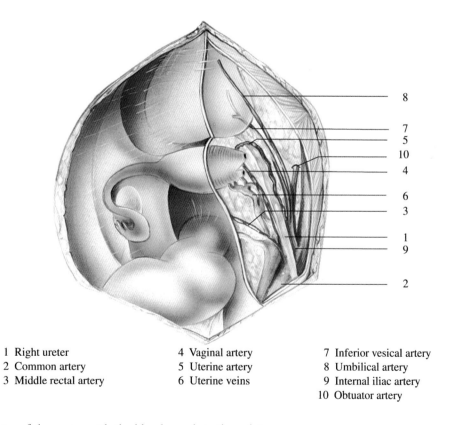

1 Right ureter	4 Vaginal artery	7 Inferior vesical artery
2 Common artery	5 Uterine artery	8 Umbilical artery
3 Middle rectal artery	6 Uterine veins	9 Internal iliac artery
		10 Obtuator artery

Figure 2 Relationships of the ureter with the blood vessels in the pelvis

and the obturator vein below. Its distal part is opposite the obturator lymph nodes. The *middle rectal artery* goes down medially towards the lateral side of the rectum, into the lateral rectal ligament. The *internal pudendal artery* accompanies the pudendal nerve in the perineum. After leaving the pelvis through the greater sciatic foramen, passing round the sciatic spine, penetrating the ischiorectal fossa and travelling along the pudendal canal, it ends in two branches, the deep artery and the dorsal artery of the clitoris.

The posterior branch of the internal iliac artery has parietal branches, the iliolumbar artery, the lateral sacral artery and the superior gluteal artery.

The *ovarian artery* emerges from the abdominal aorta at the L2 level and joins the ovary by means of the infundibulopelvic ligament.

The *superior rectal artery* emerges from the inferior mesenteric artery and joins the superior rectal ligament.

At the pelvic level, there is an *efficient anastomotic arterial system* which compensates for all obstruction, even internal iliac.

An important arterial relationship to be aware of is the *median sacral artery*. It emerges from the posterior side of the aorta just above its bifurcation and descends against the anterior side of L4, L5 and the sacrum. It vascularizes the posterior side of the rectum. During surgical intervention for genital prolapse, we perform vaginal vault sacrofixation. During strip fixation using tackers at the L4–L5 level or promontory, there is always a risk of arterial injury and that is why efficient coagulation of the fixation zone is necessary. One must also take great care not to injure the anterior sacral roots which emerge on each side.

Venous relationships

The pelvic veins are essentially drained by the internal iliac veins and secondarily by the external iliac, common iliac, superorectal and ovarian veins. The internal iliac vein does not contain valves and emerges from the superior side of the greater sciatic foramen and connects to the external iliac vein at the promontory level, to form the common iliac vein. The tributary veins are satellites of the arteries and drain the pelvic venous plexus.

The ureter and its relationships

The *lumbar ureter* lies on the psoas muscle on each side of the rachis and is only seen in gynecology by specialists who perform para-aortic lymphadenectomy. It then passes through the superior pelvic strait and becomes pelvic. The right ureter crosses the right external iliac artery in front, near its origin. The left ureter is situated in front of the end of the common iliac artery. On each side, it maintains a close relationship with the infundibulopelvic ligament which crosses it (Figure 3). It is therefore vulnerable when hemostasis of this ligament is carried out and during reperitonealization, which are pointless anyway. Laterally,

it is situated opposite the internal iliac vein and next to the obturator nerve and obturator, umbilical, uterine and vaginal vessels. In a thin patient, it is easy to identify under the peritoneum by its characteristic peristaltic motion. In an obese patient, it is necessary to search for it and dissect it in order not to injure it.

The *retroligamentary ureter* runs forwards and medially, along the posteromedian side of the uterine artery, approaching the uterosacral ligament origin. This course may be modified in case of attraction to endometriosis, sequelae of infection or previous surgery. It can then come into contact with the ovary or the uterosacral ligament and its identification is indispensable before continuing the dissection further. The distance between the ureter and the uterosacral homolateral ligament and the infundibulopelvic ligament is small but significantly greater on the left side. The ureter is located about 1–3 cm from the uterosacral ligament and the infundibulopelvic ligament.

The *intraligamentary ureter* is of even more concern to the surgeon as it is invisible. It crosses the vessels and the lateral ligaments of the uterus from back to front to join the bladder (Figures 2 and 4). In fact, in crossing under the uterine artery loop, it passes between the parametrium and the paracervix.

The ureter, however, remains clearly independent of the uterine artery, since the crossing occurs behind the artery, 15 mm from the isthmus and 10 mm from the lateral vaginal fornix. It then joins the vesical extremity of the vesicouterine ligament which attaches above the ureteral meatus (*retrovesical ureter*).

Knowing that the ureter is at some distance from the isthmus and the vaginal fornix is not enough to guarantee safe surgery. It is necessary to know exactly how to dissect and shelter it. Mobilizing the uterus, it is possible to display the ascending segment of the uterine artery without modifying the position of the ureter, which remains at some distance from the vascular section. One can also use the uterine artery as a guide, cutting it at the isthmus level and, by moving aside its parietal stump laterally, the ureter is effectively protected. Another way is to open the vesico-uterine space and remove the vesico-uterine ligament laterally and with it the retrovesical ureter which runs alongside.

Ureteral vascularization (Figure 5) merits a brief reminder. It derives from the renal, ovarian, common iliac and uterine arteries. These ureteral branches divide into a T-shape on ureteral contact to form a rich adventitial network whose anastomotic system compensates for vascular interruption, thus allowing dissection over a long distance.

Digestive system

After moving the bowels upwards, out of the way, the only other awkward digestive elements in laparoscopy are the *sigmoid* and the *rectum*. The rectal peritoneum extends forwards to the vagina to form the recto-uterine pouch.

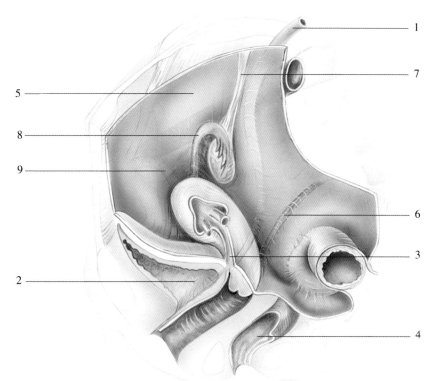

1 Right ureter: crossing at the pelvic brim	3 Broad ligament	5 Peritoneum	7 Infundibulopelvic ligament
2 Bladder	4 Rectum	6 Uterosacral ligament	8 Fallopian tube
			9 Round ligament

Figure 3 Relationships of ureter with other pelvic organs

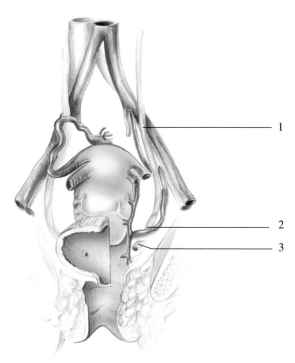

1 At the crossing with the iliac vessels   3 At the angle of the vaginal fornix
2 At the crossing with the uterine artery

Figure 4 Localization of ureteric injuries

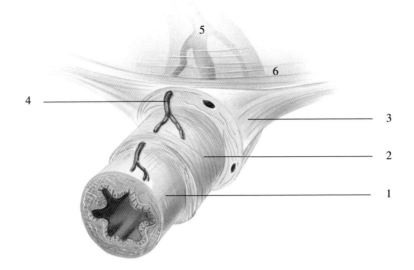

1 Mucosa with urothelium
2 Medial muscular layer
3 Adventitial sheath

4 Arteriole between musculosa and adventitial sheath
5 Ureteral artery
6 Peritoneum

Figure 5 Anatomy of the ureter

The lateral sides of the rectal peritoneum extend, with the pelvic wall peritoneum, to form the pararectal fossae which proceed obliquely towards the recto-uterine pouch. Injury is rare in gynecology but possible in some operations which require a prior intestinal wash-out, such as cases of *rectovaginal adenomyosis* resection by laparoscopy. It is difficult and perilous surgery reserved for experienced surgeons because it requires not only gynecological knowledge but also knowledge of the particular behavior of endometriosis and of digestive surgery. Rectal effraction is a constant risk and, if any doubt exists, a diagnostic test by air or dye injection in the rectum may be necessary. On the other hand, the spread of these lesions can be considerable, not only on the rectal mucous membrane but also more laterally towards the pelvic wall, sometimes leading to ureteral stenosis and even invasion of the muscle elevator ani.

The rectum can also pose a danger in cancer surgery. Its invasion can make its approach dangerous during dissection. There is another gynecological procedure that is risky for the rectum, namely vaginal vault *sacrospino-fixation*, described by Richter in prolapse surgery. It consists of fixing the vagina to the sacrospinal ligament through a vaginal approach. Without a wide opening of the pararectal fossa, the ligatures are placed blindly and a rectal or pudendal nerve injury is possible.

Nervous elements

Pelviperineal innervation is both somatic and vegetative. The peripheral nervous system of the pelvis includes the sacral and pudental plexus. The first, which consists of roots L4, L5, S1, S2 and S3 goes to the inferior limbs and the pelvis. The second, coming from roots S2, S3 and S4, is responsible for the innervation of the perineum and the viscera. These two plexi are closely linked with the vegetative nervous system from the superior and inferior hypogastric plexus. This association between the somatic and vegetative nervous system exists in all the great visceral functions of the organism, but is more intense at the level of the pelvic viscera.

The laparoscopic surgeon safely avoids, contrary to the abdominal surgeon, section of the anterior branch of the *ilio-hypogastric* and *ilio-inguinal* nerves which may lead, although reversible, to cutaneous anesthesia of the pubic region, the inside of the thigh and the labium majus, as well as injury to the *femoral nerve*, which extends along the lateral side of the psoas and which may be in danger of compression by the autostatic valves during laparotomy.

The nervous elements which are important to know in laparoscopy are primarily the *genitofemoral* nerve which emerges from spinal nerves L1 and L2 and crosses the psoas to extend in its sheath behind the ureter and the peritoneum. It then continues along the lateral side of the external iliac artery. Its genital branch provides sensitive innervation to the labia majora and the neighboring areas. Its injury is very rare in laparoscopy.

The *obturator nerve* (L2, L3, L4) emerges in the pelvis between the external and internal iliac vessels. It extends against the lateral wall opposite the ovarian fossa, before entering the obturator foramen. It can be affected at this level by endometriosis or adnexal infection, leading to obturator neuralgia on the superomedial side of the thigh and the knee.

Surgical injury to these nerves can be observed during lymphadenectomy but the functional consequences are minor.

ANATOMICAL BASIS OF PELVIC AND PERINEAL PAIN AND THERAPEUTIC APPLICATIONS

Anatomical description

The perineum receives its innervation from the pudendal plexus. This plexus also supplies visceral nerves, which are of variable number. They extend forwards towards the lateral walls of the pelvic viscera to the bladder, the rectum and the internal genital organs, either directly, or by the intermediary of the hypogastric plexus. Through these branches, the nervous impulses controlling micturition, defecation and sensory innervation of the pelvic viscera proceed. Vegetative innervation of the pelvic viscera derives essentially from the inferior hypogastric plexi, but also from the superior hypogastric plexus and the ovarian plexus.

The *superior hypogastric plexus* is situated facing L5 and the promontory and is the origin of the left and right hypogastric nerves, which connect to the corresponding inferior hypogastric plexus. This plexus used to be resected according to Cotte's procedure but the mediocre results obtained have now made this method obsolete.

The *inferior hypogastric plexus*, or *Lee and Frankenhauser's* ganglion is a collection of afferent and efferent fibers going towards the pelviperineal viscera. It is symmetrically paired in the form of a nervous quadrilateral lamina of 4 cm in length and 3 cm in height. It is located in the lateral part of the uterosacral ligament, surrounded by the lateral side of the rectum on the inside and the visceral venous plexus on the outside. Its superior edge is in contact with the ureter, its inferior edge with the pelvic floor, its posterior edge with the sacrum and its anterior edge with the posterior bladder wall. This inferior hypogastric plexus is the central point of a considerable number of nervous branches aimed at all the organs inside the pelvis.

Each inferior hypogastric plexus receives afferent branches: the hypogastric nerve originating from the superior hypogastric plexus, sacral splanchnic nerves, and pelvic splanchnic nerves (nervi erigentes). Efferent branches make up the pelvic visceral plexus: the uterovaginal plexus, the rectal plexus and the vesical plexus (vesical nerves, when cut during extended hysterectomies, can account for bladder hypotonia).

The *ovarian plexus* supplies innervation to the ovaries and the distal half of the Fallopian tubes. It originates from the aortic plexus. The parasympathetic fibers come from the pneumogastric nerve, which could explain vagal digestive reactions during adnexal torsion.

These plexi contain orthosympathetic and parasympathetic fibers. The pelvic orthosympathetic centers are located inside the *intermedio-lateralis columnae* of the medulla, from the 10th thoracic verbebra to the 3rd lumbar vertebra. The efferent branches, whose positioning is segmental, provide nerve supply to the pelvic viscera. The fibers follow the vessels, leading them to the viscera.

The sacral parasympathetic nucleus is located at the level of the S2–S4 segments, on the basal part of the ventral horn, and takes charge of all pelvic elements except the ovaries. Concerning the orthosympathetic system, the sensitive fibers are individualized and carry influx such as nociception. Thereafter, they join the closest somatic nerve and account for abdominal wall pain originating from visceral discomfort. Concerning the parasympathetic fibers, their sensitive role is still in question, even if their existence itself cannot be disputed.

The motor response to nociceptive perceptions correlates with the anatomy: the parietal pain experienced during acute salpingitis is, in fact, pain from a viscus transmitting painful information through the closest somatic nerve into the corresponding iliac fossa. Motor cells under orthosympathetic influence may account for abdominal wall contracture on clinical examination.

Another example of these sensitive functions is the pain experienced by patients who suffer from adenomyotic nodules of the rectovaginal septum. These are caused by stimulation of the orthosympathetic fibers inside the rectovaginal septum; through the inferior hypogastric plexus, they carry their nociceptive information to the superior centers. The sympathetic motor cells then induce a reflex contraction of the pelvic diaphragm, closing the vagina and making intercourse even more painful.

Although such pain is no indication for laparoscopic treatment, it is important to evoke the anatomic basis of *chronic perineal neuralgia* and the role of the *pudendal nerve* which leads to pain, whose etiologic diagnosis is sometimes difficult, and often considered as having a psychiatric origin. These patients suffer pain in the area of the pudendal nerve, either uni- or bilaterally, and this pain is exacerbated, if not provoked, by the sitting position. The positional character of this pain in a given area leads us to investigate a compression syndrome of the nerve stem.

These pains can be urogenital, anal or mixed. They involve women in two-thirds of cases and manifest themselves as burning sensations, torsions, heaviness or even intravaginal or intrarectal foreign bodies. They are not satisfactorily treated by different local therapeutic approaches and can be exacerbated by a proctological, urological or gynecological surgical procedure.

The pudendal nerve generally issues from S3 and can intercept contingents from adjoining roots S2 and S4. Emerging in the ventral sacral area, it rapidly penetrates, together with its vessels, the gluteal area under the piriformis muscle, in ligamentary claws formed from the sacrotuberous and sacrospinous ligaments (Figure 6). It passes round the sciatic spine between the superior rectal nerves on the inside and the pudendal vessels on the outside. In the perineal area, the nerve lies on the medial side of the internal obturator muscle in the pudendal canal (described by Alcock), formed by a split in the aponeurosis. In the posterior part of this canal, it crosses over the falciform process of the sacrotuberous ligament, which is a fibrous lamina with a sharp superior edge, concave above, and parallel to the medial side of the ischium. Medially, the abundant fat of the ischio-anal fossa occupies all the posterior perineum. Observation of the course of this nerve, as described above, highlights several possible areas of conflict:

(1) In the *ligamentary claws* near the sciatic spine, the nerve is pressed between the sacrotuberous and sacrospinous ligaments;

(2) The *falciform process of the sacrotuberous ligament* can emerge very high and come into contact with the nerve which overlaps it;

(3) The *fascia of the internal obturator* muscle, when it splits, can be thickened and thus become a potential site of conflict.

Several studies have shown that a sitting position provokes an ascent of the ischio-anal fat which presses the sacrotuberous ligament falciform process laterally and brings it closer to the nerve stem.

Therapeutic applications

(1) *LUNA (laser uterine nerve ablation)*: this is the practical application of the anatomy of the inferior hypogastric plexus. Uterosacral ligament ablation by laser interrupts the vegetative fibers and thus leads to a diminution in dysmenorrhea and dyspareunia. Some authors believe that the beneficial effect of LUNA is due more to the treatment of endometriosis of the uterosacral ligament than the fiber ablation itself.

(2) *Torus uterinus ablation:* according to the same principle, surgery consists of ablation of the area which joins the isthmic origin of the two uterosacral ligaments.

(3) *Rectovaginal septum adenomyosis:* apart from ablation of the adenomyotic lesion, surgery also effects suppression of vegetative fibers which provoke pain at the level of the rectovaginal septum.

(4) *Chronic perineal pain:* surgical liberation of the pudendal nerve, described by R. Robert, gives excellent results when anesthetic infiltrations fail. Of course, this type of surgery requires perfect knowledge of the regional anatomy. The principle is very simple: by a transgluteal approach, the gluteus maximus muscle is incised in the direction of its fibers, on both sides of a transverse line passing at the

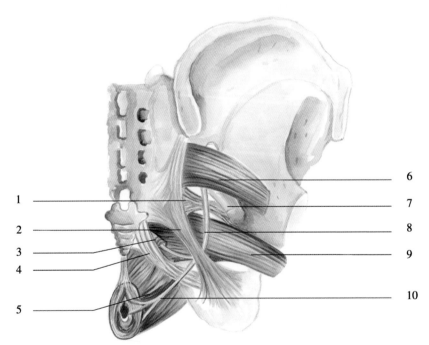

1 Sacro-spinous ligament	4 Falciform process of the sacro-tuberous ligament	7 Sciatic nerve
2 Sacro-tuberous ligament	5 Levator ani muscle	8 Pudendal nerve
3 Pudendal canal	6 Piriformis muscle	9 Internal obturator muscle
		10 Inferior rectal nerve

Figure 6 Posterior view of the deep gluteal area

level of the coccyx and thus the sciatic spine. The muscular attachments of the posterior side of the sacrotuberous ligament are removed over 2–3 cm. The pudendal pedicle then appears to cross the sacrospinous ligament behind. The latter is sectioned and the nerve can then be transposed forwards to the sciatic spine, gaining precious centimeters. Dissection of the nerve in the pudendal canal is easy and the internal obturator muscle fascia is incised and the nerve stem and its branches are freed over 3–4 cm. Section of a threatened falciform process is performed if necessary. It is then easy to release the nerve stem in this simple way.

DANGEROUS RELATIONSHIPS DURING ILIAC AND AORTIC LYMPHADENECTOMY BY LAPAROSCOPY

Because of the anatomic complexity and technical difficulty of lymphadenectomy, we devote an entire chapter to this subject. In fact, rare are those gynecologists who perform lymphadenectomy by laparoscopy, because vascular and nervous relationships of pelvic lymph nodes make dissection extremely delicate. The advantages of the laparoscopic approach are the absence of trauma and a decreased risk of adhesions, for the price of specialized

training, but without any diminution in the quality of samples taken.

Cancer work-ups and pelvic or lumbar lymphadenectomy require thorough knowledge of these lymph nodes (Figure 7). The indications are essentially diagnostic and prognostic. Lymphadenectomy is the surgical removal of an entire cellulo-lymph node area.

Occasionally present *pelvic lymph nodes* are situated near the viscera and are drained by the external iliac, obturator, interiliac, internal iliac, common iliac and lumbar nodes. The paravesical nodes are situated in the lateral ligaments of the bladder. The parauterine nodes are found in the parametrium near the uterine artery loop. The paravaginal nodes are located in the paracervix. The pararectal nodes are situated in the lateral ligaments of the rectum.

External iliac nodes are eight to ten in number; they are found along the external iliac vessels, and they include three groups:

(1) The lateral group outside the external iliac vessels;

(2) The intermediate group on the external iliac vein or between the artery and the vein. They drain the inguinal nodes and the medial external iliac nodes towards the common iliac nodes;

(3) The medial group are situated under the vein and against the pelvic wall, so it is necessary to lift the

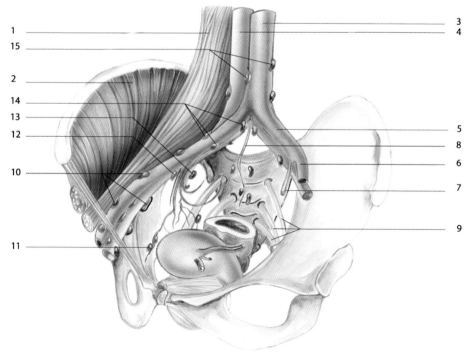

1 Psoas muscle	5 Common iliac artery	9 Sacral plexus	13 Internal iliac nodes
2 Iliacus mucle	6 External iliac artery	10 External iliac nodes	14 Common iliac nodes
3 Abdominal aorta	7 Internal iliac artery	11 Obturator nodes	15 Lumbar nodes
4 Inferior vena cava	8 Median sacral artery	12 Inter iliac nodes	

Figure 7 Anterior view of the lymph nodes of the pelvis

vein to reach them. This group receives the lymph vessels of the bladder, the pelvic ureter, the uterus and the vagina.

The *obturator nodes* are situated against the obturator pedicle and the internal obturator muscle. They receive the lymph vessels of the bladder, the ureter, the uterus and the vagina.

The *interiliac nodes* are situated at the bifurcation of the internal and external iliac vessels. They drain the obturator and external iliac nodes. The also receive the lymph vessels of the bladder, the uterus and the vagina.

The *internal iliac nodes* are found between the internal iliac artery branches. One can distinguish the sacral nodes, situated along the lateral sacral artery, which receive the lymph vessels of the rectum and the cervix, and the gluteal nodes, which lie on the piriformis muscle, and drain the lymph vessels of the rectum, the deep area of the perineum and the gluteal area.

The *common iliac nodes* are situated against the common iliac vessels, and drain the external, internal and intermediate iliac nodes. They include five groups:

(1) The lateral group: on the lateral sides of the common iliac artery at the level of the iliolumbar fossa;

(2) The intermediate group: under the common iliac vessels, against the obturator nerve, the ascending lumbar vein and the lumbosacral trunk;

(3) The medial group: situated against the medial side of the right common iliac artery and the right and left common iliac veins;

(4) Promontory nodes;

(5) Subaortic nodes.

The *lumbar nodes* are found around the aorta, the inferior vena cava and between these two vessels.

Lymphadenectomy is performed according to several techniques in laparoscopy: either by a transperitoneal approach to the paravesical fossa, or an extraperitoneal approach, by careful detachment of the peritoneum, beginning with the retropubic space and then the prevascular and preperitoneal areas. Insufflation through the trocar detaches the preperitoneal area.

Lymphadenectomy can be extended to several levels:

(1) *Level I* describes the angle defined by the common iliac artery bifurcation. It removes the medial and intermediate external iliac nodes, obturator and interiliac. These are the sentinel lymph nodes of the front line of the uterine cervix which can first be identified by the sentinel lymph node technique during surgery for cervical cancer. This level is sufficient for small cervical tumors and endometrial cancers. The risk during dissection of this area is to the inferior obturator vein, the internal iliac vein branches and the obturator vessels.

(2) *Level II* is astride the pelvis and the abdomen, limited above by the angle of the aortic bifurcation. It includes the common iliac nodes, the lateral external iliac nodes which are not affected by the first level, the promontory and the subaortic nodes. The risk during lateral external iliac node removal is injury to the genitofemoral nerve which runs alongside the psoas and, particularly, the sometimes present psoic artery, which emerges from the external iliac artery. The epigastric vessels must also be respected near the deep inguinal ring. On the other hand, the retrocrural nodes described by Cloquet are removed. During promontory node dissection, care must be taken with regard to the middle sacral pedicle, the presacral veins and, particularly, the left common iliac vein.

(3) *Level III* is lower aortic, defined above by the emergence of the inferior mesenteric artery. It is bordered laterally by the lumbar ureters, and behind by the iliac vessels, the sympathetic ganglions and psoas attachment. These elements are generally well visible and complications are rare if the dissection is carefully performed.

(4) *Level IV*, infrarenal, does not generally involve laparoscopy and is rarely carried out.

Increasingly, removal of the cellular lymph node tissue of the distal part of the paracervix, known as *paracervical lymphadenectomy*, is performed. Its purpose is to supplant the removal of the distal part of the paracervix. The affected tissue is removed, preserving the nerves and vessels of the paracervix. It is necessary, at this level, to identify the middle rectal artery at the back and the vegetative nerves in order to protect them.

ANATOMIC BASIS OF URINARY STRESS INCONTINENCE AND THERAPEUTIC APPLICATIONS

Stress incontinence is a frequent and complex symptom in women. It is caused by obstetric trauma to the urogenital perineum, but also dystrophic modifications of the menopause. Finally, it can be the consequence of surgery or radiotherapy to the bladder or urethra. The principal anatomic structures implicated in stress continence are the retropubic space, the base and cervix of the bladder, the urethra and its sphincter.

The *retropubic space* described by Retzius is situated in the preperitoneal space. It is bordered in front by the pubis symphysis, the pubovesical ligaments, the tendinous arch of the pelvic fascia and the retropubic branches of the obturator and pudendal vessels. Laterally is the superior branch of the pubis and a thickening of the periosteum, the pectineal or Cooper's ligament, implicated in pectineal colposuspension described by Burch. Behind, is the inferolateral side of the bladder as well as the urethra and the pelvic vagina. This area is closed below by the pelvic diaphragm. It is full of loose tissue, infiltrated by fat and easily cleavable during laparoscopy.

The *vesical base* includes the trigone of the bladder and the retrotrigonal fossa, whose depth increases with age, which is a factor in post-micturition dribble.

The *vesical cervix* is essential for urinary continence. It is situated 25 mm from the pubic symphysis and 10 mm above the horizontal, passing along its inferior side. Its anterior fixity is assured by the pubovesical ligaments. The normal urethrovesical angle is 90–100°.

The *urethra* includes three segments: supradiaphragmatic, diaphragmatic and infradiaphragmatic. It is situated obliquely below and in front, and at an angle of 30° from the vertical. The supradiaphragmatic urethra is supported by the pubovesical ligament; the infradiaphragmatic urethra is supported by the pubo-urethral ligament and suspensory ligament of the clitoris.

Micturition requires absolute synergy between the bladder, the urethra and abdominal pressure.

During the *repletion phase*, abdominopelvic pressure constitutes a passive occlusion force of the urethra. It opposes urogenital diaphragmatic resistance against which the urethra pushes. The resultant force exerted by the abdominopelvic pressure and the resistance of the urogenital diaphragm makes its way forward, perpendicularly to the perineal membrane, which constitutes the essential static structure of diaphragmatic urethral occlusion.

Techniques using a perineal sling in urinary stress incontinence surgery illustrate perfectly the biomechanics of the urogenital diaphragm. The TVT method (tension-free vaginal tape), in particular, is among those which, by their physiological and almost non-invasive approach, currently give very good results. This sling exerts retrourethral resistance whose orientation adjoins that of the pubis. The resultant abdominopelvic pressure and tape resistance is then perpendicular to the perineal membrane. During any effort, abdominopelvic pressure, oriented towards the posterior perineum, leads to a posterior transfer of the supradiaphragmatic urethra. On the other hand, the diaphragmatic urethra opposes the resistance of the tape and bends. Moreover, TVT allows, according to Enhorning's theory, which claims that intra-abdominal pressure is cancelled when the vesical cervix remains in the manometric abdominal enclosure, re-integration of the junction in this enclosure.

During the *micturition phase*, the association of both intravesical pressure and intraparietal tension created by detrusor contraction is directed to an area of weak resistance, the vesical cervix. The tonus of the urethra yields and the urethra opens.

In *urinary stress incontinence*, there is ptosis of the urethrovesical region, and shortening and horizontalization of the urethra. The surgeon's objective is to replace the vesical cervix so it will maintain its anatomic position, while preserving cervical and urethral flexibility.

BIBLIOGRAPHY

Bradley WE. Neural control of urethrovesical function. *Clin Obstet Gynecol* 1978;21:653–67

Carter JE. Surgical treatment for chronic pelvic pain. *J Soc Laparoendosc Surg* 1988;2:129–39

Dargent D, Salvat J. *L'envahissement Ganglionnaire Pelvien.* Paris: Medsi, 1989

Dargent D. Laparoscopic surgery in gynecologic oncology. *J Gynecol Obstet Biol Reprod Paris* 2000;29:282–4

Enhörning G. Simultaneous recording of intravesical and intravertebral pressure. A study on urethral closure pressure in normal and stress incontinent woman. *Acta Chir Scand* 1961;(Suppl):276

Faucheron JL. Surgical anatomy of pelvic nerves. *Ann Chir* 1999;53:985–9

Fauconnier A, Delmas V, Lassau JP, et al. Ventral tethering of the vagina and its role in the kinetics of urethra and bladder-neck straining. *Surg Radiol Anat* 1996;18:81–7

Jacquetin B. Use of TVT in surgery for femal urinary incontinence. *J Gynecol Obstet Biol Reprod Paris* 2000;29:242–7

Kamina P. Petit bassin et périnée. *Rectum et Organes Uro-génitaux.* Vol. 1 and 2. Paris: Maloine, 1995

Lazorthes G. Le système nerveux périphérique. *Description, Systématisation, Exploration Clinique Abord Chirurgical.* Chapter XXII. Paris: Masson, 1955

Nezhat CH, Nezhat F, Brill AI, et al. Normal variations of abdominal and pelvis anatomy evaluated at laparoscopy. *Obstet Gynecol* 1999;94:238–42

Querleu D. *Techniques Chirurgicales en Gynécologie.* 2nd edn. Paris: Masson, 1998

Richter K, Dargent D. La spino-fixation dans le traitement des prolapsus du dôme vaginal après hystérectomie. *J Gynecol Obstet Biol Reprod* 1986;15:1081–8

Robert R, Brunet C, Faure A, et al. Surgery of the pudendal nerve in various types of perineal pain: course and results. *Chirurgie* 1993–94;119:535–9

Robert R, Prat-Pradal D, Labat JJ, et al. Anatomic basis of chronic perineal pain: role of the pudendal nerve. *Surg Radiol Anat* 1998;20:93–8

Roberts WH, Hunt GM, Henken HW. Some anatomic factor having to do with urinary continence. *Anat Rec* 1968;162:341–8

Shafik A. Pudendal canal syndrome as a cause of vulvodynia and its treatment by pudendal nerve decompression. *Eur J Obstet Gynecol Reprod Biol* 1998;80:215–20

Testut L, Latarjet A. *Traité d'Anatomie Humaine.* 9th edn. Vol 3, Book 7; Vol 5, Books 12 and 13. Paris: G. Doin & Cie, 1949

Ulmsten U, Falconer C, Johnson P, et al. A multicenter study of tension-free vaginal tape (TVT) for surgical treatment of stress urinary incontinence. *Int Urogynecol J Pelvic Floor Dysfunc* 1998;9:210–13

SECTION I
Laser operative laparoscopy

Part I
Endometriosis

Peritoneal endometriosis: evaluation of typical and subtle lesions

5

M. Nisolle, F. Casanas-Roux and J. Donnez

Endometriosis most commonly affects the pelvic peritoneum close to the ovaries, including the uterosacral ligaments, the peritoneum of the ovarian fossa and the peritoneum of the cul-de-sac. The increased diagnosis of endometriosis at laparoscopy can be explained by the increased experience and ability of the surgeon to detect such lesions. The greatest change has been in the case of 'subtle' lesions, the diagnosis of which increased from 15% in 1986 to 65% in 1988[1-6]. The diagnosis of peritoneal endometriosis at the time of laparoscopy is often made by the observation of typically puckered black or bluish lesions. There are, in addition, numerous subtle appearances of peritoneal endometriosis; these lesions, frequently non-pigmented, were diagnosed as endometriosis following biopsy confirmation by Jansen and Russell in 1986[2].

TYPICAL LESIONS

The typical black peritoneal endometriotic lesion (Figure 1) results from tissue bleeding and retention of blood pigment, producing brown discoloration of tissue. Puckered black lesions are a combination of glands, stroma and intraluminal debris (Figure 1c).

Evolution

The macroscopic appearance of ectopic endometrium is probably dependent upon the longevity of the process. Viable cells may implant and the initial appearance may be an irregularity or discoloration of the peritoneal surface – the earliest sign being hemosiderin staining of the peritoneal surfaces. Initially, these lesions may appear hemorrhagic, but menstrual shedding from a viable endometrial implant initiates an inflammatory reaction which provokes a scarification process; this, in turn, encloses the implants. The presence of entrapped menstrual debris is responsible for the typical black or bluish appearance. If the inflammatory process obliterates or devascularizes the endometrial cells, eventually this discoloration disappears. A white plaque of old collagen is all that remains of the ectopic implant. Scarring of the peritoneum around endometrial implants is a typical finding. In addition to encapsulating an isolated implant, the scar may deform the surrounding peritoneum or result in the development of adhesions.

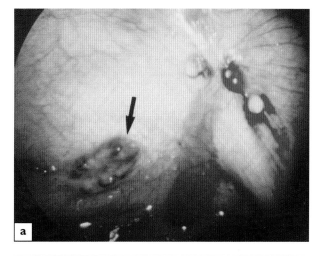

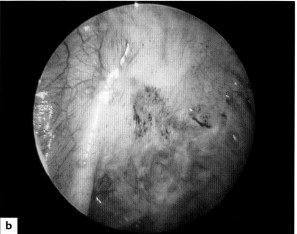

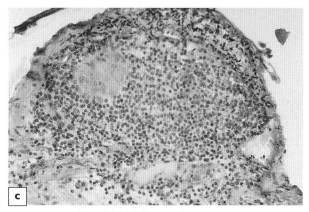

Figure 1 Puckered black lesion, laparoscopic aspect: (a) black lesion without and (b) with fibroids; (c) histology: presence of endometrial glands and typical stroma. Note the presence of intraluminal debris (Gomori's trichrome × 110)

SUBTLE APPEARANCES

Sometimes the subtle endometriotic lesions can be the only lesions seen at laparoscopy. The subtle forms are more common and may be more active than the puckered black lesions (Table 1).

Table I Different appearances of peritoneal endometriosis

Color	Description
Black	typical puckered black lesions
Red	red flame-like lesions[2]
	glandular excrescences[2]
	petechial peritoneum[7]
	areas of hypervascularization[7]
White	white opacification[2]
	subovarian adhesions[2]
	yellow-brown peritoneal patches[2]
	circular peritoneal defects[1]

The non-pigmented endometriotic peritoneal lesions include the following:

(1) White opacification of the peritoneum (Figure 2a), which appears as peritoneal scarring or as circum-scribed patches, often thickened and sometimes raised. Histologically, white opacified peritoneum is due to the presence of an occasional retroperitoneal glandular structure and scanty stroma surrounded by fibrotic tissue or connective tissue (Figure 2b and c).

(2) Red flame-like lesions of the peritoneum (Figure 3a) or red vesicular excrescences, more commonly affecting the broad ligament and the uterosacral ligaments. Histologically, red flame-like lesions and vesicular excrescences are due to the presence of active endometriosis surrounded by stroma (Figure 3b–d).

(3) Glandular excrescences on the peritoneal surface (Figure 4a), which in color, translucency and consistency closely resemble the mucosal surface of the endometrium seen at hysteroscopy. Biopsy reveals the presence of numerous endometrial glands (Figure 4b).

(4) Subovarian adhesions (Figure 5a) or adherence between the ovary and the peritoneum of the ovarian fossa, which are distinctive from adhesions characteristic of previous salpingitis or peritonitis. Histologically, connective tissue with sparse endometrial glands is found (Figure 5b).

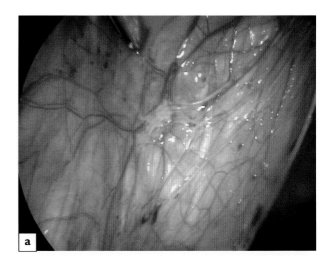

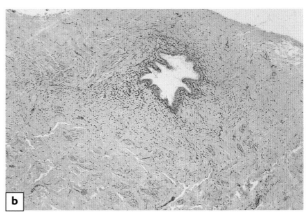

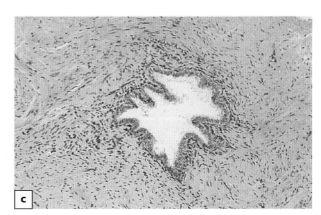

Figure 2 White opacification of the peritoneum: (a) laparoscopic aspect; (b) and (c) histology: rare retroperitoneal glandular structure and scanty stroma surrounded by fibrotic tissue (Gomori's trichrome × 56, × 110)

(5) Yellow-brown peritoneal patches (Figure 6a) resembling 'café au lait' patches. The histological characteristics are similar to those observed in white opacification, but, in the yellow-brown patches, the presence of the blood pigment hemosiderin among the stromal cells produces the 'café au lait' color (Figure 6b).

(6) Circular peritoneal defects (Figure 7a) as described by Chatman[1]. Serial section demonstrates the presence of endometrial glands in more than 50% of cases (Figure 7b).

(7) Areas of petechial peritoneum (Figure 8a) or areas with hypervascularization (Figure 9a), which were diagnosed as endometriosis in our recent study[6,7].

These lesions resemble the petechial lesions resulting from manipulation of the peritoneum or from hypervascularization of the peritoneum. They most generally affect the bladder and the broad ligament; histologically, red blood cells are numerous and endometrial glands are very rare (Figures 8b and c, 9b).

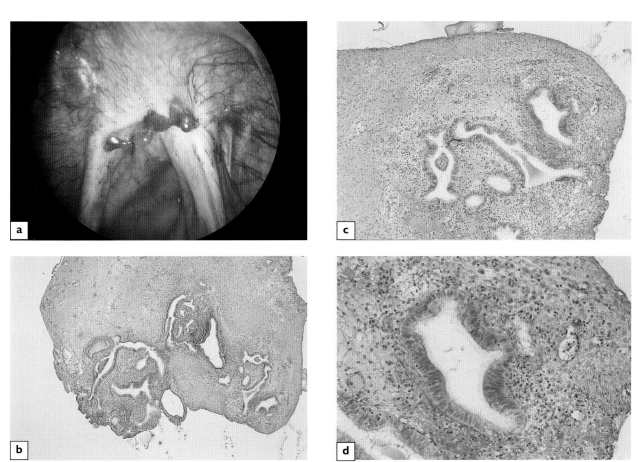

Figure 3 Red flame-like lesion of the peritoneum: (a) laparoscopic aspect; (b)–(d) histology: active endometriotic glands surrounded by stroma (Gomori's trichrome × 25, × 56, × 110)

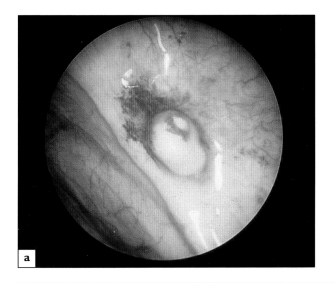

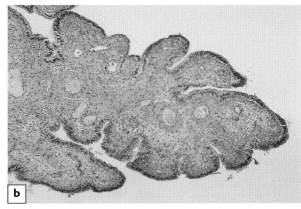

Figure 4 Glandular excrescences on the peritoneal surface: (a) laparoscopic aspect; (b) histology: presence of numerous endometrial glands (Gomori's trichrome × 56)

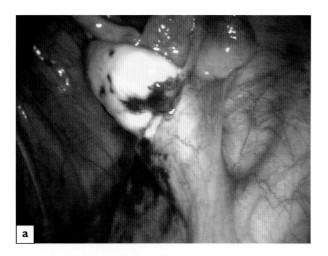

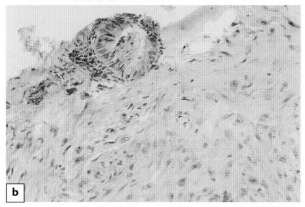

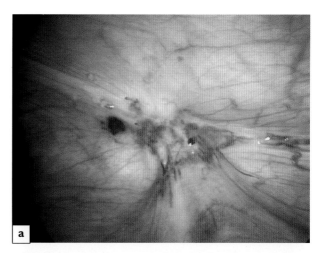

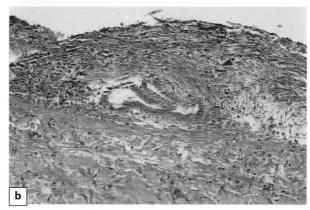

Figure 5 Subovarian adhesions: (a) laparoscopic aspect: adherence between ovary and peritoneum of the ovarian fossa; (b) histology: connective tissue with sparse endometrial glands (Gomori's trichrome × 110)

Figure 6 Yellow-brown peritoneal patches of the peritoneum: (a) laparoscopic aspect; (b) histology: the presence of blood pigment (hemosiderin) among the stroma cells produces the 'cafe au lait' color (Gomori's trichrome × 110)

HISTOLOGICAL STUDY OF PERITONEAL ENDOMETRIOSIS

Typical lesions

The morphological characteristics of peritoneal endometriosis were studied in 109 biopsies with histologically proved endometriosis[6] (Table 2). An endometriotic lesion was considered 'active' when typical glandular epithelium appeared as either proliferative or completely unresponsive to hormones, with typical stroma. Such a lesion was found in 76% of cases. Areas of oviduct-like epithelium with ciliated cells were demonstrated in 55% of peritoneal endometriotic foci. The epithelial height and the mitotic index were calculated in typical glandular epithelium. Epithelial height was measured with a micrometer and the mitotic index was calculated by counting mitotic figures per 2000 epithelial cells, as previously described[8]. Their values were 14.8 ± 3.2 µm and 0.6‰, respectively.

Table 2 Morphological characteristics of peritoneal endometriosis

Biopsies (n = 109)	Number
Typical glandular epithelium and stroma	109 (100%)
Active endometriosis	83 (76%)
Oviduct-like epithelium	46 (55%)
Epithelial height (µm)	14.8 ± 3.2
Mitotic index (‰)	0.6

Subtle lesions

Confirmation of endometriosis in subtle lesions was made by Jansen and Russell[2]. Endometriosis was confirmed in 81% of white opacified lesions, 81% of red flame-like lesions, 67% of glandular lesions, 50% of subovarian adhesions, 47% of yellow-brown patches and 45% of circular

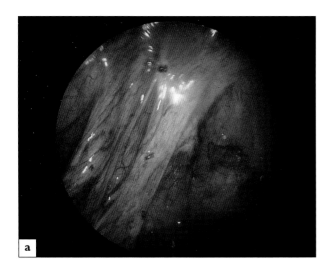

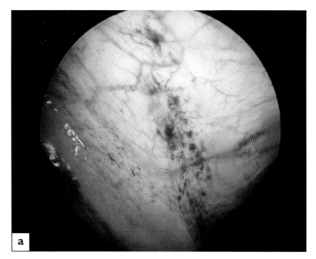

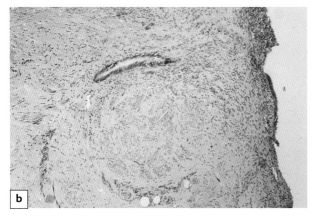

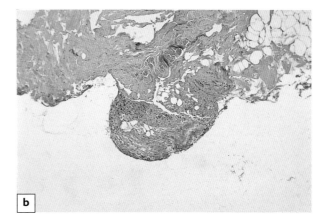

Figure 7 Circular peritoneal defects: (a) laparoscopic aspect; (b) histology: the typical endometrial glands are found in more than 50% of cases (Gomori's trichrome × 25)

peritoneal defects. Later, Stripling and colleagues[4] confirmed endometriosis in 91% of white lesions, 75% of red lesions, 33% of hemosiderin lesions and 85% of other lesions. In our study, we confirmed the presence of endometriosis in non-pigmented lesions of the peritoneum in more than 50% of cases.

Unsuspected peritoneal endometriosis

In a recent study[6], biopsies were taken from visually normal peritoneum of 32 women undergoing laparoscopy for infertility, in whom neither typical nor subtle appearances of endometriosis were found (group II). In another group of 52 women with apparent endometriosis, biopsies were also taken from visually normal peritoneum (group I).

The peritoneum was considered normal if no lesion, as previously described, was seen. A biopsy was taken from the normal peritoneum of the uterosacral ligaments. Histological study revealed the presence of endometriotic tissue in two cases (6%) in the group of 32 infertile women

Figure 8 Areas of petechial peritoneum: (a) laparoscopic aspect; (b) and (c) histology: note the typical endometrial glands and stroma (Gomori's trichrome × 25, × 56)

without endometriosis. This rate was less than one-half the rate (13%) observed in normal peritoneum taken from women with visible endometriosis (Table 3).

Identification of endometriosis in biopsy specimens from areas of normal peritoneum in patients with known endometriosis was reported by Murphy and colleagues[9]. By scanning electron microscopy, 25% of their specimens, which appeared normal by gross inspection, were found to

Table 3 Peritoneal endometriosis and infertility; biopsies were taken from the peritoneum of women with (group I) and without (group II) apparent endometriosis; all the women were undergoing laparoscopy for infertility

	Group I (n = 52)	Group II (n = 32)
Number of biopsies		
from visible endometriotic lesions*	86	—
from normal-appearing peritoneum*	52	32
Histological proof of endometriosis		
in visible lesions*	80/86 (93%)	—
in normal-appearing peritoneum*	7/52 (13%)	2/32 (6%)

*, Refers to the macroscopic appearance

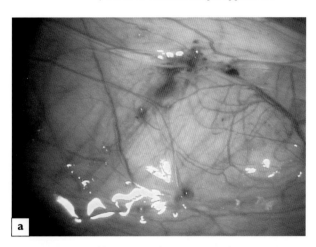
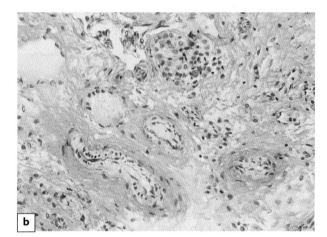

Figure 9 Areas of hypervascularization: (a) laparoscopic aspect; (b) histology: red blood cells are numerous and endometrial glands are very rare (Gomori's trichrome × 110)

contain evidence of endometriosis. In our study, by light microscopy, we reported a rate of 13%[6]. Moreover, histological study of biopsies from visually normal peritoneum in infertile women without any typical or 'subtle' endometriotic lesions revealed the presence of endometriosis in 6% of cases[6]. Unsuspected peritoneal endometriosis can thus be found in the visually normal peritoneum of infertile women, with or without known associated endometriosis. Although the rate (13%) in women with visible endometriosis was twice the rate observed in women without endometriosis, the difference was not significant. The size of the endometriotic lesions in visually normal peritoneum ($313 \pm 185 \, \mu m$) probably explains why the peritoneum had a normal aspect and why the lesion was not visible, even though a meticulous inspection was made to identify small and non-hemorrhagic lesions[6].

As recently demonstrated in infertile women, the diagnosis of endometriosis at laparoscopy has increased.

However, our data confirm that the operating surgeon did not make the diagnosis in at least 6% of cases, despite the significant increase in the diagnosis and documentation of endometriosis.

Hormonal independence

Using qualitative histochemistry, the microscopic changes[10] present in endometrium have been observed in ectopic implants, but endometrial implants do not demonstrate the characteristic ultrastructural changes of normal endometrium[11]. The fact that endometrial implants can undergo cyclical histological changes, similar to those found in normal endometrium, demonstrates that ectopic endometrium responds to gonadal hormones. But the majority of implants do not demonstrate histological changes synchronous with the comparable uterine endometrium[12]. Some of the reasons[13] may be:

(1) The deficiency in steroid receptors;

(2) The influence of the surrounding scarification process;

(3) The pressure atrophy; and

(4) The hormonal independence of ectopic endometrial glands.

The evaluation of steroid receptors in ectopic endometrial implants could be difficult because of the small number of glandular and stromal cells within the implant, and the heterogeneity of the tissue. While most implants can be demonstrated to possess progesterone receptors[14], only 30% have estrogen receptors. In the ovary, implants have far fewer estrogen and progesterone receptors than does normal epithelium[15,16]. Castration, menopause, pregnancy, or therapeutic suppression of gonadal function can dramatically alter the pattern of the disease. We have recently shown[17] that hormonal treatment is unable to eradicate endometriosis. Indeed, both in peritoneal endometriosis and in ovarian endometriosis, microscopic examination of specimens (taken after 6 months of therapy) revealed a high incidence of active endometriosis, without signs of degeneration. Mitotic activity was found, and this suggested the presence of hormonally independent glands in endometriotic foci.

MORPHOMETRIC STUDY OF THE VASCULARIZATION

Vascularization

Vascularization of endometriotic implants is probably one of the most important factors in the growth and invasion of endometrial glands into other tissue. A stereometric analysis was applied in order to study, precisely, the vascularization in peritoneal endometriotic foci[18,19].

Vascularization of typical and subtle lesions

We histologically evaluated the vascularization of typical peritoneal endometriosis and its modifications, according to the macroscopic appearance of peritoneal endometriosis.

Methods

In a series of 135 women who were undergoing laparoscopy for infertility, 220 peritoneal biopsies of 3–5 mm in size were taken from areas of the pelvic peritoneum bearing foci of endometriosis, with a biopsy punch forceps (26-175 DH, Storz, Tuttlingen, Germany). In all cases, a biopsy was taken from the typical (puckered black) endometriotic implants ($n = 135$, group Ia). Laparoscopy and biopsy were systematically carried out during the early luteal phase.

In the same series, a peritoneal biopsy was taken from an area with subtle appearances. The different subtle appearances of endometriosis were classified as red lesions: vesicular lesions, red flame-like lesions and glandular excrescences (group Ib, $n = 35$); and white lesions: white opacification, yellow-brown patches and circular peritoneal defects (group Ic, $n = 150$).

All biopsy specimens were fixed in formaldehyde and embedded in paraffin; 4-μm serial sections were stained with Gomori's trichrome and examined on a blind basis with a Leitz Orthoplan microscope (Leitz, Wetzlar, Germany). A two-dimensional image analysis program set on a Vidas computer (Kontron Bildanalyse GmBH, Eching, Germany) was completed by the interactive counting of 262 144 points.

All endometriotic lesions ($n = 220$) were analyzed, field by field, using the objective x 40 of an Axioskop light microscope (Zeiss, Oberkochen, Germany) and a television camera (Dage-MTI, Michigan City, IN, USA). The histological features were displayed on a television monitor and stored in the memory for processing by the measuring program. The mean of fields analyzed in each case was 13.3 ± 6.7. Histological structures of interest, such as the stroma, the glandular epithelium and lumen, the capillaries and the lymphocytes, were drawn by moving a cursor (Figure 10a). Each different structure was discriminated and gray-level images were transferred to binary images (Figure 10b). The interactive measurements of the selected parameters (number of structures, area and perimeter of the structures per field) were appended and stored at the end of an existing database.

Data management and evaluation were checked according to specific search criteria on the Videoplan (Kontron Bildanalyse GmBH, Eching, Germany), and displayed on the television monitor and printed. In all cases, the mitotic index was calculated as previously described[8], by counting mitotic figures (prometaphase, metaphase, anaphase and telophase) for 2000 epithelial cells per biopsy. This is the only method available for women because administration of colchicine or tritiated thymidine is not ethical. The contingency table method, the χ^2 (chi-square) test, the t test and the median test were used for statistical analysis.

Results

Biopsies taken from typical puckered black or bluish peritoneal lesions showed the presence of endometrial elements (glands and stroma) in all cases (100%).

The results concerning the capillaries are shown in Table 4. The number of capillaries per mm^2 of stroma, their mean surface area and the surface area ratio (capillaries/stroma) were calculated. In group Ia, the number of capillaries per mm^2 of stroma was 243. Their mean surface area was 118 ± 84 μm^2 and the ratio of capillaries/stroma surface area was 2.4%.

When compared to group Ia, a significant difference in the number of capillaries per mm^2 of stroma was observed in groups Ib and Ic ($p < 0.001$ and $p < 0.05$, respectively). Both the mean surface area and the ratio of capillaries/stroma surface area found in group Ic were significantly reduced when compared to groups Ia and Ib ($p < 0.001$). The capillary mean surface area was significantly higher ($p < 0.001$) in group Ib, compared to group Ia.

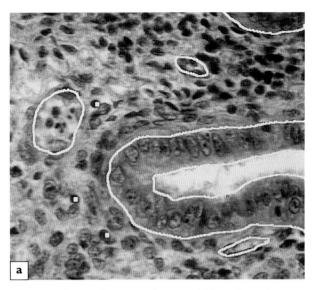
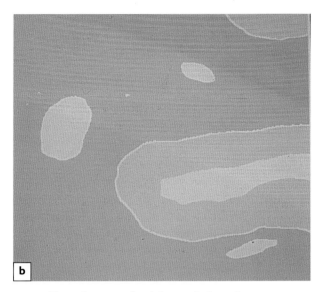

Figure 10 A two-dimensional image: (a) histological structures are traced by a digitizer: glandular epithelium, lumen, stroma and capillaries; (b) gray-level image of the same field

The contingency table method was used in order to compare the surface area occupied by the capillaries in each field. In group Ia, the surface area per field occupied by the capillaries reached 3000 μm². However, in group Ic, the surface area did not exceed 500 μm². The difference in values is statistically significant ($p < 0.05$). Not only the capillary mean surface area, but also the surface area per field occupied by the capillaries was significantly reduced in group Ic, when compared to group Ia.

The mitotic index was calculated in glandular epithelium and its value was 0.1‰ and 0.61‰ in groups Ia and Ib, respectively. In group Ic (white lesions), no mitosis was observed.

Influence of GnRH agonist on the vascularization

The vascularization of typical peritoneal endometriosis was evaluated in 45 patients after gonadotropin releasing hormone (GnRH) agonist therapy. The results concerning the capillaries are shown in Table 4. The number of capillaries per mm² of stroma, their mean surface area and the surface area ratio (capillaries/stroma) were calculated. There was no significant difference in the number of capillaries per mm² of stroma between the treated and untreated patients. However, in the treated group, their mean surface area (71 ± 40 μm²) was significantly different ($p < 0.001$) from the value observed in the untreated group (118 ± 84 μm²). The capillaries/stroma ratio was significantly lower ($p < 0.002$) in the treated group (1.4%) than in the untreated group (2.4%).

Comments on vascularization

The method of descriptive and computerized interactive morphometry for different tissue was applied to the study of endometriotic foci, in order to evaluate the stromal vascularization[19]. Our study demonstrated significant differences between the typical (black or bluish) lesion and the 'subtle' lesion. Subtle lesions were classified as red lesions (vesicular, red flame-like and glandular excrescences) and white lesions (white opacification, yellow-brown patches and circular peritoneal defects). When compared to typical lesion data, the vascularization was found to be significantly higher in red lesions and significantly lower in white lesions. This change was due to an increase (red) or a decrease (white) in the volume occupied by the vessels, as proved by both the mean capillary surface area and the ratio of capillaries/stroma surface area. This change was more evident in the group of red lesions, where the number of capillaries/mm² was significantly lower than in the other subgroups.

Thus, in the red lesions, the increased level of vascularization is due to a greater number of larger vessels than in the other groups. In white lesions, there was a greater number of smaller vessels; the number of capillaries was higher than in red lesions.

The mitotic index was also significantly different in the three groups. Mitotic processes permit the maintenance and growth of peritoneal endometriosis. The absence of mitosis in white lesions proves their low 'activity'[6,18,19].

According to our data, we can suggest that there are probably different types of peritoneal endometriotic lesions, in different stages of development. Red flame-like lesions and glandular excrescences are probably the first stage of early implantation of endometrial glands and stroma.

The growth and aggressiveness of endometrial glands in the stroma have recently been demonstrated by a three-dimensional evaluation[18]. Indeed, in this group, a higher incidence of glands with ramifications was observed when compared to typical and white lesions. The significantly

Table 4 Morphometric study of the stromal vascularization

	Typical lesions (black) group Ia (n = 135)	Red lesions group Ib (n = 35)	White lesions group Ic (n = 50)	Treated typical lesions group Id (n = 45)
Number of capillaries/mm² stroma	243	147*†	206†	225
Capillary mean surface area (μm²)	118 ± 84	234 ± 192*†	78 ± 43†	71 ± 40†
Capillaries/stroma relative surface (%)	2.4	3.2*†	1.5†	1.4†

*, Significantly different from groups Ic and Id ($p < 0.05$); †, significantly different from group Ia ($p < 0.001$)

higher stromal vascularization and epithelial mitotic index could be responsible for the invasion of ectopic sites by glands and stroma.

Thereafter, menstrual shedding from viable endometrial implants could initiate an inflammatory reaction, provoking a scarification process which encloses the implant. The presence of intraluminal debris is responsible for the typical black coloration of the same lesion. This scarification process is probably responsible for the reduction in vascularization, as proved by the significant decrease in the capillaries/stroma relative surface area. Thereafter, the inflammatory process devascularizes the endometriotic foci, and white plaques of old collagen are all that remain of the ectopic implant.

Concerning the white lesions, our study demonstrated the absence of mitosis, and poor vascularization, although a similar number of capillaries were found when compared to typical lesions. Our hypothesis is that white opacification and yellow-brown lesions are latent stages of endometriosis. They are probably non-active lesions which could be quiescent for a long time[18,19].

Some morphological changes in endometriotic foci after hormonal therapy have been described previously[17]. The mitotic index has been found to be significantly reduced. One of our hypotheses concerning the mechanism of action was the reduction in the vascularization of glandular epithelium after GnRH agonist therapy. Macroscopically, preoperative hormonal therapy results in the reduction of pelvic vascularity and inflammation diagnosed at the time of the second-look laparoscopy.

Our results demonstrated that there was a significant decrease in the vascularization of the endometriotic foci after GnRH agonist therapy[19]. This change was due, not to a reduction in the number of capillaries in the lesion, but to a decrease in the area of the vessels. Indeed, in the treated patients (group II), a predominance of smaller vessels was observed when compared with the untreated patients (group I). This vascularization decrease, observed histologically, was in accordance with the observations made by laparoscopy after hormonal therapy. Vascular

effects of the GnRH agonist on the uterine arteries have also been demonstrated by Doppler[20]. The hypoestradiol state induced by GnRH agonist therapy could also have an effect on the vascularization of the endometriotic stroma.

The reduction in the vascularization after hormonal therapy could account for the decrease in the inflammatory reaction observed around the endometriotic foci.

In conclusion, the evaluation of the stromal vascularization permitted the differentiation and classification of the different appearances of peritoneal endometriosis, according to their vascularization level. Our study proves that the 'activity' of peritoneal endometriosis is related to the vascularity. This concept must be taken into account in the further discussions of the American Fertility Society Endometriosis Classification. Typical, red and white lesions are three different stages of the peritoneal disease and their relative relation to infertility probably also differs.

THREE-DIMENSIONAL ARCHITECTURE OF ENDOMETRIOSIS

In order to further elucidate the biological characteristics of peritoneal endometriotic lesions – for example, how they stereologically develop *in vivo*, and how glandular epithelium and stroma are related to the surrounding tissue – a recently advanced stereographic computer technology[18] was applied for the investigation of the three-dimensional architecture of peritoneal endometriosis.

Methods

All biopsy specimens were fixed in formaldehyde and embedded in paraffin; 6-μm serial sections were stained with Gomori's trichrome and examined on a blind basis, with a Leitz Orthoplan microscope (Leitz, Wetzlar, Germany). The histological features of the sections were displayed using an Axioskop microscope (Zeiss, Oberkochen, Germany) through a CCD 72 E camera (Dage-MTI, Michigan City, IN, USA) on a monitor, on which two-dimensional figures drawn with a digitizer were superimposed using a computer (Vidas, Kontron Bildanalyse GmBH, Eching, Germany). Computer-assisted reconstruction of three-dimensional (3-D) models was developed with two main aims in mind: to generate a complete multicolored model of a complex structure which can be rotated and viewed from any angle or orientation; and to calculate the volumes and surfaces within the 3-D model automatically.

The major features of the program[18] include:

(1) Input of serial section data by manual tracing, or automatic contour finding;

(2) Alignment of sections;

(3) Editing and reassignment of contours of individual sections;

(4) Storing contour data in a file;

(5) Selecting a range of sections and/or a range of elements to be used for reconstruction;

(6) Reconstructing models in a wire frame and/or a solid modelling mode by using parallel projection;

(7) Rotating the reconstruction in the x, y and z planes at variable magnifications;

(8) Viewing inside a model by cutting away part of the reconstruction using an 'electronic knife';

(9) Calculating surfaces and volumes; and

(10) Plotting the reconstruction on a matrix or laser printer.

With this program, outlines of glandular structure and endometrial stroma in the serial histological sections were traced by the digitizer, sections were aligned and contour data were stored in a file; once all the serial outlines had been digitized and stored, reconstructed (3-D) image models of these *in vivo* structures were displayed on the television monitor. The 3-D reconstruction could generate a complete multicolored model of the complex structure, which could be rotated and viewed from any angle or orientation.

Volumes of the reconstructed glandular and stromal structures were obtained by a calculation function in the same program. Lumen volume was also calculated. Ratios of lumen volume/epithelial volume/stromal volume were determined for each specimen. The χ^2 test was used for statistical analysis.

Results

In 42 women who were undergoing laparoscopy for infertility, peritoneal biopsies of 3–5 mm in size were taken from areas of the pelvic peritoneum bearing foci of endometriosis, with a biopsy punch forceps (26-175dh, Storz, Tuttlingen, Germany). Biopsies were taken from the typical (puckered black) endometriotic implants in all cases.

Group I consisted of 26 women with peritoneal endometriosis who had not previously received any hormonal therapy. All of them underwent laparoscopy during the early luteal phase.

Group II consisted of 17 women who had received GnRH agonist therapy (Zoladex, Zeneca, Cambridge, UK) for 12 weeks before biopsy. After an initial stimulation of estradiol (E_2) secretion, GnRH agonist administration resulted in a range of levels of postmenopausal E_2 secretion (15 ± 6 pg/ml).

Histologically, all the biopsy specimens showed typical epithelium and stroma of the endometrial type. The reconstructed 3-D image models of the structures in the peritoneal endometriotic lesions were displayed, and a pink color was applied for the stroma (Figure 11a), a green color for the epithelium (Figure 11b) and a blue color for the lumen (Figure 11c).

The 3-D image models were usually shown as a solid structure (Figure 11); however, models could be displayed as a transparent structure, when they were simultaneously shown with their stromal and epithelial structures (Figure 12).

Stereographically, two types could be easily recognized and classified. The first type (Figure 13) was composed of cylinder-like glands without ramifications. The lesion showed a regular distribution of the glandular epithelium in the stromal structure, which was also regular. The second type (Figure 14) was composed of glands with ramifications.

Luminal structures were interconnected (Figure 15). Epithelial structures appeared like fingers and seemed to invade the stroma. The distribution of glandular structures in the stroma was not regular. Many glandular structures formed inside luminal structures, whose diameter varied from 22 to 185 µm.

In all groups, the 'external' stromal surface was regular. Like normal uterine epithelial structures, the glandular epithelium had a markedly regular luminal surface. In some cases, the lumen was dilated; in others, especially when the ramifications were numerous, the lumen was narrow. The incidence of the first type was 44% in group I and 46% in group II. The incidences of the second type were 56% and 54%, respectively. The volumes of epithelial, stromal and luminal structures were measured separately by computer stereometry, and the results are shown in Table 5. The stroma/lesion ratios were 62.2% and 51.8% in groups I and II, respectively. Although there was a decrease in stroma/lesion ratio in group II as compared to group I, the difference was not significant. The epithelium/lesion ratios were 19.9% and 14.9%, respectively. The lumen/lesion ratio was 13.2% in group I and 25.2% in group II. These values were significantly different ($p < 0.01$).

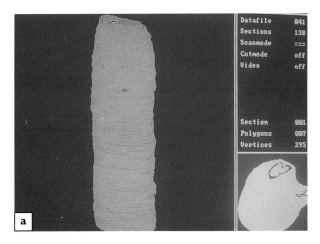

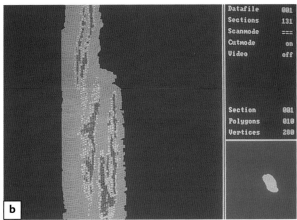

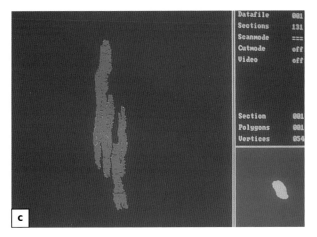

Figure 11 Reconstructed three-dimensional image models of the elements of a peritoneal endometriotic lesion indicated as a solid structure: (a) stroma (pink); (b) epithelium (green); (c) lumen (blue)

Comments

Recently, computer stereographic studies of skin tissues[21–23] have been reported describing the advantages of the computer-generated 3-D models of tissue structures. As far as we know, there has been no publication on the subject of endometriosis, using computer graphic mechanical methods of reconstruction.

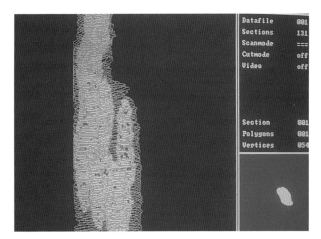

Figure 12 The three-dimensional image models displayed as a transparent structure; the stromal, epithelial and luminal structures are shown simultaneously

Table 5 Stereometry of volumes of three-dimensional structures: percentage of the lesion attributed to the epithelium, stroma or lumen

Ratio	Group I (n = 26)	Group II (n = 16)
Epithelium/lesion	19.9%	14.9%
Stroma/lesion	62.2%	51.8%
Lumen/lesion	13.2%	25.2%

When compared with the 3-D models demonstrated in other studies, the present 3-D models seemed to be much better and to show more realistic appearances of structures, since the structures of the reconstructed models were colored. Furthermore, the transparent display of our 3-D models was excellent for the observation of their interior structures. The present study demonstrates that two different types of peritoneal endometriotic lesions can be differentiated: a first type without ramification of the glands, and a second type in which glands are ramified and connected (Figures 13 and 14). Further studies are needed in order to evaluate whether the two different types could be correlated either to the different degree of 'aggressiveness' or to the different appearances of peritoneal endometriosis.

From the present stereographic findings, one may consider that the apparently multifocal occurrence (in two-dimensional views) of glandular epithelium in one lesion is not confirmed by the 3-D study. Indeed, in each peritoneal lesion, epithelial glands are interconnected by luminal structures. It is probable that, in each peritoneal lesion, epithelial structures occur in a single focus of the stroma, and then may gradually develop, elongate and swell, forming luminal structures, occasionally with

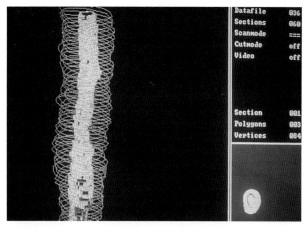

Figure 13 Cylinder-like gland; regular distribution of the glandular epithelium in the stroma

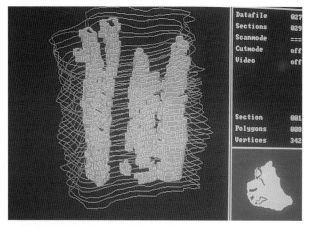

Figure 14 Glands with ramifications; luminal structures are interconnected (three-dimensional)

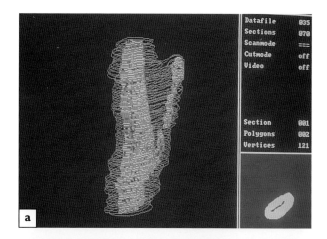

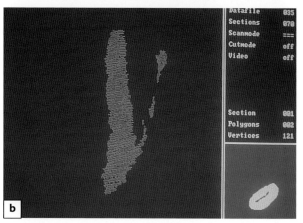

Figure 15 (a) and (b) Luminal structures are interconnected

endometrial debris inside. During the expansion, all glands are connected and no peripheral epithelial structures become independent by loss of interconnection.

Since each of the peritoneal lesions, stereographically reconstructed in the present study, was only a part of the peritoneal endometriosis of one patient, it is far too soon to reach any conclusion; however, in the future, the 3-D analysis of stereographically reconstructed lesions could contribute to the understanding of the *in vivo* development of endometriosis.

This stereometric study of volumes of 3-D structures revealed the volume distribution in peritoneal endometriosis. The ratios of epithelium, stroma and lumen/lesion observed in groups I and II indicate a more powerful effect of the GnRH agonist therapy on the stroma than on the epithelium. This effect could be due to the reduction in stromal vascularization, induced by the GnRH agonist. The stromal capillary network can also be reconstructed in 3-D. In active lesions, the 3-D evaluation of the capillary network reveals the presence of a great number of larger vessels (Figure 16). After GnRH agonist

therapy (as well as in white lesions), the network is composed of smaller vessels (Figure 17).

The present stereographic and stereometric study has shown some new characteristics of peritoneal endometriosis. Further studies are under way to investigate the variations in the 3-D architecture of peritoneal endometriotic lesions among different patients, patients of differing ages, and patients with different types of peritoneal endometriosis, before and after hormonal therapy.

HYPOTHESES

Our morphologic and morphometric data allow us to suggest that eutopic endometrium and red peritoneal lesions are similar tissues, with red lesions being recently implanted and regurgitated endometrial cells[24,25]. These data constitute an argument in favor of the transplantation theory for peritoneal endometriosis (Figure 18). After endometrial tissue transplantation, the factors that regulate the attachment phase, and thereafter initiate ectopic growth, are not known. Red lesions are located consistently on the surface of the peritoneum, which consists histologically of a thin layer of loose connective tissue

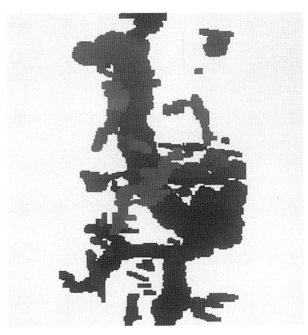

Figure 16 The three-dimensional evaluation of the capillary network; a great number of larger vessels can be seen

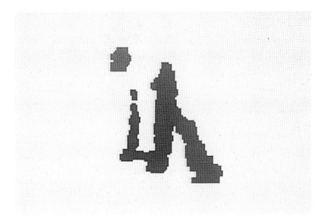

Figure 17 The three-dimensional evaluation of the capillary network; smaller vessels are seen after gonadotropin releasing hormone agonist therapy or in white lesion

covered with a layer of mesothelium. There is a rich supply of subperitoneal blood vessels and lymphatics[26].

In our opinion, vascularization of endometriotic implants is probably one of the most important factors of growth and invasion of other tissue by endometrial glands[19,27]. Thereafter, detachment of glands from viable red endometrial implants, explained by the presence of matrix metalloproteinases (MMPs), could initiate their implantation in other peritoneal sites, as in a 'metastatic' process[28]. Preliminary data from our group[28] revealed the presence of MMPs in the stroma of red lesions throughout the menstrual cycle, although, in eutopic endometrium, MMPs are detected only during the marked decline in progesterone.

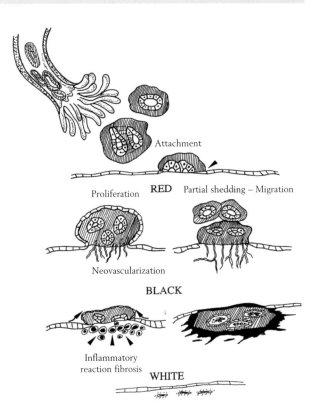

Figure 18 Hypothesis of peritoneal endometriotic lesion evolution

After this partial shedding, the remaining red lesion always regrows constantly until the next shedding, but menstrual shedding finally induces an inflammatory reaction, provoking a scarification process that encloses the implant. The enclosed implant becomes a 'black' lesion because of the presence of intraluminal debris. This scarification process is probably responsible for the reduction in vascularization, as proved by the significant decrease in the relative surface areas of the capillaries and stroma[19].

In some cases, the inflammatory process and subsequent fibrosis totally devascularize the endometriotic foci, and white plaques of old collagen are all that remain of the ectopic implant[24,25]. White opacification and yellow-brown lesions are latent stages of endometriosis[19]. They are probably inactive lesions that could be quiescent for a long time.

In agreement with Brosens[29], we regard red lesions as early endometriosis and black lesions as advanced endometriosis[19,30,31]. White lesions are believed to be healed endometriosis or quiescent or latent lesions[19,31].

REFERENCES

1. Chatman DL. Pelvic peritoneal defects and endometriosis; Allen–Masters syndrome revisited. *Fertil Steril* 1981;36:751

2. Jansen RPS, Russell P. Non-pigmented endometriosis: clinical laparoscopic and pathologic definition. *Am J Obstet Gynecol* 1986;155:1154

3. Redwine DB. The distribution of endometriosis in the pelvis by age groups and fertility. *Fertil Steril* 1987;47:173–5

4. Stripling MC, Martin DC, Chatman DL, *et al.* Subtle appearances of pelvic endometriosis. *Fertil Steril* 1988;49:427

5. Martin DC, Hubert GD, Van der Zwaag R, *et al.* Laparoscopic appearances of peritoneal endometriosis. *Fertil Steril* 1989;51:63

6. Nisolle M, Paindaveine B, Bourdon A, *et al.* Histologic study of peritoneal endometriosis in infertile women. *Fertil Steril* 1990;53:984–8

7. Donnez J, Nisolle M. Appearances of peritoneal endometriosis. In *Proceedings of the IIIrd International Laser Surgery Symposium*, Brussels, 1988

8. Donnez J, Casanas-Roux F, Caprasse EJ, *et al.* Cyclic changes in ciliation, cell height, and mitotic activity in human tubal epithelium during reproductive life. *Fertil Steril* 1985;43:554–9

9. Murphy AA, Green WR, Bobbie D, *et al.* Unsuspected endometriosis documented by scanning electron microscopy in visually normal peritoneum. *Fertil Steril* 1986;46:552

10. Brosens I, Vasquez G, Gordts S. Scanning electron microscopic study of the pelvic peritoneum in unexplained infertility and endometriosis. *Fertil Steril* 1984;41:215

11. Lox CD, Word L, Heine MW. Ultrastructural evaluation of endometriosis. *Fertil Steril* 1984;41:755

12. Roddick JW, Conkey G, Jacobs EJ. The hormonal response of endometriotic implants and its relationship to symptomatology. *Am J Obstet Gynecol* 1960;79:1173–7

13. Donnez J, Nisolle M, Casanas-Roux F, *et al.* Endometriosis: rationale for surgery. In Brosens I, Donnez J, eds. *The Current Status of Endometriosis Research and Management.* Carnforth, UK: Parthenon Publishing, 1993:385–96

14. Jänne O, Kauppila A, Kokko E. Estrogen and progestin receptors in endometriosis lesions: comparison with endometrial tissue. *Am J Obstet Gynecol* 1981;141:562–6

15. Bergqvist A, Rannevik G, Thorell J. Estrogen and progesterone cytosol receptor concentration in endometriotic tissue and intrauterine endometrium. *Acta Obstet Gynecol Scand* 1981;101:53–8

16. Tamaya T, Motoyaha T, Ohono Y. Steroid receptor levels and histology of endometriosis and adenomyosis. *Fertil Steril* 1979;31:394–400

17. Nisolle M, Casanas-Roux F, Donnez J. Histologic study of ovarian endometriosis after hormonal therapy. *Fertil Steril* 1988;49:423

18. Donnez J, Nisolle M, Casanas-Roux F. Three dimensional architectures of peritoneal endometriosis. *Fertil Steril* 1992;57:980

19. Nisolle M, Casanas-Roux F, Anal V, *et al.* Morphometric study of the stromal vascularization in peritoneal endometriosis. *Fertil Steril* 1993;59:681

20. Matta WHM, Stabille I, Shaw RS, *et al.* Doppler assessment of uterine blood flow changes in patients with fibroids receiving the GnRH agonist Buserelin. *Fertil Steril* 1988;49:1083

21. Braverman MS, Braverman IM. Three-dimensional reconstructions of objects from serial sections using a microcomputer graphic system. *J Invest Dermatol* 1986;86:290–4

22. Marchevsky AM, Gil J, Jeanty H. Computerized interactive morphometry in pathology: current instrumentation and methods. *Hum Pathol* 1987;18:320–31

23. Ito M, Yokoyama H, Ikeda K, *et al.* Stereographic analysis of syringomas. *Arch Dermatol Res* 1990;282:17–21

24. Nisolle M. *Peritoneal, ovarian and rectovaginal endometriosis are three distinct entities.* Thèse d'Agrégation de l'Enseignement Supérieur. Louvain, Belgium: Université Catholique de Louvain, 1996

25. Nisolle M, Donnez J, eds. *Peritoneal, Ovarian and Rectovaginal Endometriosis: The Identification of Three Separate Diseases.* Carnforth, UK: Parthenon Publishing, 1996

26. Bloom W, Fawcett DN. *A Textbook of Histology.* Philadelphia: WB Saunders, 1978:186–7

27. Donnez J, Nisolle M. L'endométriose péritonéale, le kyste endométriotique ovarien et le nodule de la lame rectovaginale sont trois pathologies différentes (éditorial). *Réf Gynécol Obstét* 1995;3:121–3

28. Kokorine I, Nisolle M, Donnez J, *et al.* Expression of interstitial collagenase (matrix metalloproteinase-1) is related to the activity of human endometriotic lesions. *Fertil Steril* 1997;68:246–51

29. Brosens IA. Is mild endometriosis a disease? Is mild endometriosis a progressive disease? *Hum Reprod* 1994;9: 2209–11

30. Donnez J, Casanas-Roux F, Nisolle M. Peritoneal endometriosis: new histological aspects. In Brosens IA, Donnez J, eds. *The Current Status of Endometriosis. Research and Management.* Carnforth, UK: Parthenon Publishing, 1993:75–87

31. Nisolle M, Donnez J. Peritoneal endometriosis, ovarian endometriosis and adenomyotic nodules of the rectovaginal septum are three different entities. *Fertil Steril* 1997;68:585–96

Douglasectomy – torus excision – uterine suspension

6

J. Donnez, J. Squifflet and M. Nisolle

INTRODUCTION

The correlation between the severity of pain (dyspareunia and dysmenorrhea) and the extent of disease (stage of endometriosis) has not been proved[1-3]. It is important to distinguish between psychological pelvic pain and pain due to organic pathology in order to orientate treatment: psychiatric orientation or surgical orientation. In a report from a psychiatric center, only 48% of women with pelvic pain had organic pathology while 64% reported childhood sexual abuse. Even if the studies did not show any relation between the extent of the disease and the severity of pain, it is true that there is a relation between the fluid concentrations of CA-125, the placental protein, and the peritoneal location of the lesions[4].

The American Fertility Society, in their staging concerning the classification of endometriosis, has established an association between pelvic pain, dyspareunia and moderate or severe dysmenorrhea in patients suffering from infertility. Severe dysmenorrhea is highly predictive of endometriosis.

To understand the mechanism of pain in endometriosis, it was suggested by Sturgis and All[5] that proliferation of functional glands, as well as a fibrotic reaction, are necessary to understand this mediation. It is a fact that endometriosis causes pain and tenderness in a significant number of women but it is more problematic to claim that chronic pelvic pain is just due to endometriosis. Indeed, a psychosomatic approach shows that endometriosis is not commonly a main component of the pain.

The treatment of pelvic pain has undergone various changes during the past 30 years, reflecting new developments in medicine and surgery. For many years, presacral neurectomy was performed on patients with untreatable dysmenorrhea but yielded disappointing results with failure rates of about 11–15% in primary dysmenorrhea and 25–40% in secondary dysmenorrhea. In 1952, White[6] pointed out that the nerve supply to the cervix is not usually interrupted by the presacral neurectomy procedure and for this reason, and with the development of new drugs to suppress ovulation, the procedure was abandoned by most gynecologists.

ALLEN–MASTERS SYNDROME

The Allen–Masters syndrome[7] was first described in 1955 in 28 patients, all of whom had uterine retroversion. This syndrome also included broad ligament lacerations, hyper-

mobility of the cervix and enlargement and engorgement of the uterus. Allen and Masters treated their patients with an operation that included repair of the broad ligament defects ('windows') and uterine suspension, with good relief from symptoms. However, many gynecologists doubt the existence of the syndrome. In our clinic, no patients have been operated upon for a preoperative diagnosis of the Allen–Masters syndrome. The 'windows' are presently vaporized with the Swiftlase in 'defocused' mode in order to shrink the 'pocket' where, very frequently, small lesions of endometriosis are discovered[8].

DYSMENORRHEA

Primary dysmenorrhea is not related to uterine position. It occurs in the anteverted, as well as the retroverted, uterus. Retroflexion of the uterus interferes with venous drainage from the myometrium and broad ligaments and is a factor in dysmenorrhea. Relative stenosis at the internal cervical os can increase dysmenorrhea. Menstrual discomfort may take the form of cramps or sacral backache.

DYSPAREUNIA

In some patients with deep dyspareunia, uterine retroversion or retroflexion may be the only finding in some indications, either if conservative measures have failed to relieve the pain, or if the dyspareunia disappears with the uterus in the anterior position, for example, when a Smith–Hodge pessary has been placed to hold the uterus in anteflexion. But pelvic examination usually reveals significant pelvic pathology, such as endometriosis of the uterosacral ligaments. The uterus may also be retroverted or retroflexed. If an operation is performed to treat the endometriosis, the uterus should be suspended.

INFERTILITY

The finding of a retroposed uterus in a woman complaining of infertility is not an indication that the position of the uterus is directly related to the problem. Although infertility may be more common among women with retrodisplacement of the uterus, the relationship is difficult to prove, except in cases when other associated pathology, such as pelvic endometriosis or chronic salpingitis, exists.

PELVIC CONGESTION SYNDROME

Pelvic congestion syndrome has often been associated with uterine retroversion. In Taylor's original description of the syndrome in 1949, only 35% of patients were found to have uterine retroversion[9,10]. Taylor believed that vascular congestion of the pelvic organs explained the fact that pelvic veins can easily become dilated because they lack valves, since the surrounding adventitial tissue in the broad ligaments is weak.

Taylor did not recommend hysterectomy or uterine suspension for these patients. He recognized the frequency with which his patients also suffered from psychosomatic and psychiatric complaints. It is not known how many patients with vascular congestion of pelvic organs are asymptomatic. Recently, some authors have recommended embolization of pelvic veins as treatment for pelvic congestion syndrome. Others, like Manhes (personal communication), have suggested photocoagulating the veins in order to shrink them.

INDICATIONS FOR UTERINE SUSPENSION

Since the nineteenth century, uterine suspension has been practised to relieve pelvic pain, dyspareunia and infertility. Numerous methods and variations have been described in the medical literature, wherein the round ligament has been folded, plaited, ligated, transplanted, banded and shirred[11]. Uterine suspension has been suggested to be very effective in the relief of deep dyspareunia or pelvic pain due to uterine retroversion.

Primary suspension of the retroverted uterus is not necessary for adequate gynecologic practice. Uterine suspension is most often indicated in connection with such conservative operations as those carried out for endometriosis or tubal pregnancy, or with microsurgical tubal reconstruction procedures for relief of infertility. The goal is to avoid leaving the uterus of an infertile patient in the cul-de-sac, where tubal adhesions may recur, while performing other conservational procedures.

The presence of uterine retrodisplacement alone in an asymptomatic patient is not an indication for prophylactic uterine suspension.

Symptomatic anatomic vaginal wall relaxation and uterine descensus are rarely associated with uterine retroversion. In such cases, we prefer to perform laparoscopic uterine sacrofixation (see Chapter 28).

Mild pelvic pain with dyspareunia is described as mild abdominal discomfort and fullness on intercourse, while moderate pelvic pain with dyspareunia is described as mild tolerable pain and the patient still enjoys the sexual act.

Pelvic examinations are systematically performed to evaluate the uterine position, degree of misalignment of the uterus and the severity of adhesions. We also try to reproduce the pelvic pain and dyspareunia by palpation of the retroverted uterus. Ultrasound is performed to confirm the initial findings and to rule out myomas, adenomyosis, or any uterine or ovarian abnormalities.

CHOICE OF OPERATION

To a great extent, choice of operative technique depends on the patient's desire for future pregnancy. The modified Gillian suspension is a good technique for suspending the uterus while preserving the possibility of pregnancy.

The modified Gillian suspension procedure[12] draws each round ligament through an aperture in the peritoneum near the internal inguinal ring and brings each ligament beneath the anterior rectus sheath. Although some patients experience transient round ligament pain with vigorous physical activity or uterine enlargement, there is no evidence that the suspension is detrimental to a subsequent pregnancy.

In the Olshausen operation[13], for example, the uterus is fixed to the anterior abdominal wall. This procedure precludes the possibility of a future intrauterine pregnancy because the anchored uterus will produce severe abdominal pain as the uterus enlarges with advancing pregnancy. This operation should never be done.

In the Baldy–Webster procedure[14], the round ligaments are passed through the anterior and posterior leaves of the broad ligament and are sutured to the posterior surface of the uterus. The extraperitoneal technique of shortening each round ligament in the inguinal canal described by Alexander[15] and Adams[16] is no longer used in the United States, although it is still in use in some European countries. The operation is blind because the uterus is not visualized unless a laparotomy is performed. The extraperitoneal approach is its only advantage.

Some authors suggest that another procedure for providing additional support is shortening the uterosacral ligaments. This procedure is especially valuable when some descensus is present or when the cervix has been displaced anteriorly. We have never performed this procedure.

Operative technique (Figure 1)

After general anesthesia with endotracheal intubation has been established, the patient is placed in the lithotomy position or in the Trendelenburg position. The bladder is emptied with a Foley catheter. The laparoscopic trocar is introduced into the peritoneal cavity. The pelvis is then visualized. The right, and then the left, lower quadrant are transilluminated, and an avascular region is selected about 5–6 cm away from the midline incision and 2 cm above the inguinal ligament.

A laparoscopic grasping forceps may be inserted through the trocar, or a Kelly clamp may be pushed through the incisions into the peritoneal cavity. The round ligaments are grasped (Figure 2a) about midpoint and gently pulled through the fascia as the pneumoperitoneum is allowed partially to escape (Figure 2b). The round ligaments are sutured to the fascia with a Vicryl 1-0 suture material (Figure 3).

Complications of uterine suspension

Occasionally, evulsion of the round ligament may result when pulling the ligament up to the anterior rectus sheath. The resultant bleeding must be controlled. If there is undue tension placed on the round ligaments, incisional pain may result. It is usually mild and temporary and controlled with analgesics, muscle relaxants and heat.

Results (Table 1)

The operating time of both procedures is less than an hour. Although all the patients could be treated as outpatients, due to our medical health insurance policy, they are required to stay for 2–3 days as compared to the average hospital stay of 1–2 days in other developed countries.

Table 1 Age and parity of 35 patients; indications for pelviscopic uterine suspension, combined with torus excision

	Mean
Age (years)	29.5
Parity	1.8
Number of women with deep dyspareunia and chronic pelvic pain	31 (88%)
Improved	32 (91%)
Same	3 (9%)

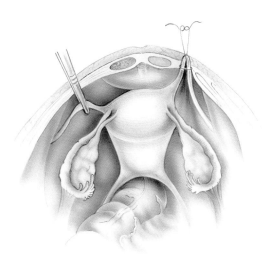

Figure 1 Technique of uterine suspension by grasping and fixation of the round ligament (ligamentum rundum)

Mild incisional pain and mild abdominal discomfort are frequently encountered and readily relieved with mild analgesics.

Although, in the study by Yoon[17], 51.5% and 18.6–45.5% felt better 6 weeks and 6 months, respectively, following surgery with no obvious causes for their deep dyspareunia or pelvic pain, all our patients (100%) experienced great improvement 6 weeks after the operation. Their sex life improved immensely.

After 6 months to 2 years of follow-up in the study by Koh and colleagues[18], 17 patients with Webster–Baldy's technique and five patients with Franke's technique (88%) enjoyed an improved sex life and the remaining three patients were lost to follow-up.

Discussion

Among the many procedures published in the medical literature are the Halben vesical suspension, Schmid–Matthiesen's suspension, Werth's interfascial

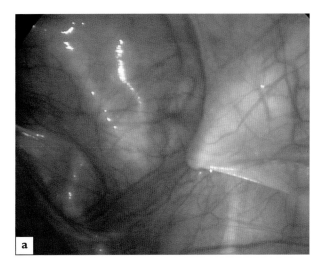

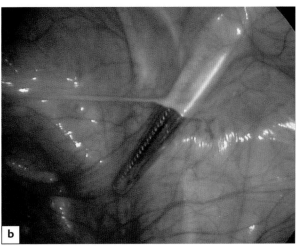

Figure 2 The forceps is introduced through a second trocar incision: (a) and (b) laparoscopic view. Care is taken to avoid injury to major blood vessels

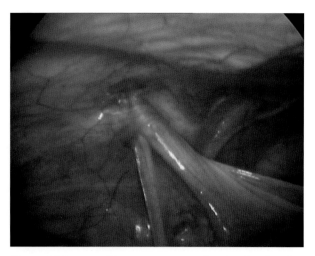

Figure 3 The round ligament is grasped and is fixed to the aponeurotic layer of the abdominal wall

plication, uterine suspension using Fallopian rings, the modified Gillian method, Mann–Stenger's suspension, and Webster–Baldy's and Franke's technique.

Laparoscopy is valuable in determining the cause of pelvic pain and, when dyspareunia and pelvic pain are caused by a retroverted uterus, we believe uterine suspension using different procedures will certainly relieve this problem.

In one study[18], the Webster–Baldy method was found to be more time-consuming, with more bleeding, but causing less kinking to the Fallopian tubes; thus this method is preferred in patients who still want to bear children. Although Franke's method is simpler, less time-consuming, with less bleeding, since it causes more kinking to the Fallopian tubes, this procedure is more appropriately performed in patients who no longer wish to become pregnant.

ASSOCIATED SURGERY

Laser uterine nerve ablation (LUNA)

Uterine neurectomy was initially performed by electrocautery but there was always concern about the spread of the electric current in this area due to the close proximity of the ureter and the uterine artery. Since 1989, we have by preference vaporized with CO_2 laser energy transmitted directly through the operating channel[19,20].

The posterior leaves of the broad ligaments are carefully inspected to try to identify the course of the ureters which usually run 1–2 cm laterally. They can usually be 'palpated' via a probe and often the characteristic peristaltic movements can be recognized beneath the peritoneal surface.

The uterosacral ligaments are pulled under tension by manipulating the uterus with an intrauterine manipulator.

The laser is set at a relatively high-power density setting of 60 W and the uterosacral ligaments are vaporized 1 cm from their attachment to the posterior aspect of the cervix over a length of 1.5 cm. The idea of the procedure is to destroy the sensory nerve fibers and their secondary ganglia as they leave the uterus; because of the divergence of these fibers in the uterosacral ligaments, they should be vaporized as close to the cervix as possible. Care must be taken to not vaporize too laterally, to avoid damage to the vessels running alongside the uterosacral ligaments.

Prospective double-blind randomized controlled studies have demonstrated that laparoscopic transection of the uterosacral ligaments close to their insertion on the posterior aspect of the cervix is an effective treatment for dysmenorrhea that has been unresponsive to drug therapy[21].

Torus excision

Another procedure is to lase deeply the posterior aspects of the cervix between the insertion of the ligaments to interrupt fibers crossing to the contralateral side. It is relatively easy to vaporize to the correct depth when the uterosacral ligaments are well formed. Sometimes their limits are poorly defined.

Douglasectomy

As previously seen (see Chapter 4), parasympathetic fibers are identified in the anterior two-thirds of the uterosacral ligaments. In some patients with deep and severe dyspareunia and secondary dysmenorrhea, or presenting with endometriosis of the uterosacral ligaments at laparoscopy or with recurrence of the symptoms after laser uterine nerve ablation, we propose a Douglasectomy by laparoscopy.

The technique starts in the same way as the LUNA, vaporizing the uterosacral ligaments as close to the cervix as possible, creating a crater about 2 cm in diameter and 1 cm deep. It is always very important to identify the course of the ureter.

Once this step is completed, the assistant manipulating the uterus will place a sponge in the posterior fornix of the vagina in order to individualize the peritoneum of the cul-de-sac of Douglas. In some cases, a 22-mm Hegar dilatator is placed in the rectum in order to identify its position.

Once the LUNA is done, we start on one side, pulling the peritoneum of the cul-de-sac of Douglas progressively with the grasping forceps and separating it from the perirectal fat and the fat below the peritoneum with the CO_2 laser until the peritoneal leaf is completely removed on the contralateral side.

If the cleavage plane between the peritoneum and the fat below has been well located, there should not be any hemostatic problems. Otherwise, careful bipolar coagulation could be carried out.

Table 2 Laser uterine nerve ablation (LUNA) results with a KTP laser (from Daniell[25])

	n	Improved (%)	Same (%)	Worse (%)
Endometriosis	80	60 (75)	17 (21)	3 (4)
Primary dysmenorrhea	20	12 (60)	6 (30)	2 (10)
Total	100	72 (72)	23 (23)	5 (5)

Forty-one laparoscopic Douglasectomies with uterosacral ligamentopexy were performed in the Department of Gynecology at the University Hospital of Caen during the period between 1990 and 1995 in patients with painful retroverted uterus[22]. The surgical endoscopic procedure, identical to the operation first promoted by Jamain and Letessier in 1976 by laparotomy, is described. Douglasectomy is the only definitive procedure for restoring normal anatomy of the pelvic floor in the case of painful uterine retroversion occurring in a setting of Masters–Allen syndrome. Additionally, it allows pathological analysis of the excised peritoneum. The results of this procedure are excellent when the indications are correctly set, particularly as concerns positive pessary testing.

Prevesical neurectomy

Resection of the presacral nerve plexus is associated with significant relief from symptoms. The pain impulses from the uterus, which travel through the inferior hypogastric plexus into the intermediate hypogastric plexus and the superior hypogastric plexus, can be interrupted by performing this procedure laparoscopically. The intermediate hypogastric plexus, which is composed of two or three trunks lying on the vertebral body of L5, is the most appropriate place for the resection. Presacral neurectomy is not appropriate treatment for relief of lateral or back pain. Patients with midline pain, however, will experience significant relief with the use of this procedure[23].

Chen and colleagues[24] compared laparoscopic presacral neurectomy and laparoscopic uterine nerve ablation for primary dysmenorrhea. One group (33 patients) underwent laparoscopic presacral neurectomy (LPSN) and the other group (35 patients) underwent laparoscopic uterine nerve ablation (LUNA). There were no complications and all the patients left hospital within 24 h of surgery. The efficacies of both surgical methods were almost the same (87.9% versus 82.9%) at the 9-month post-operative follow-up visit, but LPSN proved to be significantly more effective than LUNA (81.8% versus 51.4%) at the 12-month visit.

REFERENCES

1. Nisolle M, Casanas-Roux F, Anaf V, et al. Morphometric study of the stromal vascularization in peritoneal endometriosis. Fertil Steril 1993;59:681
2. Nisolle M, Paindaveine B, Bourdon A, et al. Histologic study of peritoneal endometriosis in infertile women. Fertil Steril 1990;53:984–8
3. Donnez J, Nisolle M, Casanas-Roux F. Three-dimensional architecture of peritoneal endometriosis. Fertil Steril 1992;57:980–3
4. Koninckx PD. Deeply infiltrating endometriosis. In Brosens I, Donnez J, eds. Endometriosis: Research and Management. Carnforth, UK: Parthenon Publishing, 1993:437–46
5. Sturgis E, All BJ. Endometriosis peritonei-relationship of pain to functional activity. Am J Obstet Gynecol 1954;68:421
6. White JC. Conduction of visceral pain. N Engl J Med 1952;156:686–90
7. Allen WM, Masters WH. Traumatic lacerations of uterine supports: the clinical syndrome and operative treatment. Am J Obstet Gynecol 1955;70:500
8. Donnez J, Nisolle M, Anaf V, et al. Endoscopic management of peritoneal and ovarian endometriosis. In Donnez J, ed. Atlas of Laser Operative Laparoscopy and Hysteroscopy. Carnforth, UK: Parthenon Publishing, 1994:63–74
9. Taylor HC Jr. Vascular congestion and hyperemia: their effect on structure and function in the female reproductive system. Am J Obstet Gynecol 1949;57:211
10. Taylor HC Jr. Vascular congestion and hyperemia. II. The clinical aspects of the congestion fibrosis syndrome. Am J Obstet Gynecol 1949;57:637
11. Fluhman CF. The rise and fall of suspension operations for uterine retrodisplacement. Bull Johns Hopkins Hosp 1955;96:59–70
12. Gillian DR. Round-ligament ventrosuspension of the uterus: a new method. Am J Obstet Gynecol 1900;41:299
13. Olshausen R. Uber ventrale operation bei prolapsus and retroversio uteri. Sbl Gynakol 1886;10:698
14. Baldy JM. Treatment of uterine retrodisplacements. Surg Gynecol Obstet 1909;8:421

15. Alexander W. Quoted by Curtis AH, ed. *Obstetrics and Gynecology*. Philadelphia: WB Saunders, 1937

16. Adams JA. Cited by Graves WP. *Gynecology*. Philadelphia: WB Saunders, 1916

17. Yoon FE. Laparoscopic ventrosuspension. A review of 72 cases. *Am J Obstet Gynecol* 1990;163:1151–3

18. Koh LM, Tang FC, Huang MH. Preliminary experience in pelviscopic uterine suspension using Webster-Baldy and Franke's method. *Acta Obstet Gynecol Scand* 1996;75:575–6

19. Donnez J, Nisolle M. Carbon-dioxide laser laparoscopy in pelvic pain and infertility. In Sutton C, ed. *Laparoscopic Surgery. Baillière's Clinical Obstetrics and Gynaecology*. London: Baillière Tindall, 1989:525–44

20. Sutton CJG. Laser uterine nerve ablation. In Donnez J, ed. *Laser Operative Laparoscopy and Hysteroscopy*. Leuven: Nauwelaerts, 1989:43–52

21. Sutton CJ, Pooley AS, Ewen SP, *et al.* Follow-up report on a randomized controlled trial of laser laparoscopy in the treatment of pelvic pain associated with minimal to moderate endometriosis. *Fertil Steril* 1997;68:1070–4

22. Von Theobald P, Barjot P, Levy G. Laparoscopic douglasectomy in the treatment of painful uterine retroversion. *Surg Endosc* 1997;11:639–42

23. Carter JE. Laparoscopic presacral neurectomy utilizing contact-tip Nd:YAG laser. *Keio J Med* 1996;45:332–5

24. Chen FP, Chang SD, Chu KK, *et al.* Comparison of laparoscopic presacral neurectomy and laparoscopic uterine nerve ablation for primary dysmenorrhea. *J Reprod Med* 1996;41:463–6

25. Daniell JF. Fibreoptic laser laparoscopy. In Sutton C, ed. *Laparoscopic Surgery. Baillière's Clinical Obstetrics and Gynaecology*. London: Baillière Tindall, 1989:477–81

Endoscopic management of peritoneal and ovarian endometriosis

7

J. Donnez, M. Nisolle, J. Squifflet, M. Smets and F. Casanas-Roux

Advanced operative laparoscopy techniques for laser adhesiolysis and vaporization of endometriotic implants have been developed, and laser surgeons are now able to remove endometriosis from the reproductive structure with precision. There are at least three advantages of laser laparoscopy over conventional operative laparoscopy: precise destruction of diseased tissue, minimal bleeding and minimal damage to the adjacent normal tissue. Tissue reaction and postoperative adhesion formation have been shown to be no greater than with conventional methods[1].

LASER SURGERY

The endoscopic use of the laser is not new in medicine, and several types of operative procedures have been carried out with the CO_2 laser laparoscope for the treatment of reproductive pathology. The most frequent indication is endometriosis, which can be vaporized by means of CO_2 laser laparoscopy with highly satisfactory postoperative pregnancy rates[2-6]. Laser surgeons have removed endometriosis with great precision from the reproductive structure. However, vaporization of the endometriotic peritoneal lesion or of the endometriotic cyst wall provokes residual carbon charring. Expensive high-power operating lasers are required for the vaporization of tissue without residual carbon charring. The SurgiTouch, which allows a char-free ablation, even when using a 30-W operating laser, will be described in this chapter.

Endoscopic techniques

From 1982 to 1991, 6250 laser laparoscopies were carried out in our department. In the series, 2912 patients underwent laparoscopy for endometriosis.

Peritoneal endometriotic implants

In general, a power setting of 40–50 W is used. The debulking of endometriotic implants is best performed using a continuous firing mode. If a lesion is overlying a vital structure such as the ureter, urinary bladder, colon, or larger blood vessels, a retroperitoneal injection of fluid (aquadissection and aquaprotection) provides safer vaporization of the lesions. This duration allows a 100–200-μm depth of vaporization, thus substantially limiting the depth of penetration. Vaporizing an endometriotic implant (Figure 1a and b) provokes the bubbling of old blood, followed by a curdy white material representing vaporiza-

tion of the stromal layer. After the endometriotic lesion has been vaporized, retroperitoneal fat is encountered, and the appearance of bubbling confirms the complete vaporization of the lesion. Absorption of the CO_2 laser by water (contained in fatty tissue) for a few seconds after the complete destruction of the implant prevents deeper penetration of the laser beam.

Ovarian endometriosis < 3 cm

Ovarian endometriosis is treated during first-look laparoscopy if a penetration of no more than 3 cm into the ovary is observed and if the cyst diameter is no larger than 3 cm (Figures 2–4).

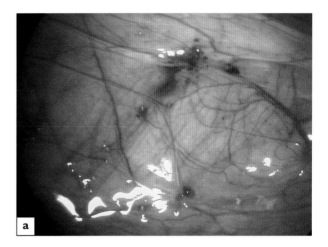

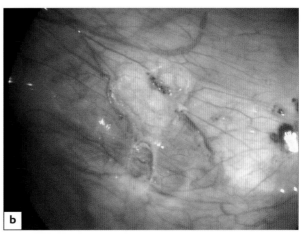

Figure 1 (a) Peritoneal endometriotic lesion, typical red lesion; (b) after vaporization with the SurgiTouch (CO_2 laser). Note the absence of carbonized areas (char-free ablation). See Chapters 1 and 2

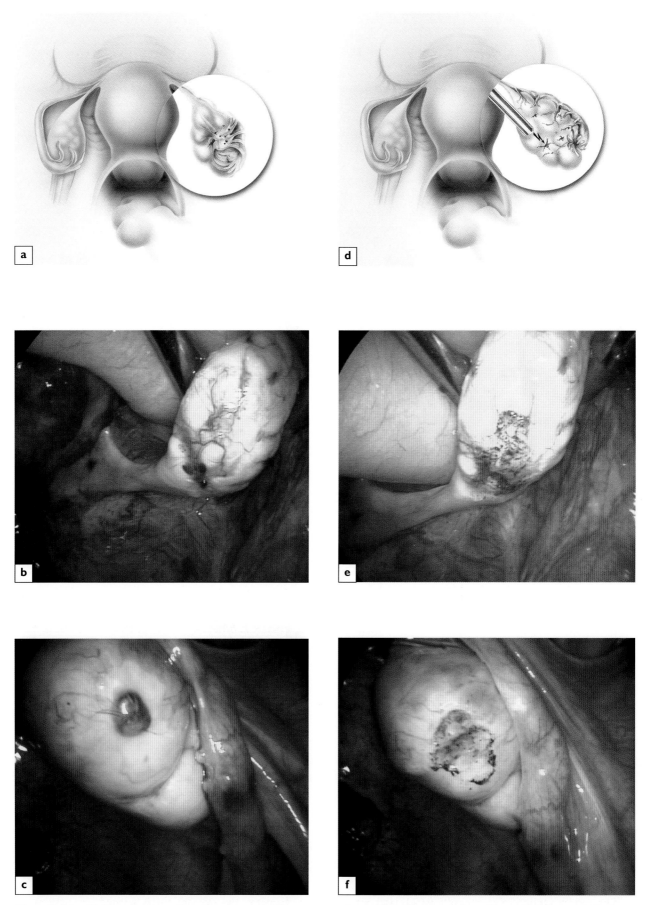

Figure 2 (a) – (c) Visualization of small and superficial ovarian implants; (d) – (f) vaporization of superficial ovarian implants

Small (< 1 cm in diameter) endometriotic implants of the ovary were vaporized until follicles containing fluid were encountered or no further pigmented tissue was seen. Large (< 3 cm in diameter) endometriomas were destroyed as follows. A 3–4-mm portion of the top of the cyst was excised, the chocolate-colored material was aspirated, and the cyst was washed out with irrigation fluid (Figure 3a and b). After washing, the interior wall of the cyst was examined carefully to confirm the absence of any intracystic lesion suspected to be malignant (ovarian cystoscopy). With a power setting of 40 W and continuous mode application, the interior wall of the cyst was then vaporized to destroy the mucosal lining of the cyst (Figure 4a and b). The vaporization continued until no further pigment could be seen. After copious irrigation, the ovaries were left open.

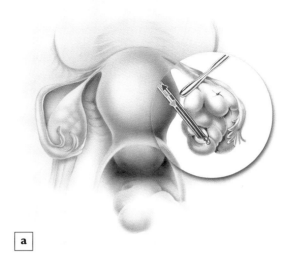

Ovarian endometriosis > 3 cm

In our series of 2912 patients with endometriosis, ovarian endometriomas larger than 3 cm in diameter (Figures 5–9) were found in 481 patients. During diagnostic laparoscopy, the endometrial cyst was washed out with irrigation fluid (saline solution), and a biopsy was taken. Then, gonadotropin releasing hormone (GnRH) agonist (Zoladex, ICI, UK) therapy was given for 12 weeks to decrease the cyst size. A decrease of 50% in cyst diameter was observed after drainage followed by a 12-week course of a GnRH agonist (Figure 5). Drainage alone (if not associated with GnRH agonist) was ineffective; indeed, 12 weeks after drainage, the ovarian cyst diameter was found to be unchanged when compared to the diameter observed before drainage.

Thereafter, a second-look laparoscopy was carried out. If the diameter of the residual endometrial cyst was < 3 cm after GnRH agonist therapy ($n = 233$), the interior wall of the cyst was vaporized as previously described. If the diameter of the residual cyst was > 3 cm after GnRH agonist therapy (Figure 6), another technique was proposed. In this series, the range of the ovarian cyst sizes was 3–8 cm. A portion of the ovarian cyst was first removed by making a circular cut over the protruded ovarian cyst portion, using the CO_2 laser. Partial cystectomy was then carried out (Figure 7). Ovarian cystoscopy (Figure 8) was performed for evaluation of the interior cyst wall, and a biopsy was taken. The residual endometrial cyst wall was then vaporized with the CO_2 laser, equipped with the SurgiTouch (Figure 9).

USE OF SURGITOUCH

The SurgiTouch (Sharplan) is a miniature optomechanical scanner compatible with any CO_2 laser. The SurgiTouch scanner consists of two almost, but not exactly, parallel folding mirrors. Optical reflections of the CO_2 laser optical beam from the mirrors cause the beam to deviate from its

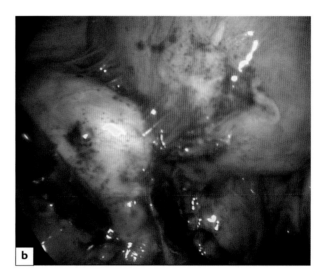

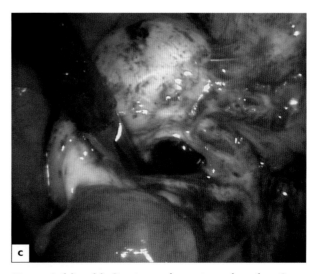

Figure 3 (a) – (c) Ovarian endometrioma less than 3 cm in diameter; the ovarian cyst is washed out with saline solution

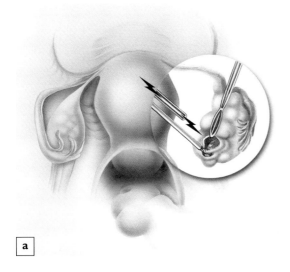

a

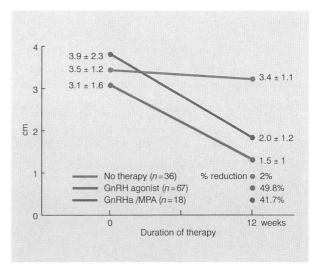

3.9 ± 2.3
3.5 ± 1.2
3.1 ± 1.6

3.4 ± 1.1

2.0 ± 1.2

1.5 ± 1

	% reduction
No therapy (n=36)	● 2%
GnRH agonist (n=67)	● 49.8%
GnRHa /MPA (n=18)	● 41.7%

cm

0   12 weeks

Duration of therapy

Figure 5 Comparative evaluation of cyst diameter after drainage alone, and after drainage followed by GnRH agonist therapy. Drainage of ovarian endometriotic cyst is ineffective if not associated with GnRH agonist. After drainage and GnRH agonist, a decrease of 50% in cyst diameter is observed

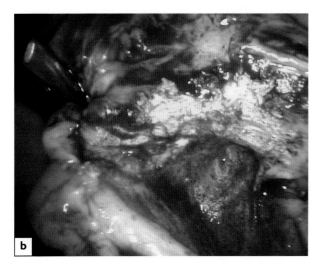

b

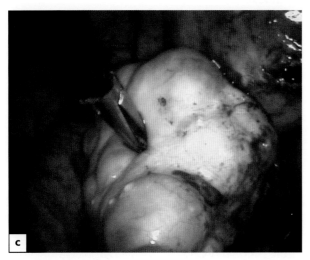

c

Figure 4 (a) – (c) The mucosal lining of the endometrial cyst is vaporized

original direction by an angle θ (see Chapter 2). The mirrors constantly rotate at slightly different angular velocities, thereby varying rapidly with time, between zero and a maximal value θ_{max}. By attaching the laparoscope focusing coupler of focal length F to the SurgiTouch, the CO_2 laser generates a focal spot which rapidly and homogeneously scans and covers a round area of diameter $2F \tan \theta_{max}$ at the distal end of the laparoscope. For a single-puncture laparoscope ($F = 300$ mm), θ_{max} was selected to provide a round treatment area of 2.5 mm in diameter. The rapid movement of the beam over the tissue ensures a short duration of exposure on individual sites within the area and very shallow ablation.

Since therapeutic CO_2 medical lasers typically generate a focused beam smaller than 0.9 mm in diameter at the laparoscope working distance, using the SurgiTouch with a laser power level of 30 W will generate an optical power density of above 50 W/mm² on tissue. This is considerably higher than the threshold for vaporization of tissue without residual carbon char (the threshold for char-free tissue ablation is about 30 W/mm²). The time required for the SurgiTouch to homogeneously cover a 2.5-mm round area is about 100 ms. During this time, the 30-W operating laser will deliver 3000 mJ to the tissue. Since the typical energy required to completely ablate tissue is about 3000 mJ/mm³, keeping the laparoscope precisely on a single site for 0.1 s will generate a clean char-free crater of 0.2 mm in depth. However, the laparoscope can be moved smoothly and evenly across an extended lesion intended for treatment, consequently ablating a tissue layer as thin as 0.05–0.1 mm.

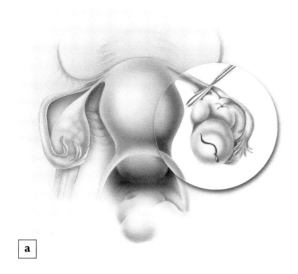

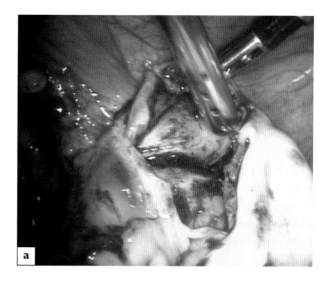

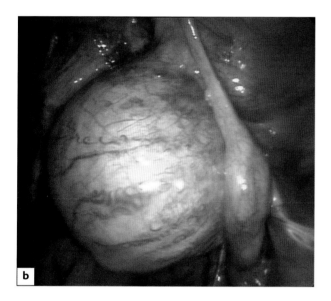

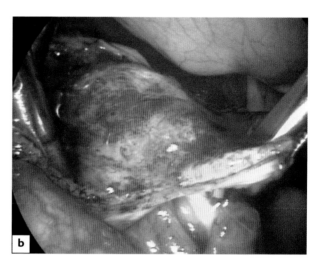

Figure 7 (a) and (b) A circular cut over the protruded ovarian cyst portion and partial cystectomy are carried out

Results

The operating time varied from 45 to 80 min. Vaporization of the mucosal lining was facilitated by the preoperative therapy (GnRH agonist administered subcutaneously)[7]. Indeed, the interior wall of the endometrial cyst seen during ovarian cystoscopy was found to be less hemorrhagic and more atrophic than before therapy. These data were confirmed by ovarian biopsy. An endometriotic lesion was considered 'active' when typical glandular epithelium was either proliferative, or completely unresponsive to hormonal therapy with typical stroma. Such a lesion was found significantly more often (84% of cases, $p < 0.001$) before GnRH agonist therapy than after such therapy (44% of cases)[3,5,7–9].

In patients with residual ovarian cysts > 3 cm in diameter, the technique was used successfully to vaporize the endometriotic ovarian lesions, and the ovary was left open;

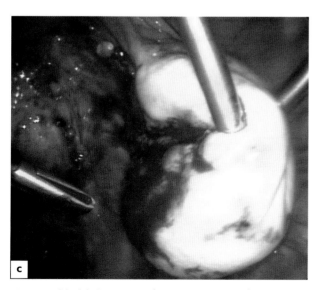

Figure 6 (a)–(c) Ovarian endometrioma more than 3 cm in diameter

3 months after the procedure, a third-look laparoscopy was performed in nine patients. Dense and fibrous adhesions between the vaporized area of the ovary and the broad ligament, the bowel, and the Fallopian tube were found in eight out of nine patients. Laparoscopic salpingo-ovariolysis was carried out.

So far, the technique has been used successfully in a series of 482 patients with endometriomas > 3 cm in diameter.

SurgiTouch

The SurgiTouch enables very rapid, homogeneous, single-layer char-free ablation, even at low power levels. Since 1992, all patients were treated with the SurgiTouch connected to the direct coupler and the laparoscope. A

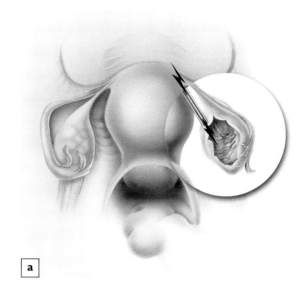

a

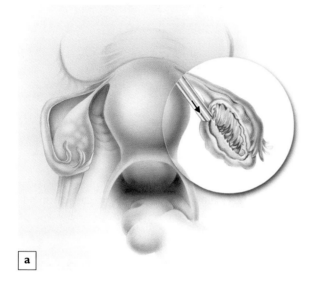

a

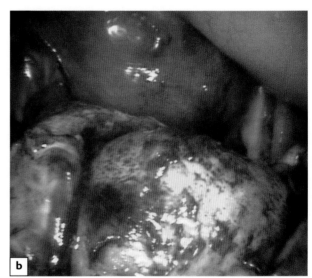

b

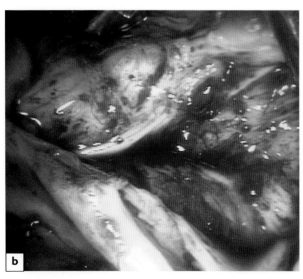

b

Figure 8 Ovarian cystoscopy: the interior wall is carefully examined

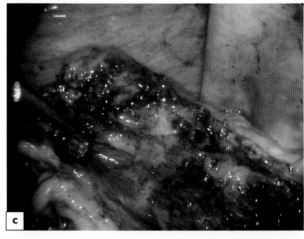

c

Figure 9 (a)–(c) Residual endometrial cyst wall is vaporized with the SurgiTouch which permits a char-free ablation, layer by layer. It reduces the carbonization and the thermal damage to the normal ovarian cortex

layer-by-layer ablation was possible and performed easily in all cases. Indeed, by moving the laparoscope smoothly, the surgeon can ablate a tissue layer as thin as 0.05–1 mm. For peritoneal endometriosis, the SurgiTouch made the vaporization procedure easier. The char-free ablation allows the surgeon to check when the endometriotic lesion has been totally vaporized by easily visualizing the retroperitoneal fat, and there is a decreased risk of thermal injury to the bowel and ureter.

In cases of ovarian endometriotic cysts more than 3 cm in diameter, GnRH agonist is used for 3 months after the cyst has been punctured and washed out. After a 3-month course of GnRH agonist therapy, the thickness of the endometrial cyst is dramatically reduced and the epithelial lining is atrophic and white. Vaporization with the SurgiTouch permits a very easy and fast vaporization of the internal wall with minimal thermal damage to the normal ovarian cortex. Indeed, histological studies have shown, in experimental studies, a char-free residual damage 0.1 mm deep[10]. Moreover, because the time required for the SurgiTouch to homogeneously cover a 2.5-mm round area is about 100 ms, vaporization of large areas of peritoneal endometriosis as well as the endometrial ovarian cyst wall is performed very fast, thus reducing the operating time. When compared to the conventional laser technique, the operating time needed to vaporize the internal wall is significantly reduced.

The reduced operating time, the better visual control (absence of carbonized particles), the reduced thermal damage (layer-by-layer ablation) and the possibility of using low-power operating lasers are the most significant advantages of this new technology.

Pregnancy rates

The cumulative pregnancy rates were analyzed (Figure 10) in a consecutive series of 407 patients with ovarian endometriosis (American Fertility Society (AFS) moderate, $n = 305$; AFS severe, $n = 102$).

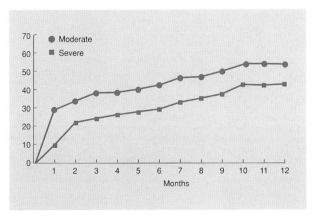

Figure 10 The cumulative pregnancy rate in cases of moderate and severe ovarian endometriosis

A pregnancy rate of more than 55% was achieved in moderate endometriosis and 44% in severe endometriosis. The majority of pregnancies occurred during the first 10 months after surgery.

OVARIAN CYSTECTOMY

Ovarian cystectomy, a frequently performed procedure, can be accomplished laparoscopically in most cases. The procedure begins with adhesiolysis. Once the cyst is mobilized, the cortex is grasped with a forceps introduced through a second trocar. The cortex is incised using laser or scissors. The cyst wall is then exposed. The incision is enlarged with scissors, and aquadissection can be used to separate the cyst wall from the ovarian stroma. If the cyst is opened and spillage occurs, peritoneal irrigation must be performed in order to remove the chocolate-colored fluid. Sometimes, ovarioscopy and careful evaluation of the internal cyst wall allow the surgeon to exclude the presence of malignant lesions. The ovary usually does not require suturing.

CONCLUSION

CO_2 laser laparoscopy offers several advantages over cautery. With the CO_2 laser, the laparoscopist is able to control the process of vaporization by seeing the three-dimensional boundaries of the lesion.

In a previous study[9], significantly different pregnancy rates according to the stage of endometriosis were found. Severe endometriosis had the poorest prognosis in terms of pregnancy rates. For this reason, a preoperative hormonal (GnRH agonist) therapy was given to patients with very large ovarian endometriomas (> 3 cm). The release of a GnRH agonist by a biodegradable implant is effective in reducing endometriotic size to a greater extent than other drugs, and permits a decrease in pelvic inflammation. Treatment by sustained release is an effective alternative to using steroid hormones before laser laparoscopy. A subcutaneous GnRH agonist implant permits a substantial reduction of large ovarian cyst diameter and a decrease in pelvic inflammation so that a second-look laser laparoscopy can be carried out for laser vaporization of residual endometriomas. During the ovarian cystoscopy, the interior ovarian wall was found to be atrophic. The cyst vascularity was decreased, and the vaporization was thus facilitated.

In cases of vaporization of very large cysts (> 3 cm), the risk of postoperative adhesions was found to be high in our study if the ovary was left open. Dense and fibrous periovarian adhesions between the vaporized area and other pelvic structures were diagnosed in eight out of nine patients who underwent a laparoscopy in the 3 months after the vaporization, although periovarian adhesions were not frequently observed after vaporization of small endometriotic implants. Our results were thus not in accordance with those of Nezhat and associates[2,6].

The SurgiTouch has been used in our department. It enables a very rapid, homogeneous, single-layer char-free ablation even at low power levels. It increases the visual control of tissue destruction and permits a layer-by-layer ablation, reducing the carbonization and the presence of carbonized particles in the tissue.

REFERENCES

1. Donnez J, Fernandez C, Willems, T, *et al.* Experimental ovarian CO_2 laser surgery. In Donnez J, ed. CO_2 *Laser in Intraepithelial Neoplasia and in Infertility*. Leuven, Belgium: Nauwelaerts Printing, 1987:25

2. Nezhat C, Crowgey SR, Garrison CP. Surgical treatment of endometriosis via laser laparoscopy. *Fertil Steril* 1986;45:778–83

3. Donnez J. CO_2 laser laparoscopy in infertile women with adhesions or endometriosis. *Fertil Steril* 1987;48:390–4

4. Donnez J, Nisolle M, Casanas-Roux F. CO_2 laser laparoscopy in infertile women with adnexal adhesions and women with tubal occlusion. *J Gynecol Surg* 1989;5:47–53

5. Donnez J, Nisolle M. Laparoscopic management of large ovarian endometrial cyst: use of fibrin sealant. *J Gynecol Surg* 1991;7:163–7

6. Nezhat C, Nezhat F, Silfen SL. Video laseroscopy: the CO_2 laser for advanced operative laparoscopy. *Obstet Gynecol Clin North Am* 1991;18:585–604

7. Donnez J, Nisolle M, Casanas-Roux F. Administration of nasal buserelin as compared with subcutaneous buserelin implant for endometriosis. *Fertil Steril* 1989;52:27–30

8. Nisolle M, Casanas-Roux F, Donnez J. Histologic study of ovarian endometriosis after hormonal therapy. *Fertil Steril* 1988;49:423-6

9. Donnez J, Nisolle M, Casanas-Roux F. Endometriosis-associated infertility: evaluation of preoperative use of danazol, gestrinone and buserelin. *Int J Fertil* 1990;42:128

10. Donnez J, Nisolle M, Gillet N, *et al.* Large ovarian endometriomas. *Hum Reprod* 1996;11:641–6

In vitro fertilization outcome after endometrioma surgery

8

C. Wyns, C. Pirard, M. Nisolle, J. Squifflet and J. Donnez

Endometriosis is frequently associated with infertility. Indeed, 30–70% of infertile women have been reported to have endometriosis[1]. A number of mechanisms for endometriosis-associated infertility have been suggested but a complete understanding of how endometriosis may affect fertility is still lacking.

Some reports in the literature suggest that ovarian endometriosis could affect the outcome of *in vitro* fertilization (IVF). Poor response to ovarian stimulation, decreased oocyte recovery rates, decreased fertilization rates and decreased implantation rates have all been implicated[2–5].

Ovarian endometriomas require surgery in infertile women. Indeed, a 50% pregnancy rate was obtained after laparoscopic management in a series of 814 cases[6]. But some reports have recently suggested that ovarian surgery in cases of ovarian endometriomas could be deleterious for the residual normal ovarian cortex. In the literature, two surgical techniques have been described:

(1) Laparoscopic ovarian cystectomy, which involves stripping the cyst wall but carries a theoretical risk of removing normal ovarian cortex because of the absence of a cleavage plane between the cyst capsule and normal tissue[6,7].

(2) Laparoscopic vaporization of the internal layers (epithelium and stroma whose thickness does not exceed 1–1.5 mm) of the endometrioma wall with

the CO_2 laser, according to the technique previously described[6,8]. For large endometriomas, drainage followed by gonadotropin releasing hormone (GnRH) agonist therapy is proposed before cyst wall vaporization in order to facilitate the laparoscopic procedure[8].

The aim of our study was to evaluate whether endometrioma surgery (cystectomy or cyst wall vaporization) could impair IVF outcome. We analyzed the ovarian response to gonadotropin stimulation conducted for IVF in women who had undergone laparoscopic surgery for endometriomas but failed to become pregnant within a year of surgery.

ANALYSIS OF 447 WOMEN

A series of 447 women (Table 1), who had undergone IVF since 1992, were analyzed. One hundred and nineteen women (group I) with laparoscopically proven endometriosis, who failed to conceive after conservative laparoscopic surgery without associated male factors, constituted the study group. No patients showed evidence of any other cause of infertility and, notably, the semen analysis of the partner was normal (sperm count $> 20.10^6$/ml; mobility $> 50\%$; normal forms according to Kruger's criteria[9] $> 13\%$).

Table I Ovarian stimulation parameters

	Endometriosis (Group I)			Non-endometriosis (Group II)	
	Peritoneal (Group Ia)	Ovarian cyst wall vaporization (Group Ib)	Endometrioma cystectomy (Group Ic)	Tubal (Group IIa)	Idiopathic (Group IIb)
n	42	57	20	193	135
Cycles	71	125	38	422	275
Ampoules	36.52 ± 13.97	41.34 ± 18.93	40.61 ± 16.20	44.17 ± 19.76	39.74 ± 19.98
Follicles	14.67 ± 8.04	15.90 ± 6.62	14.44 ± 6.41	12.96 ± 6.82	15.57 ± 9.70
Mature oocytes	9.66 ± 5.92	10.22 ± 4.91	9.29 ± 4.52	8.55 ± 6.99	9.44 ± 6.13
Estradiol peak	2339.69 ± 1148.45	2360.72 ± 1993.56	2488.34 ± 1173.10	2095.05 ± 1159.31	2282.06 ± 1252.11
Day of hCG administration	12.46 ± 1.54	12.97 ± 2.30	13.03 ± 2.31	13.08 ± 2.58	13.18 ± 2.70

hCG, human chorionic gonadotropin

This group of endometriosis patients (group I, $n = 119$) was divided into three subgroups: group Ia, 42 women with peritoneal lesions treated by laparoscopic destruction (vaporization or coagulation) who underwent 71 IVF cycles; group Ib, 57 women with ovarian endometriomas treated by cyst wall vaporization who underwent 125 IVF cycles; group Ic, 20 women with ovarian endometriomas treated by cystectomy who underwent 38 IVF cycles.

The control group (group II), which included 328 women who underwent IVF during the same period, was divided into two subgroups: group IIa, 193 women with tubal factors who underwent 422 IVF cycles; group IIb, 135 women with idiopathic infertility who underwent 275 cycles. In group II, only women whose partner's semen analysis was normal were selected.

In total, 447 women, who underwent 931 IVF cycles, were studied. The mean age was not statistically different among the different subgroups (group Ia, 32.4 ± 5.4 years; group Ib, 32.4 ± 3.8 years; group Ic, 33.9 ± 6.0 years; group IIa, 34.4 ± 5.3 years; group IIb, 33.8 ± 5.0 years). The mean duration of infertility was not statistically different either among the different subgroups (group Ia, 4.4 ± 2.3 years; group Ib, 4.5 ± 2.4 years; group Ic, 4.4 ± 3.7 years; group IIa, 4.4 ± 3.4 years; group IIb, 5.1 ± 3.1 years).

OVARIAN STIMULATION PARAMETERS AND PREGNANCY RATES

Ovarian stimulation was achieved using GnRH analogs (long protocol) (Decapeptyl® 3.75 mg, Ipsen, Paris, France) for down-regulation and human menopausal gonadotropins (hMG, Humegon®, Organon, Oss, The Netherlands; Pergonal®, Serono, Geneva, Switzerland).

For the long protocol, GnRH agonist administration was started between days 21 and 25 of the previous cycle. Sonography and estradiol (E_2) dosage were carried out 3

weeks after the beginning of GnRH agonist administration to assess the period in which the ovaries were at rest. If the ovaries were at rest and the E_2 level was < 30 pg/ml, hMG administration was begun 2 days later. Treatment was adapted according to the age of the patient, the number and size of follicles and the E_2 level.

Human chorionic gonadotropin (hCG, 10 000 IU) was administered when the E_2 level was ± 200 pg/ml per follicle ≥ 16 mm in diameter and in the presence of more than three follicles > 20 mm in diameter. Oocyte retrieval was carried out by the vaginal route under sonographic guidance using local anesthesia and sedation. Two or 3 days after oocyte retrieval, a maximum of three embryos were replaced.

The ovarian stimulation parameters are shown in Table 1. There was no significant difference among the different study subgroups in the number of gonadotropin ampules, the number of follicles, the number of follicles with a diameter > 15 mm, the number of mature oocytes, the maximum E_2 concentrations or the day of hCG administration.

The number of embryos/cycle, the number of transferred embryos/cycle, the fertilization rates, the implantation rates and the ongoing pregnancy rates are shown in Table 2. There was no significant difference among the different subgroups in the studied parameters.

In order to establish if the size of the surgically removed or vaporized endometrioma could influence IVF outcome (Table 3), certain parameters were analyzed according to the size of the endometrioma (< 3 cm vs. > 3 cm), but no statistical difference was observed between groups Ib and Ic.

Patients with unilateral endometriomas and normal contralateral ovaries were also analyzed, allowing a paired comparison for unilateral cysts (Table 4). Thirty-four women were evaluated in group Ib ($n = 57$) and 14 in group Ic ($n = 20$). The contralateral normal ovary was used

Table 2 *In vitro* fertilization outcome

	Endometriosis (Group I)			Non-endometriosis (Group II)	
	Peritoneal (Group Ia)	Ovarian cyst wall vaporization (Group Ib)	Endometrioma cystectomy (Group Ic)	Tubal (Group IIa)	Idiopathic (Group IIb)
Fertilization rate	6.81%	57.43%	64.59%	62.48%	57.99%
Embryos/mature oocytes	45.19%	41.31%	41.08%	43.50%	58.37%
Embryos/cycle	4.19 ± 4.69	4.26 ± 3.33	3.82 ± 3.09	3.72 ± 3.95	3.82 ± 3.98
Transferred embryos/cycle	2.26 ± 1.10	2.57 ± 0.92	2.63 ± 1.63	2.35 ± 1.08	2.23 ± 1.13
Implantation rate	17.72%	14.95%	25.93%	13.94%	18.05%
Pregnancy rate	32.39%	36.80%	50%	27.49%	30.18%

Table 3 *In vitro* fertilization outcome according to cyst size before surgery (< 3 cm vs. > 3 cm)

	Ovarian cyst wall vaporization (Group Ib)		Endometrioma cystectomy (Group Ic)	
	< 3 cm	> 3 cm	< 3 cm	> 3 cm
Age	31.56 ± 3.81	31.81 ± 3.50	33.14 ± 3.00	31.17 ± 4.46
Mean size	1.48 ± 0.58	5.51 ± 2.48	1.46 ± 0.67	5.96 ± 2.10
Total number of follicles	14.21 ± 6.72	17.76 ± 6.62	13.43 ± 6.70	15.92 ± 7.22
Number of follicles >15 mm	10.96 ± 5.34	13.62 ± 6.17	10.00 ± 4.45	12.62 ± 6.48

Table 4 Paired comparison for unilateral cysts: patients with unilateral endometrioma and normal contralateral ovary were analyzed

	Ovarian cyst wall vaporization (Group Ib) (n = 57 cycles)		Endometrioma cystectomy (Group Ic) (n = 20 cycles)	
	Normal ovary	Endometrioma	Normal ovary	Endometrioma
Age	31.53 ± 3.61	31.53 ± 3.61	32.14 ± 3.47	32.14 ± 3.47
Mean cyst size	—	2.66 ± 1.83	—	3.69 ± 2.71
Total number of follicles	8.29 ± 4.17	6.82 ± 3.66	6.57 ± 5.80	7 ± 4.90
Number of follicles >15 mm	6.50 ± 3.91	4.94 ± 3.16	4.07 ± 4.98	5.28 ± 3.93
Number of oocytes	5.31 ± 3.02	4.39 ± 2.91	3.64 ± 3.24	4.51 ± 3.37

as a control for paired analysis. The number of follicles > 15 mm in size, the total number of follicles and the number of oocytes were similar in the treated ovary and the normal contralateral ovary.

COMMENTS

Appropriate surgical management of endometriotic cysts remains a subject of debate and discussion. Some authors recently suggested that cystectomy could provoke loss of normal ovarian tissue either by removing ovarian stroma with oocytes together with the capsule or by thermal damage provoked by coagulation[6,10].

In 1991, Fayez and Vogel observed, in a series of large endometriomas, that drainage was effective in about 32% of cases[11]. In contrast, we clearly demonstrated, in a prospective randomized study, the rapid recurrence of endometriomas after drainage[8]. The persistence of active endometriotic foci and mitotic activity after 3 months of GnRH agonist therapy provides strong arguments in favor of surgical removal of endometriomas[12]. The technique of vaporization of the internal wall of endometriomas by CO_2 laser equipped with the SurgiTouch (Sharplan, Tel-Aviv, Israel) was described in 1994 and the results of the first series of 814 women with large endometriomas were published in 1996[6,13]. A pregnancy rate of 50% and a recurrence rate of 8% were observed. Some authors who

reported higher recurrence rates after fenestration and coagulation probably coagulated the cyst wall lining insufficiently and thus the quick 'recurrence' could well be due to the persistence of non-treated areas[14].

On the other hand, Canis and co-workers described the technique of laparoscopic cystectomy with removal of the cyst and its fibrotic capsule, with a pregnancy rate of 44.2% in a series of 92 women with endometriomas > 3 cm in size[7]. The recurrence rate was 7.6%.

Others reported similar pregnancy and recurrence rates for fenestration and coagulation vs. cystectomy[10]. Hemmings and colleagues correlated the faster conception and better pregnancy rates observed in patients treated by cyst wall coagulation compared to cystectomy with the less considerable loss of ovarian tissue[10]. Back in 1996, we suggested that endometrioma stripping may result in loss of viable cortex during surgery[6]. In a histological study[6,13], we demonstrated the absence of a plane of cleavage, making stripping of the cyst wall difficult and giving rise to the possibility of bleeding at the hilus, requiring extensive coagulation. According to the metaplasia theory of invaginated mesothelium, oocytes are found closely surrounding the endometrioma capsule and there is a theoretical risk of removing oocytes together with the endometrioma capsule[1,15]. By carrying out serial sections of excised endometriomas, we demonstrated that oocytes are present in the excised tissue[1,15]. Saleh and Tulandi, however, failed to demonstrate the presence of follicles after histopathologic evaluation of excised endometriomas, but serial sections were not performed in their study[14].

As one can see in the literature, data are controversial and there is a need to correlate the ovarian response in terms of production of follicles after gonadotropin stimulation with the type of surgical technique (cystectomy vs. vaporization).

Most studies have reported the ovarian response to stimulation in non-surgically treated endometriomas[16–18]. Only a few have analyzed data from women who underwent surgical management of endometriomas. In these studies, however, the surgical techniques were not clearly described. Only Loh and colleagues demonstrated that post-cystectomy ovaries reduced follicular response in natural and clomiphene citrate-stimulated cycles, but produced a comparable number of follicles to normal ovaries when stimulated with gonadotropins[19].

In the present study, we thus compare the results obtained using two different techniques (cystectomy vs. vaporization). Our results for ovarian stimulation suggest that both cystectomy and cyst wall vaporization allow preservation of a good ovarian response to stimulation by gonadotropins. This is in accordance with the findings of Loh and co-workers who found that post-cystectomy ovaries produced a comparable number of follicles to normal ovaries when stimulated by gonadotropins[19].

To further the comparison, a second analysis was performed on patients with unilateral endometriomas, whereby a paired comparison was made between the post-cystectomy or post-vaporization ovary and the contralateral normal ovary of the same patient. To our knowledge, this is the first time that, using the contralateral normal ovary as a control, a normal ovarian response was demonstrated in post-surgery ovaries in cases of endometriomas, regardless of surgical technique: cystectomy or vaporization. This proves that vaporization and cystectomy, when carefully performed in experienced hands, do not affect the ovarian response in terms of production of mature oocytes, providing indirect evidence of the persistence of viable ovarian cortex, similar to a normal ovary. Even if the size (< or > 3 cm) of the endometrioma is taken into account, no difference in ovarian stimulation is observed.

Numerous studies have compared IVF outcome (in terms of fertilization rate, embryo development, implantation and pregnancy rates) in women with endometriosis with other diagnostic entities, but comparisons with treated endometriosis are scarce in the literature. Published studies are almost exclusively retrospective and observational. Their results are highly dependent on proper selection of subjects and controls.

In our study, we selected women with *one* pathology (endometriosis, tubal or idiopathic) and excluded women with mixed pathologies or whose partner's semen analysis was not normal. Our results demonstrated a similar fertilization rate among the different subgroups (varying from 57.4 to 64.9%). Our data do not corroborate those of the groups of Foad and Huang who observed a significantly

lower fertilization rate in endometriosis patients compared to women with tubal factors[20,21]. It could be that the removal or destruction of endometriomas restores a normal anatomy and ovarian structure. Some authors have reported a reduction in oocyte quality and thereby a decrease in fertilization rates[4,5,22–24]. They suggest that ovarian endometriomas produce substances that are toxic to maturing oocytes and these compounds may adversely affect cleavage of oocytes after fertilization.

Our study clearly demonstrated that the fertilization rate is not affected in women with endometriosis or at least that endometrioma surgery does not interfere with the fertilization rate. Therefore, if the fertilization rate is found to be impaired in women with endometriomas, as some authors claim, it can be normalized by surgery[4,5,22–24]. Moreover, implantation rates and ongoing pregnancy rates were found to be similar in all subgroups, disputing the findings of other authors who reported a consistently high risk of spontaneous abortion[25].

We therefore conclude, first, that vaporization of the internal cyst wall does not impair ovarian function in terms of IVF parameters and outcome; second, that theoretical risks of loss of viable ovarian tissue during cystectomy exist but may be avoided by a 'microsurgical' laparoscopic technique, taking care to preserve the normal residual ovarian cortex; and, third, that, after removal or destruction of endometriomas, IVF outcomes are similar in endometriosis patients when compared to women with tubal factor or idiopathic infertility.

REFERENCES

1. Nisolle M, Donnez J. Peritoneal endometriosis, ovarian endometriosis and adenomyotic nodules of the rectovaginal septum are three distinct entities. *Fertil Steril* 1997;68:585–96
2. Arici A, Oral E, Bukulmez O, et al. The effect of endometriosis on implantation: results from the Yale University *in vitro* fertilization and embryo transfer program. *Fertil Steril* 1996;65:603–7
3. Cahill DJ, Wardle PG, Maile LA, et al. Ovarian dysfunction in endometriosis-associated and unexplained infertility. *J Assist Reprod Genet* 1997;14:554–7
4. Yanushpolsky EH, Best CL, Jackson KV, et al. Effects of endometriomas on oocyte quality, embryo quality, and pregnancy rates in *in vitro* fertilization cycles: a prospective case-controlled study. *J Assist Reprod Genet* 1998;15:193–7
5. Pal L, Shifren JL, Isaacson KB, et al. Impact of varying stages of endometriosis on the outcome of *in vitro* fertilization-embryo transfer. *J Assist Reprod Genet* 1998;15:27–31
6. Donnez J, Nisolle M, Gillet N, et al. Large ovarian endometriomas. *Hum Reprod* 1996;11:641–6

7. Canis M, Mage G, Wattiez A, *et al.* Second look laparoscopy after cystectomy of large ovarian endometriomas. *Fertil Steril* 1992;58:617–19

8. Donnez J, Nisolle M, Gillerto S, *et al.* Ovarian endometrial cysts: the role of gonadotropin-releasing hormone agonist and/or drainage. *Fertil Steril* 1994;62:63–6

9. Kruger TF, Menkveld R, Stander FSH, *et al.* Sperm morphologic features as a prognostic factor in *in vitro* fertilization. *Fertil Steril* 1986;46:1118–23

10. Hemmings R, Bissonnette F, Bouzayen R. Results of laparoscopic treatments of ovarian endometriomas: laparoscopic ovarian fenestration and coagulation. *Fertil Steril* 1998;70:527–9

11. Fayez JA, Vogel MF. Comparison of different treatment methods of endometriomas by laparoscopy. *Obstet Gynecol* 1991;78:660–5

12. Nisolle M, Casanas-Roux F, Donnez J. Immunohistochemical analysis of proliferative activity and steroid receptor expression in peritoneal and ovarian endometriosis. *Fertil Steril* 1997;68:912–19

13. Donnez J, Nisolle M, Anaf V, *et al.* Endoscopic management of peritoneal and ovarian endometriosis. In Donnez J, Nisolle M, eds. *An Atlas of Laser Operative Laparoscopy and Hysteroscopy*. Carnforth, UK: Parthenon Publishing, 1994:53–74

14. Saleh A, Tulandi T. Reoperation after laparoscopic treatment of ovarian endometriomas by excision and by fenestration. *Fertil Steril* 1999;72:322–4

15. Nisolle M, Casanas-Roux F, Donnez J. Large ovarian endometriomas: new perspectives in histogenesis. *Ref Gyn/Obst* 1996;4:381–8

16. Stewart EA, Jackson KV, Friedman AJ, *et al.* The effect of baseline complex ovarian cysts on *in vitro* fertilization outcome. *Fertil Steril* 1992;52:1274–8

17. Isaacs JD Jr, Hines RS, Sopelak VM, *et al.* Ovarian endometriomas do not adversely affect pregnancy success following treatment with *in vitro* fertilization. *J Assist Reprod Gen* 1997;14:551–3

18. Segal S, Shifren JL, Isaaacson KB, *et al.* Effect of a baseline ovarian cyst on the outcome of *in vitro* fertilization-embryo transfer. *Fertil Steril* 1999;71:274–7

19. Loh F-H, Tan AT, Kumar J, *et al.* Ovarian response after laparoscopic ovarian cystectomy for endometriotic cysts in 132 monitored cycles. *Fertil Steril* 1999;72:316–21

20. Foad A, Lessing JB, Geva E, *et al.* Patients with stages III and IV endometriosis have a poorer outcome of IVF-ET than patients with tubal infertility. *Fertil Steril* 1999;72:1107–9

21. Huang H-Y, Lee C-L, Lai Y-M, *et al.* The outcome of *in vitro* fertilization and embryo transfer therapy in women with endometriosis failing to conceive after laparoscopic conservative surgery. *J Am Assoc Gynecol Laparosc* 1997;4:299–303

22. Wardle PC, Mitchell JD, McLaughlin EA, *et al.* Endometriosis and ovulatory disorder: reduced fertilization *in vitro* compared with tubal and unexplained infertility. *Lancet* 1985;2:236–9

23. O'Shea RT, Chen C, Weiss T, *et al.* Endometriosis and *in-vitro* fertilization. *Lancet* 1985;2:723

24. Simon C, Gutierrez A, Vidal A, *et al.* Outcome of patients with endometriosis in assisted reproduction: results from *in vitro* fertilization and oocyte donation. *Hum Reprod* 1994;9:725 9

25. Oehringer S, Acosta AA, Kreiner D, *et al. In vitro* fertilization and embryo transfer (IVF/ET): an established and successful therapy for endometriosis. *J In Vitro Fert Embryo Transf* 1988;5:249–56

Laparoscopic treatment of rectovaginal septum adenomyosis

9

J. Donnez, M. Nisolle, J. Squifflet and M. Smets

INTRODUCTION

It is generally believed that endometriosis is caused by the implantation of retrograde menstrual endometrial cells, or by metaplasia. In the pelvis, three different forms of endometriosis must be considered[1–4]:

(1) Peritoneal[5];

(2) Ovarian[6,7];

(3) Rectovaginal septum[1–4,8–11].

The early manifestations of the disease are believed to be subtle or non-colored lesions such as white lesions (white opacification, yellow-brown patches or hemosiderin patches). The presence of a lower mitotic activity in white lesions[1] suggests that this type of lesion is a patent form of the disease. The presence of a scanty stroma and poor stromal vascularization are two other arguments. Red lesions (red vesicles, polypoid lesions, flame-like lesions, hypervascularized areas or even peritoneal petechiae) are more active forms of the disease. Recent experimental studies in the baboon[5] have suggested that these lesions undergo active remodelling, some disappearing while other new lesions are formed.

In women, our hypothesis is that red lesions are more aggressive and progress to the so-called typical or black lesions which must be considered as an enclosed implant surrounded by fibrosis. Red lesions have recently been proved to be a very active form of the disease.

Ovarian chocolate-colored fluid cysts are, according to the hypothesis of Hughesdon[6], the consequence of the invagination of superficial implants into the ovary. Endometriomas can also develop in the ovaries and this type of cystic ovarian endometriosis must be considered to be another severe form of endometriosis, often related to infertility.

A third form of the disease is adenomyosis of the rectovaginal septum as defined by Donnez and colleagues[8–11] and Nisolle and colleagues[3]. Sampson[12] defined cul-de-sac obliteration as 'extensive adhesions in the cul-de-sac, obliterating its lower portion and uniting the cervix or the lower portion of the uterus to the rectum; with adenoma of the endometrial type invading the cervical and the uterine tissue and probably also (but to a lesser degree) the anterior wall of the rectum' (Figures 1 and 2). Cul-de-sac obliteration implies the presence of deep fibrotic retrocervical adenomyosis beneath the peritoneum (Figure 3). Treatment options for pain or infertility secondary to cul-de-sac obliteration include ovarian suppression therapy with danazol or gonadotropin releasing hormone agonists, or surgery[13].

For existing infertility or the preservation of fertility, reconstructive surgery can be considered either via laparotomy, microsurgery or laparoscopy, depending on the skill and experience of the surgeon.

Deep fibrotic retrocervical adenomyosis is commonly managed by bowel resection, assuming that the major portion of the lesion infiltrates the anterior rectum. In such cases, the deep fibrotic lesion is mobilized, starting with the posterior uterus and progressing downward to the rectum where it appears to be attached. However, the endoscopic technique has been developed[8–11,13–18].

MATERIALS AND METHODS

Our series of 1125 cases of rectovaginal septum adenomyosis treated by laparotomy is presented here (Table 1). The main symptom was pelvic pain. About 25% suffered pelvic pain and infertility. In all cases of infertility, an evaluation of ovulation, cervical mucus–sperm interaction (postcoital test) and male factor (defined as < 15 million sperm/ml using a Makler counting chamber) was undertaken. Preoperative radiography of the colon was carried out in order to evaluate the involvement of the rectal surface. Profile radiography offers the best evaluation of infiltration of the anterior rectal wall (Figure 4).

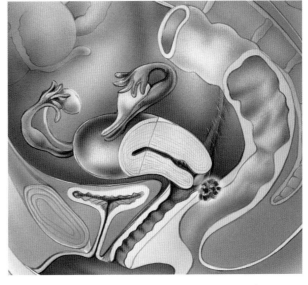

Figure 1 Adenomyotic nodule of the rectovaginal septum

Table I Rectovaginal adenomyosis ($n = 1146$)

	n	%
Laparoscopic adenomyotic nodule excision	1125	98.2
Laparotomy: nodule excision with bowel (sigmoidal or rectal) resection and anastomosis in cases of bowel substenosis and menstrual rectal bleeding	21	1.8

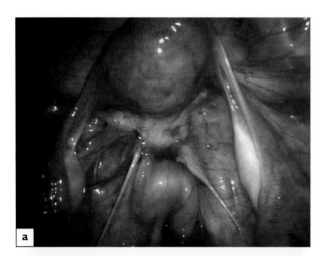

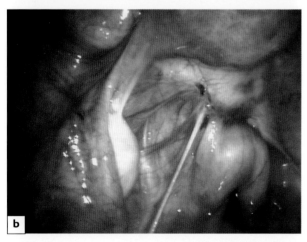

Figure 2 (a) and (b) Laparoscopic view. Note that the ovaries are normal and free of adhesions. Peritoneal endometriosis is minimal. Ninety percent of the lesion is located in the retroperitoneal space

The surgical techniques have evolved gradually but all of them involve the separation of the anterior rectum from the posterior vagina and the excision or ablation of the endometriosis in that area. Aquadissection, scissor dissection and electrosurgery with an unmodulated (cutting) current are used by some authors[14,17], while others[8–11,15,16] prefer the use of the CO_2 laser.

CO_2 laser dissection is currently used in our department. At present, all treatment modes have been used to

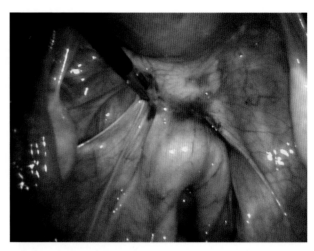

Figure 3 The rectosigmoid is clearly attached to the posterior part of the cervix (arrow)

some extent in most cases. Whenever extensive involvement of the cul-de-sac was suspected preoperatively, either because of the clinical presentation or from another physician's operative record, a mechanical bowel preparation was administered orally before surgery to induce brisk, self-limiting diarrhea that rapidly cleanses the bowel without disrupting the electrolyte balance. In cases of lesions of the anterior rectal wall (diagnosed by radiography or by echography (Figure 5)), a bowel preparation was proposed as for conventional bowel resection (2 days).

CLINICAL AND LAPAROSCOPIC ASPECTS

Clinical aspects and diagnosis

Examination with a speculum reveals either a normal vaginal mucosa or a protruded bluish nodule in the posterior fornix (Figure 6). By palpation, the diameter of the lesion can be evaluated. Palpation is very often painful and the presence of the nodule accounts for symptoms like deep dyspareunia and dysmenorrhea.

Laparoscopic aspects (Table 2)

To determine the diagnosis of cul-de-sac obliteration, a sponge on a ring forceps was inserted into the posterior vaginal fornix (Figures 7 and 8). A dilator (Hegar 25) on a rectal probe was systematically inserted into the rectum (Figure 9). Complete obliteration was diagnosed when the outline of the posterior fornix could not be seen through the laparoscope (Figure 10).

Cul-de-sac obliteration was partial when rectal tenting was visible but a protrusion of the sponge in the posterior vaginal fornix was identified between the rectum and the inverted U of the uterosacral ligaments. However, sometimes a deep lesion of the rectovaginal septum is only barely visible by laparoscopy. We believe that this type of lesion is not actually endometriosis, but a specific disease called adenomyosis, which is characterized by the presence of abundant muscular tissue invaded by glandular epithelium covered with a scanty stroma (see below). This type of 'adenomyosis' must be clearly differentiated in the new classification.

Table 2 Rectovaginal adenomyosis operated on by laparoscopy (n = 1125)

Technical aspects	
Duration (min)	65 (35–186)
Hospitalization (days)	2.8 (2–5)
Laparoscopic bowel resection*	0
Complications	
Rectal perforation	7 (0.6%)
Delayed hemorrhage (< 24 h postoperation)	3 (0.3%)
Ureteral injury	1 (0.1%)
Urinary retention	6 (0.5%)
Fecalis peritonitis	1 (0.1%)

* In 21 cases, bowel resection was carried out by laparotomy (these cases are not included in this series of 1125) (see Table 1)

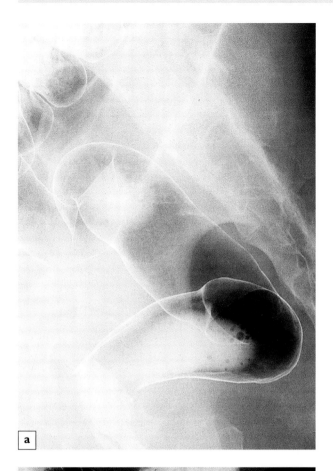
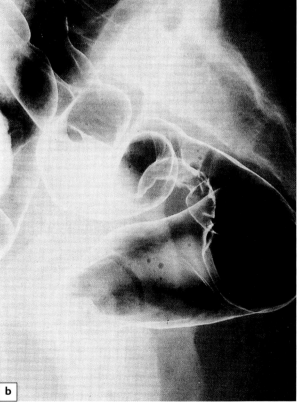
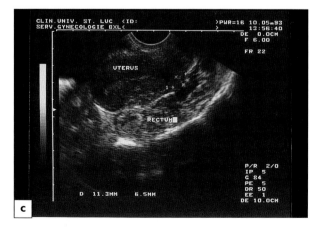

Figure 4 Profile radiography offers the best evaluation of the infiltration of the anterior rectal wall; (a) no signs of infiltration; (b) typical 'endometriotic' infiltration of the anterior rectal wall without stenosis, intact mucosa; (c) the same patient showing evaluation of rectal infiltration by vaginal echography

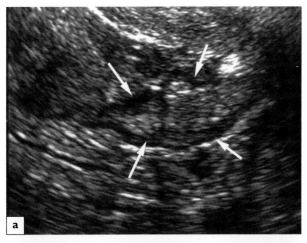

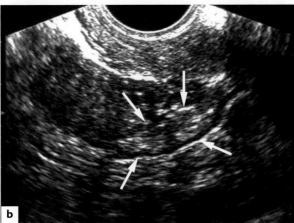

Figure 5 (a) Vaginal and (b) rectal echography reveal the infiltration by the adenomyotic disease

HISTOLOGY

Deep vaginal adenomyosis associated with pelvic endometriosis can take the form of nodular or polypoid masses involving the posterior vaginal fornix. The differential diagnosis of vaginal endometriosis, particularly of the superficial type, includes vaginal adenosis of the tubo-endometrial variety, but the latter lacks endometrial stroma and the characteristic inflammatory response of endometriosis. In the body of the uterus, adenomyosis is a common condition characterized pathologically by the presence of endometrial glands and stroma within the myometrium. Microscopically, there are endometrial glands and stroma within the myometrium. The lower border of the endometrium is irregular and dips into the superficial myometrium.

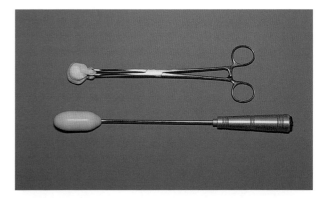

Figure 7 Sponge grasped by forceps (top); rectal probe (bottom)

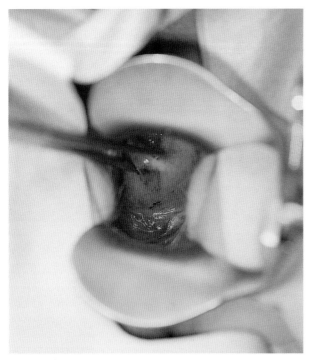

Figure 6 Speculum examination: sometimes a bluish lesion is seen protruding in the vaginal fornix

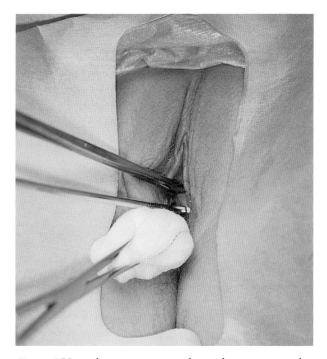

Figure 8 Vaginal sponge is inserted into the vagina in order to see the cleavage plane between the rectum, the vagina and the nodule

Adenomyosis exhibits a varied functional response to ovarian hormones. Proliferative glands and stroma are generally observed in the first half of the menstrual cycle. Adenomyosis may not respond to physiological levels of progesterone, and secretory changes are frequently absent or incomplete during the second half of the cycle. Similar histological observations are made at the level of rectovaginal nodules. Like adenomyoma, it is a circumscribed, nodular aggregate of smooth muscle, endometrial glands and, usually, endometrial stroma.

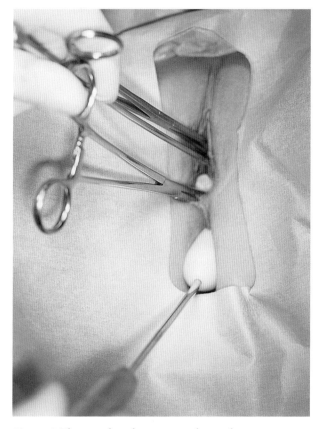

Figure 9 The rectal probe is inserted into the rectum

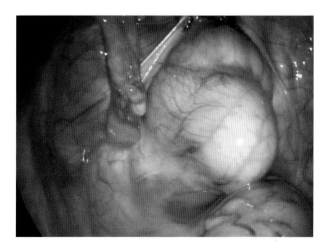

Figure 10 Laparoscopic view of the rectal probe which allows visualization of the rectum and of the cleavage plane

Histologically, scanty endometrial-type stroma and glandular epithelium are disseminated in muscular tissue. These very similar histological descriptions have led to the suggestion that the so-called endometriotic nodule of the rectovaginal septum is, in fact, just like an adenomyoma or an adenomyotic nodule. By three-dimensional evaluation, the reconstructed endometriotic lesion has the appearance of a unique 'gland' with multiple ramifications. Here also, as in the peritoneal 'red' lesion, the apparent multifocal aspect of the glands is not confirmed by three-dimensional evaluation. Sometimes, the invasion of the muscle by a very active glandular epithelium proved that the stroma is not necessary for invasion in this particular type of pathology called adenomyosis. Invasion of the vaginal musculature by the glandular epithelium is not rare.

SURGICAL TECHNIQUE

All the laparoscopic procedures were performed using general anesthesia. A 12-mm operative laparoscope was inserted through a vertical intraumbilical incision. Three other puncture sites were made: 2–3 cm above the pubis in the midline, and in the areas adjacent to the deep inferior epigastric vessels, which were visualized directly.

Deep fibrotic nodular adenomyosis involving the cul-de-sac required an excision of the nodular tissue from the posterior vagina, rectum, posterior cervix and uterosacral ligaments. As described by Reich and colleagues[14] and Donnez and colleagues[8–11], attention was first directed toward a complete dissection of the anterior rectum throughout its area of involvement until the loose tissue of the rectovaginal space was reached. A sponge on a ring forceps was inserted into the posterior vaginal fornix and a dilator (Hegar 25) was placed in the rectum. In addition, a cannula was inserted into the endometrial cavity to markedly antevert the uterus. The peritoneum covering the cul-de-sac of Douglas was opened between the 'adenomyotic' lesion (Figure 11) and the rectum.

We used a technique of first freeing the anterior rectum from the loose areolar tissue of the rectovaginal septum, prior to excising and/or vaporizing visible and palpable deep fibrotic endometriosis. This approach was possible even when anterior rectal muscle infiltration was present. Careful dissection was then carried out using the aquadissector, and the CO_2 laser for sharp dissection, until the rectum was completely freed and identifiable below the lesion (Figure 12).

Excision of the fibrotic tissue on the side of the rectum was attempted only after the rectal dissection was complete (Figure 13). A partial rectal resection was never performed in our series. In cases of deep lesions, the vaginal wall was more or less penetrated by the adenomyosis and excision of a part of the vagina was essential (Figure 14).

Dissection was performed accordingly, not only with the removal of all visible adenomyotic lesions, but also the vaginal mucosa with at least a 0.5-cm disease-free margin

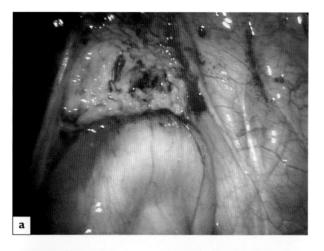

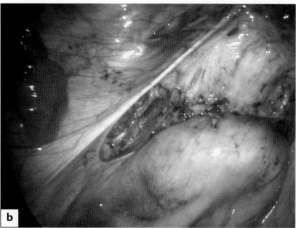

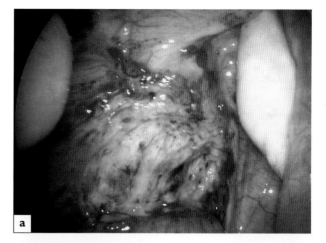

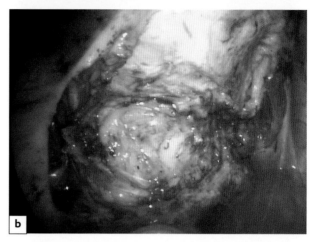

Figure 12 (a) and (b) After the rectum has been freed, the vaginal wall is opened below the adenomyotic lesion

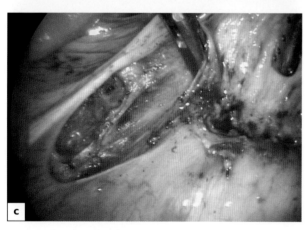

Figure 11 (a) Dissection with the CO_2 laser until the rectum is completely freed and identifiable below the lesion. (b) and (c) Lateral dissection and section of the uterosacral ligament lateral to the rectum

(laterally). Lesions extending totally through the vagina were treated with en bloc laparoscopic resection from the cul-de-sac to the posterior vaginal wall (Figures 15 and 16); the pneumoperitoneum was maintained and the posterior vaginal wall was closed vaginally (Figure 17).

The anterior rectum can be reperitonealized by plicating the uterosacral ligaments and lateral rectal peritoneum

across the midline using 4-0 Polydioxanone Tissucol® or Interceed® (Figure 18)[8–11]. Deep rectal muscle defects can be closed with suture. Full-thickness rectal lesion excisons were successfully repaired with suture in the series of Reich and associates[14].

In our series of 1125 cases, laparoscopic dissection was performed successfully in all cases, even when the radiography of the colon showed bowel involvement. Bowel resection is usually unnecessary, except in cases of bowel occlusion and rectal bleeding. Then, resection of the rectosigmoid junction must be carried out. In our series of 1125 cases, laparoscopic rectal perforation occurred in seven cases. All perforations were diagnosed at the time of the laparoscopy. In three cases, the rectum was repaired by laparotomy and, in the others, by colpotomy.

During the same period, 21 patients who had rectal endometriosis with stenosis and rectal bleeding were operated on by laparotomy. A bowel resection with anastomosis was then carried out.

When a ureter is close to the lesion, its course can be traced starting at the pelvic brim. The peritoneum overlying the ureter can be opened to confirm the ureteral position deep in the pelvis.

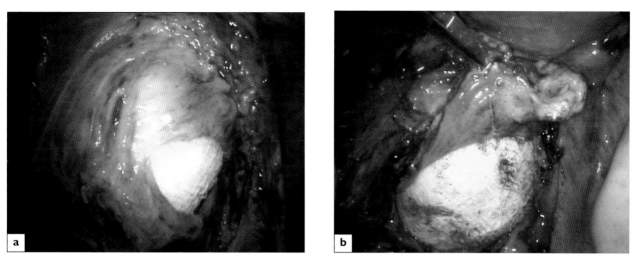

Figure 13 (a) and (b) The vaginal sponge is clearly visible and avoids loss of pneumoperitoneum

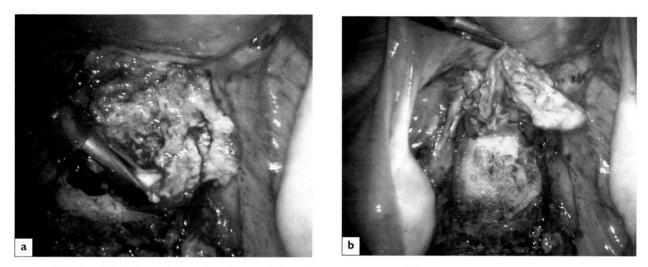

Figure 14 (a) and (b) The nodule is then dissected from the posterior part of the cervix

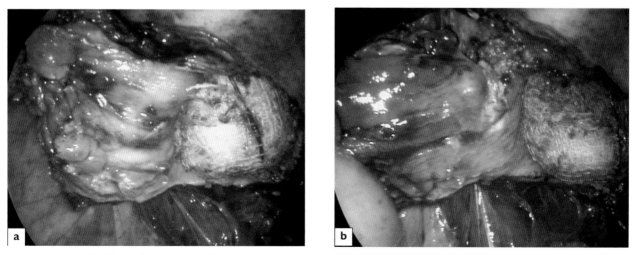

Figure 15 (a) The bluish lesion is visible on the vaginal mucosa. (b) By laparoscopy, the margins of the resection can be defined

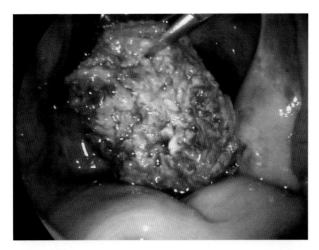

Figure 16 The adenomyotic nodule has been completely resected

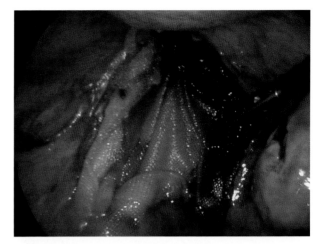

Figure 18 The deperitonealized area is covered with Interceed

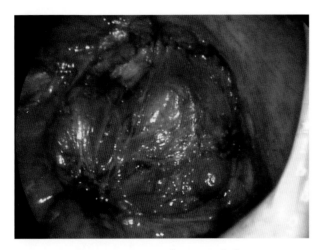

Figure 17 Laparoscopic view after vaginal closure

Bipolar forceps were used to control arterial and venous bleeding. A final copious irrigation with saline solution was carried out and all clots were aspirated directly. Reich and co-workers[14] suggest leaving at least 2 l of Ringer's solution in the abdomen to separate the raw surfaces during early healing. In our department, Interceed was employed as an antiadhesion agent (Figure 18). All the women were discharged either the next day or 2 days after surgery.

The surgical objectives of laparoscopic treatment are similar: to remove all evident endometriosis by excising large superficial and deep lesions and vaporizing smaller deposits. With our approach, first the anterior rectum was freed; this was possible even when anterior rectal infiltration was present.

LONG-TERM RESULTS

Table 3 shows the number of patients followed for more than 3 years in our department. We thus excluded patients who were referred by foreign centers and followed in other countries. We have analyzed the long-term (3–10 years) results (Table 4). Recurrence rates of dysmenorrhea, deep dyspareunia and nodules were noted according to the surgical technique used.

The recurrence rate of dysmenorrhea was, respectively, 9%, 17% and 26% in the three groups, but, if severe dysmenorrhea was chosen as a criterion, the recurrence rate was significantly lower when excision of the nodule was carried out together with resection of the posterior fornix. The same conclusion could be drawn if the recurrence rate of severe dyspareunia is analyzed.

In our opinion, the better results found in group II are explained by the wide resection of the posterior vaginal fornix, including the resection of the sympathetic nerves situated between the cervix and the uterosacral ligaments (torus uterinum).

It is very important to note that the recurrence rates of dysmenorrhea, dyspareunia and nodules were lower in group II (excision of nodules + posterior fornix) when compared to group III (bowel resection, no vaginal resection). It proves again that very aggressive surgery, including bowel resection, does not prevent recurrence.

Large debulking surgery must be considered more appropriate than extensive surgery including bowel resection. Vaginal fornix resection must be considered as the first choice. Bowel resection must be indicated only in cases of rectal bleeding or in cases of sigmoidal or rectal stenosis.

DISCUSSION

In some lesions, the main feature is a bowel which is retracted over the lesion, which thus becomes deeply situated in the rectovaginal septum, although not really infiltrating it. Another type of lesion is the deepest and most severe. It is spherically shaped, situated deep in the recto-

Table 3 More than 3-year follow-up of rectovaginal 'adenomyotic' nodule excision ($n = 437$)

Group I ($n = 150$) (34%)	excision of the nodule without resection of the vaginal mucosa (laparoscopy)
Group II ($n = 272$) (62.5%)	excision of the nodule with resection of the posterior vaginal fornix (laparoscopy)
Group III ($n = 15$) (3.5%)	excision of the nodule and bowel resection because of bowel substenosis (laparotomy)

Table 4 Recurrence of dysmenorrhea, deep dyspareunia and nodules according to the surgical technique used

	Group I ($n = 150$)*	Group II ($n = 282$)†	Group III ($n = 15$)§
Recurrence of dysmenorrhea	43 (29%)	46 (17%)	4 (26%)
severe	21 (14%)	20 (7.5%)	3 (20%)
mild or moderate	22 (15%)	26 (9.5%)	1 (6%)
Deep dyspareunia	29 (19%)	35 (13%)	4 (26%)
severe	22 (15%)	20 (7.5%)	3 (20%)
mild or moderate	7 (4%)	15 (5.5%)	1 (6%)
Severe pelvic pain	24 (16%)	27 (10%)	3 (20%)
Recurrence of nodules	26 (17.3%)	10 (3.7%)**	3 (20%)
Average delay	4.9 years (3–10 years)	3.8 years (3–6 years)	4.1 years (3–10 years)

* Excision of the nodule without resection of the vaginal mucosa (laparoscopy); † excision of the nodule with resection of the posterior vaginal fornix (laparoscopy); § excision of the nodule and bowel resection because of bowel substenosis (laparotomy); ** significantly different from other groups ($p < 0.05$)

vaginal septum, and is often visible only as a small typical lesion at laparoscopy. This lesion is often more palpable than visible.

For us, there are two different types of deep endometriosis:

(1) True infiltrating endometriosis causes the invasion of a very active peritoneal lesion deep in the retroperitoneal space. In cases of lateral peritoneal invasion, the uterosacral ligaments are involved.

(2) Adenomyosis of the rectovaginal septum which originates from the tissue of the rectovaginal septum and consists essentially of smooth muscle with active glandular epithelium and scanty stroma[19].

Kelly and Diamond[20], reporting on a series of 68 women who underwent laparotomy for endometriosis, found that it was rarely necessary to penetrate the bowel lumen to excise the endometriosis; colonic endometriosis was vaporized down to normal tissue, as proved by palpation and viewing with magnification.

In two of the largest series published in the literature[10,11], deep fibrotic tissue assumed to contain adenomyosis was excised or vaporized from the anterior rectum with the aid of multiple rectovaginal examinations. Cul-de-sac dissection was followed by excision of deep fibrotic adenomyosis, with or without cul-de-sac reconstruction. In seven cases, the bowel lumen was entered.

A comprehensive laparoscopic procedure, while not eradicating all the endometriosis, may result in considerable pain relief or a desired pregnancy. While we recognize that bowel resection may be necessary in rare cases (1.8%), it seems prudent to curtail, rather than encourage, the widespread use of an aggressive, potentially morbid procedure.

In conclusion, deep adenomyosis should be considered as a specific disease, different from mild or minimal endometriosis and ovarian cystic endometriosis. We suggest that this disease be called 'rectovaginal adenomyosis'.

REFERENCES

1. Donnez J, Nisolle M, Casanas-Roux F. Three-dimensional architectures of peritoneal endometriosis. *Fertil Steril* 1992;57:980–3

2. Nisolle M, Donnez J. Peritoneal endometriosis, ovarian endometriosis, and adenomyotic nodules of the rectovaginal septum are three different entities. *Fertil Steril* 1997;68:585–96

3. Donnez J, Nisolle M. Appearances of peritoneal endometriosis. In *Proceedings of The 3rd International Laser Surgery Symposium*, Brussels, 1988

4. Nisolle M, Paindaveine B, Bourdon A, *et al.* Histologic study of peritoneal endometriosis in infertile women. *Fertil Steril* 1990;53:984–8

5. Nisolle M, Casanas-Roux, Anaf V, *et al.* Morphometric study of the stromal vascularization in peritoneal endometriosis. *Fertil Steril* 1993;59:681–4

6. Hughesdon PE. The structure of endometrial cysts of the ovary. *J Obstet Gynaecol Br Empire* 1957;64:481–7

7. Donnez J, Nisolle M, Gillet N, *et al.* Large ovarian endometriomas. *Hum Reprod* 1996;11:641–6

8. Donnez J, Nisolle M, Casanas-Roux F, *et al.* Laparoscopic treatment of rectovaginal septum endometriosis. In Donnez J, Nisolle M, eds. *An Atlas of Laser Operative Laparoscopy and Hysteroscopy*. Carnforth, UK: Parthenon Publishing, 1994:75–85

9. Donnez J, Nisolle M. Advanced laparoscopic surgery for the removal of rectovaginal septum endometriotic and adenomyotic nodules. *Baillieres Clin Obstet Gynecol* 1995;9:769–74

10. Donnez J, Nisolle M, Casanas-Roux F, *et al.* Rectovaginal septum endometriosis or adenomyosis: laparoscopic management in a series of 231 patients. *Hum Reprod* 1995;10:630–5

11. Donnez J, Nisolle M, Gillenot S, *et al.* Rectovaginal septum adenomyotic nodules: a series of 500 cases. *Br J Obstet Gynaecol* 1991;104:1009–13

12. Sampson JA. Intestinal adenomas of endometrial type. *Arch Surg* 1922;5:217

13. Donnez J, Nisolle M, Casanas-Roux F. Endometriosis-associated infertility: evaluation of preoperative use of danazol, gestrinone and buserelin. *Int J Fertil* 1990;35:297–301

14. Reich H, McGlynn F, Salvat J. Laparoscopic treatment of cul-de-sac obliteration secondary to retrocervical deep fibrotic endometriosis. *J Reprod Med* 1991;36:516

15. Koninckx PD. Deeply infiltrating endometriosis. In Brosens I, Donnez J, eds. *Endometriosis: Research and Management*. Carnforth, UK: Parthenon Publishing, 1993:437–46

16. Nezhat C, Nezhat F, Pennington E. Laparoscopic treatment of lower colorectal and infiltrative rectovaginal septum endometriosis by the technique of video laparoscopy. *Br J Obstet Gynaecol* 1992;99:664–7

17. Canis M, Wattiez A, Pouly JL, *et al.* Laparoscopic treatment of endometriosis. In Brosens I, Donnez J, eds. *Endometriosis: Research and Management*. Carnforth, UK: Parthenon Publishing, 1993:407–17

18. Donnez J, Nisolle M, Casanas-Roux F, *et al.* Endometriosis: rationale for surgery. In Brosens I, Donnez J, eds. *Endometriosis: Research and Management*. Carnforth, UK: Parthenon Publishing, 1993:385–95

19. Zaloudek C, Norris HJ. Mesenchymal tumors of the uterus. In Kurman R, ed. *Blaustein's Pathology of the Female Genital Tract*. New York, 1987:373–408

20. Kelly R, Diamond MP. Laparotomy in infertile patients (use of CO_2 laser). *J Reprod Med* 1989;34:25

Ureteral endometriosis: a complication of rectovaginal adenomyosis

10

J. Donnez and M. Nisolle

INTRODUCTION

Despite thousands of scientific reports in the literature on endometriosis, its prevalence in the general population is unknown. In women with pelvic pain and/or infertility, high prevalences, ranging from 20 to 80–90%, have been reported[1–4].

Usually, endometriosis involves the peritoneum, the ovaries or the rectovaginal septum, and three distinct entities have recently been described[4]. Ureteral endometriosis is relatively uncommon and is estimated to occur in about 0.08–1% of patients with endometriosis[5,6]. The prevalence of 1% observed in the study by Nezhat and colleagues[6] was considered to be somewhat overestimated according to Donnez and Brosens, who observed six cases in a series of 6285 patients (0.1%). It was suggested, in 1997, that there was a more frequent association of obstructive uropathy with rectovaginal adenomyosis[7].

A distinction must be made between extrinsic and intrinsic ureteral endometriosis[8,9]. Indeed, intrinsic ureteral endometriosis, characterized by the presence of endometriotic glands and stroma in the ureteral wall, is a very rare entity. However, extrinsic ureteral endometriosis, caused by extra-ureteral disease, is more frequent.

The late consequence of ureteral endometriosis is the silent loss of renal function caused by the progressive 'enclosure' of the lower part of the ureter by the adenomyosis.

PATIENTS

We evaluated prospectively the prevalence of ureteral lesions in a series of 306 patients treated for rectovaginal adenomyotic nodules between March 1998 and July 2000. The patients were classified according to the size of the nodule (< 2 cm, > 2 cm and < 3 cm, and > 3 cm). The size of the nodule was evaluated by palpation on the posterior fornix of the vagina during vaginal examination and vaginal echography. Intravenous pyelography (IVP) was performed in all patients, prior to surgery. Care was taken to analyze the lower segment of the ureter. The stenosis was judged partial or complete (Figure 1a and b). The degree of uterohydronephrosis was evaluated according to ureteral diameter. In cases of cortical atrophy (Figure 2), kidney scintigraphy (Tc99-DMSA) (Figure 3) was performed preoperatively and postoperatively in order to evaluate renal function. Fourteen cases of ureteral endometriosis were observed during this period.

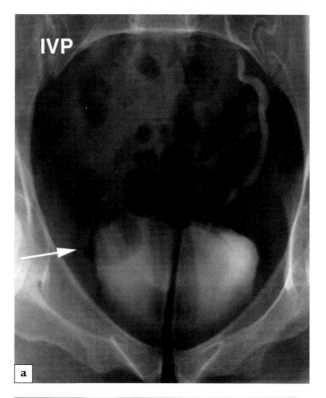

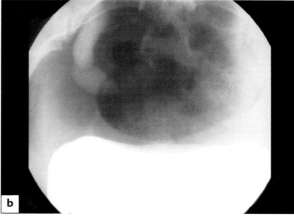

Figure 1 Intravenous pyelogram (IVP): (a) partial stenosis with ureteronephrosis; (b) complete stenosis with subsequent cortical atrophy

The preoperative characteristics of patients with ureteral endometriosis are shown in Table 1. They ranged in age from 21 to 39 years (mean 28.7 years). In the majority of patients, the main symptoms were severe pelvic pain, severe dysmenorrhea and severe dyspareunia. Only three patients suffered pelvic pain and infertility.

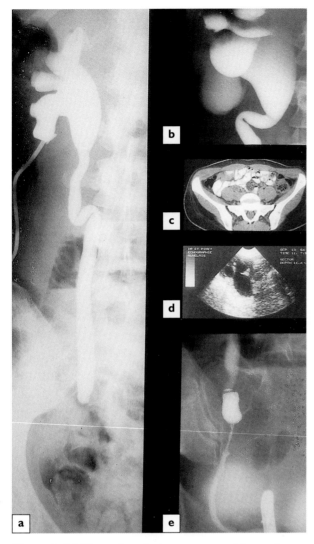

Figure 2 (a) Ureteral occlusion was proved by pyelography; ureteral dilatation was diagnosed by (b) intravenous pyelography, (c) computerized tomography scan and (d) renal echography; (e) retrograde catheterization of the uterer indicated the level of occlusion

Preoperative CA-125 levels ranged from 16 to 100 IU/ml (mean 50.8 IU/ml).

OPERATIVE SURGERY

In all cases but one, conservative surgery without ureteral resection was carried out by laparoscopy. Under general anesthesia, an umbilical incision was made and a 12-mm laparoscope (Sharplan, Tel Aviv, Israel) was introduced. Three suprapubic trocars (5 mm in size; Storz, Tuttlingen, Germany) were placed to insert instruments to perform the laparoscopic procedure. A CO_2 laser (Sharplan, Tel-Aviv, Israel) was used for dissection of the bowel, and removal of the adenomyotic lesion and vaginal pouch in cases of rectovaginal adenomyotic nodules, as previously described[10,11]. In all cases, ureterolysis was performed

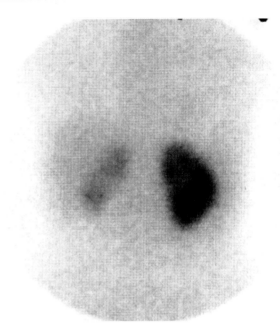

Figure 3 Kidney scintigraphy (Tc99-DMSA) demonstrates significantly decreased renal function (17% in the case showed in Figure 2)

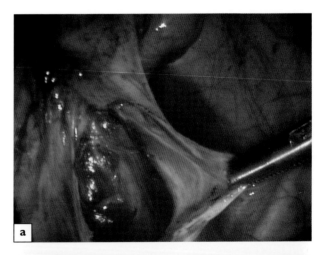

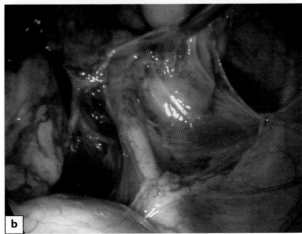

Figure 4 (a) and (b) The dissection of the ureter starts by opening the peritoneum covering the ureter, where the ureter is free of adhesions and clearly visible

Table I Preoperative characteristics of 14 patients with ureteral endometriosis

Age (years)	Parity	Associated symptoms of endometriosis	Ca-125 (IU/ml)	Ureteral stenosis at IVP	Rectovaginal adenomyotic nodule size (cm)
25	G0 P0	infertility, DIII, DD	26.7	right	4
31	G0 P0	DIII, DD	25.8	right	3
30	G0 P0	DIII, DD	100	right	3
30	G0 P0	DIII, DD	54.7	left	4
29	G0 P0	DIII, dyschesia	66.6	left	3.5
31	G0 P0	infertility, DIII	62.5	right	4
39	G0 P0	DIII, DD	42	left	3
26	G1 P1	DIII, DD, dyschesia++	53.6	left	3
37	G3 P3	DIII, DD	72	left	2–3
21	G0 P0	DIII, DD	98	bilateral	5
28	G1 P1	DIII, DD	17	left	4
21	G0 P0	DII, DD	37.7	right	4
28	G0 P0	DIII, DD	16	left	3–4
27	G1 P0	DII, DD, infertility, dyschesia	39.9	left	3

DII, moderate dysmenorrhea; DIII, severe dysmenorrhea; DD, deep dyspareunia; IVP, intravenous pyelography

before adenomyotic nodule resection. The peritoneum covering the ureter was opened with the CO_2 laser, where the ureter was free of adhesions and clearly visible (Figure 4). The dissection was progressively made in the direction of the uterosacral ligament (Figure 5). The ureter was freed from surrounding tissue using CO_2 laser section and vaporization. To facilitate this step of the procedure, a JJ stent was inserted retrogradely, by cystoscopy just before surgery in five cases. In three cases, after ureterolysis, the fibrotic stenotic ring responsible for the ureteral structure was removed without opening the ureteral lumen. The adventitial sheath was cut but the medial muscular layer was respected, as far as possible (Figure 6). Ureteral opening or resection never occurred during the laparoscopic procedure.

In six cases, voluntary section of the uterine artery was performed during ureterolysis, using titanium clips which were placed on the uterine artery crossing the lowest part of the ureter (Figure 5b and c). This procedure enabled us to free the ureter until its lowest part. At the end of the procedure, the ureter was free of disease in all cases (Figure 7).

Non-conservative surgery, including partial ureteral resection, was required in one case (Figure 8). This patient, suffering from sigmoidal endometriosis and ovarian endometriosis with extensive and dense adhesions, required laparotomy with left oophorectomy and salpingectomy and ureteral-ureterostomy with a 2-cm ureteral resection (Figure 9).

In the series described here, we did not encounter any more cases like that described in 1994 (Figure 10).

RESULTS

In a series of 306 cases of rectovaginal adenomyosis, ureteral endometriosis was encountered in 14 cases. The prevalence was thus 4.5% in our prospective study.

In the study group, severe dysmenorrhea and deep dyspareunia were experienced by all patients, but only three suffered infertility. Only one of the patients, who had ureterohydronephrosis, complained of typical pain due to obstructive uropathy.

Isolated ureteral endometriosis was never noted; it was in all cases associated with rectovaginal adenomyosis. Ovarian endometriomas were observed in three cases on the ipsilateral side of ureteral endometriosis but they were always associated with rectovaginal adenomyosis. The ureteral stenosis was not situated where the ovarian endometriomas were adherent to the broad ligament.

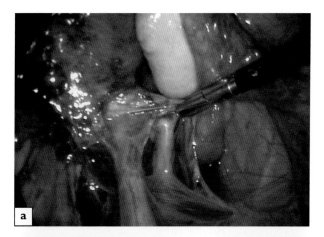

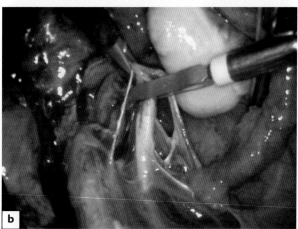

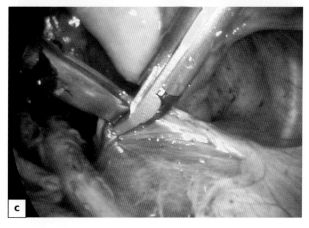

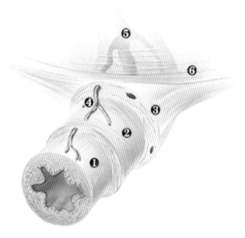

Figure 6 The ureter and its different layers. 1, Mucosa with urothelium; 2, medial muscular layer; 3, adventitial sheath; 4, arteriole between musculosa and adventitial sheath; 5, ureteral artery; 6, peritoneum

Figure 5 The dissection is progressively made in the direction of the uterosacral ligament. (a) Identification of the uterine artery; (b) coagulation of the uterine artery; (c) ligation of the uterine artery

In our prospective study, classification of patients was carried out according to the size of the rectovaginal adenomyotic nodule (Table 2). Seventy-one patients had a rectovaginal nodule of less than 2 cm in size, 119 patients had a nodule of > 2 cm and < 3 cm in size, and 116 patients had a very large rectovaginal nodule, measuring more than 3 cm. A significantly ($p < 0.05$) higher prevalence of

ureteral endometriosis (11.2%) was observed in patients with rectovaginal adenomyotic nodules of more than 3 cm in size than in patients with smaller nodules (< 2 cm: 0%; > 2 and < 3 cm: 0.8%).

In our series, all patients underwent preoperative IVP. It revealed a stricture of the lowest portion of the ureter, 2–3 cm long, with moderate to severe hydronephrosis as a consequence. Unilateral stenosis (partial or complete) and ureterohydronephrosis were detected in 13 cases (right $n = 5$; left $n = 8$) and it was bilateral in one case. Ureteral stenosis was thus right-sided in six cases and left-sided in nine cases. The prevalences of right-sided and left-sided lesions were thus, respectively, 2% (6/306) and 3% (9/306). In four cases, ureterohydronephrosis was severe (ureteral dilatation > 1.5 cm) and associated with cortical atrophy. Kidney scintigraphy (Tc99-DMSA) revealed renal function, evaluated at 18%, 19%, 29% and 42%. In cases of cortical atrophy and decreased renal function, helical computerized tomography allowed us to detect the level of ureteral occlusion (Figure 11).

Ureterolysis was performed on the right side in six cases and on the left in nine cases. During surgery, the lower part of the ureter was systematically found to be enclosed in fibrosis due to the rectovaginal adenomyotic nodule. All women underwent rectovaginal adenomyotic nodule removal during the same procedure, without segmental bowel resection. In one patient, ureteral endometriosis was found to be associated with bladder endometriosis and a rectovaginal adenomyotic nodule. After removal of the rectovaginal adenomyotic nodule and ureterolysis, the bladder endometriotic nodule was laparoscopically removed using the extramucosal approach, as recently described by Donnez and colleagues[12].

In patients with moderate or severe ureterohydronephrosis, preoperative and postoperative IVP were compared. Patent ureters and functional kidneys were

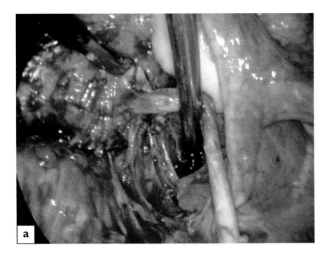

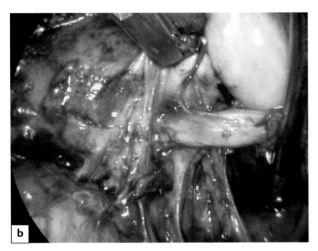

Figure 7 (a) and (b) At the end of the dissection, the ureter is free of disease

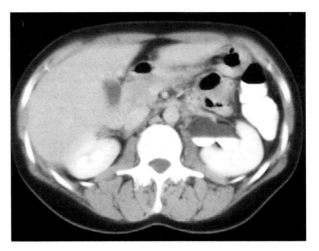

Figure 8 Computerized tomography scan: left uretero-hydronephrosis with significant dilatation of renal pelvic and renal cortical atrophy

cally demonstrated in all cases where the uterine artery was resected.

The follow-up ranged from 4 to 26 months. Relief from pain was noted in 13 women (92%). Only one patient underwent a second laparoscopy, after 9 months due to recurrence of pelvic pain. It was due to a recurrence of a nodular lesion in the Douglas pouch but, at the preoperative IVP, no recurrent ureteral dilatation was observed.

Two of the three women suffering from primary infertility became pregnant a few months after surgery.

DISCUSSION

Ureteral endometriosis is infrequent, accounting for less than 0.3% of all endometriotic lesions. Ureteral lesions are relatively rare but they are a very serious condition because they may cause silent loss of renal function. There are two types of ureteral endometriosis, extrinsic and intrinsic[7–9]. Intrinsic ureteral obstruction is characterized by the presence of endometriotic glands and stroma in the ureteral wall due to primary endometriotic involvement of the ureteral wall. This type of ureteral endometriosis is less common, however, than ureteral obstruction, caused by external compression by surrounding endometriosis, which is known as extrinsic ureteral endometriosis. According to Stanley and colleagues[13], endometriosis of the ureter usually arises by extension from pelvic foci, and ovarian endometriosis is a prerequisite of ureteral involvement.

In a retrospective study from 1988 to 1997, the prevalence of ureteral endometriosis was estimated to be less than 0.1% in cases of endometriosis[7]. In women suffering from rectovaginal adenomyosis, it was found to be 0.9% (6/711).

In this prospective study, we report 14 cases of ureteral endometriosis. Among the 14 patients, 13 (92%) presented with pure extrinsic ureteral endometriosis.

observed in all of them. Recovery of the ureteral diameter was also observed in all cases, as well as disappearance of pyelic dilatation. Patients who underwent preoperative or intraoperative retrograde stent placement kept the catheter in place for 3 months ($n = 5$). After that period, the JJ stent was removed and IVP demonstrated the absence of any ureteral stricture (Figure 12).

Kidney scintigraphy (Tc99-DMSA) was performed pre- and postoperatively in four patients who had severe pyelic dilatation and cortical atrophy. The association of complete ureterolysis and administration of gonadotropin releasing hormone analog therapy for 3 months led to a significant recovery of ureteral diameter but the postoperative kidney scintigraphy revealed only a slight improvement (from 2 to 5%) in renal function.

Histological study of peri-ureteral resection specimens revealed the presence of endometriotic glands in contact with the uterine artery, and the ureter itself (Figure 13). Serial sections demonstrated hyperplasia of the smooth muscle, invading the retroperitoneal space. Scanty stroma and glandular epithelium were found. Peri-artery invasion by the retroperitoneal adenomyotic disease was histologi-

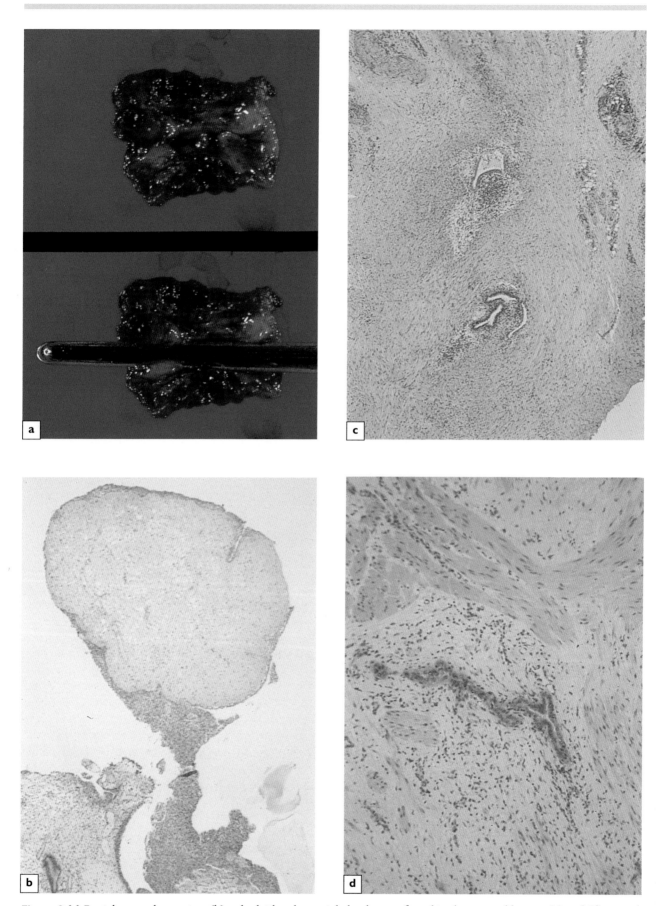

Figure 9 (a) Partial ureteral resection; (b) polyploid endometrial glands were found in the ureteral lumen; (c) and (d) typical endometrial epithelium and stroma were found invading the ureteral wall

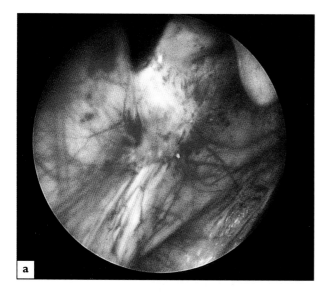

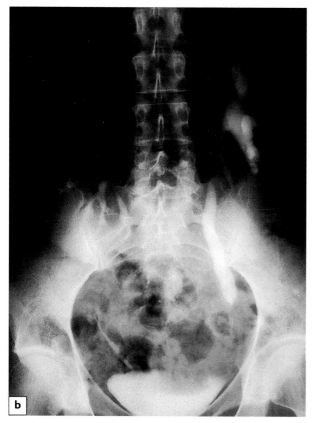

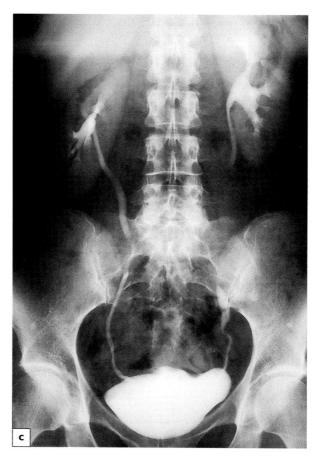

Figure 10 (a) Ureteral pseudo-occlusion provoked by endometriotic peritoneal lesion covering the ureter; (b) preoperative intravenous pyelography (IVP) showing the dilatation of the left ureter; (c) postoperative IVP showing the recovery of the left ureter 3 months after CO_2 laser laparoscopic removal of the peritoneal lesion covering the ureter (a)

Surrounding endometriotic lesions responsible for external ureteral compression, without histological evidence of endometriotic glands and stroma in the ureteral wall, are thus mostly the consequence of lateral extension of rectovaginal adenomyotic nodules. These patients also showed another localization of endometriosis, but ovarian endometriomas were never considered solely responsible for ureteral endometriosis because they were always associated with rectovaginal adenomyosis. One patient with a rectovaginal adenomyotic nodule of 3 cm in size had an associated 3-cm bladder adenomyotic nodule. Nezhat and co-workers described concomitant bowel endometriosis in 62% of cases (13/21), requiring bowel resection and anastomosis in three cases[6]. In our series, bowel resection was never needed.

In one case (8%), extrinsic and intrinsic ureteral endometriosis were mixed. Histological analysis of the removed ureteral segment revealed the presence of glands in the ureteral wall as far as the lumen (Figure 9).

The concept of adenomyosis of the retroperitoneal space should thus cover not only the rectovaginal space and the vesicovaginal space but also the area extending laterally in the direction of the cardinal ligaments[9–12,14].

In a large review of the literature on retrospective series of ureteral endometriosis, the proportion of lesions located on the left was found to be significantly higher than on the right[15]. In our study, a higher proportion was also found on the left (nine cases versus six cases), but the difference was not significant, the prevalences being, respectively, 3% and 2%. In the series of Nezhat and colleagues, a non-significant prevalence of ureteral endometriosis was observed between left and right sides[6].

Table 2 Incidence of ureteral endometriosis according to the size of the rectovaginal adenomyotic nodule (in the prospective study of 306 patients)

Rectovaginal adenomyotic nodule size (cm)	Number of patients	Number of patients with ureteral endometriosis	Prevalence of ureteral endometriosis (%)
< 2	71	0	0
> 2 and < 3	119	1	0.8
> 3	116	13	11.2*
Total	306	14	4.5

* The prevalence of ureteral endometriosis is significantly higher in this group of patients than in the other groups ($p < 0.05$)

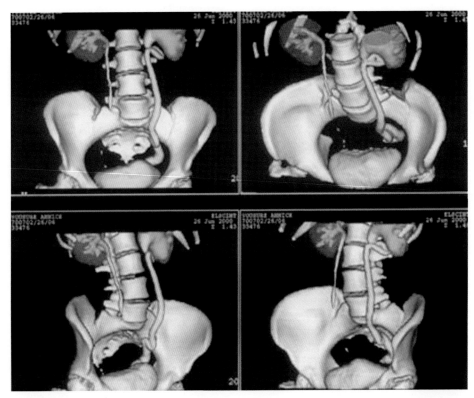

Figure 11 Helical computerized tomography: detection of the level of ureteral occlusion in cases of complete stenosis with very severe ureterohydronephrosis and cortical atrophy

In a recent publication by Vercellini and colleagues[15], six cases of ureteral endometriosis were described as being associated with ovarian endometriomas and, in the opinion of the authors, neither the coelomic metaplasia, nor the embryonic cell rests theory could explain such a clear-cut difference in frequency of distribution of ovarian and ureteral lesions between the two pelvic sites. On the contrary, in our study, adenomyotic disease of the retroperitoneal space, originating from metaplasia of Müllerian remnants, was obviously the cause of extrinsic ureteral endometriosis. It was proved by clinical examination and by histological serial sections.

In our series, all the patients had suffered from chronic pelvic pain, severe dysmenorrhea, or deep dyspareunia. We recommend clinically investigating the presence of a nodular adenomyotic lesion, either in the posterior vaginal fornix or the anterior vaginal fornix, in all patients suffering from chronic pelvic pain and/or severe dysmenorrhea or deep dyspareunia[10,11]. In cases of large (> 3 cm) rectovaginal adenomyotic nodules, IVP should be performed in all patients considered at risk of obstructive uropathy before proceeding with the laparoscopic procedure, including ureterolysis and removal of associated adenomyotic lesions, thus avoiding the risk of progressive hydronephrosis and silent loss of renal function. Indeed, surprisingly, only one patient complained of lumbalgia during the cycle or menstruation, leading us to suggest that ureteral stricture and stenosis are the consequence of very slightly progressive disease.

The management of ureteral endometriosis is controversial. Successful medical therapy (progestin or danazol) of ureteral obstruction secondary to pelvic endometriosis has been reported in the literature[16,17]. Conservative

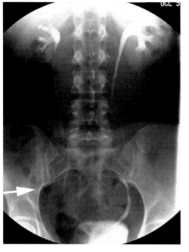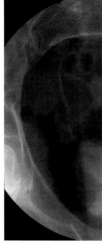

Figure 12 Postoperative (3 months) intravenous pyelogram (IVP) demonstrating an absence of ureteral stricture after ureterolysis

surgery with relief of ureteral obstruction and removal of adenomyosis or endometriosis should be the management of choice. In 1996, Nezhat and colleagues described a series of 17 cases of partial ureteral obstruction[6]. Laparoscopic ureterolysis was performed in ten women, but seven out of 17 women (41%) required partial wall resection. More recently, Nezhat and colleagues reported the laparoscopic vesicpsoas hitch for infiltrative ureteral endometriosis to obtain tension-free anastomosis to the bladder[18]. The case report described one case of 'recurrent ureteral endometriosis' after partial laparoscopic ureteral resection and ureteroneocystectomy. This approach should be considered only in cases of intrinsic ureteral endometriosis involving a long segment of the ureter, to avoid a laparotomy.

According to our results, conservative surgery should be proposed to the majority of patients. Indeed, we recommend performing laparoscopic ureterolysis and removal of the adenomyotic lesions responsible for the ureteral stenosis even in cases of moderate or severe pyelic dilatation. In the majority of cases, ureteral dissection, with or without uterine artery ligation, is sufficient to free the ureter. In all cases, ureterohydronephrosis was found to be decreased after this procedure. Resection of a part of the ureter should only be performed in exceptional cases. In our series, only one case required ureteral resection. Even when some part of the muscle was resected, the lumen was not entered in 13 out of 14 cases.

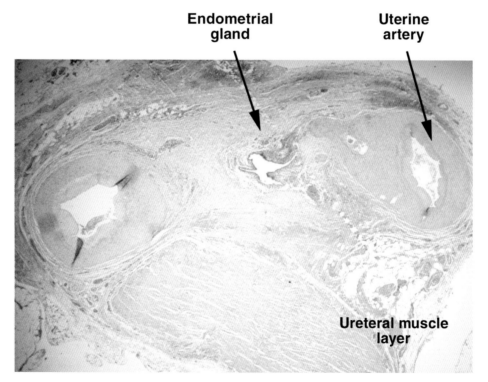

Figure 13 Histology of extrinsic endometriosis invading the ureter wall: adenomyotic-like lesion surrounding the uterine artery and the ureter wall

In cases of ureteral stenosis and pyelic dilatation, kidney scintigraphy (Tc99-DMSA) should be performed. If only a small part of functional kidney remains (scintigraphy less than 10–15%), a nephrectomy is usually recommended because of the lesser chance of recovery after surgery. However, if the kidney scintigraphy reveals that more than 15% of the renal parenchyma is functional, conservative treatment should be proposed. In our series, four patients who needed a kidney scintigraphy because of cortical atrophy, showed only a slight improvement in the kidney parenchymal function after ureterolysis.

In conclusion, obstructive uropathy is more frequently provoked by 'extrinsic' rather than 'intrinsic' endometriosis. The approximate ratio of four cases of extrinsic to one case of intrinsic disease, as previously described, has to be re-evaluated according to our study[6]. Obstructive uropathy should be suspected in patients with a rectovaginal adenomyotic nodule of more than 3 cm because of its high prevalence (11.2%). In this group of patients, there is a need to perform non-invasive urinary tract exploration to detect obstructive uropathy and prevent silent loss of renal function.

REFERENCES

1. Donnez J, Thomas K. Incidence of the luteinized unruptured follicle syndrome in fertile women and in women with endometriosis. *Eur J Obstet Gynecol Reprod Biol* 1982;14:187–90

2. Strathy JH, Molgaard GA, Coulam CB, *et al.* Endometriosis and infertility: a laparoscopic study of endometriosis among fertile and infertile women. *Fertil Steril* 1982;38:667–72

3. Haney AF. Endometriosis: pathogenesis and pathophysiology. In Wilson EA, ed. *Endometriosis*. New York: Alan R Liss, Inc., 1987:23–51

4. Nisolle M, Donnez J. Peritoneal endometriosis, ovarian endometriosis and adenomyotic nodules of the rectovaginal septum are three different entities. *Fertil Steril* 1997;68:585–96

5. Stillwell TJ, Kramer SAZ, Lee RA. Endometriosis of the ureter. *Urology* 1986;26:81–5

6. Nezhat C, Nezhat F, Nezhat C, *et al.* Urinary tract endometriosis treated by laparoscopy. *Fertil Steril* 1996;66:920–4

7. Donnez J, Brosens I. Definition of ureteral endometriosis? *Fertil Steril* 1997;68:178–9

8. Donnez J, Nisolle M, Casanas-Roux F. Endometriosis: rationale for surgery. In Donnez J, Nisolle M, eds. *An Atlas of Laser Operative Laparoscopy and Hysteroscopy*. Carnforth, UK: Parthenon Publishing, 1994:53–62

9. Clement PB. Disease of the peritoneum. In Kurman RJ, ed. *Blaustein's Pathology of the Female Genital Tract*. New York: Springer-Verlag, 1994:647–703

10. Donnez J, Nisolle M, Casanas-Roux F, *et al.* Rectovaginal septum endometriosis or adenomyosis: laparoscopic management in a series of 231 patients. *Hum Reprod* 1995;10:630–5

11. Donnez J, Nisolle M, Gillerot S, *et al.* Rectovaginal septum adenomyotic nodules: a series of 500 cases. *Br J Obstet Gynaecol* 1997;104:1014–18

12. Donnez J, Spada F, Squifflet J, *et al.* Bladder endometriosis or adenomyosis. *Fertil Steril* 2000;74:1175–81

13. Stanley Ke Jr, Utz DC, Dockerty MB. Clinically significant endometriosis of the urinary tract. *Surg Gynecol Obstet* 1965;120:491–502

14. Donnez J, Nisolle M, Casanas-Roux F, *et al.* Endometriosis: rationale for surgery. In Brosens I, Donnez J, eds. *The Current Status of Endometriosis and Management*. Carnforth, UK: Parthenon Publishing, 1993:385–95

15. Vercellini P, Pisacreta A, Pesole A, *et al.* Is ureteral endometriosis an asymmetric disease? *Br J Obstet Gynaecol* 2000;107:559–61

16. Gantt PA, Hunt JB, McDonough PG. Progestin reversal of ureteral endometriosis. *Obstet Gynecol* 1981;57:665–7

17. Rivlin ME, Krueger RP, Wiser WL. Danazol in the management of ureteral obstruction secondary to endometriosis. *Fertil Steril* 1985;44:274–6

18. Nezhat C, Nezhat F, Freiha F, *et al.* Laparoscopic vesicpsoas hitch for infiltrative ureteral endometriosis. *Fertil Steril* 1999;71:376–9

Bladder endometriosis or adenomyosis? Diagnosis and management

11

J. Donnez, M.F. Spada and M. Nisolle

INTRODUCTION

Although endometriosis is frequently encountered in females of reproductive age[1], bladder endometriosis is relatively rare, representing less than 1% of all endometriosis cases. One must take particular care, however, to define bladder endometriosis clearly as full-thickness detrusor lesions (Figure 1). Indeed, small implants and small nodules of the vesico-uterine fornix cannot be considered as bladder endometriosis. The condition was first described by Judd[2] in 1921 and a review of 200 cases was published in 1980[3]. In the literature, two distinct forms appear to exist: one is found in women without any medical history of uterine surgery (primary), the other develops after Cesarean section (iatrogenic or secondary)[4].

SYMPTOMS AND DIAGNOSIS

Prevalence

Between October 1982 and December 1999, 17 women aged 25–43 years underwent laparotomy or laparoscopy for bladder endometriosis. During the same period, more than 9200 patients were treated for endometriosis. The prevalence of this type of lesion is thus 0.2%.

It is important to underline that only full-thickness detrusor lesions (Figure 2) were taken into consideration and small subperitoneal nodules or implants of the anterior cul-de-sac were excluded.

Symptoms

In our study, nine patients presented with primary infertility (Table 1). In seven of them, endometriotic lesions (peritoneal and/or ovarian) were present. Four women had never been pregnant and had no desire to conceive. Four (23%) had undergone Cesarean section. One had suffered a spontaneous abortion and one had undergone a normal vaginal delivery.

The different symptoms that women suffering from bladder endometriosis (adenomyotic nodules) present with, beginning with the most frequent, are summarized in Table 2.

Thirteen women (76%) reported menstrual mictalgia and pollakiuria, mostly limited to the menstrual period. No germs could be isolated from the urine culture, even after several days. Dysmenorrhea and dyspareunia were experienced by 15 patients (88%). Only one (6%) reported gross

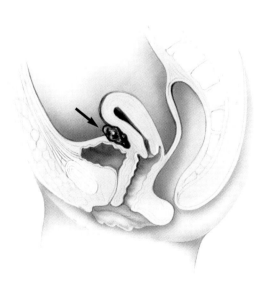

Figure 1 Bladder adenomyotic nodule: the nodule in the anterior fornix (arrow) strictly adherent to the bladder and the uterus

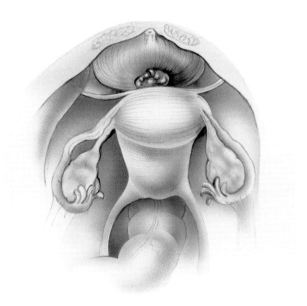

Figure 2 Schema of laparoscopic view: note the attraction of the round ligaments to the bladder nodule

Table 1 Clinical characteristics of the patients

Patient	Age (years)	Parity	Urinary symptoms during the menstrual period	Other symptoms	Size of bladder lesion (mean) (cm)	Other endometriotic localization
1	35	G1P1	mict, poll	dysmen, dyspar	3 × 3 (3)	–
2	40	G1P1	–	dysmen, dyspar	2 × 1 (1.5)	appendix peritoneal endometriosis
3	38	G2P2	mict, poll, hem	dysmen, dyspar	4 × 2 (3)	peritoneal endometriosis
4	28	G0P0	mict, poll	dysmen, dyspar	1.4 × 3 (2.2)	–
5	26	G1P0A1	mict, poll	dysmen, dyspar	3.5 × 2.3 (2.9)	–
6	25	G0P0	mict, poll	dysmen, dyspar	3 × 3 (3)	uterine sacral ligament rectovaginal adenomyotic nodule
7	29	G0P0	–	–	2.5 × 4 (3.2)	peritoneal, ovarian endometrioma
8	27	G0P0	mict, poll	–	2.1 × 2 (2)	–
9	43	G2P2	mict, poll, dysuria	dysmen	4 × 4 (4)	–
10	42	G2P2	–	dysmen, dyspar	2.9 × 1.3 (2.1)	rectovaginal adenomyotic nodule
11	26	G0P0	mict, poll, dysuria	dysmen, dyspar	4 × 2.5 (3.2)	rectovaginal adenomyotic nodule
12	27	G0P0	mict, poll, dysuria	dysmen, dyspar	3 × 3 (3)	rectovaginal adenomyotic nodule, peritoneal, ovarian endometrioma
13	27	G0P0	mict, poll	dysmen, dyspar	4.2 × 4 (4)	rectovaginal adenomyotic nodule
14	30	G0P0	–	dysmen	3 × 2.8 (2.9)	ovarian endometrioma
15	27	G0P0	mict, poll	dysmen, dyspar	2 × 2 (2)	–
16	31	G0P0	mict, poll	dysmen, dyspar	4 × 4	rectovaginal adenomyotic nodule
17	27	G0P0	mict, poll	dysmen, dyspar	2.5 × 2.5 (2.5)	peritoneal ovarian endometrioma

Mict, mictalgia; poll, pollakiuria; dysmen, dysmenorrhea; dyspar, dyspareunia; hem, hematuria

hematuria during menstruation, which was confirmed by microscopic analysis that failed to determine hematuria in all other cases.

Diagnosis

The diagnosis of bladder endometriosis can often be made by vaginal examination (Table 3). In fact, in our series, a tender nodule could be palpated in the anterior fornix of the vagina in all cases. In all cases, abdominal ultrasonography confirmed the presence of a regular heterogeneous hypo-echogenic nodule of the uterovesical septum (Figure 3) and showed an association between the endometriotic nodule and the anterior uterine wall. In our series, one patient (6%) had a 1-cm nodule, five (29%) had 2–3-cm nodules, eight (47%) had 3-cm (± 0.2 cm) nodules and three (18%) had nodules of 4-cm maximum diameter.

Table 2 Clinical aspects

	Incidence (%)
Dysmenorrhea, dyspareunia	88
Recurrent cystitis in the perimenstrual period	76
Primary infertility	50
Menstrual hematuria	6

Cystoscopy was performed in all cases in the preoperative assessment. In all patients, a protruded mass of the posterior bladder wall was visible at the level of the fundus or the trigone. It showed a typical bluish or brownish nodule, but the vesical mucosa was only ulcerated in one

Table 3 Diagnosis

Vaginal examination	tender nodule in the anterior fornix
Abdominal echography	hyperechogenic nodule
Cystoscopy	protruded bluish mass of the posterior bladder wall with intact mucosa (ulceration, $n = 1/16$)
Intravenous pyelography	extravesical nodule
Magnetic resonance imaging	nodular mass in the anterior fornix adjacent to a normal uterus

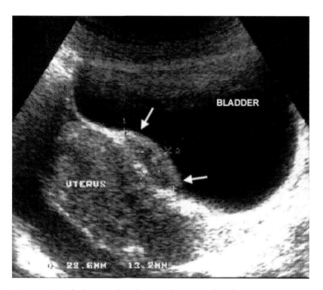

Figure 3 Abdominal echography: regular heterogeneous, hypo-echogenic nodule is clearly visible in the vesical muscularis protruding into the bladder cavity. In the majority of cases, there is no mucosal involvement

case (Figure 4a and b). This was in the patient who experienced menstrual hematuria.

Intravenous pyelography (IVP) demonstrated the typical aspect of an extravesical nodule in all cases, revealed by a filling defect (Figure 5a) in the upper part of the bladder. The vesical filling defect was more obvious on the profile picture (Figure 5b). In two cases, associated with rectovaginal adenomyotic nodules, the IVP revealed a stricture of the lower portion of the ureter 2–3 cm long with resulting moderate hydronephrosis. In these two cases, a JJ stent allowed laparoscopic ureterolysis, and was left in place for 3 months. After the JJ stent was removed, IVP demonstrated the absence of any ureteral stricture.

Magnetic resonance imaging (MRI) should be performed on all patients but, in our study, it was only performed on six. In these six patients, MRI excluded the presence of associated uterine adenomyosis and clearly revealed the presence of a nodular mass in the anterior

fornix adjacent to the uterine wall, provoking extensive compression of the posterior bladder wall (Figure 6).

Surgical technique

In the first 12 cases, the peritoneal cavity was entered by means of a suprapubic mini-laparotomy. The bladder, uterus, ovaries and peritoneum were checked for endometriotic lesions. If found, they were vaporized with the CO_2 laser (Sharplan, Tel Aviv, Israel). After dissecting the bladder from the surrounding tissue, we performed a small resection of the involved bladder wall using scissors. The vesical defect was closed in two layers, with separate submucosal stitches or a running suture of catgut 2-0 or Vicryl 2-0. To ensure the watertightness of the sutures, a solution of diluted methylene blue was injected through the vesical catheter. Bladder drainage was continued for 10 days postoperatively. Oral antibiotics were given during these 10 days to prevent bladder infection.

In the last five cases, prompted by our first anatomic analysis, which revealed an intact vesical mucosa, a laparoscopic extramucosal dissection was performed. In these cases, after classic transumbilical insufflation with a Verres needle, the peritoneal cavity was entered by means of one 12-mm umbilical trocar connected to a 12-mm laser laparoscope (Stortz, Tuttlingen, Germany) using a coupler system equipped with the Swiftlase (Sharplan, Model 757)[5]. Three other suprapubic trocars of 5 mm were also introduced.

The first step was to check the uterus, the pouch of Douglas and the peritoneum for other endometriotic lesions. If minimal peritoneal or ovarian endometriosis was found, it was immediately vaporized. When associated with many other ovarian lesions (cysts more than 3 cm in size; $n = 4$; 23%), medical therapy (3 months of gonadotropin releasing hormone agonist (GnRH-a) therapy; Zoladex, Zeneca, Cambridge, UK) was given after drainage of the ovarian cyst, as described in a previous chapter[1,6], followed by surgical treatment, including ovarian cyst wall vaporization and segmental bladder resection, carried out either by laparotomy or laparoscopy. In seven cases (41%), a rectovaginal adenomyotic nodule

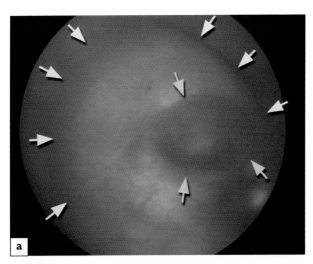
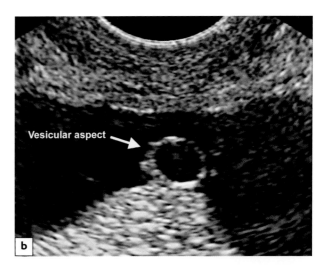

Figure 4 (a) Cystoscopy: protruding bluish vesicular nodule is clearly visible in the posterior bladder wall with an intact vesical mucosa. (b) In this case, the nodule is clearly visible in the bladder muscularis, but, in the bladder, a vesicle was detected on the bladder mucosa

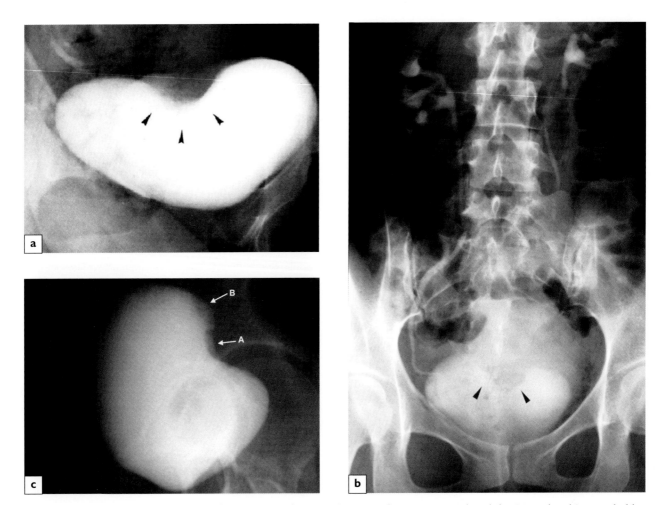

Figure 5 (a) Intravenous pyelography demonstrates the typical aspect of an 'extravesical nodule' (arrowheads), revealed by a filling defect. (b) Note the absence of ureterohydronephrosis. (c) Profile image: the bladder filling defect due to the nodule (A) must be distinguished from the normal filling defect due to an anteflexed uterus (B)

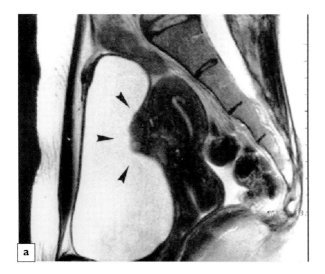

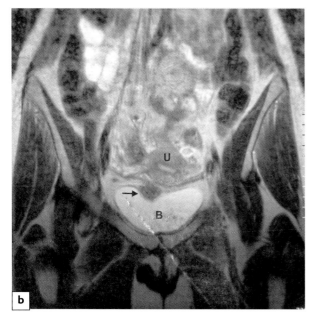

Figure 6 Magnetic resonance imaging shows a nodular mass in the anterior fornix adjacent to the uterine wall (arrowheads), causing extensive compression of the posterior bladder wall (note the absence of concomitant uterine adenomyosis). (a) Sagittal image; (b) transverse image

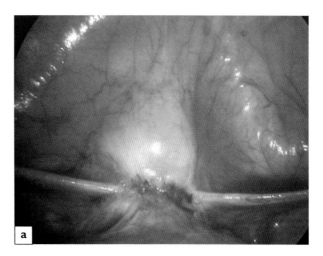

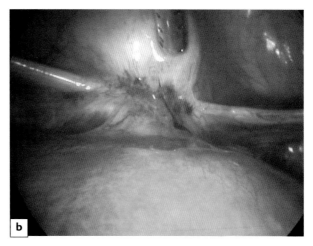

Figure 7 (a) First laparoscopic view of the bladder adenomyotic nodule; (b) first step of the dissection with the help of the CO_2 laser *(continued on next page)*

was found to be associated. In these seven cases, the rectovaginal adenomyotic nodule was removed and the associated peritoneal and/or ovarian lesions were vaporized in the first laparoscopy.

The second step was to check the vesico-uterine fornix to confirm the presence of the bladder adenomyotic nodule by retroflecting the uterus with a uterine cannula (Figure 7a). Grasping forceps were then introduced through the suprapubic trocars to expose the lesion correctly for dissection with the CO_2 laser (Figure 7b).

Deep nodular lesions involving the vesical muscularis required excision of the nodular tissue from the anterior uterine wall. Attention was first directed towards achieving

complete dissection of the uterine wall throughout its area of attachment or involvement until the loose tissue of the vesical space was reached (Figure 7c).

This could be done by cutting this area of attachment with the CO_2 laser while the uterus was retroflexed and the bladder was pulled up by grasping forceps. The peritoneum covering the bladder was opened. By gentle traction, the plane of dissection between the fibrotic nodular tissue and the normal vesical muscularis was exposed, and resection of the nodule was easily carried out, taking care not to enter the bladder and staying far away from the ureteral insertions (Figure 7d and e).

In these five cases, extramucosal dissection was successfully carried out (Figure 7f).

At the end of surgery, the vesical muscularis was closed with two or three (Vicryl-0) stitches depending on the size of the muscularis defect. Either separate stitches or a running suture were performed (Figure 7g and h). Finally, a diluted methylene blue solution was injected to ensure the watertightness of the sutures.

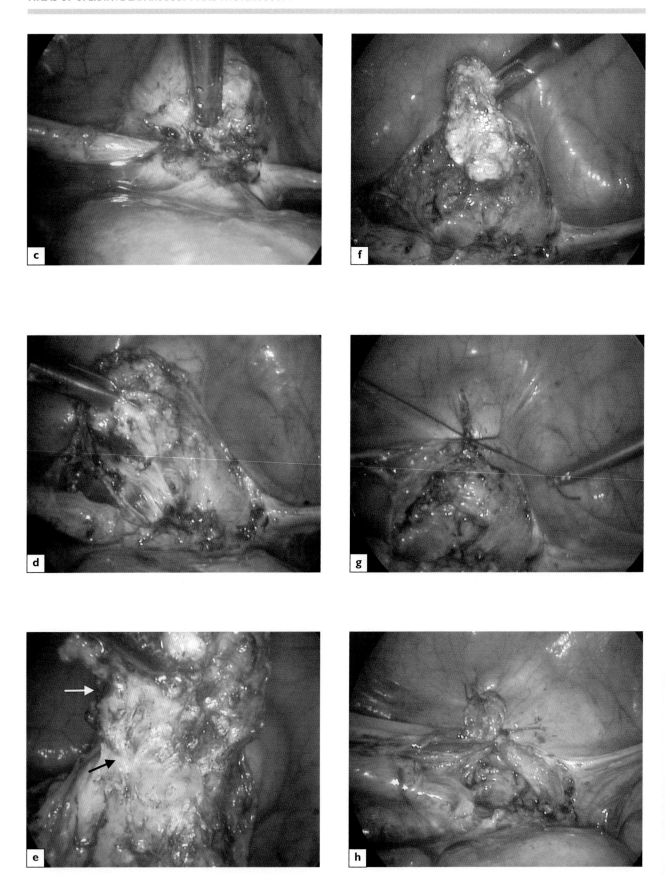

Figure 7 *Continued* (c) CO_2 laser dissection of the nodule from the uterine wall; (d) grasping forceps for dissection from the intact bladder muscularis; (e) the nodule (white arrow) is nearly dissected from the intact mucosa (black arrow); (f) complete extramucosal excision of the nodule; the bladder has not been entered; (g) extramucosal vesical suture by separate or continuous stitches of Vicryl 2-0; (h) closure of the muscularis defect

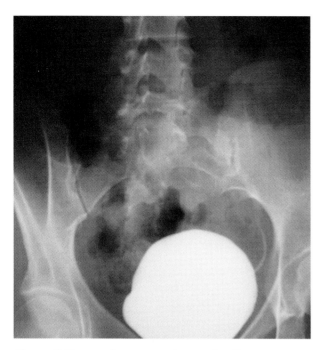

Figure 8 Retrograde cystography on day 9; no urine or contrast medium leakage is visible

In some cases, a control cystoscopy was carried out to check the intact bladder mucosa. In all cases, retrograde cystography was performed 10 days postoperatively to confirm the complete recovery of the bladder wall and to exclude any liquid leakage (Figure 8).

Histology

After surgery, the resected lesion was sent to the pathologist. Serial sections were obtained and colored by hematoxylin–eosin or analyzed to evaluate the steroid receptor (estrogen and progestogen receptors) content according to a previously described method[7]. On microscopic examination (Figure 9), the lesion was characterized by the presence of scarce glands, with active endometrial-type epithelium and scanty stroma. No secretory changes were observed, even when the patient was under progestogen therapy or during the luteal phase. More than 90% of the lesion consisted of smooth muscle hyperplasia. The bladder nodule was localized throughout the whole thickness of the bladder wall. The vesical epithelium was intact in all cases but one. By serial section, we were able to demonstrate that endometrial glands were not connected to the peritoneal serosa and were almost in the subperitoneal space. Glands sometimes appeared dilated and lined with flattened cells. However, in most of them, the epithelium was represented by a single layer of cylindrical cells with very weak mitotic activity and without any typical progesterone-induced changes. In smooth muscle, estrogen and progestogen receptors were systematically present in more than 40% of the cells.

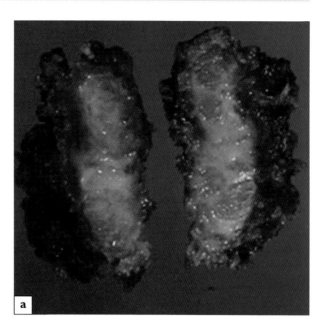

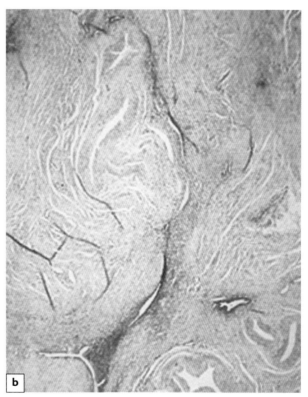

Figure 9 Vesical adenomyosis: (a) 90% of the lesion consisted of smooth muscle hyperplasia; (b) scarce glands with active endometrial-type epithelium and scanty stroma were visible

The first 12 cases now have a follow-up ranging from 2 to 18 years. No recurrence has been observed. In one case, a second-look laparoscopy was performed 3 months after the surgical procedure. Cystoscopy and laparoscopy (Figure 10a and b) confirmed complete healing without fibrosis or adhesions.

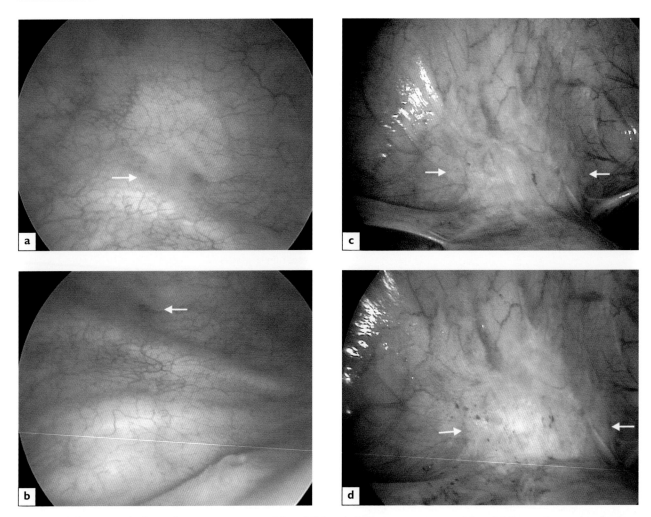

Figure 10 Three months later: the cystoscopy view (a) and (b) and the laparoscopic view (c) and (d) reveal complete healing of the bladder after resection of an adenomyotic vesical nodule. (a) and (b) Cystoscopic view: absence of intravesical lesion (the ureteral ostium is clearly visible); (c) and (d) laparoscopic view: complete healing of the bladder and vesico-uterine space

RESULTS AND DISCUSSION

Several authors have recently described two types of bladder endometriosis, the first occurring in women who have not previously undergone any uterine surgery (primary) and the second following Cesarean section (iatrogenic or secondary)[8,9].

In this study, we report 17 cases of bladder endometriosis. Among the 17 patients, 13 (77%) presented with primary bladder lesions and the other four (23%) had secondary bladder endometriosis.

Koninckx and Martin[10] suggested that extraperitoneal endometriosis derives from endoperitoneal disease. Vercellini and colleagues[8] later proposed this theory to explain bladder endometriosis. In their opinion, peritoneal lesions are able to penetrate under the peritoneum and develop into deep-infiltrating endometriosis. If this were the case, we would have found peritoneal endometriosis in all cases. In our series, six patients (35%) had no associated endometriotic lesions. Moreover, six cases (35%) were associated with rectovaginal adenomyotic nodules, which we clearly described as a distinct retroperitoneal entity[1,11]. Indeed, the rectovaginal septum nodule was described, like the adenomyoma, as a circumscribed nodular aggregate of smooth muscle and endometrial glands, surrounded by scanty stroma. As in the 'uterine adenomyoma'[12] and in rectovaginal adenomyotic nodules[1,11], secretory changes were absent in 'adenomyotic' bladder nodules. Sometimes, there was invasion of the muscle by very active glandular epithelium without stroma, which proved that stroma is not mandatory for invasion in this particular type of pathology. We have previously suggested that the recto-vaginal nodule may be the consequence of the metaplasia of Müllerian remnants. Not surprisingly, the bladder nodule was exactly the same as the rectovaginal nodule when viewed microscopically.

Not only the frequent association, but also the similar histological findings observed in our study, strongly lead us to propose that bladder endometriosis is actually bladder adenomyosis, and also the consequence of metaplasia of

Müllerian remnants, which can be found in the recto-vaginal septum as well as the vesicovaginal septum[1] (Figure 11).

Moreover, the invasion of smooth muscle fibers by active glandular epithelium without stroma proves that in the vesical nodule, as well as the rectovaginal nodule, stroma is not mandatory for invasion; the bladder nodule is thus different from peritoneal endometriosis, in which epithelial glands are surrounded by endometrial-type stroma. These metaplastic changes of Müllerian rests into endometriotic glands involving the uterovesical septum are responsible for the striking proliferation of smooth muscle, creating an adenomyomatous appearance similar to that of uterine adenomyosis and the rectovaginal adenomyotic nodule.

One of the hypotheses advanced by Fedele and colleagues[4], claiming that detrusor endometriosis could result from the extension of adenomyotic lesions from the anterior uterine wall to the bladder, is not supported by our study. Indeed, although the adenomyotic vesical nodule was systematically found to be adherent to the uterine wall, no adenomyotic nodules of the anterior uterine wall were found. These data, observed at surgery,

were corroborated by the absence of uterine adenomyosis at echography and MRI, when available.

Moreover, on histological examination, we noted that there was no continuity between the endometrial glands and the mesothelium, proving that the bladder nodule is a retroperitoneal disease. A further argument to support this view is the intact vesical mucosa observed in 94% of cases.

Concerning the therapy, although medical therapy has proven effective in relieving symptoms, the quick recurrence of irritative urinary symptoms after cessation of therapy indicates that surgery is required. So far in the literature, partial cystectomy (or segmental bladder resection) has been considered the treatment of choice[9,13,14]. Subsequent to our histological findings, extramucosal resection of bladder adenomyosis must be seriously considered. Indeed, the vesical mucosa was intact, as proven by serial histological sections, and did not need to be resected. This is why we proposed extramucosal bladder resection of the adenomyotic nodule in the last five cases.

In conclusion, so-called primary bladder endometriosis must be considered as a retroperitoneal adenomyotic nodule which is the consequence of metaplasia of Müllerian rests and which can be resected using an extra-mucosal laparoscopic approach[15].

REFERENCES

1. Nisolle M, Donnez J. Peritoneal endometriosis, ovarian endometriosis and adenomyotic nodules of the rectovaginal septum are three different entities. *Fertil Steril* 1997;68:585–96
2. Judd ES. Adenomyomata presenting as a tumor of the bladder. *Surg Clin North Am* 1921;1:1271–8
3. Fianu S, Ingelman-Sundberg A, Nasiell K, *et al.* Surgical treatment of post abortum endometriosis of the bladder and postoperative bladder function. *Scand J Urol Nephrol* 1980;14:151–5
4. Fedele L, Piazzola E, Raffaeli R, *et al.* Bladder endometriosis: deep infiltrating endometriosis or adenomyosis? *Fertil Steril* 1998;69:972–5
5. Donnez J, Nisolle M, Anaf V, *et al.* Endoscopic management of peritoneal and ovarian endometriosis. In Donnez J, Nisolle M, eds. *An Atlas of Laser Operative Laparoscopy and Hysteroscopy.* Carnforth, UK: Parthenon Publishing, 1994:63–74
6. Donnez J, Nisolle M, Gillerot S, *et al.* Ovarian endometrial cysts: the role of gonadotropin-releasing hormone agonist and/or drainage. *Fertil Steril* 1994;62:63–6
7. Nisolle M, Casanas-Roux F, Wyns Ch, *et al.* Immunohistochemical analysis of estrogen and progesterone receptors in endometrium and peritoneal endometriosis: a new quantitive method. *Fertil Steril* 1994;62:751–9

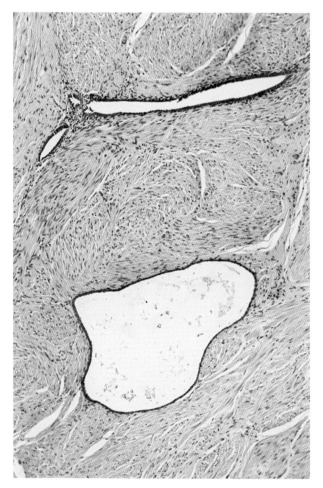

Figure 11 Histology reveals the presence of a flattened epithelium typical of Müllerian remnants which are present in the adenomyotic vesical nodule

8. Vercellini P, Meschia M, De Giorgi O, *et al*. Bladder detrusor endometriosis: clinical and pathogenetic implication. *J Urol* 1996;155:84–6

9. Brosens IA, Puttemans P, Deprest J, *et al*. The endometriosis cycle and its derailments. *Hum Reprod* 1994;9:770–1

10. Koninckx PR, Martin D. Deep endometriosis: a consequence of infiltration or retraction or possible adenomyosis externa. *Fertil Steril* 1992;85:924–8

11. Donnez J, Nisolle M, Smoes P, *et al*. Peritoneal endometriosis and 'endometriotic' nodules of the rectovaginal septum are two different entities. *Fertil Steril* 1996;66:362–8

12. Dubuisson JB, Chapron C, Aubriot FX, *et al*. Pregnancy after laparoscopic partial cystectomy for bladder endometriosis. *Hum Reprod* 1994;9:730–2

13. Zaloudek C, Norris HJ. Mesenchymal tumors of the uterus. In Kurman R, ed. *Blaustein's Pathology of the Female Genital Tract*. New York: Springer-Verlag, 1987:373–408

14. Nezhat C, Nehzat F. Laparoscopic segmental bladder resection for endometriosis: a report of two cases. *Obstet Gynecol* 1993;81:882–4

15. Donnez J, Spada F, Squifflet J, *et al*. Bladder endometriosis must be considered as bladder adenomyosis. *Fertil Steril* 2000;74:1175–81

The concept of retroperitoneal adenomyotic disease is born

12

J. Donnez, O. Donnez, J. Squifflet and M. Nisolle

The notion that peritoneal endometriosis, ovarian endometriosis and adenomyotic nodules of the recto-vaginal septum are three different entities was clearly demonstrated by Nisolle and Donnez in 1997[1]. In other words, peritoneal and ovarian endometriosis are diseases of the 'intraperitoneal' space but the adenomyotic recto-vaginal nodule is retroperitoneal disease. If we agree that the most widely accepted theory, the transplantation theory proposed by Sampson in 1927[2], can explain the pathogenesis of peritoneal endometriosis, there is strong evidence that the adenomyotic nodule is of extraperitoneal origin.

We now suggest that one should consider the retroperitoneal space as the origin of this adenomyotic disease, and banish the concept of deep-infiltrating endometriosis.

Back in 1922, Cullen described adenomyoma of the vaginal septum[3]. Because of the success of Sampson's theory[2], Cullen's theory was forgotten for decades. Even the concept of deep-infiltrating endometriosis described by Koninckx and Martin in 1992 could not explain the adenomyotic nodule[4].

On the other hand, the concept of metaplasia from Müllerian rests, suggested by Nisolle and Donnez in 1997 and strongly supported by biological and histological studies, appears to explain retroperitoneal adenomyosis[1].

ARGUMENTS IN FAVOR OF RETROPERITONEAL DISEASE

(1) The significantly greater increase in the prevalence of rectovaginal nodules when compared to the prevalence of peritoneal and ovarian endometriosis has remained stable for the last 10 years (Table 1).

(2) In 28% of cases, the rectovaginal adenomyotic nodule is not associated with peritoneal endometrio-

sis. In such cases, the hypothesis of deep invasion by a peritoneal lesion, with the subsequent formation of a retroperitoneal nodular lesion, is obsolete.

(3) The histological continuum between Müllerian remnants and glandular epithelium and stroma of adenomyotic lesions (Figure 1) proves the metaplasia theory of Müllerian remnants located in the retroperitoneal space.

(4) Similar histological observations made at the level of the rectovaginal adenomyotic nodule, which is, like an adenomyoma, a circumscribed nodular aggregate of smooth muscle (Figure 2), endometrial glands and, usually, endometrial stroma[5-7]. The similarity of histological descriptions of uterine adenomyosis and rectovaginal adenomyosis has led us to suggest that the so-called endometriotic nodule of the recto-vaginal septum is the same as an adenomyoma or adenomyotic nodule.

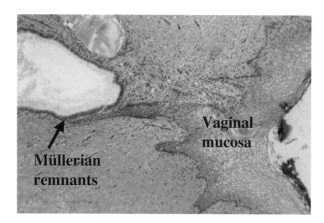

Figure 1 Histological continuum between Müllerian remnants and glandular epithelium and stroma of adeno-myotic lesions

Table 1 Increasing prevalence of adenomyotic nodules among the 'endometriosis' population

	1986–1993 8 years	1994–1996 4 years	1997–2000 4 years
Endometriosis	2214	1389	1513
Peritoneal and ovarian endometriosis	2116	1077	931
Adenomyotic nodules	98 (4.5%)	312 (22.4%)	582 (38.4%)

(5) Uterine adenomyosis exhibits a varied functional response to ovarian hormones. Proliferative glands and stroma are usually observed in the first half of the menstrual cycle. Adenomyosis may not respond to physiological levels of progesterone, and secretory changes are frequently absent or incomplete during the second half of the menstrual cycle.

(6) This lesion originates from the tissue of the recto-vaginal septum (Figure 2) and consists essentially of smooth muscle with active glandular epithelium and scanty stroma. The consistently observed prolifera-tion and fibrosis of smooth muscle are responsible for the nodular aspect of endometriosis located in the rectovaginal septum. The clinical diagnosis is made only when smooth muscle proliferation is sufficient to be felt on vaginal examination.

(7) Invasion of smooth muscle by active glandular epithelium without stroma (Figure 3) proves that the stroma is not mandatory for invasion and that the nodule is different from peritoneal endometriosis, in which epithelial glands are surrounded systemati-cally by endometrial-type stroma[8,9].

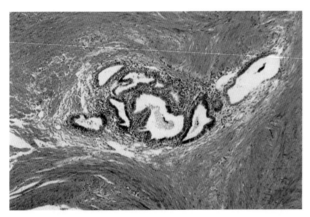

Figure 2 This lesion originates from the tissue of the recto-vaginal septum and consists essentially of smooth muscle with active glandular epithelium and scanty stroma

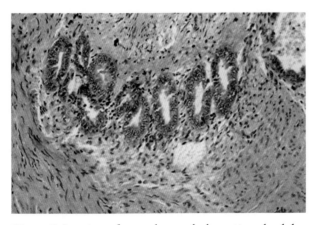

Figure 3 Invasion of smooth muscle by active glandular epithelium without stroma

(8) The co-expression of vimentin and cytokeratin in rectovaginal nodules indicates a close relationship with their mesodermal Müllerian origin[7–9] (Figure 4). The significantly lower vimentin expres-sion in the epithelium of nodules, compared to black lesions and eutopic endometrium, has led us to suggest, as we have for red peritoneal lesions, that low expression of vimentin can be related to a trend towards hyperplasia[7,10]. When endometriotic glands affect the rectovaginal septum, which contains smooth muscle, smooth muscle proliferation can take place and the nodule thus develops[11].

(9) Variations in the estrogen receptor (ER) and proges-terone receptor (PR) content of nodules throughout the cycle suggest that they are probably not regu-lated by steroids. In our study, the very low gland-ular epithelial and stromal ER content during the follicular phase can explain the absence of any secre-tory changes in the glandular epithelium of the nodule[7,8,12]. A recent study suggested that a low ER level was the key factor in explaining the out-of-phase endometrium despite normal progesterone levels, but the reduction in PR could also cause resis-tance to progesterone action and result in inadequate secretory transformation[13]. The absence of response to progesterone levels suggests that the different regulatory mechanisms of endometriotic steroid receptors result in deficient endocrine dependency or that the receptors are present but biologically inactive[14,15].

(10) The low mitotic activity observed in this pathology may account for the relatively slow evolution of the adenomyoma and the weak response to medical therapy, necessitating surgical excision[16,17].

(11) Hyperplasia of smooth muscle present in the septum provokes perivisceritis (Figure 5), visible at radiogra-phy, because of the inflammatory process and

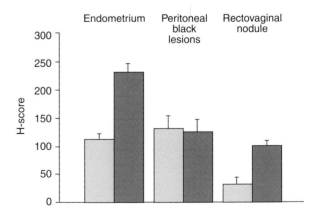

Figure 4 The lower vimentin expression in the epithelium of nodules compared to black lesions and ectopic endometrium

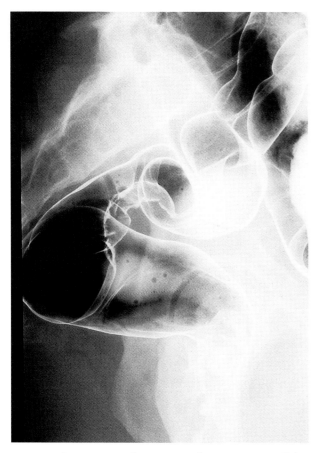

Figure 5 Perivisceritis due to secondary retraction of the rectal wall

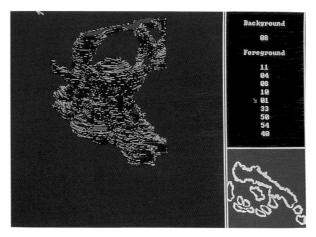

Figure 6 By three-dimensional evaluation, the reconstructed adenomyotic lesion has the appearance of a 'nodule' with multiple ramifications

secondary retraction of the rectal serosa. The absence of evolution of the rectal lesion after removal of the nodule supports our hypothesis concerning its purely rectovaginal septal origin[16,18].

(12) Three-dimensional evaluation reveals that a reconstructed lesion has the appearance of a nodular lesion with lateral and multiple ramifications (Figure 6).

In recent studies, we described the differences observed between peritoneal and nodular lesions and suggested that the nodule is not the consequence of deep-infiltrating endometriosis, but is the same as an adenomyotic nodule, which develops from Müllerian rests by metaplasia[7–9,18]. In rectovaginal nodules, the hyperplasia of the smooth muscle present in the septum provokes perivisceritis, visible at radiography, because of the inflammatory process and secondary retraction. This perivisceritis phenomenon is not an endometriotic rectal lesion or invasion of the rectal wall by the endometriotic process, as has been suggested by many investigators. In our opinion, it is only the consequence of serosal retraction caused by the inflammatory process and fibrosis on the anterior wall of the rectum. The absence of evolution of the rectal lesion after removal of the nodule supports our hypothesis concerning its rectovaginal septal origin, and strongly suggests that it is

not necessary to excise the anterior wall of the rectum in such circumstances.

IS THE ADENOMYOTIC NODULE LIMITED TO THE RECTOVAGINAL SPACE?

Müllerian rests are not only present in the rectovaginal space but also in the vesico-uterine space and in the cardinal ligaments[4,6].

Bladder endometriosis must also be considered as retroperitoneal disease. Indeed, in one of our recent studies, 35% of bladder adenomyosis cases had no associated peritoneal endometriotic lesions, but they were associated with rectovaginal adenomyosis in 45% of cases[19].

The theory that extraperitoneal endometriosis, such as bladder endometriosis, derives from endoperitoneal disease[3,20] can, therefore, not be proposed to explain bladder endometriosis. Indeed, the bladder adenomyotic nodule is also a circumscribed nodular aggregate of smooth muscle and endometrial glands surrounded by scanty stroma (Figure 7). As in the 'uterine adenomyoma'[21] and in recto-vaginal adenomyotic nodules[4,7], secretory changes are absent in 'adenomyotic' bladder nodules. Sometimes, we observed invasion of the muscle by very active glandular epithelium without stroma, which proved that stroma is not mandatory for invasion in this particular type of pathology. Not only the frequent association with adenomyotic rectovaginal nodules, but also the similar histological findings observed in our study[19], have led us to suggest strongly that bladder endometriosis is actually bladder adenomyosis and also the consequence of metaplasia of Müllerian remnants, which can be found in the rectovaginal septum as well as the vesicovaginal septum[4].

One of the hypotheses advanced by Fedele and colleagues[22], claiming that detrusor endometriosis could result from the extension of adenomyotic lesions from the

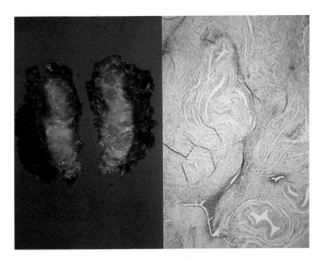

Figure 7 Bladder adenomyotic nodule

anterior uterine wall to the bladder, is not supported by our study[19]. Indeed, although the vesical adenomyotic nodule was systematically found to be adherent to the uterine wall, no adenomyotic nodules of the anterior uterine wall were found. These data, observed at surgery, were corroborated by the absence of uterine adenomyosis at vaginal echography and magentic resonance imaging[19].

Moreover, on histological examination, we noted that there was no continuity between the endometrial glands and the mesothelium, proving that the bladder nodule constitutes retroperitoneal disease. A further argument to support this view is the intact vesical mucosa observed in 94% of cases[19].

Side-wall endometriosis and ureteral endometriosis are the consequences of retroperitoneal adenomyotic disease.

The concept of adenomyosis of the retroperitoneal space should thus cover not only the rectovaginal space[19] and the vesicovaginal space[23] but also the area extending laterally in the direction of the cardinal ligaments. From our experience, we recommend clinically investigating the presence of a nodular adenomyotic lesion, either in the posterior vaginal fornix or the anterior vaginal fornix, in all patients suffering from chronic pelvic pain and/or severe dysmenorrhea or deep dyspareunia. In cases of recto-vaginal adenomyotic nodules or nodules developed more extensively laterally, and in cases of large uterosacral endometriotic nodules (> 2.5 cm), patients should system-atically undergo preoperative diagnosis of ureteral endometriosis. Lateral extension from the rectovaginal space to the side wall through the cardinal ligaments also happens in the retroperitoneal space, sometimes provoking ureteral stenosis, erroneously called ureteral endometriosis (Figure 8).

The notion that ureteral endometriosis is the compli-cation of lateral extension from a rectovaginal nodule has been discussed earlier (Chapter 10) in this review of gyne-cologic endoscopy devoted to retroperitoneal disease.

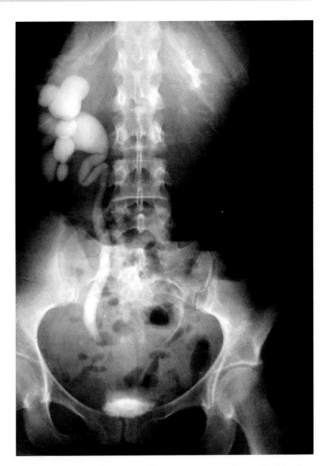

Figure 8 Ureteral stenosis (intravenous pyelography) is due to the lateral extension from the rectovaginal space to the side wall through the cardinal ligament

CONCLUSION

In conclusion, we strongly suggest considering the retroperitoneal space as the origin of this retroperitoneal adenomyotic disease and banishing the concept of deep-infiltrating endometriosis. The concept of 'retroperitoneal adenomyotic disease (RAD)' is born.

REFERENCES

1. Nisolle M, Donnez J. Peritoneal endometriosis, ovarian endometriosis, and adenomyotic nodules of the rectovaginal septum are three different entities. *Fertil Steril* 1997;68:585–96

2. Sampson J. Peritoneal endometriosis due to menstrual dissemination of endometrial tissue into the peritoneal cavity. *Am J Obstet Gynecol* 1927;14:422–69

3. Cullen TS. Adenomyoma of the rectovaginal septum. *J Am Med Assoc* 1916;67:401–6

4. Koninckx PR, Martin D. Deep endometriosis: a consequence of infiltration or retraction or possible adenomyosis externa? *Fertil Steril* 1992;58:924–8

5. Nakamura M, Katabuchi H, Toya TR, *et al.* Scanning electron microscopic and immunohistochemical studies of pelvic endometriosis. *Hum Reprod* 1993;8:2218–26

6. Donnez J, Nisolle M. L'endométriose péritonéale, le kyste endométriotique ovarien et le nodule de la lame rectovaginale sont trois pathologies différentes [éditorial]. *Réf Gynécol Obstét* 1995;3:121–3

7. Donnez J, Nisolle M, Smoes P, *et al.* Peritoneal endometriosis and 'endometriotic' nodules of the rectovaginal septum are two different entities. *Fertil Steril* 1996;66:362–8

8. Nisolle M. Peritoneal, ovarian and rectovaginal endometriosis are three distinct entities. [Thèse d'Agrégation de l'Enseignement Supérieur]. Louvain, Belgium: Université Catholique de Louvain, 1996

9. Nisolle J, Donnez J, eds. *Peritoneal, Ovarian and Rectovaginal Endometriosis: the Identification of Three Separate Diseases.* Carnforth, UK: Parthenon Publishing, 1996

10. Nakopoulou L, Minaretzia D, Tsionou C, *et al.* Value of immunohistochemical demonstration of several epithelial markers in hyperplasia and neoplastic endometrium. *Gynecol Oncol* 1990;37:346–53

11. Nisolle M, Casanas-Roux F, Donnez J. Peritoneal endometriosis, ovarian endometriosis and adenomyotic nodules of the rectovaginal septum: a different histopathogenesis? *Gynaecol Endosc* 1997;6:203–9

12. Haining RE, Cameron IT, Van Pajendorps C, *et al.* Epidermal growth factor in human endometrium: proliferative effects in culture and immunocytochemical localization in normal and endometriotic tissues. *Hum Reprod* 1991;6:1200–5

13. Hirama Y, Ochiai K. Estrogen and progesterone receptors of the out-phase endometrium in female infertile patients. *Fertil Steril* 1995;63:948–8

14. Laatikainen T, Andersson B, Karkkainen J, *et al.* Progestin receptor levels in endometriomas with delayed or incomplete changes. *Obstet Gynecol* 1983;62:595

15. Spirtos NY, Yurewicz EC, Moghissi KS, *et al.* Pseudocorpus luteum insufficiency: a study of cytosol progesterone receptors in human endometrium. *Obstet Gynecol* 1985;65:535–40

16. Donnez J, Nisolle M, Casanas-Roux F, *et al.* Rectovaginal septum endometriosis or adenomyosis: laparoscopic management in a series of 231 patients. *Hum Reprod* 1995;2:630–5

17. Donnez J, Nisolle M, Gillerot S, *et al.* Recto-vaginal septum adenomyotic nodule: a series of 500 cases. *Br J Obstet Gynaecol* 1997;104:1014–18

18. Donnez J, Nisolle M, Casanas-Roux F, *et al.* Stereometric evaluation of peritoneal endometriosis and endometriotic nodules of the rectovaginal septum. *Hum Reprod* 1995;11:224–8

19. Donnez J, Spada F, Squifflet J, *et al.* Bladder endometriosis must be considered as bladder adenomyosis. *Fertil Steril* 2000;74:1175–81

20. Vercellini P, Meschia M, De Giorgi O, *et al.* Bladder detrusor endometriosis: clinical and pathogenetic implication. *J Urol* 1996;155:84–6

21. Dubuisson JB, Chapron C. Pregnancy after laparoscopic partial cystectomy for bladder endometriosis. *Hum Reprod* 1994;9:730–2

22. Fedele L, Piazzola E, Raffaeli R, *et al.* Bladder endometriosis: deep infiltrating endometriosis or adenomyosis? *Fertil Steril* 1998;69:972–5

23. Stanley KE Jr, Utz DC, Dockerty MB. Clinically significant endometriosis of the urinary tract. *Surg Gynecol Obstet* 1965;120:491–502

Part 2
Tubal pathology and ovarian pathology

13

Fertiloscopy

A. Watrelot

INTRODUCTION

The diagnosis of the cause of infertility is not easy, especially when it is necessary to establish the status of the Fallopian tubes and the relationship between the tubes and the ovaries. Hysterosalpingography (HSG) is often performed for this purpose, but this examination is of value only when it shows complete tubal blockage. In other cases, the rate of false negatives, and even false positives, is very high, as shown by laparoscopy. Swart and co-workers[1], in a meta-analysis of HSG, found a point estimate of 0.65 for sensitivity and of 0.83 for specificity. They underline the fact that HSG was not suitable for the evaluation of peri-adnexal adhesions.

In contrast, laparoscopy is considered as the gold standard for exploring tubo-peritoneal infertility. Nevertheless, laparoscopy is very often performed without discovering any significant pathology.

Unfortunately, laparoscopy presents some risks which can be very serious, as recently shown in the French register of laparoscopic accidents, where six major injuries during diagnostic laparoscopies are recorded[2]. The results are either a delay in carrying out laparoscopy, which can be prejudicial to the patient, for instance if an *in vitro* fertilization (IVF) procedure is decided on the basis of a wrong diagnosis, or the conducting of a great number of normal laparoscopies, with the potential risks that accompany such procedures.

Other diagnostic procedures, such as hysterosonography or falloposcopy, are not sufficiently accurate to support a therapeutic strategy. Culdoscopy could have been an alternative method but was abandoned in the 1970s in its classical version in favor of laparoscopy.

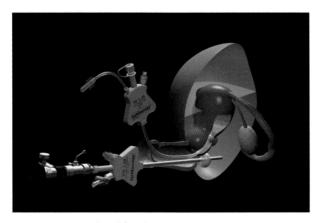

Figure 1 Principle of fertiloscopy

More recent improvements have been suggested, such as the use of dorsal decubitus[3], the use of hydroflotation[4], and transvaginal hydrolaparoscopy, which provides very good imaging of the pelvis[5].

Following this initial work, we have defined the concept of 'fertiloscopy'[6–8] as the combination, at the same time, of transvaginal hydropelviscopy, a dye test, a salpingoscopy, a microsalpingoscopy and, lastly, an hysteroscopy performed under strict local anesthesia (Figure 1).

TECHNIQUE

Instrumentation

Single-use introducers

Fertiloscopy uses specific instrumentation of single-use type. The other equipment is the same as that used for gynecological laparoscopy, even though a special scope is required in order to make use of all the possibilities given by fertiloscopy.

Specially designed introducers are the key to performing fertiloscopy. They are disposable. They come in a kit which is composed of two introducers, one for the uterine cavity, the other for the pouch of Douglas (Figure 2).

The uterine introducer (FH 1-29 Soprane, France) is fitted with a balloon to provide a good seal during the dye test. It also has a smooth mandrel to allow easy insertion into the uterine cavity. Once in place, the mandrel is removed and, due to the flexible nature of the introducer, it can be fixed to the patient's thigh using the Velcro provided.

The Douglas introducer (FTO 1-40 Soprane, France) has three channels. The central channel is fitted with a sharp mandrel for insertion into the pouch of Douglas. It is then replaced by the telescope. The second channel allows the balloon, located at the tip of the introducer, to be inflated. The balloon is of paramount importance: first, it prevents the introducer from slipping involuntarily out of the abdominal cavity; second, by pulling on the introducer, the pouch of Douglas can be stretched in order to have a better view of it; third, the balloon acts as a ball joint from which the telescope can be directed in every direction. The last lumen is an operative channel allowing the use of 5 French instrumentation as an outflow channel (Figure 3).

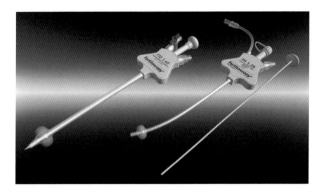

Figure 2 Fertiloscopy® introducers

Verres needle

A Verres needle is necessary and can either be disposable or reusable. The important point is to be sure that the safety mechanism works normally.

Fertiloscope

To practice fertiloscopy, it is necessary that the telescope has a diameter not greater than 4 mm and a 30° lens. In practice, the use of the Hamou II telescope (K. Storz, Germany) is strongly recommended for several reasons: its 2.9-mm diameter, the 30° for oblique vision and its 120 times magnification make it the only telescope capable of performing microsalpingoscopy (Figure 4).

Additional instrumentation

The Douglas introducer has an operative channel allowing the use of 5 French instrumentation. Biopsy forceps, grasping forceps and scissors are used (Figure 5a and b).

Bipolar coagulation (which is the only electrical option in saline medium) is also useful by means of electrode or bipolar forceps.

Lay-out of room

The patient has to be in a gynecological position. The Trendelenburg position is not required and a slight procubitus is even recommended. A monitor and cold light are installed on a mobile videocart located at the left side of the patient. Saline solution is provided on the right side through a standard infusion set-up.

Technique

The technique of fertiloscopy is simple. Nevertheless, it has to be very precise if problems are to be avoided.

Preparation of the patient

Preparation of the colon is useful in order to deflate the colon and thus to increase the safety space in the pouch of

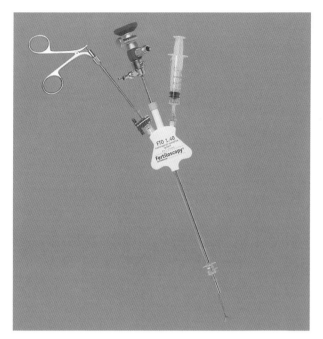

Figure 3 FTO 1-40 device with Hamou II telescope, syringe and grasping forceps

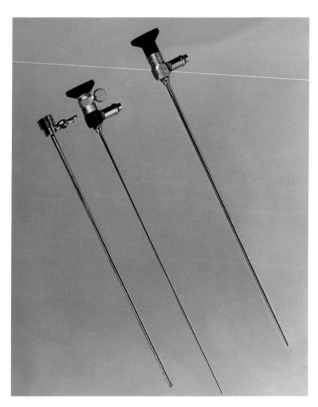

Figure 4 Hamou II telescope, with its sheath

Douglas. In practice, a mini-enema, such as Normacol®, is very useful.

A careful vaginal examination must be performed prior to fertiloscopy in order to detect any obstructive pathology of the pouch of Douglas, such as pelvic mass prolapsed in

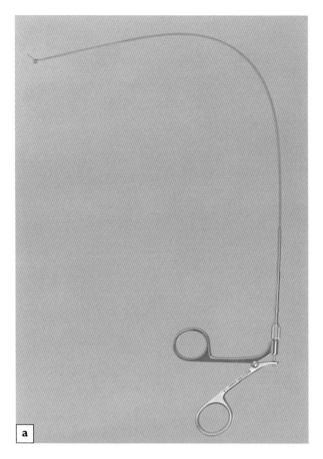

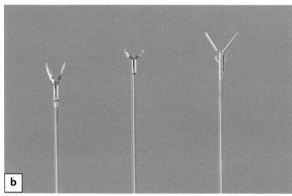

Figure 5 (a) Special atraumatic grasping forceps; (b) 5 French instrumentation; from left to right: scissors, biopsy forceps and grasping forceps

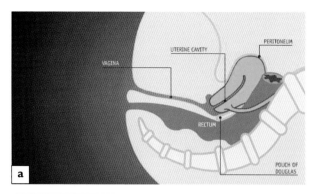

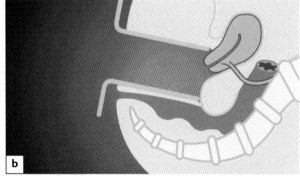

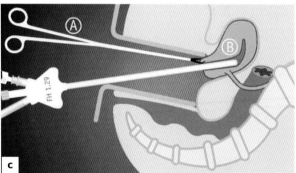

Figure 6 (a) Sagittal section of the pelvis; (b) exposition of the cervix; (c) a Pozzi forceps (A) is attached at 8 o'clock and a uterine introducer (B) is inserted (FH 1-29) *(continued on next page)*

the cul-de-sac, or endometriosis of the rectovaginal septa, which are contraindications to the technique (Figure 6).

Anesthesia

Fertiloscopy can be performed either under general anesthesia or under strict local anesthesia without any general sedation. We describe here the technique using local anesthesia: we start by inserting an anesthetic gel in the fornix (Emla®, Asta Medica). Ten minutes later, the local anesthesia can be induced, using Xylocaine® 1% without

epinephrine, without any painful sensation for the patient; 4–5 cm³ of Xylocaine are then injected in the vaginal vault, close to the uterosacral ligaments.

Introduction of the 'Uterine Fertiloscope®'

The cervix is first exposed by means of a Colin speculum, inserted deeply in the vagina, in order to expose the posterior cul-de-sac. It is important to use a Colin speculum, because it is the only one which can be removed while instruments are still in the vagina. A Pozzi tenaculum is fixed at 8 o'clock on the cervix. Then, the intrauterine balloon fertiloscope® (FH 1-29 Soprane, France) is inserted into the cervix. If needed, a gentle dilatation of the cervix is performed with Hegar dilators. Once in the uterine

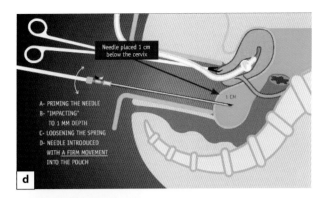
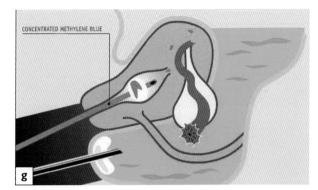
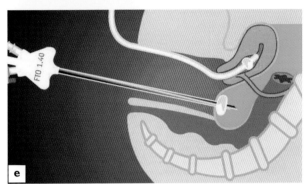
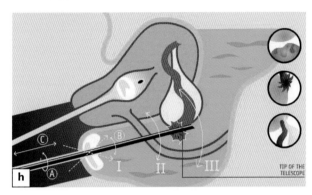
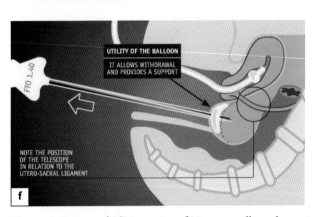
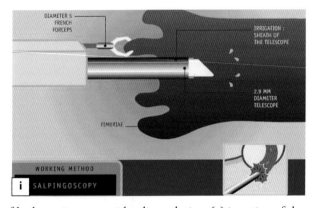

Figure 6 *Continued* (d) Insertion of Verres needle and creation of hydroperitoneum with saline solution; (e) insertion of the Douglas introducer (FT 1-40); (f) the fertiloscope is introduced; (g) dye test; (h) the three necessary movements for a complete view; (i) salpingoscopy

cavity, the mandrel is removed and the balloon is inflated with 2–3 cm³ of air.

It is important not to overinflate the balloon when the procedure is performed under local anesthesia because dilatation of the uterine cavity may be rather painful for the patient. The introducer is lastly attached to the patient's thigh, with the adhesive provided.

Hydroperitoneum

In order to create a safety space for the introduction of the Douglas fertiloscope®, a Verres needle is used.

The point of entry is located 5–10 mm below the cervix. To avoid the Verres needle sliding on the vaginal mucosa, it is necessary, at the start, to retract the safety

obturation while pushing the tip of the needle into the first millimeter of mucosa. Then, the safety mechanism is released and the Verres needle is inserted with a firm movement. The axis of penetration has to take into account the position of the uterus. In the case of a retroverted uterus, the axis has to be parallel to the inferior blade of the speculum. In the case of an anteverted uterus, the axis has to be horizontal. As during laparoscopy, the tactile sensation of transfixing the vaginal wall and the peritoneum is easily acquired with practice. Once in the right space, the tap of the Verres needle is opened and, therefore, the preheated (35–36°C) isotonic saline solution can penetrate freely into the pouch of Douglas. About 200 cm³ of saline solution are injected before the next step, which is the insertion of the Douglas introducer.

Introduction of the 'Douglas fertiloscope®'

The Douglas fertiloscope® (FTO 1-40 Soprane, France) is then inserted in the same place and along the same axis as the Verres needle, which is now removed. If the introducer is in the correct position, and after removing the mandrel, usually, some saline will flow out and, therefore, the balloon can now be inflated. If no liquid appears, it is better to check the position of the introducer through the scope. The visualization of the intraperitoneal structure allows inflation of the balloon at that time with 4–5 cm³ of air.

The telescope is introduced by unscrewing the valve located at the proximal end of the main channel and irrigation is continued through the sheath of the scope. Observation can now start.

Use of the operative channel

A red tap on the introducer closes the operative channel. When opened, it allows the passage of additional 5 French instrumentation. It is necessary to rotate the introducer until the red tap is located on the left side. In doing so, the operative channel will be above the main scope channel and, therefore, the instrument can be seen through the 30° lens of the telescope. The operative channel is also useful as a saline outflow channel. It is important when blood is present in the pouch of Douglas, to be able to rinse the cavity in order to increase the quality of vision.

Operative procedure

The view obtained is inverted in comparison with that obtained by laparoscopy. Therefore, some time is necessary to become familiar with the fertiloscopic view. However, the learning curve is short for any laparoscopic surgeon.

Exploration of the pelvis

As in many procedures, it is important to have a systematic method (Figure 7). The first element to find is the posterior part of the uterus. This is the roof of the explored

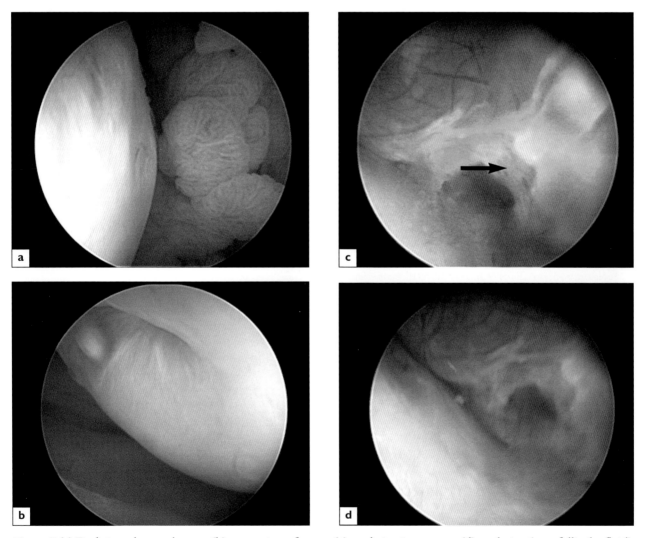

Figure 7 (a) Fimbria and normal ovary; (b) zoom view of ovary; (c) ovulation in progress; (d) ovulation (note follicular fluid) *(continued on next page)*

ATLAS OF OPERATIVE LAPAROSCOPY AND HYSTEROSCOPY

space. Then going alternately from one side to the other, it is possible to find the origins of the adnexae: the utero-ovarian ligament and the tubal isthmus. In following the utero-ovarian ligament, the ovary can be visualized, and every part of the ovary must be examined. The upper part of the ovary can be seen, with the 30° lens of the telescope,

by entering the space between the ovary and fossa ovarica and rotating the scope on its axis.

The tube can be followed from the isthmus to the ampulla and the fimbria. Due to the inverted vision, the tube appears to be located internally to the ovary, which can be disorientating at first.

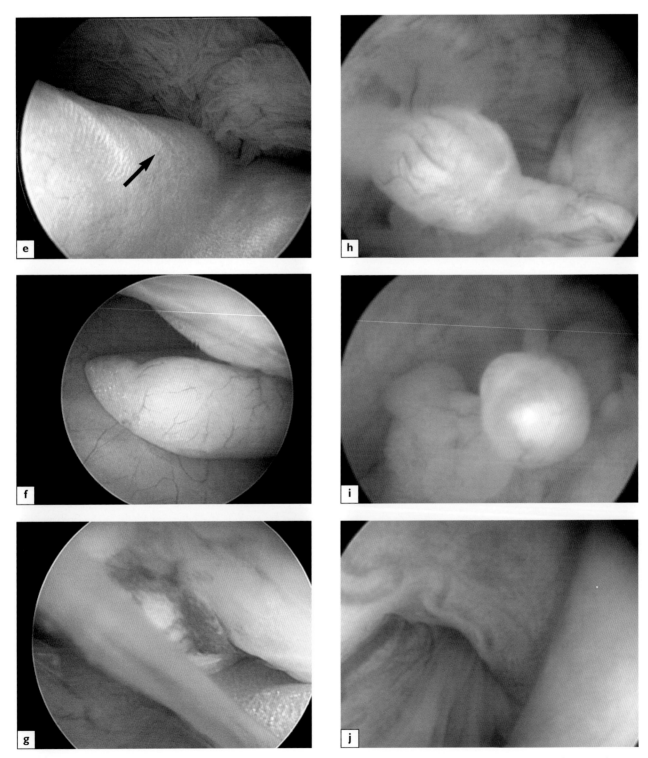

Figure 7 *Continued* (e) Right uterosacral ligament and fimbria; (f) appendix; (g) corpus luteum; (h) accessory tube; (i) paratubal cyst; (j) phimosis (under increased magnification)

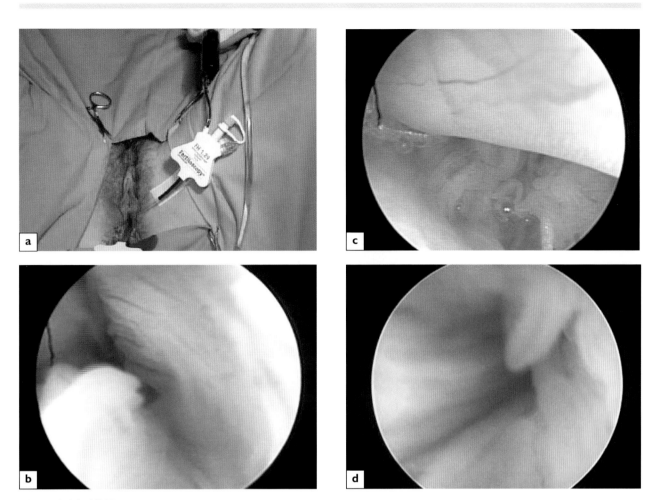

Figure 8 (a)–(d) Dye test

If the view of any structure is difficult, it is necessary to wait until more liquid has been instilled, which will improve the view. It is also necessary to move the telescope in all directions, not forgetting forward and backward motion.

The dye test

When all genital structures have been recognized, the dye test can be performed (Figure 8). The dye is instilled through the appropriate channel of the uterine introducer. A 20-cm³ syringe is connected and dye must be infused gently in order to avoid tubal spasms. The dye is seen at the fimbria and it is necessary to move from one side to the other to be sure of bilateral patency.

Salpingoscopy

Salpingoscopy is known as a very useful means of investigating the Fallopian tube[9]. Brosens and co-workers[10], for instance, clearly demonstrated the pathological results of intratubal adhesion. Brosens and Puttemans have described a salpingoscopic score which is useful for classifying the findings. Nevertheless, routine salpingoscopy is rarely performed during laparoscopy because it is necessary to

use a second telescope and an additional cold light source, video camera, monitor and irrigation. In contrast, salpingoscopy is very easily practiced during fertiloscopy with the same telescope due to the position of the fimbria and the use of a small telescope (Figure 9). The technique is simple; it consists of stabilizing the fimbria by means of grasping forceps introduced into the operative channel. Then, by pushing the telescope gently in the fimbria, it is possible to enter the ampulla and reach the isthmo-ampullary junction. During the whole procedure, it is necessary to irrigate the tube through the sheath of the telescope. A tap located on the sheath allows for in-flow adjustment to avoid pressure becoming too high in the ampulla. By rotating the telescope on its axis and due to the 30° lens, each portion of the ampulla can be examined. All pathological findings can be identified, such as intra-ampullary adhesions or flattened folds. These findings are of great importance when deciding whether surgical repair of a damaged tube is possible or whether IVF is a better option.

Microsalpingoscopy

As we have seen, salpingoscopy is of great value when a tube is blocked in discovering whether it can be repaired

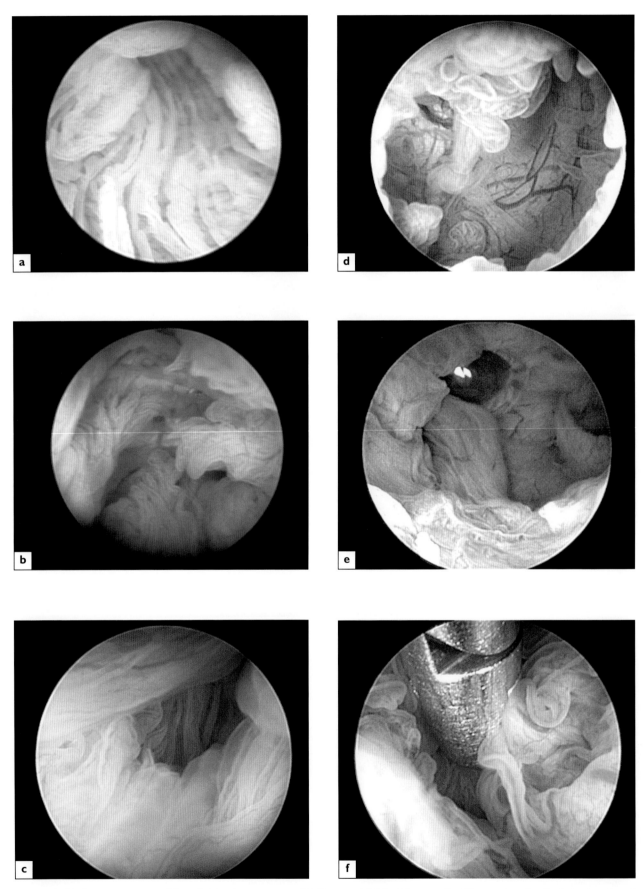

Figure 9 (a) Panoramic view; (b) and (c) salpingoscopy; (d) flattened folds; (e) ampulla; (f) grasping the fimbria *(continued on next page)*

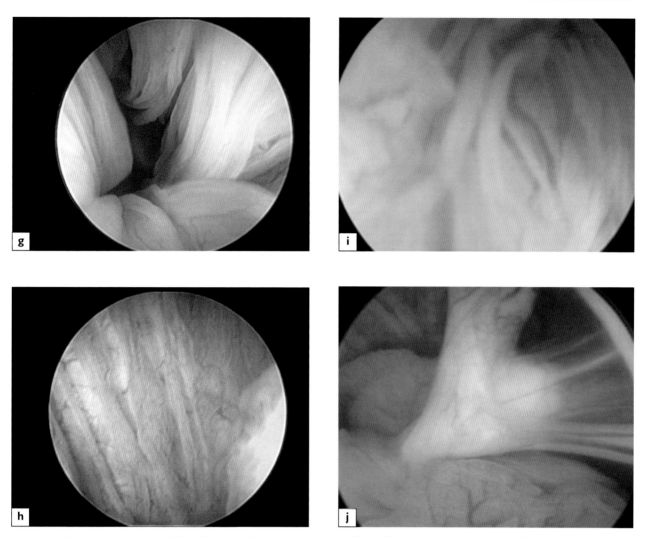

Figure 9 *Continued* (g) Major folds; (h) minor folds; (i) intra-ampullary adhesions; (j) intra-fimbrial adhesion

or not. More often, patent tubes are discovered at the time of fertiloscopy. In these cases, and according to the work of Marconi and Quintana[11], it is very interesting to have a more precise evaluation of the tubal epithelium. This can be obtained by performing microsalpingoscopy (Figure 10).

Microsalpingoscopy is possible thanks to the Hamou II telescope (K. Storz, Germany) which allows magnification up to × 180 by rotating the wheel near the eyepiece. Microsalpingoscopy is performed after the dye test. It is, therefore, possible to examine the number of dye-stained nuclei on the tubal epithelium, which are either intermediary cells on the epithelium or inflammatory cells (mastocytes) in the middle of the tubal folds. According to Marconi and Quintana, the number of dye-stained nuclei allows classification of the tubes into four stages, from normal (stage 1), where no nuclei are dye-stained, to pathological (stage 4), where a great number of cells appear to be dye-stained. This can be confirmed by taking a microbiopsy using the 5 French biopsy forceps available.

Hysteroscopy

Hysteroscopy is the last step of the procedure (Figure 11). It is practiced using the same scope. Endometrial biopsy is performed at this time if any pathology is suspected.

Operative fertiloscopy

Even if the main aim of fertiloscopy is diagnostic, operative fertiloscopy is a new challenge. At present, a few procedures are possible such as ovarian drilling, limited adhesiolysis and biopsy. All these procedures are performed thanks to the 5 French operative channel. They are, therefore, limited by the small diameter of the instrumentation (5 French has a diameter of 1.5 mm) and also by the fact that the instrumentation follows a co-axial approach without the triangulation obtained in laparoscopy.

Nevertheless, in the future, better adapted instrumentation will allow more operative procedures to be performed. Ovarian drilling is very easily performed during

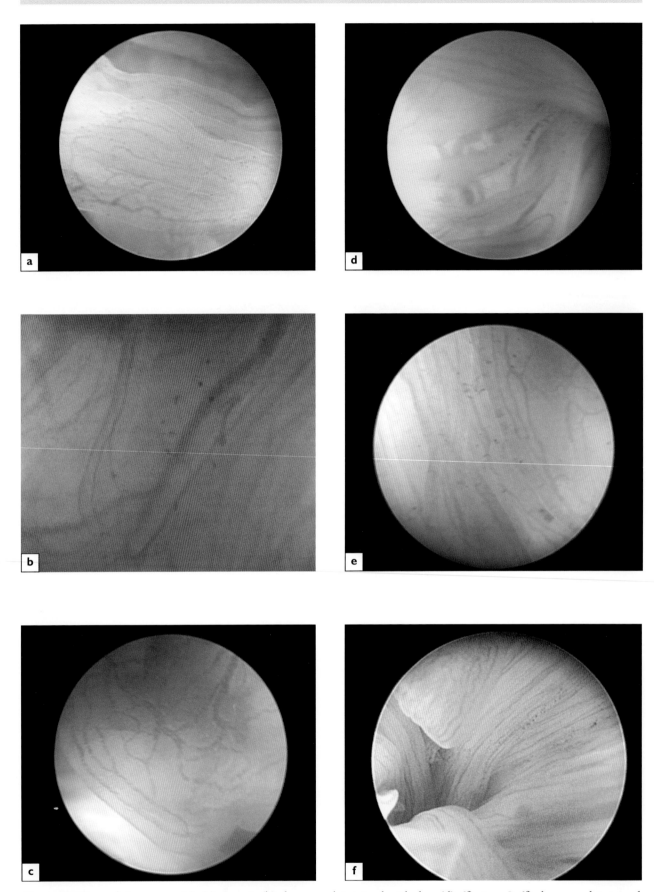

Figure 10 Microsalpingoscopy: (a)–(c) stage 1, (b) shows nuclei stained with dye; (d)–(f) stage 2, (f) shows nuclei stained with dye, these are sometimes visible in simple salpingoscopy without magnification *(continued on next page)*

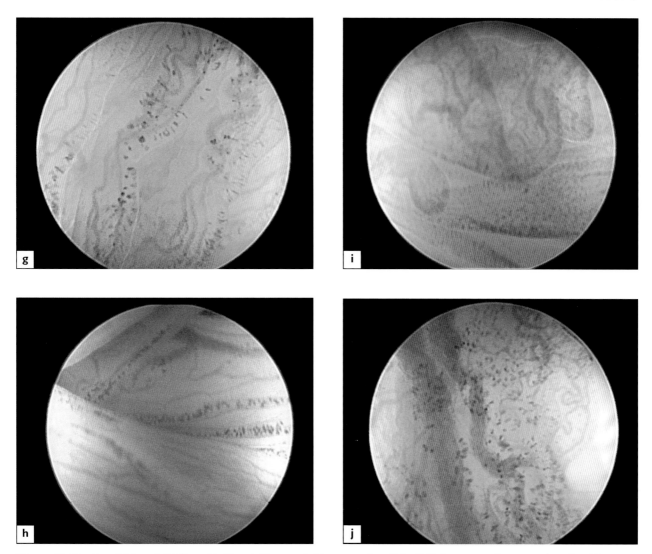

Figure 10 *Continued* (g) and (h) Stage 3; (i) and (j) stage 4, (i) every edge of the folds has many dye-stained nuclei; (j) masto-cytes (between the mucosal folds) and epithelial cells (on the fold edges) are dye-stained

fertiloscopy (Figure 12). Proposed by Fernandez and Alby, in the treatment of women with polycystic ovarian syndrome (PCOS)[12], after failure of clomiphene citrate, fertiloscopic drilling has proved to be as effective as laparoscopic drilling and in a very mini-invasive way. A 5 French bipolar probe is used, either disposable (Versapoint®, Gynecare, USA) or reusable (Ovadrill®, Erbé-Soprane, Germany/France). Ten to 15 holes are made on each ovary after visualization of the ovarian ligament, which is the landmark of a proper ovarian drilling. The operative procedure is very fast (less than 15 min) and is performed as an ambulatory procedure.

Biopsies are also performed. They are used in the tubes to correlate the microsalpingoscopic findings with the histologic results.

Adhesiolysis is also possible using the combination of bipolar probe and scissors (Figure 13). Of course, it is only possible when the adhesions are limited (i.e. when adhesions affect the tubo-ovarian area).

It is also possible to open closed tubes as in hydrosalpinx, not in order to treat the obturation but to enable salpingoscopy to be performed to select the best therapeutic option (salpingoplasty or salpingectomy and IVF). Lastly, treatment of minimal or mild endometriosis is possible but the numbers practised today are too limited to be sure of the effectiveness of such procedures.

End of the procedure

At the end of the procedure, the telescope is removed and the liquid can drain out freely. It is not important to remove all the saline instilled, because it is well known that the remaining saline will be reabsorbed over the following hours. No stitches are required on the vaginal scar.

The patient can be discharged immediately if fertiloscopy has been practiced under local anesthesia and in the following hours if general anesthesia was used. The only recommendation for the patient is to avoid sexual intercourse and the use of tampons for a period of 6 days.

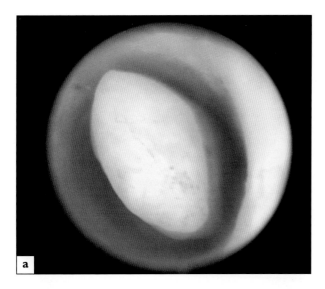

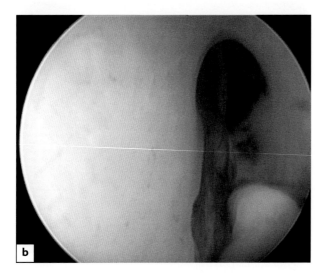

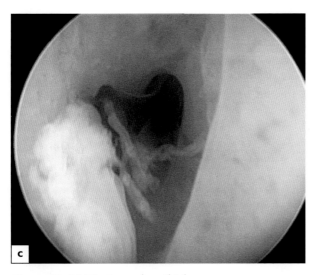

Figure 11 (a) Uterine polyp; (b) hysteroscopy – mucous plug in the tubal ostium; (c) hysteroscopy – the dye previously injected is not an obstacle to clear hysteroscopic vision

Contraindications

There is only one real contraindication: the obstruction of the pouch of Douglas either by a fixed retroverted uterus or by a myoma or an endometriosis of the rectovaginal septum. It is easy to detect an obstructive pathology of the pouch of Douglas either by ultrasonography or by a careful vaginal examination. Where there is any doubt, fertiloscopy must not be performed.

RESULTS

Between July 1997 and July 2000, we have performed 521 diagnostic fertiloscopies and 58 operative fertiloscopies. For the diagnostic fertiloscopies, we have divided our results into three periods. Between July 1997 and October 1997, a preliminary study of the first 21 cases assessed the value of fertiloscopy. For this purpose, fertiloscopy was coupled with a laparoscopy. Results show a very good correlation and, therefore, fertiloscopy was introduced on a routine scheme in our practice. At that time, we created the name of 'fertiloscopy'.

Between November 1997 and December 1998, we performed 268 fertiloscopies. The third period, between January 1999 and July 2000, was when microsalpingoscopy was systematically added and 211 fertiloscopies were achieved. Overall, we had 11 false routes where insertion of the scope was made under the peritoneum. These cases occurred mostly in the first two periods and we have observed no more false routes since the injection of local anesthetic has been performed not on the central line but laterally in the sacral ligaments. These events were probably due to a dissection created by injection between the peritoneum and the vaginal vault. Another means of preventing false routes was to insert the Verres needle firmly and to be sure that the flow of saline was spontaneous.

The only complications observed were two cases of rectal injury ($2/500 = 0.4\%$), easily recognized with the scope. In these two cases, due to a lack of experience, the contraindications had not been respected and insertion was attempted in a pathologic cul-de-sac. However, it is very important to note that the perforations took place at a site located beneath the peritoneum. The treatment of such an injury is conservative, needing only antibiotics for some days. Of course, everything must be done to avoid such problems, and strict respect of contraindications is the best means of prevention.

The characteristics of the patients are summarized in Table 1; this also shows that fertiloscopy findings appeared to be normal in 62.6% of cases. In 27 (8.2%) cases (Table 2), the salpingoscopy finding was abnormal, and the patients were referred for IVF for this reason. When microsalpingoscopy was performed (last period since January 1999, Table 3) it was considered as stage 3 or 4 of Marconi and Quintana[11] in 37% of cases. So these patients

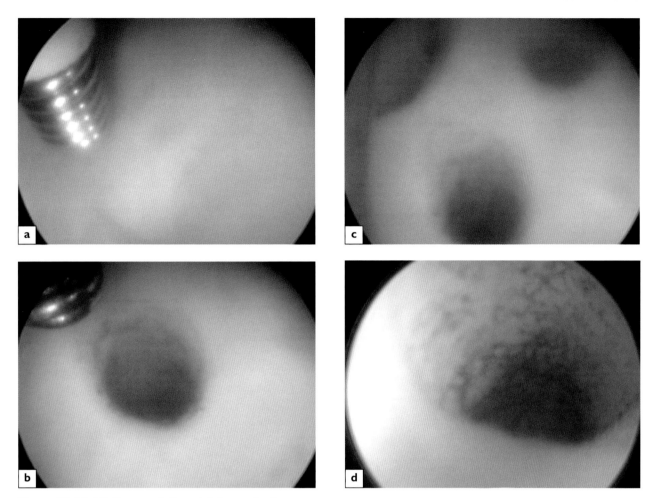

Figure 12 (a)–(d) Ovarian drilling, (a) shows the first step

Table 1 Global results of 500 fertiloscopies in women of mean age 33.3 years (range 22–42 years), whose mean duration of fertility was 4.1 years

	n	%
Primary infertility	358	71.6
Nulliparous	405	81.0
Failure	11	2.2
Complications	2	0.4
Normal fertiloscopy	313	62.6
Endometriosis	95	19.0
Post-PID lesions	79	15.8
Total	500	

PID, pelvic inflammatory disease

Table 2 Results of microsalpingoscopy procedures for the last two periods (n = 500)

	n	Normal	Abnormal
Phimosis	25 (5%)	12	17 (68%)
Hydrosalpinx	6 (1.2%)	1	5 (83%)
Adhesions	48 (9.5%)	15	33 (68%)
Endometriosis	95 (19%)	79	16 (16%)
No pathology	326 (65.2%)	299	27 (8.2%)
Total	500		98 (19.6%)

were directly referred for IVF. When microsalpingoscopy was normal, intrauterine insemination (IUI) was the chosen option.

Endometriosis was discovered in 19% of cases, and post-pelvic inflammatory disease lesions occurred in 15.8% of cases. Further laparoscopies were performed in cases of abnormalities, except in six cases where a micro-surgical anastomosis was performed for proximal tubal obstruction. It is interesting to notice that, in every case where pathology was found at the time of fertiloscopy, it was confirmed at the laparoscopy. Only some lesions located above the uterus were not correctly appreciated.

Fifty-eight operative fertiloscopies were also performed. In 41 cases, ovarian drilling was performed in cases of PCOS. Results are summarized in Table 4 and seem comparable to those obtained by laparoscopy if the

Table 3 Results of microsalpingoscopy procedures for the last period ($n = 211$)

	n	Stage 1–2	Stage 3–4
Phimosis	12	2	10
Hydrosalpinx	1	0	1
Adhesions	20	8	12
Endometriosis	38	33	5
No pathology	140	87	53 (37%)
Total	211	130	81 (38%)

Table 4 Results of fertiloscopic ovarian drilling ($n = 41$)

	n	%
Spontaneous ovulation	20	48.7
Ovulation with stimulation	9	21.9
Total ovulation	29	70.6
Pregnancy	13	31.0

length of the follow-up (between 3 and 6 months) is considered.

In 17 cases, tubo-ovarian adhesiolysis was performed. Five pregnancies occurred in the following 6 months, but the series is too short to conclude anything.

DISCUSSION

The concept of fertiloscopy was originally designed as a diagnostic tool for the infertile patient. We developed the name 'fertiloscopy' to indicate the global quality of this examination, which allows access to the uterine cavity (thanks to the hysteroscopy), the outside of the tube and the tuboperitoneal environment, and the inside of the tube (thanks to the salpingoscopy and microsalpingoscopy), all in the same procedure[6]. Therefore, fertiloscopy is an alternative to other existing diagnostic tools.

Classically, hysterosalpingography (HSG) has been performed and, in cases of abnormalities, diagnostic laparoscopy (lap and dye) is proposed. Nevertheless, the high rate of false negatives observed in HSG (up to 40%)[1] leads to many pathological situations, such as endometriosis and post-pelvic inflammatory disease lesions being missed. As a result, such patients are directed straight to IVF with the diagnosis of 'unexplained' infertility. Should their pathology be discovered, some of these patients could become pregnant without artificial reproductive techniques. Therefore, many surgeons propose performing a diagnostic laparoscopy systematically before IVF. However, due to the risks involved with this tech-

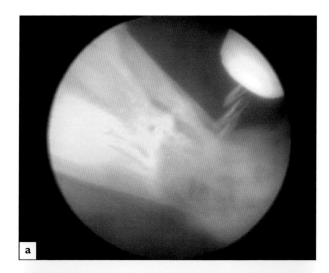

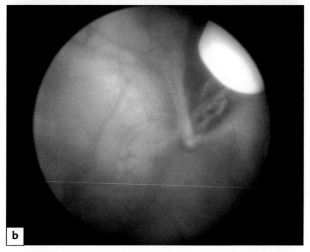

Figure 13 (a) and (b) Adhesiolysis *(continued on next page)*

nique, laparoscopy is practiced late in the infertility work-up. Some other teams, for the same reason, propose laparoscopy only in those cases where there is a strong suspicion of tubo-ovarian pathology. In contrast, due to its simplicity and ease, fertiloscopy under strict local anesthesia can be proposed very early in the diagnostic sequence.

Fertiloscopy, therefore, now replaces HSG and diagnostic laparoscopy. If tubal distal pathology or peritoneal disease is discovered, one has to decide what is the best therapeutic option, laparoscopic surgery or IVF. In these situations, we think that laparoscopy is mandatory because, when fertiloscopy is abnormal, it is not always possible to have a complete evaluation of the lesions, due to the limits of fertiloscopy, which gives a perfect view only of the pelvis and not of the whole abdominal cavity.

When the dye test is negative, one can expect a proximal pathology. In this situation, we perform HSG because this examination is pertinent for the interstitial parts of the tubes. If a blockage is observed, a tentative selective salpingographic desobstruction can be tried. If this fails, a microsurgical anastomosis is possible in the second step.

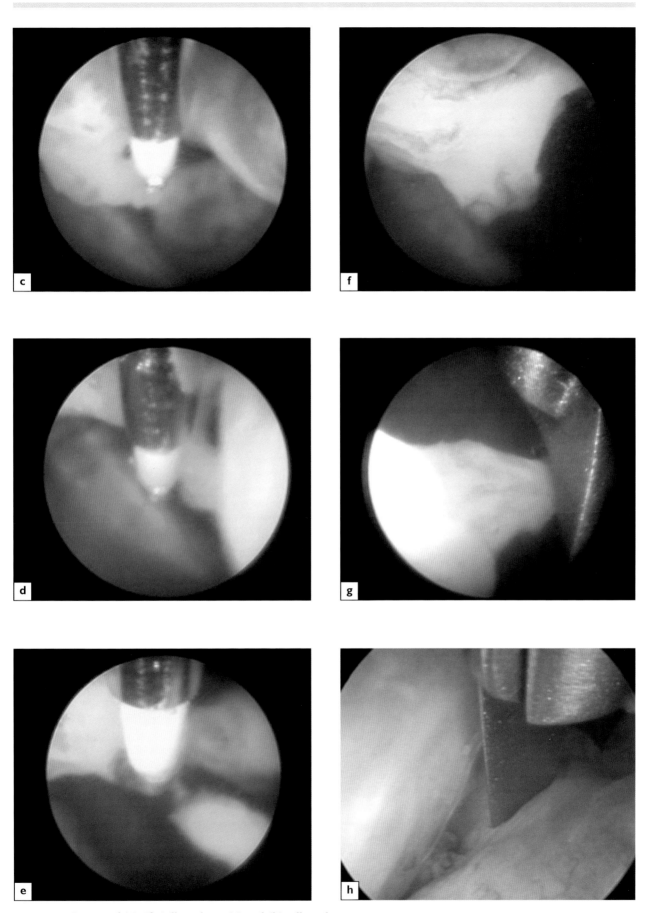

Figure 13 *Continued* (c)–(f) Adhesiolysis; (g) and (h) adhesiolysis using microscissors

In practice, the first explorations for infertile couples are semen analysis, evaluation of ovulation, echography and postcoital test. If everything is normal, we propose fertiloscopy. Thus, there is no delay in the recognition of tubo-ovarian or peritoneal disease. Of course, if a severe male problem is encountered, intracytoplasmic sperm injection will be required, and there is no necessity to practice fertiloscopy. In every other case, fertiloscopy appears to be a major element in deciding the therapeutic option.

The last development of diagnostic fertiloscopy is microsalpingoscopy, which allows a better evaluation of the tubal mucosa. It is interesting to notice that, in about 30% of cases, even if the tubal patency and the salpingoscopic findings are perfect, the microexamination of the tubal mucosa shows abnormalities (i.e. numerous dye-stained nuclei). The simplicity of tubal cannulation by fertiloscopy is probably one of the greatest advantages of the technique. The interest of salpingoscopy[9,10] and of microsalpingoscopy[11] have been clearly demonstrated. Due to the complexity of these technique during laparoscopy, they are very rarely practiced as a routine. In contrast, they are an integral part of fertiloscopy and allow a better evaluation of tubal function.

In cases of abnormal salpingoscopy, we are conducting a pilot study where patients with abnormal microsalpingoscopy are given antibiotics (Minocycline 100 mg daily for 2 months) to see if there is some kind of reversibility. A second-look fertiloscopy is then performed. First results show reversibility (i.e. normal microsalpingoscopy) in about 50% of cases in a short series. These results need to be confirmed in the future.

Concerning operative fertiloscopy, it represents a new challenge for this technique. Already ovarian drilling is possible, with results similar to those of laparoscopic drilling, but in a safe and mini-invasive way thanks to the Ovadrill® (Erbe-Soprane) developed for this indication. Adhesiolysis is also possible, but the aim of fertiloscopy is not to compete with operative laparoscopy, which will remain the only option for complex surgery. The operative channel of the fertiloscope is co-axial and limits the number of procedures possible.

Nevertheless, tubal sterilization by this route seems to have a real advantage if it is possible to perform it without increasing the diameter of the fertiloscope. Actually, prototypes of 5 French memory alloy bipolar forceps are currently being for this purpose and should be proposed in the near future.

REFERENCES

1. Swart P, Mol BW, Van Beurden M, *et al.* The accuracy of hysterosalpingography in the diagnosis of tubal pathology: a meta-analysis. *Fertil Steril* 1995;64: 486–91

2. Chapron C, Querleu D, Bruhat MA, *et al.* Surgical complications of diagnostic and operative gynaecologic laparoscopy: a series of 29,966 cases. *Hum Reprod* 1998;13:867–72

3. Mintz M. Actualisation de la culdoscopie transvaginale en décubitus dorsal. Un nouvel endoscope à vision directe muni d'une aiguille à ponction incorporée dans l'axe. *Contr Fertil Sex* 1987;15:401–4

4. Odent M. Hydrocolpotomie et hydroculdoscopie. *Nouv Press Med* 1973;2:187

5. Gordts S, Campo R, Rombauts L, *et al.* Transvaginal hydrolaparoscopy as an outpatient procedure for infertility investigation. *Hum Reprod* 1998;13: 99–103

6. Watrelot A, Gordts S, Andine JP, *et al.* Une nouvelle approche diagnostique: la Fertiloscopie. *Endomag* 1997;21:7–8

7. Watrelot A, Dreyfus JM, Andine JP. Fertiloscopy; first results (120 cases report). *Fertil Steril* 1998;70(Suppl):S-42

8. Watrelot A, Dreyfus JM, Andine JP. Evaluation of the performance of fertiloscopy in 160 consecutive infertile patients with no obvious pathology. *Hum Reprod* 1999;14:707–11

9. Surrey E. Microendoscopy of the human fallopian tube. *J Am Assoc Gynecol Lap* 1999;6,:383–90

10. Brosens I, Campo R, Gordts S. Office hydrolaparoscopy for the diagnosis of endometriosis and tubal infertility. *Curr Opin Obstet Gynecol* 1999;11: 371–7

11. Marconi G, Quintana R. Methylene blue dyeing of cellular nuclei during salpingoscopy, a new *in vivo* method to evaluate vitality of tubal epithelium. *Hum Reprod* 1998;13:3414–17

12. Fernandez H, Alby JD. De la culdoscopie à la fertiloscopie opératoire. *Endomag* 1999;21:5–6

CO$_2$ laser laparoscopic surgery: fimbrioplasty, salpingoneostomy and adhesiolysis

14

J. Donnez, M. Nisolle, J. Squifflet and M. Smets

New perspectives have emerged in the management of distal tubal occlusion from the tremendous advances gained in the field of assisted reproduction technology and in operative endoscopy techniques. With regard to surgery, it has been demonstrated on numerous occasions that classic microsurgery[1-3] and laparoscopic surgery[4-9] show comparable results in terms of pregnancy rates. There is no doubt that the crucial issue in the surgical management of distal tubal occlusion is the proper selection of the patient according to a set of strict criteria, which have a prognostic value in determining the chances of postoperative conception.

PHYSIOPATHOLOGY OF THE HYDROSALPINX

To understand the physiopathological events associated with the development of distal tubal occlusion, an experimental model has been created in the rabbit by ligating the uterotubal junction and the ampullofimbrial junction[10]. This model closely reproduces the natural clinical hydrosalpinx, observed in 10–15% of all infertile patients. The size of the experimental hydrosalpinx can reach up to 2 cm 6 months after the ligature. Morphologically, only the epithelium of the ampulla is affected by a significant deciliation process, which appears in the 2 months after the induction of the experimental hydrosalpinx; epithelial height is seen to be decreased and the stroma thickens because of submucosal edema and fibrosis. After 6 months, primary mucosal folds become scarce and atrophic, whereas secondary folds in the ampulla completely disappear (Figure 1).

Ampullary muscularis is typically invaded by fibrosis, and the size of the capillaries in the tubal wall is significantly decreased; this decrease in the ampullary vascularization probably explains the deciliation process. It should be pointed out that the muscularis layer also shares a role in the transportation of the fertilized egg, since intrauterine pregnancies have been described in Kartagener's syndrome[11].

In addition, there is a generalized adrenergic denervation of the tubal wall, this feature being more prominent on the isthmic portion than at the level of the ampulla where the innervation is minimal in the healthy tube[12]. All these lesions induced by the hydrosalpinx in the muscularis layer are permanent and explain the high failure rate associated with the surgical restoration of tubal patency. The increase in the fluid volume of the hydro-salpinx is probably the result of the depolymerization of the fluid components and a subsequent transudation from the underlying chorion. It could also result from a slowing down in secretion of fluid by the epithelial cells combined with the complete absence of drainage[10-12].

The experimental hydrosalpinx of the rabbit and the hydrosalpinx observed in infertile women have similar patterns: distension associated with the unfolding of the mucosal folds and the degeneration of the epithelial cells. As will be discussed later, the deciliation index investigated on fimbrial biopsies and the degree of dilatation are correlated, and both serve as physiopathological prognostic factors for the success of a salpingoneostomy; indeed, from hydrosalpinx specimens obtained at hysterectomy, it seems that the occurrence of dilatation of the tube results in the adrenergic denervation and fibrosis of the muscular layer, exactly in accordance with the observations made in the experimental model[10,11].

DIAGNOSIS OF THE HYDROSALPINX

The presence of hydrosalpinx can be diagnosed by hysterosalpingogram (Figure 2) or by laparoscopy with or without chromopertubation. A meta-analysis of all the studies comparing hysterosalpingography to the gold standard of laparoscopy with chromopertubation showed the hysterosalpingogram to have a sensitivity of 65% in the diagnosis of tubal obstruction and a specificity of 83%[13,14].

Transvaginal ultrasonography has also been used to evaluate pelvic structures. Normal Fallopian tubes can only be recognized in the presence of pelvic fluid. Transvaginal ultrasonography is very specific in the diagnosis of hydrosalpinx, but its sensitivity is poor[15]. Occasional longitudinal folds in the ampullary portion of the Fallopian tube can be seen[16] by transvaginal ultrasonography. A study by Atri and colleagues[15] evaluated the accuracy of endovaginal sonography in the detection of Fallopian tube blockage and found the specificity of transvaginal ultrasonography to be 100%, with a sensitivity of only 34%. Methods using the passage of air or fluid to visualize the tubes sonographically have also been described. The same principle makes sono-hysterosalpingography a useful tool in the diagnosis of hydrosalpinx[17-19]. Color Doppler ultrasonography has also been used in evaluating tubal patency and diagnosing hydrosalpinx[20,21]. Other diagnostic methods include salpingoscopy or falloscopy[22-24].

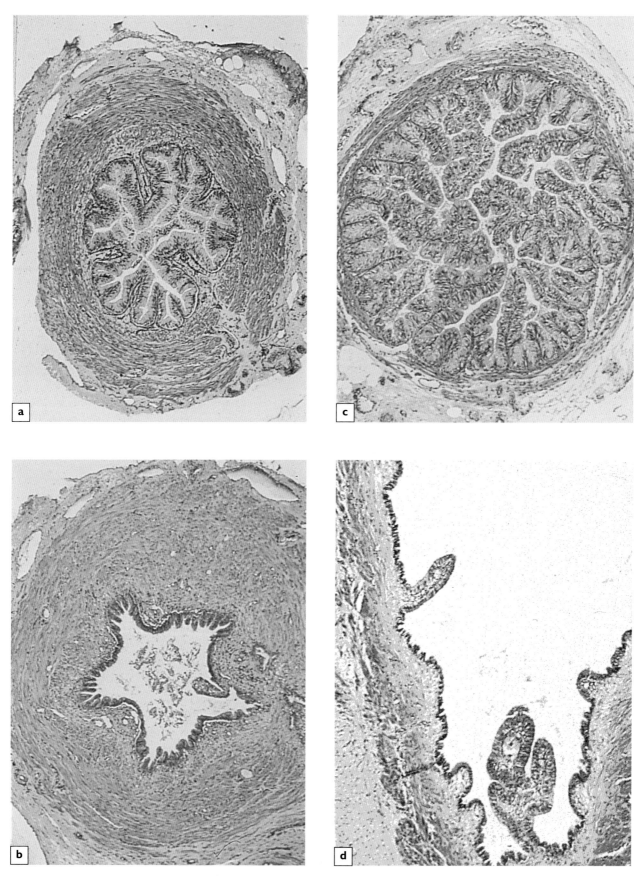

Figure 1 Experimental hydrosalpinx: (a) normal isthmus; (b) dilated isthmus after induction of experimental hydrosalpinx; (c) normal ampulla; (d) dilated ampulla after induction of experimental hydrosalpinx. Note reduction in number and in size of ampullary folds and flattened epithelium between the ampullary folds

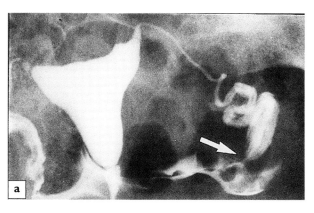
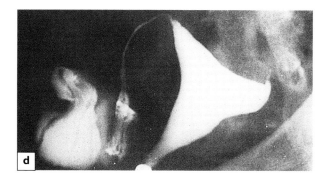
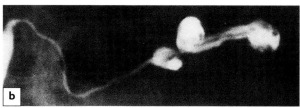
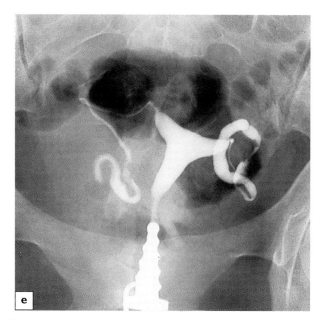
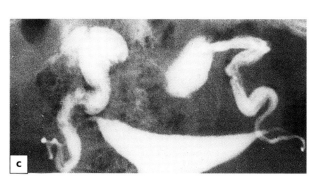

Figure 2 Classification of tubal occlusion according to our classification. (a) Degree I: phymotic ostium with preserved tubal patency; (b) degree II: total distal occlusion without ampullary dilatation; (c) degree III: ampullary dilatation < 2.5 cm, ampullary folds well-preserved; (d) degree IV: hydrosalpinx simplex dilatation more than 2.5 cm, well-preserved ampullary folds; (e) degree V: thick-walled hydrosalpinx, absence of ampullary folds

DEFINING THE PROGNOSTIC FACTORS FOR SUCCESSFUL TUBAL SURGERY

In the management of distal tubal infertility, *in vitro* fertilization (IVF) and tubal surgery should not be considered as competitive but rather as complementary modalities[25]. When feasible, with a good chance of success, surgery should always be attempted; IVF should only be considered when the fertility prognosis associated with conservative surgery is too poor. The conditions for surgical feasibility are based on the thorough evaluation of prognostic factors, usually obtained preoperatively and at the time of laparoscopy; this will orientate the patient towards the best therapeutic alternative. Factors contributing to the establishment of a prognosis for surgery can be subdivided into two groups: tubal and extratubal factors. The information collected during the evaluation phase is usually included in various scoring systems, with the aim of better defining the chances of conception if a surgical approach is selected.

Tubal factors

Inflammation following pelvic infection during surgery leads to tubal damage which is observed, described and eventually scored through different investigational procedures. Tubal factors to be considered are:

(1) Ampullary dilatation;

(2) Preservation of the ampullary folds;

(3) Detection of intratubal adhesions;

(4) Macroscopic and microscopic mucosal tubal status.

Ampullary dilatation

Ampullary dilatation is best assessed and measured at the time of the hysterosalpingogram. Indeed, we, like others[26], are convinced that a well-performed hysterosalpingography (Figure 2) remains one of the best investigational examinations of the infertile patient. Hysterosalpingography provides clear information on the normality of the uterine cavity and the endocervical canal, the patency and status of the intramural/interstitial portion of the tube, the patency, possible dilatation, rigidity and anatomy of the ampullar segment and, finally, the suspicion of peritubal adhesions, although the predictive value of the latter remains poor compared to direct visualization by laparoscopy.

We have proposed a hysterosalpingographic classification of distal tubal occlusion[27], based on the extent of occlusion combined with the preservation of the ampullary folds (Table 1, Figure 2). From a series of 215 infertile women with bilateral distal tubal disease operated on by microsurgery[27], it was concluded that ampullary dilatation, as determined by laparoscopy and hysterosalpingography, influences the postoperative pregnancy rate. After fimbrioplasty for occlusion of degree I and salpingostomy for occlusion of degree II, the term pregnancy rate averaged 50%, whereas salpingoneostomies performed for occlusions of degree III and IV resulted in term pregnancy rates of 25% and 22%, respectively. Singhal and colleagues[28] found that microsurgical salpingostomy results drop if the dilatation is either less or more than 2 cm. The prognostic grading system elaborated by the American Fertility Society (AFS)[29] clearly follows the

same lines, stating that an ampullary diameter over 3 cm gives a poor pregnancy outcome.

A prospective study by Vasquez and co-workers[30], investigating tubal mucosal lesions and fertility in hydrosalpinges, recently concluded that there was a significantly better outcome following surgery of thin-walled hydrosalpinges of less than 1 cm in size, compared to moderate (1–2 cm) and large hydrosalpinges (> 2 cm). However, size should not be considered without close examination of the thickness of the ampullary wall, as thick-walled hydrosalpinges, usually a moderate dilatation, have the worst prognosis[27].

Preservation of the ampullary folds

The presence of ampullary folds can be observed by hysterosalpingography, endovaginal echography, hysterosalpingosonography and falloscopy. Hysterosalpingography is still considered as a reference for the description of the inner architecture of the ampulla and is included in several tubal scoring systems[31] (Table 2). A number of other examinations have recently been proposed as alternative investigational procedures.

Endovaginal echography has the resolution power to reveal the presence of rugae in dilated tubes (Figure 3). Compared to hysterosalpingography, endovaginal echography offers poor sensitivity in the detection of hydrosalpinges (obviously less so in the description of the tubal wall); it is estimated to be potentially useful in detecting a combination of proximal and distal tubal blockage when hysterosalpingography shows a proximal block[15].

Hysterosalpingosonography[32] was developed mainly to document tubal patency, sometimes using a color Doppler imaging system[33,34], and offers the following advantages over the classic hysterosalpingography: absence of radiation, avoidance of potential allergic reactions to iodinated contrast medium and the possibility of office use. While the results correlate well with those of hysterosalpingography and laparoscopic findings as far as tubal patency[33,34] is concerned, the technique cannot correctly delineate the inner architecture of the Fallopian tube and, therefore, is of little prognostic interest[26].

Falloscopy is the endoscopic (transhysteroscopic) exploration of the tube[24], an office procedure[35] that can indicate the tubal status. There is, at this stage, a definite

Table 1 Classification of distal tubal occlusion by Donnez and Casanas-Roux[27]

1	degree I	phymotic ostium with preserved tubal patency
2	degree II	total distal tubal occlusion without ampullary dilatation
3	degree III	ampullary dilatation inferior to 2.5 cm; ampullary folds well-preserved
4	degree IV	hydrosalpinx simplex; dilatation more than 2.5 cm; well-preserved ampullary folds
5	degree V	thick-walled hydrosalpinx; absence of ampullary folds

Table 2 Distal tubal scoring system of Mage and colleagues[31]

Tubal patency	Ampullary tubal mucosa (hysterosalpingography)	Ampullary tubal wall (laparoscopy)
Phimosis = 2	normal folds = 0	normal = 0
	decreased folds = 5	thin = 5
Hydrosalpinx = 5	no fold, honeycomb = 10	thick or rigid = 10

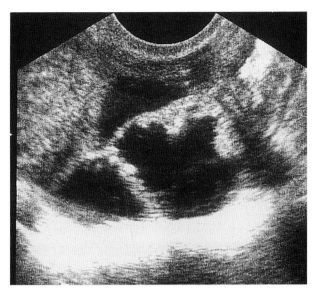

Figure 3 Vaginal echography reveals the presence of well-preserved ampullary folds

Table 3 Hydrosalpinx classification by Boer-Meisel and colleagues[39]

1	normal mucosa; regular patterns of lush mucosal folds, richly vascularized
2	hydrosalpinx with moderate attenuation of mucosal folds; patches of normal mucosa
3	absence of ampullary folds; honeycomb aspect

Detection of intratubal adhesions

Intratubal adhesions are detected only at falloscopy and/or tuboscopy. The formation of intratubal adhesions is one consequence among others of an underlying inflammatory process. It is not recognized specifically as a major prognostic factor, probably because the use of tuboscopy has not been generalized; Herschlag and co-workers[42], however, include this parameter in their tuboscopic score. No intrauterine pregnancy was reported in the presence of intratubal adhesions by De Bruyne and associates[23] in the presence of intratubal adhesions in a series of 17 patients, despite an overall intrauterine pregnancy rate of 59% in their study. Vasquez and colleagues[30] also clearly addressed this issue; in a multicenter study of 50 patients, it was concluded that mucosal adhesions in thin-walled hydrosalpinges are the most important factor in determining the fertility outcome. Indeed, presence and absence of intratubal adhesions were associated with an intrauterine pregnancy rate following surgery of 22 and 58%, respectively, differing significantly. The rate of ectopic pregnancy was 11% if adhesions had previously been discovered; this condition is seriously affected by a significant risk of ectopic gestation, as was also stressed by Marana and co-workers[44].

Evaluation of the tubal mucosa

The tubal mucosa can be assessed endoscopically and the observations are often included in various scoring classifications[6,27,29,31,39]. Apart from the various features already reviewed above, the macroscopic evaluation of the tubal mucosa attempts to determine the tubal wall thickness[31] and, also, to distinguish areas of normal-looking mucosa on the tubal wall, the inflammatory aspect of the epithelium and the underlying vascularization. We pointed out[6,10] that the smaller the area of normal mucosal surface observed under the operative microscope, the less is the incidence of intrauterine pregnancy; the difference was clearly significant when the cut-off level was chosen at 50% of normal-looking mucosal surface.

Histological data in tubal infertility are available from some authors[10,45], who have studied the histophysiopathological factors of distal tubal occlusions and correlated this with the pregnancy outcome.

lack of studies correlating this procedure with hysterosalpingographic and/or laparoscopic features, and with fertility outcome. A classification of luminal disease exists[36] but it does not explicitly consider the ampullary fold preservation as a significant parameter. The obscure and narrow view provided by these endoscopes limits the quality and the reliability of the observations, thereby somewhat restricting the importance of this examination in the evaluation of ampullary fold preservation.

If not using hysterosalpingography, mucosal folds are probably best visualized at the time of the laparoscopy, combined, or not, with salpingoscopy[22,37], or under the magnifying microscope at microsurgery. Paucity of endotubal folds is unanimously recognized as pejorative[10,27,29,31,38,39]. Boer-Meisel and colleagues[39] have proposed an endosalpingeal score as part of an overall score for distal tubal occlusions (Table 3); this endosalpingeal score was recently demonstrated by Dubuisson and co-workers[40] to correlate closely with more complex classification systems and to predict fairly the fertility outcome. In our series, complete absence of mucosal folds, often associated with thick and fibrotic tubal walls, was followed by no intrauterine pregnancy after microscopic repair. Tuboscopy has the potential to provide an excellent close-up vision of the tubal architecture. Abnormal findings can be revealed at tuboscopy in 20–30% of cases with, otherwise, normal hysterosalpingography and/or laparoscopy[41]. Herschlag and colleagues[42], attempting to correlate salpingoscopic findings (including the evaluation of the mucosal fold architecture) with histology, demonstrated a good correlation, only in the cases of mild and severe disease. Our surgical stance depends on a combination of these first two prognostic factors, i.e. the degree of distal occlusion and the preservation of ampullary folds, as assessed by hysterosalpingography[27,43].

The ciliation index. The ciliation index was proven to be valuable in the prognosis of tubal surgery[3,10,45]. In our original study in which we investigated the prognosis factors of fimbrial microsurgery on 215 patients[27], the ciliated cell percentage, as evaluated on fimbrial microbiopsy, and the pregnancy outcome were significantly decreased in cases of degree III and IV distal occlusion, when compared with degree I and II distal occlusion. In our study, the ciliation index was related to the pregnancy rate after microsurgical correction of the distal occlusion.

Fibrosis and the thickness of the tubal wall. Long-standing evolution of hydrosalpinges sometimes leads to the invasion of the muscularis by fibrosis which is responsible for a significant thickening of the tubal wall and leads, ultimately, to the so-called thick-walled hydrosalpinx. Vasquez and colleagues[30] have correlated the incidence of thick-walled hydrosalpinx with histological parameters: in thick-walled hydrosalpinges, the thickness of the tubal wall measures 2–10 mm at the thinnest part and 4–10 mm at the thickest part. The thick-walled hydrosalpinx is usually associated with other pejorative macro- and microscopic features, explaining the very poor results of fertility-promoting surgery. In our series[27], the intrauterine pregnancy rate for this type of tube was 0%, as found by some other authors[1–3,30,40]. The recommended attitude in this case is to perform a salpingectomy at the time of the laparoscopy in an attempt to enhance the results of IVF[46] and to limit the incidence of tubal gestation, reported as high as 11% in tubal infertility patients undergoing IVF[47].

Extratubal factors

Adnexal adhesions and endometriosis are sometimes included in the list of prognostic factors affecting the pregnancy rate outcome.

Periadnexal adhesions

The significance of pelvic adhesions is controversial in the prognosis determination for the patients with tubal factors. The studies from several authors[2,28,38,39] suggest that the fertility prognosis is correlated with the presence of tubal adhesions presence and degree of severity. Some investigators[48,49] restrict the negative influence of adhesions to severe cases only; actually, frozen pelvis is still considered as a contraindication to conservative surgery. Nevertheless, it should be noted that microsurgical or laparoscopic adhesiolysis alone has been shown to promote fertility[28,43,50], giving credit to the implication of adhesions in mechanical infertility.

The most recent series, however, tend to challenge the role of adhesions in impairing the promotion of fertility following surgery. Dubuisson and colleagues[40], in a series of 90 patients undergoing laparoscopic salpingostomy, failed to show any relationship between adhesion score and pregnancy outcome. Canis and co-workers[9] did not note any significant difference in their group of 87 laparoscopic tuboplasties as far as crude pregnancy and monthly fecundity rates were concerned. The implication of periadnexal adhesions has also recently been questioned by Vasquez and colleagues[30] in a prospectively designed study.

Endometriosis

Endometriosis has rarely been taken into account in the evaluation of the success of tubal surgery. The most recent study in this aspect is by Dlugi and colleagues[49] who, on treating 113 patients with tubal factors and comparing pregnancy curves, concluded that endometriosis-related tubal occlusion was less detrimental than post-pelvic inflammatory disease or post-surgical tubal distal occlusions. Obviously, treating the concomitant endometriosis at the time of tubal surgery improves the fertility outcome on its own and can modulate the actual implication of endometriosis as a prognostic factor for successful tuboplasty.

This finding agrees with a report from Nezhat and co-workers[51], who found no significantly abnormal findings with tuboscopy in a population of 100 patients with endometriosis; this might suggest a better inner tubal condition in distal tubal occlusions of endometriotic origin compared to distal tubal occlusion of inflammatory etiology, where the mucosal impairment is probably more aggressive.

TECHNIQUES AND RESULTS

Tubal occlusion: degree I

Fimbrioplasty is also carried out during laparoscopy. When fimbrial adhesions are found as the blue dye begins to spill through the open tube, these adhesions between the fimbrial folds are carefully grasped by means of the probe with a hook passed through a third-puncture trocar, and cut in a bloodless fashion with the finely focused CO_2 beam set at 40 W (Figure 4). Thereafter, a defocused beam (10 W) is used to cause blanching of the serosa (Figure 5). The SurgiTouch™ is useful for this purpose. This allows adequate eversion of the mucosa and prevents any recurrence of adhesions.

Tubal occlusion: degrees II, III and IV

Salpingostomy can be performed with the CO_2 laser and is indicated in cases of thin-walled hydrosalpinx where both proximal tubal patency and the presence of ampullary folds have been confirmed by a hysterosalpingogram (Figure 6). Two grasping forceps are introduced for traction and manipulation at the ampullary–fimbrial segment. The blocked tube is held so that the focused laser beam can be aligned at a 90° angle to the dimple (Figure 6). The laser is set on continuous mode (40 W) and two linear incisions are made (Figure 7), cutting from the anterior to the posterior region along blood vessels. As soon as the lumen is entered, the tube collapses; continuous dye injection keeps it distended. Only then is the incision enlarged. At this point, the probes and grasping forceps gently hold the incision edges and a reduced-power (10–15 W), defocused beam (SurgiTouch) is used to evert the serosal aspect of the incised edge (Figure 8).

The final aspect of the tube reveals a well-everted fimbria and, if performed, ampulloscopy reveals the presence of well-vascularized ampullary folds (Figure 9). At the end of the procedure, the peritoneal cavity is irrigated with Ringer's solution to remove carbonized particles.

Tubal occlusion: degree V

In cases of thick-walled hydrosalpinx, the ampullary folds are absent. The pregnancy rate after microsurgery[10] is 0%; for this reason, there is no indication for salpingostomy.

We propose a laparoscopic salpingectomy to the patient before an IVF procedure, in order to avoid the risk of tubal pregnancy after embryo transfer.

Table 4 describes the results we have obtained in a series of 1184 laparoscopic tubal surgery cases[43]. As has been repeatedly reported in the literature, these figures are comparable to results obtained from microsurgery and

Table 4 Laser laparoscopic management of distal occlusions: 18-month cumulative viable pregnancy rate[43]

Procedure	n	Pregnancies n	%
Fimbrioplasty	380	228	60
Salpingostomy	85	22	27
Adhesiolysis			
degree I	412	255	62
degree II	307	157	51

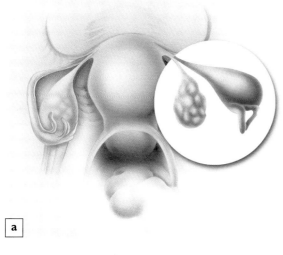

a

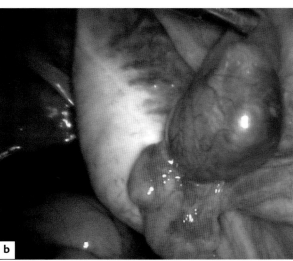

b

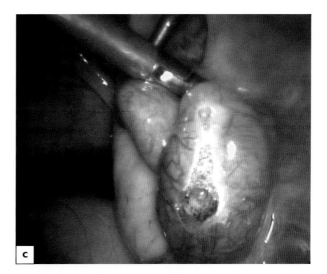

c

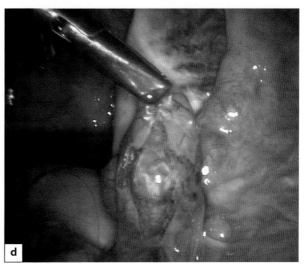

d

Figure 4 (a)–(d) Fimbrioplasty: the peritoneum covering the ostium is cut by means of the hook

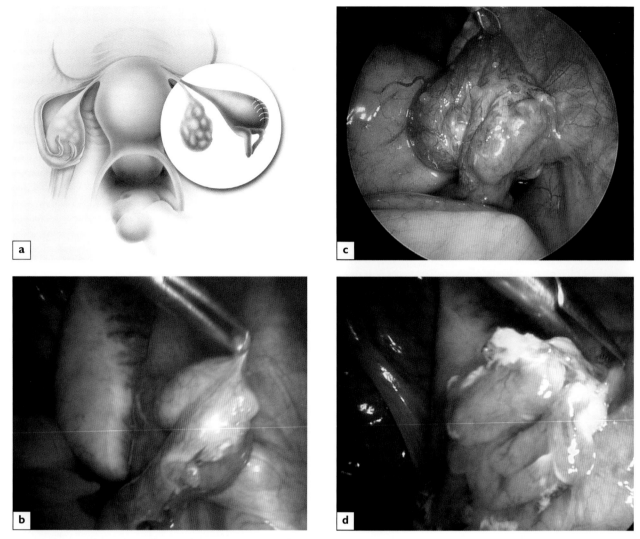

Figure 5 (a)–(d) Fimbrioplasty: adequate eversion of the mucosa is allowed by causing blanching of the serosa. The SurgiTouch is useful for this purpose

from other laparoscopic series. Indeed, the pregnancy rates are significantly different after fimbrioplasty for occlusions of degree I (60%), after salpingoneostomy for occlusions of degree III and IV. In cases of adhesiolysis, the pregnancy rates are 62% and 51% according to the type of adhesions (degree I and degree II, respectively).

Table 5 summarizes the results obtained in major series of laparoscopic salpingoneostomies; the intrauterine pregnancy rate ranges from 19% to 48% according to the inclusion criteria reported by the authors. These rates remain low and stress the fact that the tubes have probably undergone irreversible damage. The degree of the lesion influences the success of fertility-promoting surgery, so it is essential to rely on prognostic factors, the evaluation of which will help in predicting the success of a surgical approach. We have opted for the technique summarized in Figure 10 for the management of distal tubal occlusion. In degree II–IV, hysterosalpingography is systematically performed 3 months after surgery under antibiotic prophylaxis, in the absence of pregnancy.

Reocclusion is, in our opinion, an indication to remove laparoscopically the diseased tube and to direct the patient towards IVF, as the presence of hydrosalpinx is felt to impair the success rate of IVF and exposes the patient to the increased risk of ectopic gestation[46,47]. In cases of thick-walled hydrosalpinx (degree V, according to Donnez and colleagues[27]), the ampullary folds are absent. The pregnancy rate after microsurgery is 0%; for this reason, there is no indication for salpingostomy. Since 1991, we have proposed a laparoscopic salpingectomy for the patient before an IVF procedure, in order to avoid the risk of tubal pregnancy after embryo transfer (ET) and the possibility of embryotoxicity with subsequent low pregnancy rates.

HYDROSALPINX AND IVF–ET

In a recent review, Nackley and Muasher[52] analyzed the effects of hydrosalpinx in IVF–ET.

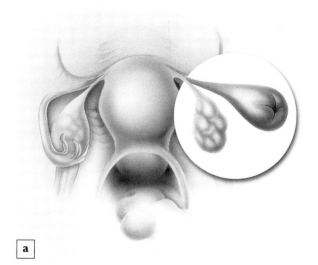

a

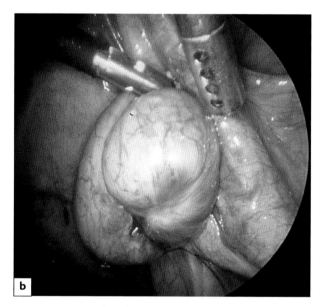

b

Figure 6 (a) Hydrosalpinx: tubal occlusion of degree IV; (b) laparoscopic view

Table 5 Intrauterine pregnancy rate obtained from laparoscopic salpingoneostomies

Author	n	Intrauterine pregnancy rate (%)
Daniell (1984)	21	19
Nezhat (1984)	33	36
Bouquet (1987)	20	25
Reich (1987)	7	29
Manhes (1987)	19	48
Donnez (1989)	25	20
Dubuisson (1990)	31	26
Larue (1990)	15	20
Henry-Suchet (1991)	28	32
McComb (1991)	22	22.7
Matvienko (1991)	50	48
Canis (1991)	87	33.3
Audebert (1992)	142	20.4
Donnez (1994)	85	27
Total	585	29.03

Sims and co-workers[53] were the first to study the effect of hydrosalpinx on IVF outcome. A retrospective case-controlled study was conducted involving 118 patients with hydrosalpinx undergoing 283 stimulations, and 823 patients with tubal factor infertility but without hydrosalpinx undergoing 1431 stimulations. A lower clinical pregnancy rate of 18%, and a higher miscarriage rate of 42% resulting in a lower ongoing pregnancy rate of 10% was discovered compared to the control group. They suggested treatment of the hydrosalpinx before IVF, such as by laparoscopic removal or peritransfer antibiotic coverage.

In a retrospective study, Strandell and colleagues[46] concluded that persistent hydrosalpinx was associated with a reduced implantation rate and an increased risk for early pregnancy loss. It was hypothesized that the removal of the hydrosalpinx by salpingectomy or salpingostomy would normalize the IVF–ET rates in this group.

Andersen and co-workers[54] reported a marked reduction in implantation rates when hydrosalpinx was visible on ultrasonography. They found the rates of implantation, pregnancy, early pregnancy loss and delivery per aspiration were significantly reduced despite a comparable number of aspirated oocytes and embryos transferred. Vandromme[55] and Vejtorp[56] and their groups also demonstrated a decreased pregnancy rate after IVF in women with hydrosalpinx. The significant decreases in implantation rate and pregnancy rate per transfer in the hydrosalpinx group suggest an unfavorable uterine environment.

We have suggested[57] that this unfavorable environment could possibly be attributable to hydrosalpingeal fluid drainage into the endometrial cavity. The possibility has been raised of a connection between the hydrosalpinx and the uterine cavity, allowing a direct flow of hydrosalpingeal fluid into the uterus, thus exposing the endometrium and embryo to potentially toxic fluid. It is postulated that the fluid in damaged tubes contains micro-organisms, debris, lymphocytes, macrophages and other toxic agents that flow into the uterus and exert a detrimental effect on the endometrium and developing embryo. There may also be substances, such as cytokines and prostaglandins, interfering with normal endometrial function[46,54].

Freeman and co-workers[58] recently suggested that not only does hydrosalpinx negatively affect endometrial receptivity during implantation, but it also exerts a negative influence over oocytes early in follicular recruitment. The presence of hydrosalpinx has also been shown to affect the implantation rates in unstimulated cycles[59].

145

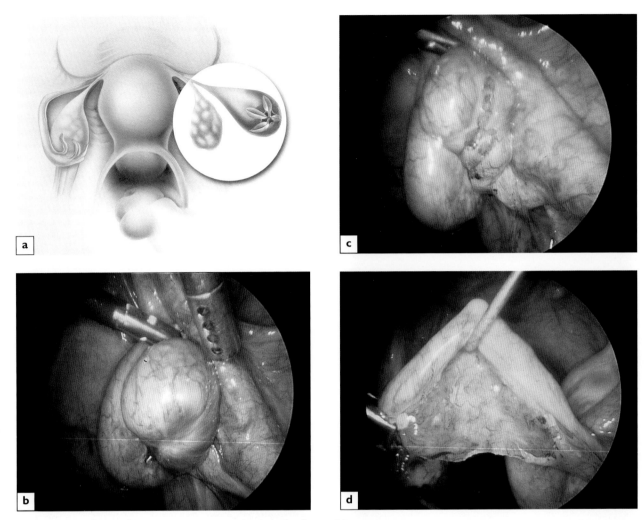

Figure 7 (a)–(d) Two linear incisions are made with the focused beam

Hydrosalpinx also predisposes patients to increased ectopic pregnancies after IVF–ET[59-61]. The first human pregnancy after IVF was, indeed, a tubal pregnancy[62]. Zouvres and colleagues[63] suggested prophylactic proximal tubal occlusion to prevent tubal pregnancy after IVF. This recommendation had also been suggested by Steptoe[64], Tucker[65] and Herman[66] and their colleagues. However, we do not recommend proximal tubal occlusion in cases of distal occlusion because of the risk of subsequent pelvic pain and inflammation due to increased intratubal pressure[57]. We prefer to recommend prophylactic salpingectomy instead of prophylactic proximal occlusion.

A study by Schenk and colleagues[67] and Mukherjee and co-workers[68] examined the effect of hydrosalpingeal fluid on embryogenesis. All samples demonstrated significant embryotoxic effects.

Although the exact mechanism by which hydrosalpinx alters intrauterine receptivity remains unclear, a marker of uterine receptivity has been established. Integrins are adhesion molecules that participate in cell–cell interactions and are present on all human cells. Lessey and associates[69] conducted an interesting study that examined endometrial integrin expression to evaluate the effects of hydrosalpinges on uterine receptivity. The expression of β-integrin, measured by immunohistochemical assays of endometrial biopsies, was assessed. Women with hydrosalpinges expressed significantly lower levels than those without hydrosalpinges[69].

REMOVAL OF HYDROSALPINX BEFORE IVF–ET

The benefit of salpingectomy before IVF–ET in patients with hydrosalpinx has been debated by Puttemans and Brosens[70]. They believe that preventive salpingectomy should not be performed without demonstration by salpingoscopy of severe pathology, specifically chronic inflammation.

On the other hand, the study by Vandromme and associates[55] sought to determine whether surgical treatment would benefit those patients with hydrosalpinx attempting IVF–ET. The ongoing pregnancy rate before surgery was 10.1%, whereas the postoperative group had an ongoing

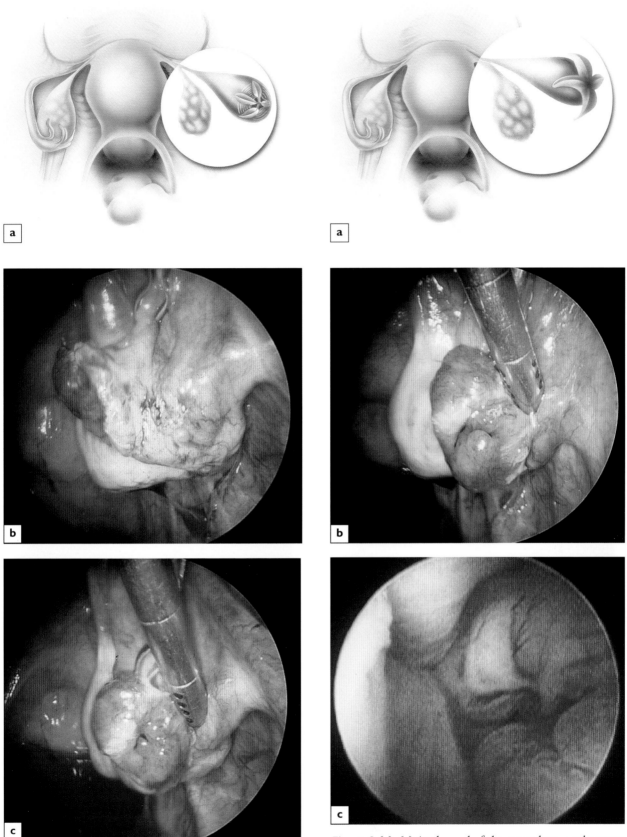

Figure 8 (a)–(c) When the incision is enlarged, the defocused beam (with the SurgiTouch™ on) is used to evert the serosal aspect of the incised edge

Figure 9 (a)–(c) At the end of the procedure, a tuboscopy is not systematically performed, but when performed, as in this case, ampulloscopy reveals the presence of well-vascularized ampullary folds

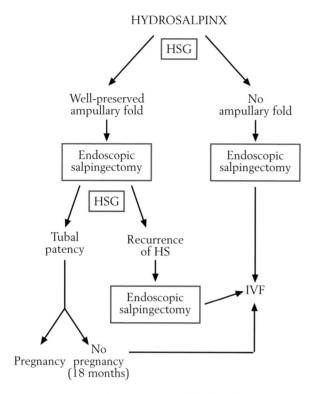

HYDROSALPINX

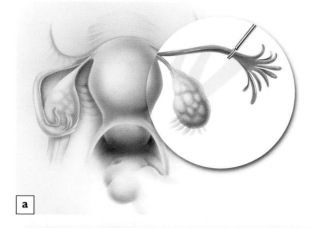

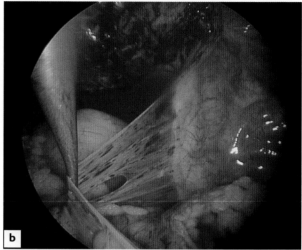

Figure 10 Proposed management of hydrosalpinx (HS) in infertility. HSG, hysterosalpingography; IVF, *in vitro* fertilization

pregnancy rate of 31%. In the control group, the rate was 21.3%. The results revealed that surgical correction by ablation of the diseased tubes restored the normal chances of success for patients with hydrosalpinges.

Shelton and colleagues[71] were the first to conduct a prospective study that demonstrated a positive impact on pregnancy rates in patients with repeated IVF failures by removing the hydrosalpinges. Fifteen patients with unilateral or bilateral hydrosalpinges with a history of repeated IVF failures underwent laparoscopic excision of the affected tubes. Because the patients undergoing surgical excision served as their own control, the ongoing pregnancy rate per transfer was 0% pre-salpingectomy. After salpingectomy, the ongoing pregnancy per transfer rate was 25%. Improved pregnancy rates were noted for both the fresh and frozen embryo transfers after surgery.

Lessey and co-workers[69] were also successful in demonstrating an improvement of integrin status and, therefore, uterine receptivity after correction of the hydrosalpinx.

It is unclear whether salpingectomy has a detrimental effect on ovarian blood supply and neural linkage, thus affecting folliculogenesis and hormone production. Studies by Vandromme[55], Shelton[71] and Kassabji[72] and their colleagues showed no difference in ovarian response, oocyte retrieval, or fertilization rates after salpingectomy. Nevertheless, other authors[73–75] have addressed the importance of maintaining the integrity of the anastomotic

Figure 11 Three types of adhesions are distinguished: (a) and (b) type I, filmy and avascular adhesions *(continued on next page)*

vessels between the ovary and tube. McComb and Delbelke[75] evaluated the relationship between the ovary and oviduct using microsurgery to alter the structure of the Fallopian tube. The number of ovulations was reduced by ablating the vasculature transmitted through the mesosalpinx. Preservation of the anastomotic ovarian blood supply at the time of salpingectomy must be emphasized to decrease the possible effects of radical surgery on ovarian function[74]. The risk of interstitial pregnancy is not eliminated and the remote chance of uterine rupture at the site of salpingectomy exists[47,76]. Pavic and colleagues[77] were the first to report an interstitial pregnancy after bilateral salpingectomy for hydrosalpinx and IVF. Cornual resection at the time of salpingectomy does not prevent interstitial pregnancies.

ADHESIONS

Three types of adhesions must be defined:

(1) Type I (Figure 11 a and b): filmy and avascular adhesions;

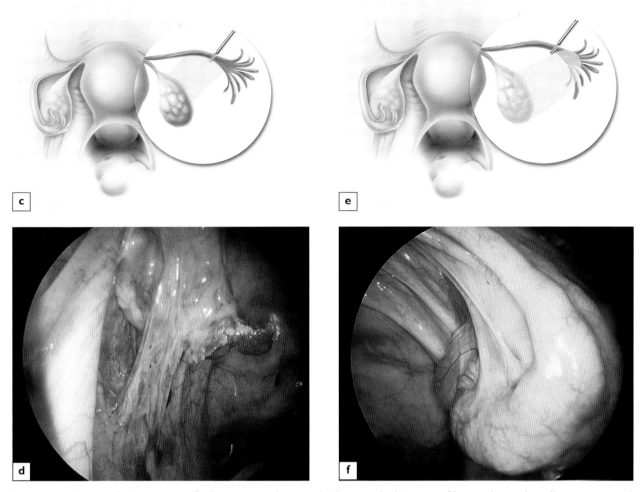

Figure 11 *Continued* Three types of adhesions are distinguished: (c) and (d) type II, filmy and vascular adhesions; (e) and (f) type III, dense, fibrous and vascular adhesions

(2) Type II (Figure 11 c and d): filmy and vascular adhesions;

(3) Type III (Figure 11 e and f): dense, fibrous and vascular adhesions.

Adhesiolysis

In many patients, postoperative or postinfectious adhesions are amenable to vaporization by laser laparoscopy[6,10,27]. When compared to the standard technique with cautery and the use of laparoscopic scissors or blunt dissection, there is probably no difference in the outcome when the adhesions are small and avascular. With more vascular adhesions or particularly thick tubo-ovarian adhesions, however, the CO₂ laser allows more precise destruction of the adhesions with minimal injury to the adjacent normal tissue. Filmy peritubal and periovarian adhesions are easily vaporized with the operative laser laparoscope. The adhesiolysis probe with its backstop should be used to make the procedure safer. Traction to adhesions must be applied by two atraumatic forceps.

The adhesion is positioned across the 'firing' platform when the laser is activated to prevent damage to any tissue distal to the adhesion. Using a power output of 40 W, adhesions can be both coagulated and incised. For beginners, single or repeat pulse modes should be used for laser vaporization of the adhesions until confidence in the technique is gained. Great care should be taken when dividing adhesions between the tube and the ovary because this area is very vascular. Adhesions of degree I (filmy and avascular) and II (dense and vascular, but not very thick) are easily vaporized with the operative laser laparoscope.

Salpingolysis is performed by applying traction to the adhesions by a suprapubic atraumatic grasping forceps and by another probe (smooth manipulating probe, hook or probe with its backstop) (Figure 12). The probe with a backstop can be used to make the procedure easier. When this probe is used, the adhesion is placed across the 'firing' platform and the laser is fired to vaporize the band. The use of the probe with a backstop eliminates the risk of inadvertent injury to intraperitoneal structures.

Using a power output of 40 W, the adhesions are coagulated and incised (Figure 13). Short exposure times are

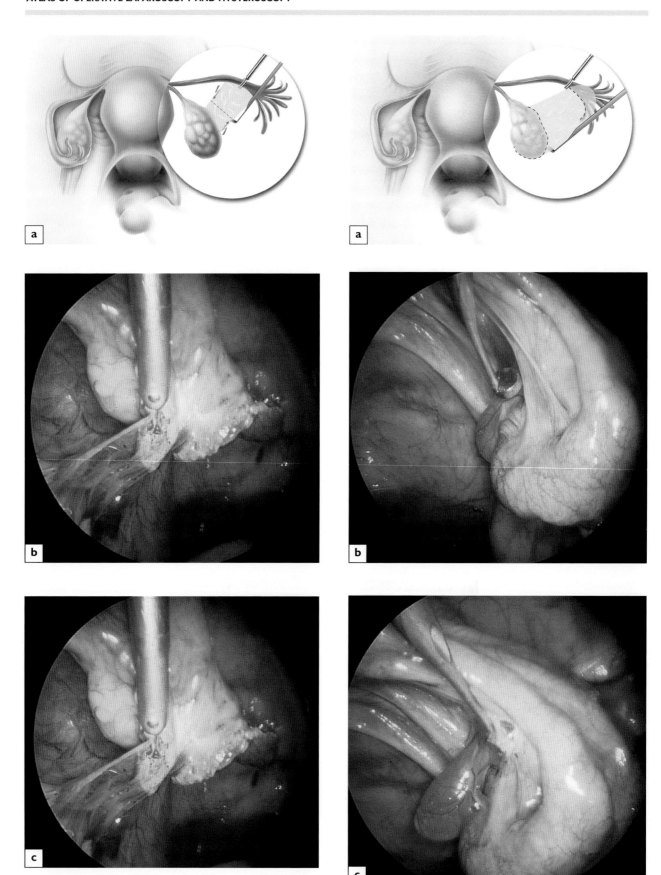

Figure 12 (a)–(c) Salpingolysis is usually performed by applying traction to adhesions by a suprapubic atraumatic grasping forceps and by one or two other probes (probe with the hook or with the backstop)

Figure 13 (a)–(c) In case of adhesions of degree III, a CO_2 laser is useful for cutting dense and fibrous adhesions *(continued on next page)*

adequate to vaporize the adhesions around the Fallopian tubes and ovaries, and will prevent the laser beam from penetrating more than 100–200 μm. In the hands of more experienced laparoscopists, continuous mode is easily used.

Ovariolysis is performed by applying torsion to the utero-ovarian ligaments with atraumatic tubal forceps (Figure 14). Elevation and rotation of the ovary are performed while continuing traction and torsion. Adhesions can easily be dissected from the ovarian surface by superficial vaporization. Care must also be taken not to apply too much traction for fear of tearing the ovarian ligament from its attachment, which can result in copious

bleeding that can only be stopped by hemostatic clips or coagulation. During adhesiolysis, the use of the probe with a backstop eliminates the risk of inadvertent injury to other intraperitoneal structures, particularly the bowel. Irrigation fluid can be introduced into the pelvis as an aquatic backstop to protect the bowel from any damage from the scatter of the laser beam.

CONCLUSION

In conclusion, the list of prognostic factors for tubal infertility is long[78]. It stresses the major role attributable to the quality of the investigational examinations performed preoperatively on the infertile patient, particularly the hysterosalpingogram and at the time of the laparoscopy, when the exploration of the tubal mucosa must be meticulous. Direct visual investigation of the tube, whether

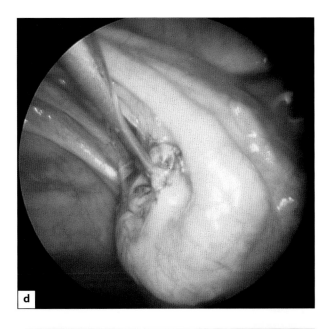
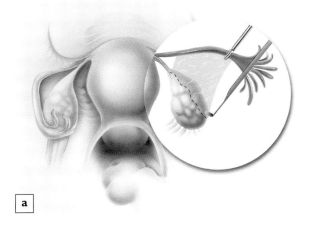
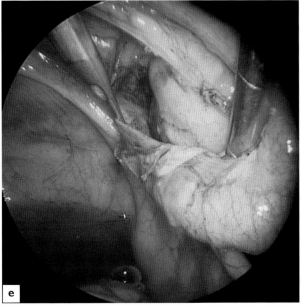
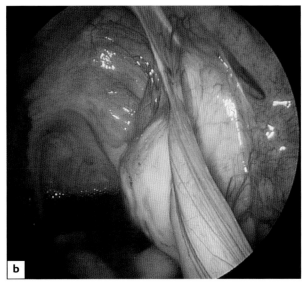

Figure 13 *Continued* (d) and (e) In case of adhesions of degree III, a CO₂ laser is useful for cutting dense and fibrous adhesions

Figure 14 (a) and (b) Ovariolysis is performed by applying traction. Elevation and rotation of the ovary are performed while continuing traction and torsion. A probe with a backstop is used to avoid damage behind the adhesion

preoperatively (falloscopy) or peroperatively (tuboscopy), enables the clear documentation of the endosalpingeal features.

Failure to be aware of these prognostic factors, and subsequent poor selection of the patient for conservative surgery, could lead to an unacceptable loss of time and of disillusionment for our patients.

REFERENCES

1. Swolin K. Electromicrosurgery and salpingostomy: long-term results. *Am J Obstet Gynecol* 1975;121:418–19
2. Gomel V. Salpingostomy by microsurgery. *Fertil Steril* 1978;34:380–5
3. Winston RML. Microsurgery of the fallopian tube: from fantasy to reality. *Fertil Steril* 1980;46:521–30
4. Gomel V. Salpingostomy by laparoscopy. *J Reprod Med* 1977;18:265–7
5. Daniell JF, Herbert CM. Laparoscopic salpingostomy utilizing the CO_2 laser. *Fertil Steril* 1984;41:558–63
6. Donnez J, Nisolle M, Casanas-Roux F. CO_2 laser laparoscopy in infertile women with adnexal adhesions and women with tubal occlusion. *J Gynecol Surg* 1989;5:47–53
7. Dubuisson JB, de Jolinière JB, Aubriot FX, *et al.* Terminal tuboplasties by laparoscopy: 65 consecutive cases. *Fertil Steril* 1990;54:401–3
8. Mettler LR, Irani S, Kapamadzija A, *et al.* Pelviscopic tubal surgery: the acceptable vogue. *Hum Reprod* 1990;5:971–4
9. Canis M, Mage G, Pouly JL, *et al.* Laparoscopic distal tuboplasties: reports of 87 cases and a 4-year experience. *Fertil Steril* 1991;56:616–21
10. Donnez J. *La trompe de Fallope: Hystopathologie Normale et Pathologique.* Nauwelaerts Printing, 1984
11. Afzelius BA, Camner P, Mossberg B. On the function of the cilia in the female reproductive tract. *Fertil Steril* 1978;29:72
12. Donnez J, Caprasse J, Casanas-Roux F, *et al.* Loss of adrenergic innervation in rabbit induced hydrosalpinx. *Gynecol Obstet Invest* 1986;21:213–16
13. Mol BWJ, Swart P, Bossuyt PMM, *et al.* Reproducibility of the interpretation of hysterosalpingography in the diagnosis of tubal pathology. *Hum Reprod* 1996;11:1204–8
14. Swart P, Mol BWJ, van der Veen F, *et al.* The accuracy of hysterosalpingography in the diagnosis of tubal pathology, a meta-analysis. *Fertil Steril* 1995;64:486–91
15. Atri M, Tran CN, Bret PT, *et al.* Accuracy of endovaginal sonography for the detection of fallopian tube blockage. *Ultrasound Med* 1994;13:429–34
16. Schiller VL, Tsuchiyama K. Development of hydrosalpinx during ovulation induction. *J Ultrasound Med* 1995;14:799–803
17. Friberg B, Joergensen C. Tubal patency studied by ultrasonography. A pilot study. *Acta Obst Gynecol Scand* 1994;73:53–5
18. Heikkinen H, Tekay A, Volpi E, *et al.* Transvaginal salpingosonography for the assessment of tubal patency in infertile women: methodological and clinical experiences. *Fertil Steril* 1995;64:293–8
19. Volpi E, Piermatteo M, Zuccaro G, *et al.* The role of transvaginal sonosalpingography in the evaluation of tubal patency. *Minvera Ginecol* 1996;48:1–3
20. Allahbadia GN. Fallopian tubal patency using color Doppler. *Int J Gynaecol Obstet* 1996;40:241–4
21. Yarali H, Gurgan T, Erden A, *et al.* Colour Doppler hysterosalpingo-sonography: a simple and potentially useful method to evaluate fallopian tube patency. *Hum Reprod* 1994;9:64–6
22. Brosens I, Boeckx W, Delattin P, *et al.* Salpingoscopy: a new pre-operative diagnostic tool in tubal infertility. *Br J Obstet Gynaecol* 1987;94:768–73
23. De Bruyne F, Puttemans P, Boeckx W, *et al.* The clinical value of salpingoscopy in tubal infertility. *Fertil Steril* 1989;51:339–40
24. Kerin J, Daykhovsky L, Grundfest W, *et al.* Falloscopy. A microendoscopic transvaginal technique for diagnosing and treating endotubal disease incorporating guide wire cannulation and direct balloon tuboplasty. *J Reprod Med* 1990;35:606–12
25. Gomel V, Taylor PJ. *In vitro* fertilization versus reconstructive tubal surgery. *J Assist Reprod Genet* 1992;9:306–9
26. Gomel V, Yarali H. Infertility surgery: microsurgery. *Curr Opin Obstet Gynecol* 1992;4:390–9
27. Donnez J, Casanas-Roux F. Prognostic factors of fimbrial microsurgery. *Fertil Steril* 1986;46:200–4
28. Singhal V, Li TC, Cooke ID. An analysis of factors influencing the outcome of 232 consecutive tubal microsurgery cases. *Br J Obstet Gynaecol* 1991;98:628–36
29. American Fertility Society. The American Fertility Society: classifications of adnexal adhesions, distal tubal occlusion, tubal occlusion secondary to tubal ligation, tubal pregnancies, Müllerian abnormalities and intrauterine adhesions. *Fertil Steril* 1988;49:944–55
30. Vasquez G, Boeckx W, Brosens I. Prospective study of tubal mucosal lesions and fertility in hydrosalpinges. *Hum Reprod* 1995;10:1075–8
31. Mage G, Pouly JL, Bouquet de Jolinière J, *et al.* A preoperative classification to predict the intrauterine and ectopic pregnancy rates after distal microsurgery. *Fertil Steril* 1986;46:807–10
32. Schlief R, Deichert U. Hysterosalpingo-contrast sonography of the uterus and fallopian tube: results of a clinical trial of a new contrast medium in 120 patients. *Radiology* 1991;178:213–15
33. Peters AJ, Coulam, CB. Hysterosalpingography with color doppler ultrasonography. *Am J Obstet Gynecol* 1991;164:1530–4

34. Stern J, Peters AJ, Coulam CB. Color Doppler ultrasonography assessment of tubal patency: a comparison study with traditional techniques. *Fertil Steril* 1992;58:897–900

35. Dunphy BC. Office falloscopic assessment in proximal tubal occlusive disease. *Fertil Steril* 1994;61:168–70

36. Kerin JF, Williams DB, San Roman GA, *et al.* Falloscopic classification and treatment of Fallopian tube lumen disease. *Fertil Steril* 1992;57:731–41

37. Cornier E, Feintuch MJ, Bouccara L. Ampullafibrotuboscopy. *J Gynecol Obstet Biol Reprod* 1985;14:459–66

38. Schlaff WD, Hassiakos DK, Damewood MD, *et al.* Neosalpingostomy for distal tubal obstruction: prognostic factors and impact of surgical technique. *Fertil Steril* 1990;54:984–90

39. Boer-Meisel ME, Te Velde ER, Habbema JDF, *et al.* Predicting the pregnancy outcome in patients treated for hydrosalpinx: a prospective study. *Fertil Steril* 1986;45:23–9

40. Dubuisson JB, Chapron C, Morice P, *et al.* Laparoscopic salpingostomy: fertility results according to the tubal mucosal appearance. *Hum Reprod* 1994;9:334–9

41. Marana R, Muscatello P, Muzii L, *et al.* Perlaparoscopic salpingoscopy in the evaluation of the tubal factor in infertile women. *Int J Fertil* 1990;35:211–14

42. Herschlag A, Seifer DB, Carcangiu ML, *et al.* Salpingoscopy: light microscopic and electron microscopic correlations. *Obstet Gynecol* 1991;7:399–405

43. Donnez J, Nisolle M, Casanas-Roux F, *et al.* CO₂ laser laparoscopic surgery: adhesiolysis, salpingostomy and fimbrioplasty. In Donnez J, Nisolle M, eds. *Atlas of Laser Operative Laparoscopy and Hysteroscopy.* Carnforth, UK: Parthenon Publishing, 1994:97–112

44. Marana R, Muzii L, Rizzi M, *et al.* Salpingoscopy in patients with contralateral ectopic pregnancy. *Fertil Steril* 1991;55:838–40

45. Brosens I, Vasquez G. Fimbrial microbiopsy. *J Reprod Med* 1976;16:171

46. Strandell A, Waldenstrom U, Nilsson L, *et al.* Hydrosalpinx reduces *in vitro* fertilization/embryo transfer pregnancy rates. *Hum Reprod* 1994;9:861–3

47. Dubuisson JB, Aubriot FX, Mathieu L, *et al.* Risk factors for ectopic pregnancy in 556 pregnancies after *in vitro* fertilization: implications for preventive management. *Fertil Steril* 1991;56:686–90

48. Laatikainen TJ, Tenhumen AK, Venesmaa PK, *et al.* Factors influencing the success of microsurgery for distal tubal occlusion. *Arch Gynecol Obstet* 1988;243:101–6

49. Dlugi AM, Reddy S, Saleh WA, *et al.* Pregnancy rates after operative endoscopic treatment of total (neosalpingostomy) or near total (salpingostomy) distal tubal occlusion. *Fertil Steril* 1994;62:913–20

50. Donnez J. CO₂ laser laparoscopy in infertile women with endometriosis and women with adnexal adhesions. *Fertil Steril* 1987;48:390

51. Nezhat F, Winer WK, Nehzat C. Fimbrioscopy and salpingoscopy in patients with minimal to moderate pelvic endometriosis. *Obstet Gynecol* 1990;75:15–17

52. Nackley AC, Muasher SJ. The significance of hydrosalpinx in *in vitro* fertilization. *Fertil Steril* 1998;69:373–4

53. Sims JA, Jones D, Butler L, *et al.* Effect of hydrosalpinx on outcome in *in vitro* fertilization (IVF). Presented at the *49th Annual Meeting of the American Fertility Society 1993*, Chicago. Program Supplement. American Fertility Society, 1993:S95

54. Andersen A, Yue Z, Meng F, *et al.* Low implantation rate after *in vitro* fertilization in patients with hydrosalpinges diagnosed by ultrasonography. *Hum Reprod* 1994;9:1935–8

55. Vandromme J, Chasse E, Lejeune B, *et al.* Hydrosalpinges in *in vitro* fertilization: an unfavorable prognostic feature. *Hum Reprod* 1995;10:576–9

56. Vejtorp M, Petersen K, Andersen AN, *et al.* Fertilization *in vitro* in the presence of hydrosalpinx and in advanced age. *Ugeskr Laeger* 1995;157:4131–4

57. Donnez J, Polet R, Nisolle M. Prognostic factors of distal tubal occlusion. *Ref Gynecol Obstet* 1993;1:94–102

58. Freeman MR, Whitworth CM, Hill GA. Hydrosalpinx reduces *in vitro* fertilization–embryo transfer rates and *in vitro* blastocyst development. Presented at the *52nd Annual Meeting of the American Society 1996*, Washington. Program Supplement. American Fertility Society, 1996:S211

59. Akman MA, Garcia JE, Damewood MD, *et al.* Hydrosalpinx affects the implantation of previously cryopreserved embryos. *Hum Reprod* 1996;11:1013–14

60. Herman A, Ron-El R, Golan A, *et al.* The role of tubal pathology and other parameters in ectopic pregnancies occurring in *in vitro* fertilization and embryo transfer. *Fertil Steril* 1990;54:79–87

61. Martinez F, Trounson A. An analysis of risk factors associated with ectopic pregnancy in a human *in vitro* fertilization program. *Fertil Steril* 1986;45:79–87

62. Steptoe P, Edwards R. Reimplantation of a human embryo with subsequent tubal pregnancy. *Lancet* 1976;1:880

63. Zouvres C, Erenus M, Gomel V. Tubal ectopic pregnancy after *in vitro* fertilization and embryo transfer: a role for proximal occlusion or salpingectomy after failed distal tubal surgery. *Fertil Steril* 1991;56:691–5

64. Steptoe PC. Pregnancies following implantation of human embryos grown in culture. Presented at the *45th Annual Meeting of the American Fertility Society 1989*, San Francisco. Program Supplement. American Fertility Society, 1989:S152

65. Tucker M, Smith D, Pike I, *et al.* Ectopic pregnancy following *in vitro* fertilization and embryo transfer. *Lancet* 1981;2:1278

66. Herman A, Ron-El R, Golan A, *et al.* The dilemma of optimal surgical procedure in ectopic pregnancies occurring in *in vitro* fertilization. *Hum Reprod* 1991;6:1167–79

67. Schenk LM, Ramey JW, Taylor SL, *et al.* Embryotoxicity of hydrosalpinx fluid. Presented at the 43rd Annual Meeting of the Society of Gynecologic Investigators 1996. *J Soc Gynecol Invest* 1996:88A

68. Mukherjee T, Copperman AB, McCaffrey C, *et al.* Hydrosalpinx fluid has embryotoxic effects on murine embryogenesis: a case for prophylactic salpingectomy. *Fertil Steril* 1996;66:851–3

69. Lessey BA, Castelbaum AJ, Riben M, *et al.* Effect of hydrosalpinges on markers of uterine receptivity and success in IVF. Presented at the *50th Annual Meeting of the American Fertility Society 1994*, New York. Program Supplement. American Fertility Society, 1994:S45

70. Puttemans PJ, Brosens IA. Preventive salpingectomy of hydrosalpinx prior to IVF. Salpingectomy improves *in vitro* fertilization outcome in patients with a hydrosalpinx: blind victimization of the Fallopian tube? *Hum Reprod* 1996;11:2079–84

71. Shelton KE, Butler L, Toner JP, *et al.* Salpingectomy improves the pregnancy rate in *in vitro* fertilization with hydrosalpinx. *Hum Reprod* 1996;11:523–5

72. Kassabji M, Sims J, Butler L, *et al.* Reduced pregnancy rates with unilateral or bilateral hydrosalpinx after *in vitro* fertilization. *Eur J Obstet Gynecol Reprod Biol* 1994;56:129–32

73. Levy MJ, Murray D, Sagoskin A. The adverse effect of hydrosalpinges on IVF success rates are reversed equally well by salpingectomy, proximal tubal occlusion and neosalpingostomy. Presented at the *Meeting of the American Society for Reproductive Medicine 1996*. Program Supplement. American Society for Reproductive Medicine, 1996:S64

74. Donnez J, Wauters M, Thomas K. Luteal function after tubal sterilization. *Obstet Gynecol* 1982;37:38

75. McComb P, Delbelke L. Decreasing the number of ovulations in the rabbit with surgical division of the blood vessels between the fallopian tube and ovary. *J Reprod Med* 1984;29:827–9

76. Sharif K, Kaufmann S, Sharma V. Heterotopic pregnancy obtained after *in vitro* fertilization and embryo transfer following bilateral total salpingectomy: case report. *Hum Reprod* 1994;9:1966–7

77. Pavic N, Neuenschwander E, Gschwind C, *et al.* Interstitial pregnancy following bilateral salpingectomy and *in vitro* fertilization–embryo transfer. *Fertil Steril* 1986;46:701–2

78. Donnez J, Nisolle M. Prognostic factors of distal tubal occlusion. In di Zerega GS, ed. *Peritoneal Surgery*. New York: Springer-Verlag, 2000:265–74

Ectopic pregnancy following assisted conception treatment and specific sites of ectopic pregnancy

15

C. Pirard, M. Nisolle and J. Donnez

ECTOPIC PREGNANCY AFTER ASSISTED REPRODUCTION AND HETEROTOPIC PREGNANCY

The first pregnancy ever conceived after *in vitro* fertilization–embryo transfer (IVF–ET) was an ectopic pregnancy[1]. Ectopic pregnancy occurs in 2–11% of all those pregnancies resulting from IVF treatment and, for unknown reasons, this incidence is much higher than that in the normal fertile population.

RISK FACTORS

Some risk factors for ectopic pregnancy are common after spontaneous pregnancy, as well as after IVF:

(1) Pelvic inflammatory disease (PID);

(2) Pre-existing tubal pathology or tubal surgery[2];

(3) Exposure to diethylstilbestrol (DES) *in utero;*

(4) The risk of ectopic pregnancy is two to 15 times higher in women with a previous ectopic pregnancy compared to women without such a history.

Some risk factors are specifically linked to the assisted conception treatment[3]. The use of clomiphene citrate for stimulation could induce a different hormonal milieu, that may interfere with tubal function, but this remains controversial. The number of patent Fallopian tubes at the time of embryo transfer, when the embryos are replaced higher than mid-cavity, and the technique of embryo transfer used could also play a role[4].

The technique of embryo transfer

The technique of embryo transfer may be implicated in the increased incidence of ectopic pregnancy after IVF.

Difficult embryo transfer

Lesny and co-workers[4] observed (in a group of oocyte donors) that a difficult embryo transfer, due to manipulation of the external rigid part of the catheter, multiple transfer attempts, change of catheter, application of a tenaculum to the cervix, and use of a uterine sound (or hegar dilators), stimulates junctional zone contractions and that strong endometrial waves in the fundal area of the uterus can move mock embryos into the Fallopian tubes. According to their findings, difficult transcervical embryo transfer should be perceived as a significant risk factor for ectopic pregnancy. Indeed, the overall risk of ectopic pregnancy is 1.5–10 times higher when the embryo transfer is difficult than when the transfer is easy.

Position of the catheter

The position of the catheter inside the uterus is also important. If the uterine fundus is reached during the transfer, fundocervical waves occur which could relocate the embryos toward the cervix or into the Fallopian tubes. It is recommended that the uterine fundus should not be stimulated and that a mid-cavitary delivery of the embryos (or keeping a minimal distance of 0.5–1 cm between the end of the catheter and the fundus) should be performed. Ultrasound measurement of uterine length is useful in patients with surgically shortened cervices.

Volume of transfer medium

Hydrostatic pressure due to a large volume of transfer medium or excessive force during embryo transfer may force migration of embryos into the tube. The catheter may also be placed into the tube itself.

HOW TO DIAGNOSE ECTOPIC PREGNANCY

The symptoms of ectopic pregnancy may be masked by symptoms frequently found after IVF (for example, ovarian hyperstimulation syndrome (OHSS) induces pain, pelvic liquid and heterogeneous adnexa at echography).

Some tests are helpful in the diagnosis of ectopic pregnancy, e.g. human chorionic gonadotropin (hCG) and transvaginal ultrasound. Early normal intrauterine pregnancies are associated with doubling of serum hCG concentrations every 1.4–2.1 days. An hCG titer of 1000–15 000 IU/l is associated with the presence of an intrauterine sac on transvaginal ultrasound.

In IVF patients, more than one embryo is generally transferred, so more trophoblastic tissue may be present to produce hCG. Thus, an extra 2 or 3 days are required for a sac to become visible. An intrauterine pregnancy, diagnosed by ultrasound, can be associated with an extra-uterine one[5,6] (see section on Heterotopic pregnancy below), or multiple extrauterine pregnancies can coexist.

IS THERE A RISK AFTER BILATERAL SALPINGECTOMY?

Some patients have indications for salpingectomy before starting an IVF program, because of severely damaged bilateral tubes, hydrosalpinges, salpingitis isthmica nodosa, and/or recurrent ectopic pregnancy. But even after bilateral salpingectomy, the risk of ectopic pregnancy still remains, even if it is reduced. Indeed, patients who undergo IVF–ET are at risk of cornual implantation.

Salpingectomy with cornual resection, performed in order to reduce the possibility of interstitial pregnancy, is not a good option, because this resection may attenuate the musculature in the cornual region, which can lead to rupture even early in the course of a subsequent pregnancy.

HETEROTOPIC PREGNANCY

Incidence and predisposing factors

Natural heterotopic pregnancy (or simultaneous intra- and extrauterine gestations) is a very rare condition. The first case was described by Duverney in 1708 at autopsy[8]. Because of the development of stimulated ovulation and IVF, the incidence of heterotopic pregnancy dramatically increased, then stabilized at approximately 1/100 pregnancies obtained by assisted reproductive technologies (ART)[4].

Fifty years ago, the incidence of spontaneous heterotopic pregnancies was estimated at 1/30 000 pregnancies, with an ectopic pregnancy rate of 0.37%. In the 1980s, the incidence of spontaneous heterotopic pregnancies reached a rate of 1/3000–1/10 000 because of the increased prevalence of PID and the frequent use of intrauterine devices. In patients treated with clomiphene citrate, the heterotopic pregnancy rate was calculated at 1/1250–1/3000.

Multiple ovulation or multiple embryo–gamete transfers, with the associated hormonal changes, have a major impact on the incidence of heterotopic pregnancies and the underlying tubopelvic pathology is contributory, mainly in assisted reproduction technology (ART) patients[4]. Nevertheless, some authors have not found any correlation between the number of embryos transferred and the rate of ectopic pregnancy after ART treatment[9]. The most important factor, however, that dramatically increased the incidence, was the induction of multiple ovulation and the exposure to multiple embryo–gamete transfers in patients consulting for infertility (some of whom have tubal damage).

Symptoms and diagnosis

The diagnosis of heterotopic pregnancy is very important because an early diagnosis allows prompt treatment, which will avoid maternal morbidity and mortality, and will also increase the chances of salvaging the associated intrauterine pregnancy.

Generally, the symptoms are abdominal pain or tenderness. Sometimes, there is also an acute abdomen and hypovolemic shock. Vaginal bleeding only occurs in 50% of patients, probably because of the coexisting intrauterine pregnancy. Vaginal bleeding (associated with abdominal pain) can lead to an erroneous diagnosis of miscarriage and be erroneously treated by dilatation and curettage (D&C). Echographic control, which will reveal an intrauterine pregnancy, is preferable before performing a D&C, especially in patients who have been treated for ovulation induction or by ART.

When the diagnosis is late, the clinical examination reveals abdominal pain, adnexal mass, signs of peritoneal irritation and an enlarged uterus.

Symptomless heterotopic pregnancies are sometimes detected due to early monitoring of pregnancy by transvaginal ultrasonography.

In the review of heterotopic pregnancy from 1971 to 1993 by Tal and colleagues[5], 59% of cases were discovered by laparotomy or laparoscopy. Sonographic detection was only possible in 41% of cases and was not always performed on first examination. Echographic diagnosis is easier when a fetal pole, with or without cardiac activity, is detected outside the uterine cavity. However, even in that case, the localization may be misconstrued if the echographist does not have enough experience (a cornual or cervical pregnancy can be misinterpreted as a second twin in an intrauterine pregnancy). The frequency of ultrasonic detection has undoubtedly increased since 1993, with the generalized use of vaginal ultrasonography. Sometimes, the diagnosis is only suspected at echography and then confirmed by surgery.

Localization

An ectopic pregnancy can be localized in the tube (in the ampullary part, in the isthmic portion, in the fimbria or cornua), on the ovary, in the cervix, or in the abdomen.

Heterotopic pregnancies with cornual or abdominal implantation can provoke diametric obstetric phenomena. The incidence of hemorrhagic shock is 2.5–5 times greater when a cornual pregnancy is detected, than in other varieties of ectopic pregnancy[10].

Bassil and co-workers[6] reported an abdominal pregnancy, detected by echography at only the 19th week of gestation, with both fetuses of corresponding size. The patient was hospitalized, tocolytics were administered until the 34th week, and two viable babies were delivered by laparotomy.

Treatment

Surgical treatment

Surgical treatment consists of laparotomy or laparoscopy. In most cases, salpingectomy is preferable to salpingotomy because conservative treatment requires control of the hCG decrease, which is impossible if the intrauterine pregnancy survives.

Total or partial ovariectomy is the surgical procedure performed to remove the ectopic gestation when it involves the ovary. The differential diagnosis from a ruptured and bleeding corpus luteum is not always easy.

Cervical pregnancy can be treated by curettage or suturing of the profusely bleeding cervix, but the chances of a surviving intrauterine pregnancy are very low[5]. In 2000, Carreno and colleagues[11] reported a case of heterotopic cervical and intrauterine pregnancy which was successfully managed by transcervical puncture of the cervical embryo and ended in a healthy newborn.

According to Habana and colleagues[12], cornually implanted ectopic pregnancy can be evacuated by uterine section and suture. Because of the expected continuation of the intrauterine pregnancy, this operation must be performed by laparotomy, which allows better suture of a uterus that is supposed to continue its growth and preserve further fertility. This type of surgery is nevertheless questionable. The question of KCl injection, at least as first-line therapy, must be discussed. In this case, laparotomy should be reserved in case of failed KCl injection.

Removal of an abdominal pregnancy by laparotomy is possible during pregnancy or, exceptionally, at the time of the Cesarean, when both fetuses continue to develop normally. Bassil and colleagues reported a case of delivery by laparotomy at 34 weeks of gestation[6].

If uncontrollable bleeding occurs, or if uterine tissue damage is extensive, hysterectomy remains the only option to save the mother's life.

During the operation, careful surgical handling is mandatory to avoid endangering the intrauterine pregnancy. But a complete check of the whole pelvis must be carried out because multiple ectopic pregnancies, even in both tubes, have been described[5].

Non-surgical management

Non-surgical management of early ectopic pregnancy has been described. Salpingocentesis with a long needle allows injection of KCl with or without methotrexate. The safety of this technique for the intrauterine pregnancy has not been proved. Active substances may enter the uterine circulation and damage the intrauterine pregnancy. Experience in transvaginal ultrasound-guided puncture is also needed to reduce the risk of miscarriage. In 1996, Fernandez and Benifla[13] reported their experience of the management of cornual pregnancy with methotrexate. In

their series of 15 cases, three were heterotopic pregnancies. Complete resolution was obtained in 13 cases (86.6%) with local injection of methotrexate (1 mg/kg) or KCl under transvaginal ultrasound guidance (*n* = 7) or a laparoscopic procedure (*n* = 6).

In some cases, salpingectomy is necessary after failed non-surgical management.

Spontaneous resolution of ectopic pregnancy under expectant management has also been encountered, but only three cases were described in the review by Tal and co-workers[5].

Conclusion

There is a very important question of ethics associated with the treatment of heterotopic pregnancy. The mother's life is involved but also the future of two or more babies, whose chances of being delivered alive are not equal. Approximately two-thirds of intrauterine pregnancies are delivered alive after treatment[5].

SPECIFIC SITES OF ECTOPIC PREGNANCY

Cornual pregnancy

Introduction

Cornual ectopic pregnancy is a rare entity, found in 2–4% of all ectopic pregnancies, with an estimated incidence of one in every 2500–5000 deliveries[14]. Correct diagnosis of cornual pregnancy in early gestation is difficult. Usually, uterine bleeding, pelvic pain and rupture occur later in pregnancy, compared with ectopic pregnancies located more distally in the Fallopian tube. Transvaginal echography can reveal the gestational sac in a very lateral position in the uterine cavity. Figure 1 demonstrates a case of pseudocornual pregnancy. Indeed, the gestational sac was found in the left uterine horn of an as yet undiagnosed

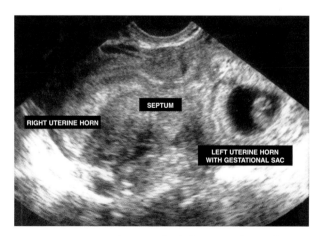

Figure 1 Gestational sac in the left uterine horn of an as yet undiagnosed bicornual uterus

bicornual uterus. In some instances[15] (see later), magnetic resonance imaging (MRI) can confirm a suspected cornual pregnancy.

However, rupture of cornual pregnancies may cause severe bleeding because they are located so close to the uterine blood supply and, in the literature, some cases of hysterectomy have been described because uterine disruption was extensive.

Treatment by surgical management

Laparotomy. Cornual ectopic pregnancy is the least common of the four tubal sites for ectopic gestations to be located. These ectopic gestations are most often treated by surgical excision, which at times necessitates removal of a portion of the myometrium as well. This raises concerns for possible uterine rupture if a subsequent pregnancy is achieved; thus, the mass of tissue excised must be kept to a minimum.

Laparoscopy. The possibility of laparoscopic management of cornual gestations has been demonstrated in several case reports (Table 1). The initial procedures that were described, however, did not preserve tubal continuity. For example, Hill and colleagues[17] described a patient who presented at 10 weeks' gestation with a large unruptured cornual pregnancy. The authors, after placing an endoloop (Ethicon) around the cornua, were able to evacuate the pregnancy using a unipolar current and blunt removal. In contrast, both Tulandi[19] and Reich[16] and their colleagues used laparoscopic cornual excision to manage interstitial pregnancy. Cornual excision has also been useful for the treatment of ruptured interstitial pregnancy[18].

A less extensive laparoscopic procedure was performed by Pasic and Wolfe[20]. They visualized a small cornual pregnancy which was evacuated through a 1-cm salpingostomy. Subsequent hemostasis was maintained with electrocoagulation. A similar procedure was successfully used by Pansky and colleagues[22]. Conservative laparoscopic management was also advocated by Gleicher and colleagues[21]. In their report, a twin gestation visualized on ultrasound, but small enough not to be seen at laparoscopy, was removed from the cornua by salpingostomy. It has been confirmed that

Table 1 Summary of the reported cases of laparoscopic management of cornual pregnancy

Reference	Operation	β-hCG (mIU/ml)	Diameter (cm)	Rupture	Estimated gestational age (weeks)	Vasopressin
Reich et al.[16]	CE	NA	NA	no	14	yes
	CE	NA	NA	no	NA	yes
	CE	NA	NA	no	NA	yes
Hill et al.[17]	S	NA	NA	no	10	yes
Reich et al.[18]	CE	16 300	NA	yes	NA	no
Tulandi et al.[19]	CE	6 000	3	no	6	yes
	CE	14 500	4	no	NA	yes
	CE	12 000	5	no	10	yes
	CE	4 700	5	no	6	yes
	S	8 000	4	no	6	yes
Pasic and Wolfe[20]	S	4 400	2	no	6	yes
Gleicher et al.[21]	S	7 704	0	no	NA	yes
Pansky et al.[22]	S	3 000	NA	no	7	yes
	S	2 600	NA	no	9	yes
Grobman and Milad[23]	S	32 827	4.5	no	7	yes
Donnez and Nisolle[24]	S	6 200		no	NA	yes + MTX
	S	7 000		no	NA	yes + MTX
	S	11 200		no	NA	yes + MTX
	S + CE	18 250		yes	NA	yes + MTX

MTX, methotrexate; CE, cornual excision; S, salpingotomy; NA, not available

conservative laparoscopic surgery could also be used successfully for larger cornual pregnancies[19].

A linear incision is made with monopolar electro-surgery parallel to the axis of the Fallopian tube, in order to minimize bleeding, or perpendicular, in order to mini-mize extension into the tube. After copious irrigation and suction, removal of the product of conception can be performed by laparoscopy. Cornual injection of diluted vasopressin (5 IU/20 ml saline solution) and coagulation of the implantation site are often necessary to stop the bleed-ing in this highly vascular region of the uterus. An injection of methotrexate (20 mg) in the implantation site can be administered only in cases of cornual pregnancy where the site of implantation is the distal portion of the intramural tube[24]. The question of the sutured closure of the cornual defect is still unresolved. Some authors use electrocoagula-tion with closure by secondary intention, and others make a sutured closure of the cornual defect.

In our series of ectopic pregnancies, we treated four cases of cornual pregnancy by laparoscopy according to the following technique:

(1) Injection of diluted vasopressin (2–5 IU/20 ml saline);

(2) Linear incision (Figure 2);

(3) Removal of trophoblast;

(4) Reducing coagulation to a minimum;

(5) Injection of 20 mg methotrexate in the implantation site;

(6) In one of the four cases, closure of the defect was carried out with one stitch (Vicryl 2.0).

Some authors recently published other modalities which probably do not offer any advantages over the previously described methods. In 1999, Rahimi[25] described the successful management of an interstitial ectopic pregnancy using three endoloops. In 2000, Moon and colleagues[26] reported a new approach to the endoscopic management of interstitial pregnancies (endoloop and encircling suture methods) without the uterine rupture encountered in the pregnancies subsequent to these methods of endoscopic

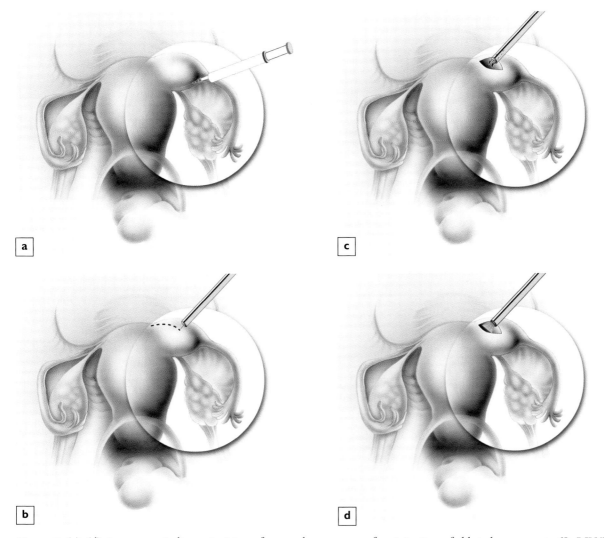

a   b   c   d

Figure 2 (a)–(d) Laparoscopic linear incision of cornual pregnancy after injection of diluted vasopressin (2–5 IU/20 ml saline) and subsequent injection of a mixed solution of methotrexate

management. Laparoscopy-controlled hysteroscopic removal of interstitial pregnancy and expectant management have also been described[27]. Most authors generally suggest that interstitial pregnancies larger than 4 cm in size may be better managed by cornual excision.

Non-surgical management: methotrexate

Methotrexate is generally preferred but, as already discussed, in case of heterotopic pregnancy, KCl injection could also be recommended. Different modalities of treatment with methotrexate exist: systemic, puncture and injection under laparoscopic or ultrasonographic guidance.

In 1996, Fernandez and Benifla[13] reported their experience of the management of cornual pregnancy with methotrexate. Complete resolution was obtained in 13 cases out of 15 (86.6%) with local injection of methotrexate (1 mg/kg) or KCl under transvaginal ultrasound guidance or during a laparoscopic procedure. In this series, three of the 15 cases were heterotopic pregnancies. However, Agarwal and colleagues[28] reported only one successful methotrexate treatment in a series of four cases of cornual pregnancies. Transvaginal utrasound-guided puncture has been proposed for the treatment of cornual pregnancy. However, risks of ectopic rupture and profuse bleeding following needle extraction still exist, even if potentially safer routes for puncture and injection of cornual pregnancies are used, as recommended by Timor-Tritsch and co-workers[29].

In 1997, Batioglu and colleagues[30] reported a case of cornual pregnancy which was successfully treated with two doses of methotrexate under laparoscopic and ultrasonographic guidance.

Anecdotal: triplet cornual pregnancy

We reported a case of triplet cornual pregnancy in a woman who underwent IVF–ET[15]. Transvaginal echography performed 35 days after embryo transfer showed three gestational sacs with heart beats in a very lateral position in the uterine cavity and also asymmetric development of the right uterine horn. MRI confirmed the sonographic suspicion of the localization of the three gestational sacs in the right uterine horn (Figure 3). Laparoscopy confirmed the cornual pregnancy with a very enlarged hypervascularized uterine horn without rupture (Figure 4). Immediate laparotomy permitted conservative treatment and uterine horn reconstruction.

Anecdotal: intramyometrial implantation

We encountered a case of intramyometrial implantation diagnosed after laparoscopy. Indeed, because of suspected ruptured tubal pregnancy (raised hCG and intraperitoneal hemorrhage), laparoscopy was carried out which detected a myometrial and serosal defect on the posterolateral side of the uterus. Because the patient had undergone a D&C

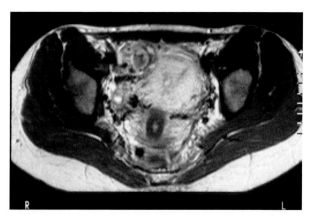

Figure 3 Triplet cornual pregnancy: magnetic resonance imaging confirmed the cornual localization of the three gestational sacs in the right uterine 'horn'

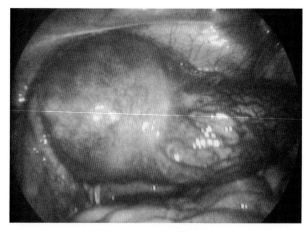

Figure 4 Laparoscopic view: very enlarged hypervascularized uterine horn of the case described in Figure 3

7 days before, perforation was suspected. Coagulation was performed and, after removal of blood clots and peritoneal lavage, methotrexate was injected into this area. There was a substantial decrease in the hCG level. Hysterosalpingography, carried out 2 months later, revealed a diverticulum in the myometrium (Figure 5).

Two years later, the patient experienced a recurrence of implantation in this 'myometrial' diverticulum. A laparoscopy performed because of hemoperitoneum with an hCG level of 2082 mIU/ml showed a suspected ovarian pregnancy which was not confirmed according to the criteria of ovarian pregnancy (see section on Ovarian pregnancy). The myometrial defect was visible (Figure 6) but, at the time, intramyometrial pregnancy was not suspected. The hCG levels increased over the following days and vaginal echography revealed an intramyometrial pregnancy (Figure 7) with only a 2-mm distance between the sac and the serosa. This sac was not visible on the day of the laparoscopy. Methotrexate (40 mg) was administered and hCG levels decreased rapidly, proving the efficacy of

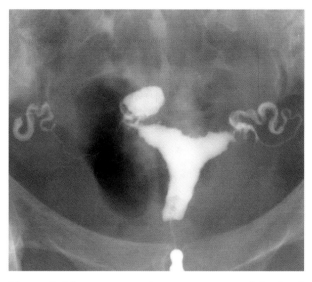

Figure 5 After myometrial pregnancy treated by local injection of methotrexate, hysterosalpingography carried out 2 months later revealed a diverticulum in the myometrium

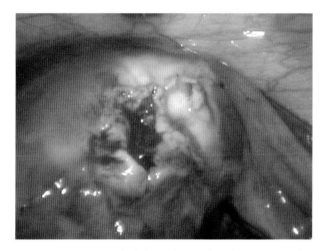

Figure 6 Myometrial defect observed at laparoscopy for diagnosis of suspected extrauterine pregnancy. The pregnancy was again located in the myometrial defect

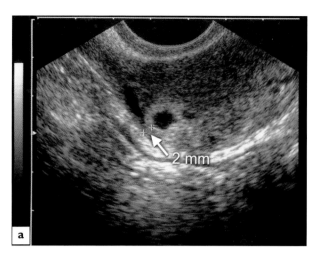

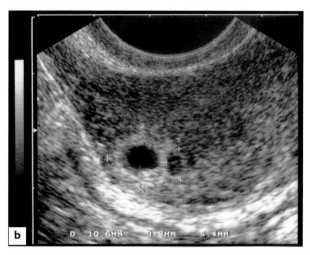

Figure 7 Vaginal echography: intramyometrial pregnancy (a) is obvious with only a 2-mm distance (b) between the sac and the serosa

methotrexate. After an increase to 5648 mIU/ml (day 3 post-methotrexate), hCG levels decreased (Figure 8). A second methotrexate injection (40 mg) was then given.

Results from a review by Lau and Tulandi[31]

In 1999, Lau and Tulandi[31] carried out a review of 41 patients with interstitial pregnancy who were treated either with methotrexate, or by a conservative laparoscopic technique, or with KCl injection (in case of heterotopic pregnancy). Methotrexate had a success rate of 83%. Conservative laparoscopic techniques had a success rate of 100% (n = 22). In cases of heterotopic pregnancy, after treatment (KCl or conservative surgery), 67% of coexisting intrauterine pregnancies resulted in successful deliveries.

There is insufficient evidence to recommend any single treatment modality, and the decision should be based on such factors as clinical presentation, the surgeon's expertise, side-effects, overall cost and the mother's wish to conceive again. Cornual resection by laparotomy should no longer be the first-line treatment for a hemodynamically stable patient with an interstitial pregnancy. Whatever treatment is chosen, the patient must be informed that any subsequent pregnancy must be followed very carefully because of the risk of future complications, such as recurrence or uterine rupture. Indications for Cesarean at term, prior to the onset of labor, must be decided before the next pregnancy occurs.

Ovarian pregnancy

Incidence and risk factors

The incidence of ovarian pregnancy is approximately 1/2000–1/7000 deliveries[32], i.e. less than 3% of all ectopic pregnancies, following natural conception. But the incidence of ovarian pregnancy after IVF–ET increases to 11% of all ectopic pregnancies. Apart from several reports on ovarian pregnancies following IVF–ET[32–36] or gamete intrafallopian transfer (GIFT)[37], only two cases after intrauterine insemination[38,39] have been reported so far. The common feature of all these cases is an enlargement of the ovary due to stimulation with gonadotropins, often with several hemorrhagic lutein cysts or corpora lutea. The increased vulnerability and vascularity of the ovary constitutes a higher risk of rupture with serious bleeding and, possibly, hemorrhagic shock. This considerably complicates manipulation of the ovary for diagnosis and therapy during operation, and even localization of the pregnancy in cases without rupture may be difficult[40]. Some cases will not be diagnosed because they can be mistaken for ruptured corpus luteum during laparoscopy or because of the use of medical management without performing prior laparoscopy.

According to Spiegelberg[41], the distinction between primary ovarian pregnancy and distal tubal pregnancy, a condition that can secondarily involve the ovary on its surface (secondary ovarian implantation), is based on four criteria:

(1) The Fallopian tubes with their fimbriae should be intact and separated from the ovary;

(2) The gestation should occupy the normal position in the ovary;

(3) The gestation should be connected to the uterus by the utero-ovarian ligament;

(4) Ovarian tissue must be present in the specimen attached to the gestational sac.

The risk factors are controversial. Globally, they are the same as those for ectopic pregnancy, except that the woman must have at least one patent tube, or a fistula which allows the sperm, or the embryo, to pass. The use of an intrauterine contraceptive device could be a more important risk factor than for other ectopic pregnancies[42].

Diagnosis

Ovarian pregnancy still presents problems of diagnosis, both in cases of ovarian stimulation and after natural conceptions.

Most of the time, the diagnosis of ectopic pregnancy is suspected by the clinical presentation of hCG levels and an empty uterus found on vaginal echography (with or without signs of adnexal mass or fluid in the pouch of Douglas) (Figure 9), but, in most cases, the localization of the pregnancy is not known exactly before performing the operation. Vaginal echography can lead to the incorrect diagnosis of an ovarian cyst (corpus luteum, endometrioma) and threatened abortion.

When a patient undergoes IVF–ET or ovulation stimulation, the ultrasonic aspect of the ovaries changes, which increases the risk of misdiagnosis. However, even during laparoscopy, it is not easy to localize a pregnancy when it is surrounded by several corpora lutea[40,43]. If a gestational sac has been clearly identified on vaginal echography, intraoperative transvaginal ultrasonography can be helpful after filling the lower pelvis with saline solution, but laparoscopy remains the gold standard for the diagnosis of ovarian pregnancy (Figure 10). In some cases, definitive diagnosis must await histological confirmation, which will show microscopic ovarian tissue around the gestational sac. However, this is not always possible, due to coagulation artefacts and the small tissue volume available.

Etiology

Three mechanisms can explain ovarian implantation:

(1) Fertilization occurs normally and implantation in the ovary follows reflux of the conceptus from the tube;

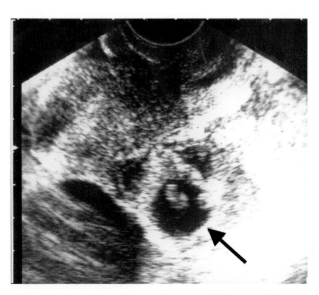

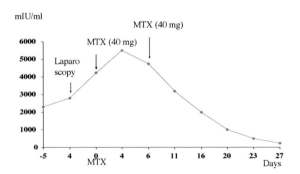

Figure 8 Evolution of intramyometrial pregnancy: hCG level following intramuscular injection of 40 mg methotrexate (MTX)

Figure 9 Vaginal echography revealed an embryonic ovarian pregnancy. The arrow shows the embryonic ectopic pregnancy

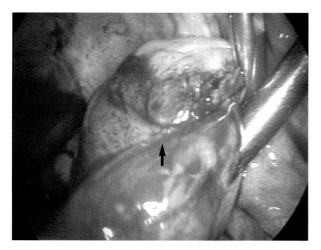

Figure 10 Laparoscopic view of ovarian pregnancy

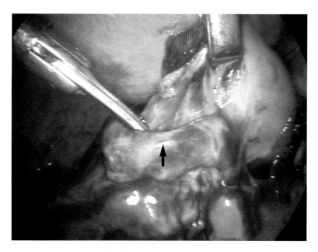

Figure 11 Removal of ovarian pregnancy

(2)   Various disturbances in ovum release are responsible for ovarian implantation;

(3)   Intrauterine insemination could push some spermatozoa all the way to the ovarian surface and lead to ovarian implantation[39].

Treatment by surgical management

Compared to laparotomy, laparoscopy has the advantage of reducing morbidity, hospitalization and probably the risk of postoperative adhesion formation, which is important to women of childbearing age[43].

Van Coevering and Fisher[44] were the first, in 1988, to report a laparoscopic approach used at an early stage of ovarian pregnancy. In fact, they removed what they believed to be a hemorrhagic corpus luteum cyst, but pathological examination showed an ovarian pregnancy.

After performing laparoscopy, copious pelvic lavage of the hemoperitoneum is carried out to facilitate the exploration of the pelvis and both ovaries. The pregnancy can be removed using biopsy forceps or enucleation (Figure 11). Deeper trophoblastic invasion of the ovarian stroma requires aggressive thermal coagulation for hemostasis. We prefer to use bipolar coagulation with 2 mm-wide bipolar forceps for hemostasis of the placental site, because extensive thermal damage could cause undesired superficial ovarian injury. Moreover, the site of the ovarian implantation causes a relative defect of the ovarian surface which could lead to adhesion formation. In order to avoid this type of complication, the ovary may be covered with a piece of Interceed (Johnson and Johnson, NY, USA) The use of a CO_2 laser has also been described[45] in order to vaporize the placental site.

Partial ovariectomy (ovarian wedge resection), including the site of implantation, or ovarian cystectomy must be performed if possible. Ovariectomy or adnexectomy is performed when a more conservative treatment is not possible. In all cases, one must take into consideration the

patient's desire for future pregnancy, and the operative feasibility.

Medical management

Medical management of ovarian pregnancy has been reported by some authors. They described the use of methotrexate[46], prostaglandin, prostaglandin and estrogen, and mifepristone. We believe that, as laparoscopy is generally needed to confirm the diagnosis, surgical treatment must be carried out at the same time.

Methotrexate is, in our opinion, only indicated as a secondary option for organ-preserving operations with primary incomplete resection or trophoblast persistence, as shown by the disappointing decrease in hCG level after the operation.

Cervical pregnancy

Incidence

The incidence of cervical pregnancy ranges from 1/2400 to 1/50 000 pregnancies; it occurs in 0.15% of all ectopic pregnancies and in 0.1% of IVF pregnancies.

Diagnosis

When an embryo implants and grows within the endocervical canal, it can lead to life-threatening bleeding. Previously, diagnosis was often made only at the time of D&C when extensive hemorrhage occurred.

Early diagnosis is now facilitated by the use of transvaginal ultrasound. Sonographic criteria of cervical pregnancy include endocervical localization of the gestational sac and trophoblastic invasion. Differential diagnosis from Naboth eggs (Figure 12) must be considered. MRI can be performed to eliminate any doubt and to confirm the ectopic location of the implantation site.

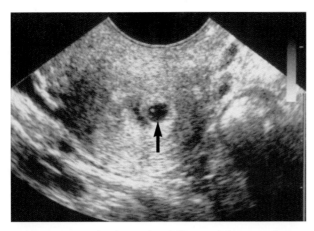

Figure 12 Vaginal echography: differential diagnosis from a Naboth egg (arrow) is not always easy

Etiology and risk factors

The pathogenesis of cervical pregnancy is poorly understood. Prior surgical uterine manipulation and tubal disease are implicated as risk factors for cervical pregnancy, but it remains unclear. In certain cases of IVF, reflux of the embryo into the cervix after transfer or trauma to the cervix during embryo transfer are two possible contributory factors[47].

Treatment by non-conservative surgical technique

Before 1979, hysterectomy was performed to save the life of the patient in about 90% of cases. This type of surgery has now become obsolete thanks to conservative (surgical and medical) procedures.

Treatment by conservative surgical techniques

In order to preserve women's fertility, conservative surgical techniques have been developed. The main problem of conservative treatment is life-threatening hemorrhage after pregnancy evacuation. Cervical curettage can be followed by intracervical balloon tamponade, cervical cerclage or local prostaglandin instillation. Angioembolization of the uterine artery and bilateral ligation of the hypogastric arteries are other possibilities for hemorrhage control when the previously described techniques have failed. In a review by Ushakov and colleagues[48], the use of cervical canal tamponade with a Foley catheter balloon after pregnancy evacuation led to reliable hemostasis in 92.3% of cases.

Ash and Farrell[49] have reported a case of hysteroscopic resection of a 6-week cervical pregnancy.

Non-surgical treatment techniques

In 1998, Hung and colleagues[50] reported a review of 52 cases of cervical pregnancy primarily treated by methotrexate (locally, systemic, or both). The overall success rate was 61.5% (32/52): 90.9% (20/22) and 40% (12/30) for cervical pregnancy without or with embryonic cardiac activity, respectively.

From the pooled data derived from the literature review[51], factors that increased the risk for unsatisfactory primary methotrexate treatment were:

(1) Gestational age ≥ 9 weeks;

(2) hCG ≥ 10 000 mIU/ml;

(3) Embryonic cardiac activity;

(4) Crown–rump length of > 10 mm.

In this review[50], the number of previous D&Cs, previous Cesareans and the maximal diameter of the gestational sacs did not influence the results. In some cases, two techniques can be associated to improve results. Concomitant feticide (with intracardiac KCl injection) and methotrexate can be performed to minimize the potential risk of methotrexate failure, if embryonic cardiac activity is evident. In their series, failure of methotrexate treatment was noted in a total of 20 cases. Causes for abdominal interventions included massive or uncontrollable bleeding ($n = 6$), rise in serum β-hCG levels ($n = 6$), persistent cervical ectopic gestations ($n = 7$) and the appearance or persistence of embryonic cardiac activity ($n = 7$). Out of these 20 patients, 15 were successfully treated with one of the following additional therapeutic modalities:

(1) Systemic methotrexate administration;

(2) Intra-amniotic methotrexate instillation;

(3) Intracardiac injection of KCl (feticide);

(4) D&C;

(5) Embolization of uterine arteries;

(6) Conservative abdominal surgery.

The five remaining patients needed more than one additional operation. Among them, three underwent hysterectomy due to uncontrollable bleeding.

Conclusions

Whatever treatment was used, they were all associated with some degree of failure. Combination of treatments was possible. Sometimes after treatment, rapid and massive bleeding from the uninvolutive and atonic cervix may occur unexpectedly and lead to hysterectomy.

Conservative treatment with methotrexate (followed or not by other conservative treatment) carries a 91% success rate for preservation of the uterus[51,52].

Ectopic pregnancy in a Cesarean section scar

This entity must be distinguished clearly from cervical pregnancy[53]. Pregnancy developing in a previous Cesarean section scar is the rarest type of ectopic pregnancy. The risk involved in this type of pregnancy is that of uterine rupture and hemorrhage, requiring emergency hysterectomy[54–56]. As an explanation for this entity, the most reasonable hypothesis is that the conceptus enters the myometrium through a microscopic dehiscent tract of the Cesarean section scar. In 1993, a case was diagnosed by echography and required hysterectomy due to rupture and extensive bleeding at week 24 of gestation[55]. In 1995, another case was treated conservatively by methotrexate but laparotomy was required 2 weeks after injection because of extensive bleeding[57]. Still more recently, hysterectomy was performed to accomplish pregnancy termination[58].

In our report[53,59], the first case of ectopic pregnancy developing in a previous Cesarean section scar diagnosed by vaginal echography and MRI was treated successfully by local injection of KCl and methotrexate. This minimally invasive non-surgical approach can preserve fertility without any major risk to the mother.

Since the advent of endovaginal echography (Figure 13) and MRI (Figure 14), it has been possible to make the diagnosis earlier in the gestation and to use a more conservative approach. Strict imaging criteria must be used to assess the diagnosis: empty uterus, empty cervical canal, development of the sac in the anterior part of the isthmic portion, and an absence of healthy myometrium between the bladder and the sac. This last criterion allows us to differentiate a pregnancy implanted in a Cesarean scar from cervical or cervicoisthmic pregnancy.

At 9 weeks of amenorrhea, the embryo had a crown–rump length of 24 mm and persistent cardiac activity. No myometrium was visible between the bladder and the sac, which obviously bulged in a 'prerupture' stage (Figure 13). The uterine cavity remained empty. To confirm the diagnosis, MRI was carried out. The uterine cavity was empty, although trophoblastic tissue and an embryo were seen on a transverse section in the anterior portion of the cervix (Figure 14) outside the endocervical canal, in a previous Cesarean section scar.

Because of the risk of uterine rupture, it was decided to interrupt the pregnancy. Under the guidance of endovaginal sonography, a 22-gauge needle was introduced transvaginally into the gestational sac through the cervix, 8 Meq KCl (2 Meq/ml) was injected directly into the fetal thorax to stop cardiac motion and 60 mg of methotrexate was injected into the sac and the surrounding myometrium.

The subsequent course was characterized by a steady progressive resorption of the pregnancy, as demonstrated by the decrease in the hCG level. The hCG levels were 62 000, 39 800, 11 900, 552 and 114 mIU/ml on days 0, 5, 12, 23 and 45, respectively. It was finally undetectable on day 82 (Figure 15). Sonographic findings showed a rapid disappearance of the fetal pole, with persistent amorphous echoes. On day 96, an ultrasound examination demonstrated a normal non-gravid uterus and cervix. There was no change in either liver function or bone marrrow suppression. Bleeding and uterine cramps were intermittent and minimal.

The patient experienced menstrual bleeding 16 weeks after the methotrexate injection. A hysterosalpingography was performed and demonstrated a dehiscent Cesarean section scar. Because of the very low risk of recurrence of an ectopic pregnancy in this site, it was decided that the patient could attempt to conceive. She delivered a healthy baby 14 months later by Cesarean section performed at 38 weeks.

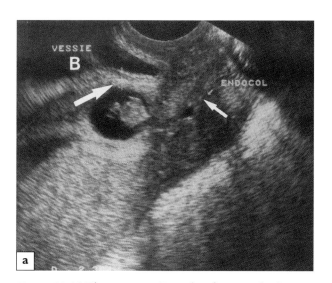 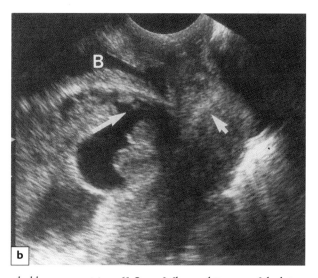

Figure 13 (a) The gestation (7 weeks of amenorrhea) was surrounded by myometrium (1.2 mm) (long white arrow) bulging from the serosal surface of the uterus. Short white arrow, endocervical canal; B, bladder. (b) At 9 weeks of amenorrhea, the embryo had a crown–rump length of 24 mm. No myometrium (long white arrow) was visualized between the sac and the bladder. Short white arrow, endocervical canal; B, bladder

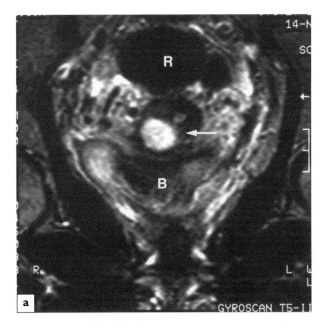

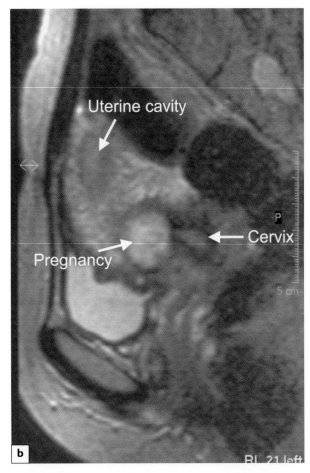

Figure 14 (a) Magnetic resonance imaging (MRI): transverse section clearly demonstrated the pregnancy (arrow) implanted in the anterior portion of the cervix, outside the endocervical canal. R, rectum; B, bladder. (b) Sagittal section demonstrated the pregnancy implanted in the anterior portion of the cervix. The cervical canal as well the uterine cavity are clearly visible

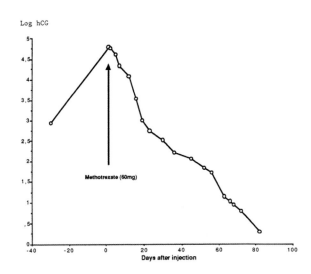

Figure 15 Cesarean scar pregnancy: evolution of hCG levels following intrauterine methotrexate administration

REFERENCES

1. Steptoe PC, Edwards RG. Reimplantation of the human embryo with subsequent tubal pregnancy. *Lancet* 1976;1:880

2. Marcus SF, Brinsden P. Analysis of the incidence and risk factors associated with ectopic pregnancy following *in-vitro* fertilization, and embryo transfer. *Hum Reprod* 1995;10:190

3. Abusheikha N, Salha O, Brinsden P. Extra-uterine pregnancy following assisted conception treatment. *Hum Reprod Update* 2000;6:80

4. Lesny P, Killick SR, Robinson J, *et al.* Transcervical embryo transfer as a risk factor for ectopic pregnancy. *Fertil Steril* 1999;72:305

5. Tal J, Haddad S, Godon N, *et al.* Heterotopic pregnancy after ovulation induction and assisted reproductive technologies: a literature review from 1971 to 1993. *Fertil Steril* 1996;66:1

6. Bassil S, Pouly JL, Canis M, *et al.* Advanced heterotopic pregnancy after *in-vitro* fertilization and embryo transfer, with survival of both the babies and the mother. *Hum Reprod* 1991;6:1008

7. Inovay J, Marton T, Urbancsek J, *et al.* Spontaneous bilateral cornual uterine dehiscence early in the second trimester after bilateral laparoscopic salpingectomy and *in-vitro* fertilization. *Hum Reprod* 1999;14:2471

8. Reece EA, Petrie RH, Sirmans MF, *et al.* Combined intrauterine and extrauterine gestations: a review. *Am J Obstet Gynecol* 1983;146:323

9. Verhulst G, Camus M, Bollen N, *et al.* Analysis of the risk factors with regard to the occurrence of ectopic

pregnancy after medically assisted procreation. *Hum Reprod* 1993;8:1284

10. Felmus LB, Pedowitz P. Interstitial pregnancy: a survey of 45 cases. *Am J Obstet Gynecol* 1953;66:1271

11. Carreno C.A, King M, Johnson MP, *et al.* Treatment of heterotopic cervical and intrauterine pregnancy. *Fetal Diagn Ther* 2000;15:1

12. Habana A, Dokras A, Giraldo JL, *et al.* Cornual heterotopic pregnancy: contemporary management options. *Am J Obstet Gynecol* 2000;182:1264

13. Fernandez H, Benifla JL. Medical treatment of cornual pregnancy? *Fertil Steril* 1996;66:862

14. Thompson JD, Rock JA. *Te Linde's (1997) Operative Gynecology*, 8th edn. Philadephia: JB Lippincott, 1997

15. Bassil S, Gordts S, Nisolle M, *et al.* A magnetic resonance imaging approach for the diagnosis of a triplet cornual pregnancy. *Fertil Steril* 1995;5:1029

16. Reich H, Johns DA, DeCaprio J, *et al.* Laparoscopic treatment of 109 consecutive ectopic pregnancies. *J Reprod Med* 1988;33:885–90

17. Hill GA, Segars JH, Herbert CA. Laparoscopic management of interstitial pregnancy. *J Gynecol Surg* 1989;5:209–12

18. Reich H, McGlynn F, Budin R, *et al.* Laparoscopic treatment of ruptured interstitial pregnancy. *J Gynecol Surg* 1990;6:135–8

19. Tulandi T, Vilos G, Gomel V. Laparoscopic treatment of interstitial pregnancy. *Obstet Gynecol* 1995;85:465–7

20. Pasic R, Wolfe WM. Laparoscopic diagnosis and treatment of interstitial ectopic pregnancy: a case report. *Am J Obstet Gynecol* 1990;163:587–8

21. Gleicher N, Karande V, Rabin D, *et al.* Laparoscopic removal of twin cornual pregnancy after *in vitro* fertilization. *Fertil Steril* 1994;61:1161–2

22. Pansky M, Bukovsky I, Golan A, *et al.* Conservative management of interstitial pregnancy using operative laparoscopy. *Surg Endosc* 1995;9:515–16

23. Grobman WA, Milad MP. Conservative laparoscopic management of a large cornual ectopic pregnancy. *Hum Reprod* 1998;13:2002

24. Donnez J, Nisolle M. Endoscopic management of ectopic pregnancy. *Bailliere's Clin Obstet Gynaecol* 1994;8:707

25. Rahimi MA. A new laparoscopic approach for the treatment of interstitial ectopic pregnancy. *J Am Assoc Gynecol Laparosc* 1999;6:205

26. Moon HS, Choi YJ, Park YH, *et al.* New simple endoscopic operations for interstitial pregnancies. *Am J Obstet Gynecol* 2000;182:114

27. Woodland MB, DePasquale SE, Molinari JA, *et al.* Laparoscopic approach to interstitial pregnancy. *J Am Assoc Gynecol Laparosc* 1996;3:439

28. Agarwal SK, Wisot AL, Garzo G, *et al.* Cornual pregnancies in patients with prior salpingectomy under-

going *in vitro* fertilization and embryo transfer. *Fertil Steril* 1996;65:659

29. Timor-Tritsch IE, Monteagudo A, Lerner JP. A 'potentially safer' route for puncture and injection of cornual ectopic pregnancies. *Ultrasound Obstet Gynecol* 1996;7:353

30. Batioglu S, Haberal A, Yesilyurt H, *et al.* Successful treatment of cornual pregnancy by local injection of methotrexate under laparoscopic and transvaginal ultrasonographic guidance. *Gynecol Obstet Invest* 1997;44:64

31. Lau S, Tulandi T. Conservative medical and surgical management of interstitial ectopic pregnancy. *Fertil Steril* 1999;72:207

32. Riethmuller D, Sautiere JL, Benoit S, *et al.* Ultrasonic diagnosis and laparoscopic treatment of an ovarian pregnancy. A case report and review of the literature. *J Gynecol Obstet Biol Reprod Paris* 1996;25:378

33. Rizk B, Lachelin CL, Davies MC, *et al.* Ovarian pregnancy following *in-vitro* fertilization and embryo transfer. *Hum Reprod* 1990;5:763–4

34. Marcus SF, Brinsden PR. Primary ovarian pregnancy after *in vitro* fertilization and embryo transfer: report of seven cases. *Fertil Steril* 1993;60:167–9

35. Ranieri DM, Vicino MG, Simonetti S, *et al.* Gravidanza eterotopica ovarica dopo fertilizzazione in vitro ed embryo transfer e gravidanza tubarica controlaterale dopo trasferimento intratubarico dei gameti. *Minerva Ginecol* 1994;46:365–8

36. Shibahara H, Funabiki M, Shiotani T, *et al.* A casc of primary ovarian pregnancy after *in vitro* fertilization and embryo transfer. *J Assist Reprod Genet* 1997;14:63–4

37. Lehmann F, Baban N, Harms B, *et al.* Ovarialgravidität nach Gametentransfer (GIFT), Ein Fallbericht. *Geburtshilfe Frauenheilkd* 1991;51:945–7

38. El-Lakany NEH, Hock YL, Boyd NRH. Primary ovarian pregnancy following intra-uterine insemination. *J Obstet Gynecol* 1995;15:182–3

39. Bontis J, Grimbizis G, Tarlatzis BC, *et al.* Intrafollicular ovarian pregnancy after ovulation induction/intrauterine insemination: patho-physiological aspects and diagnostic problems. *Hum Reprod* 1997;12:376–8

40. Einenkel J, Baier D, Horn LC, *et al.* Laparoscopic therapy of an intact primary ovarian pregnancy with ovarian hyperstimulation syndrome: case report. *Hum Reprod* 2000;15:2037–40

41. Spiegelberg O. Zur kasuistick der ovarialschwangerschaff. *Arch Gynekol* 1878;13:73

42. Ercal T, Cinar O, Mumcu A, *et al.* Ovarian pregnancy; relationship to an intrauterine device. *Aust N Z J Obstet Gynaecol* 1997;37:362

43. Seinera P, Di-Gregorio A, Arisio R, *et al.* Ovarian pregnancy and operative laparoscopy: report of eight cases. *Hum Reprod* 1997;12:608

44. Van Coevering RJ, Fisher JE. Laparoscopic management of ovarian pregnancy. A case report. *J Reprod Med* 1988;33:774

45. Godenberg M, Bider D, Maschiach S, *et al.* Laparoscopic laser surgery of primary ovarian pregnancy. *Hum Reprod* 1994;9:1337

46. Chelmow D, Gates E, Penzias AS. Laparoscopic diagnosis and methotrexate treatment of an ovarian pregnancy: a case report. *Fertil Steril* 1994;62:879

47. Ginsburg ES, Fox JH, Frates MC. Early diagnosis and treatment of cervical pregnancy in an *in vitro* fertilization program. *Fertil Steril* 1994;61:966

48. Ushakov FB, Elchalal U, Aceman PJ, *et al.* Cervical pregnancy: past and future. *Obstet Gynecol Surv* 1997;52:45

49. Ash S, Farrell SA. Hysteroscopic resection of a cervical ectopic pregnancy. *Fertil Steril* 1996;66:842

50. Hung TH, Shau WY, Hsieh TT, *et al.* Prognostic factors for an unsatisfactory primary methotrexate treatment of cervical pregnancy: a quantitative review. *Hum Reprod* 1998;13:2642

51. Kung FT, Chang SY, Tsai YC, *et al.* Subsequent reproduction and obstetric outcome after methotrexate treatment of cervical pregnancy: a review of original literature and international collaborative follow-up. *Hum Reprod* 1997;12:591

52. Kung FT, Chang SY. Efficacy of methotrexate treatment in viable and nonviable cervical pregnancies. *Am J Obstet Gynecol* 1999;181:1438

53. Godin PA, Bassil S, Donnez J. An ectopic pregnancy developing in a previous Caesarian section scar. *Fertil Steril* 1997;67:398

54. Herman A, Weinraub Z, Avrech O, *et al.* Follow-up and outcome of isthmic pregnancy located in a previous caesarean section scar. *Br J Obstet Gynaecol* 1995;102:839–41

55. Wehbe A, Ioan A, Allart JP, *et al.* A case of cervico-isthmic pregnancy with delayed development. *Rev Fr Gynecol Obstet* 1993;88:439–44

56. Rempen A, Albert P. Diagnosis and therapy of an in the caesarean section scar implanted early pregnancy. *Geburtshilfe Pertinatol* 1990;194:46–8

57. Lay YM, Lee JD, Lee CL, *et al.* An ectopic pregnancy embedded in the myometrium of a previous caesarean section scar. *Acta Obstet Gynecol Scand* 1995;74:573–6

58. Valley MT, Pierce JC, Daniel TB, *et al.* Cesarean scar pregnancy: imaging and treatment with conservative surgery. *Obstet Gynecol* 1998;91:838

59. Donnez J, Godin PA, Bassil S. Successful methotrexate treatment of a viable pregnancy within a thin uterine scar. *Br J Obstet Gynaecol* 1997;104:1255

Medical treatment: the place of methotrexate

16

J. Donnez, C. Pirard and M. Nisolle

METHOTREXATE AS FIRST-LINE THERAPY

Since the first reports by Stovall and colleagues in 1989[1,2], methotrexate (MTX) has been extensively studied and may offer an alternative to laparoscopic surgery. This treatment can be proposed when a diagnosis of unruptured ectopic pregnancy (EP) is made.

MTX allows effective treatment of unruptured EP at low cost, but the question is, how can one establish that the EP is not ruptured, or that there is no active bleeding, without performing a laparoscopy? Also, if laparoscopy is needed to confirm the diagnosis of unruptured pregnancy, it is then less expensive and more logical to treat it by laparoscopy.

The rupture rate of tubal pregnancies, confirmed by laparoscopy, is 18–36% (42% in 1991)[3]. According to Mol and colleagues[4], abdominal pain, rebound tenderness on abdominal examination, fluid in the pouch of Douglas at transvaginal ultrasound and a low serum hemoglobin level are independent predictive factors for tubal rupture and/or active bleeding. But the most sensitive predictor factor is abdominal pain (sensitivity of 95%). Surprisingly, they found that pregnancy obtained by *in vitro* fertilization–embryo transfer (IVF–ET) and the presence of an ectopic gestational sac or an ectopic mass at echography reduced the risk of tubal rupture.

Fernandez and colleagues[5–9] have proposed using a predictive pre-therapeutic score for the medical treatment of EP.

Six criteria are assessed and graded on a scale of 1 to 3:

(1) Gestational age;

(2) Level of human chorionic gonadotropin (hCG);

(3) Progesterone level;

(4) Presence of abdominal pain;

(5) Echographic evaluation of hemoperitoneum volume;

(6) Hematosalpinx diameter.

The success rate of medical treatment is more than 90% when the pre-therapeutic score is less than 13 (which represents ± 30–40% of patients with EP).

Different means of administration are described: systemic (intramuscular or intravenous), oral, locally injected at laparoscopy or under ultrasound guidance. There is also a great heterogeneity in the use of MTX at doses ranging from 0.4 to 1 mg/kg per day given one to four times. Single-dose MTX (1 mg/kg) seems to be as effective as the multidose regimen[8,9].

Injection under ultrasonic guidance

Transvaginal ultrasound aims to localize the EP. The procedure is carried out without anesthesia, with an 18-gauge needle inserted into a needle introducer. First, the gestational sac is aspirated and then the MTX is injected (1 mg/kg). In some cases, this technique allows confirmation of the diagnosis by histological examination. In fact, it constitutes an association between mechanical and medical management.

In a study by Fernandez and colleagues[8], MTX was administered into the sac in 29 women, and was given intramuscularly to 22 women whose sac could not be safely or easily punctured. Patients followed up by telephone were aware of the possibility of treatment failure, which was defined by the persistence of high hCG concentrations or by the onset of abdominal pain, or both. In such cases, patients were treated either by laparoscopy or by a second injection of MTX when the patients were asymptomatic. The success rate (88.2%) obtained after MTX injection was similar to the rate after laparoscopic salpingotomy (95.9%)[9].

There were no statistical differences between local and intramuscular administration of MTX. Nevertheless, it is important to note that four of the six failures occurred among patients who received an intramuscular injection.

In conclusion, local MTX treatment under ultrasound guidance was associated with high tissue MTX concentrations with fewer systemic side-effects than after intramuscular administration. The study by Fernandez and colleagues[8] demonstrates that, when the ectopic sac is easily visualized by echography, direct puncture and injection of a minimal dose of 1 mg/kg MTX are as effective as systemic treatment, with no side-effects for the patients. However, side-effects were rare in their study[8,9]. An initial rise in hCG plasma levels after medical treatment might reflect an increase in hCG metabolism due to intracellular polyglutamation of MTX and/or trophoblastic cell necrosis, with release of hCG into the maternal circulation.

Injection at laparoscopy

In 1993, Pansky and associates[10] published a study of 77 unruptured EPs treated by laparoscopic injection of MTX (12.5 mg or 25 mg), and concluded that local MTX injection does not modify tubal or pelvic anatomy and does not impair subsequent reproductive performance, compared with laparoscopic salpingotomy. We do not fully agree, however. Indeed, we consider that, when an ectopic sac is found at laparoscopy, a linear salpingotomy to remove the trophoblast or a salpingectomy should be performed immediately. During laparoscopy, local injection of MTX should be indicated only in cases of cornual ectopic pregnancy or in cases of large tubal pregnancy with embryos with cardiac activity.

Systemic treatment (Table 1)

In 1994, it was concluded that, when echo-guided local injection of MTX looks difficult or is not readily available, systemic MTX injection (1 mg/kg, intramuscularly) should be administered[8]. Systemic MTX therapy is associated with a prolonged duration of treatment, potential drug toxicity, pain during treatment and the need for scrupulous follow-up. Repeat injection of MTX (or laparoscopic treatment) is required only when the hCG level increases above the normal regression curve. Many authors (see the review by Morlock and colleagues[11]) have proposed the systemic approach as first-line therapy. The selection criteria are those already described, involving determination of the pre-therapeutic score[5-9].

Following the first reports[1,2], a review by Morlock and colleagues in 2000[11] clearly analyzed the pros and cons of this approach.

Resolution rates of women treated by laparoscopy and single-dose methotrexate used in the baseline model were analyzed. The published resolution rates of studies with laparoscopy ranged from 72% to 100%[12-25], whereas the overall resolution rates for MTX therapy ranged from 75% to 90%[10,28-34]. The average rate of laparoscopic resolution was 90%. The average resolution rate in studies whose reports included first- and second-dose MTX resolution rates was 84%. This has placed the medical treatment of

EP securely within the therapeutic options of general practice gynecologists because of the ease of application and the low incidence of serious side-effects. However, the high success rates reported by Stovall and Ling[35] have been difficult to reproduce in other studies. Many believe that randomized clinical trials are required before MTX treatment can be considered anything other than second-line or experimental therapy[36].

In terms of fertility sparing, laparoscopy successfully resolves pregnancies more than 90% of the time, with relatively low complication rates.

Follow-up

Regression of the hCG level must be followed until it reaches the assay detection limit. The timing of regression is well known and regression curves are often used.

It is interesting to note that, after injection of MTX, there is, initially, an increase in hCG (between day 1 and 4), which might reflect an increase in hCG metabolism, as stated earlier in this chapter. The hCG resolution time is shorter when a salpingotomy is performed than when MTX is used[37].

Failure of treatment

When non-surgical treatment does not succeed, even after repeat MTX injection, surgical management must be decided upon. The most frequent reason to perform laparoscopy is unusual abdominal pain, an inadequate decrease in hCG plasma levels, an acute hemoperitoneum and an increase in hematosalpinx observed by echography. Conservative laparoscopic treatment is then advocated.

Table 1 Success rates of systemic methotrexate

Study	Number of women	Type of protocol	Success rate n (%)
Lipscomb et al.[38]	352	single intramuscular dose	322 (91.5)
Stovall et al.[2]	100	multiple intramuscular doses	96 (96.0)
Henry and Gentry[34]	61	single intramuscular dose	52 (85.2)
Hajenius et al.[15]	51	multiple intramuscular doses	44 (86.3)
Thoen and Creinin[30]	47	single intramuscular dose	43 (91.5)
Stika et al.[31]	50	single intramuscular dose	39 (78.0)
Corsan et al.[32]	44	single intramuscular dose	33 (75.0)
Schafer et al.[39]	40	various single intravenous doses	37 (92.5)
Saraj et al.[37]	38	single intramuscular dose	36 (94.7)
Lecuru et al.[13]	37	single intramuscular dose	34 (91.9)
Glock et al.[33]	35	single intramuscular dose	30 (85.7)
Fernandez et al.[9]	22	single intramuscular dose	18 (47.4)
Total	877		784 (89.4)

Discussion

In 1993, Stovall and Ling[35] reported a resolution rate of 94% in a series of 120 patients treated with single-dose intramuscular MTX (50 mg/m^2). Post-treatment hCG demonstrated tubal patency on the ipsilateral side in 82% of patients.

In 1999, Lipscomb and colleagues[38] reported the results of their study of 350 patients treated with intramuscular MTX according to a single-dose protocol. They observed a success rate of 91%. They concluded that the pretreatment hCG concentration was the most important factor contributing to the failure rate.

According to Morlock and co-workers[11], who carried out a cost-effectiveness comparison between single-dose MTX and laparoscopic treatment of EP, MTX is $3000 less expensive than laparoscopy, as front-line therapy for unruptured EP. In this review, they mentioned that the average resolution rate was 87% with MTX and 91% with laparoscopy.

In conclusion, MTX given intramuscularly is a valid option when laparoscopy does not offer a diagnosis and the ectopic mass is smaller than 4 cm, when the gestational sac is no longer viable, and when the ectopic pregnancy cannot be safely and easily punctured under echographic guidance. In the presence of cardiac activity in the EP, we consider MTX treatment to be contraindicated and we prefer to perform laparoscopy and salpingotomy. When cardiac activity is present, vasopressin injection in the broad ligament beneath the EP could be helpful before salpingotomy. We consider that MTX injection in the broad ligament during laparoscopy should be performed if trophoblast removal is difficult or possibly incomplete.

In a recent review published in the *New England Journal of Medicine*, Lipscomb and colleagues[40] still considered selective suction curettage as part of the algorithm for EP diagnosis. Even if some arguments are given in support of this, such as eliminating the possibility of giving MTX unnecessarily to a patient with a non-viable intrauterine pregnancy, or the decreased need for unnecessary serial monitoring of hCG levels, we disagree with this view.

Indeed, in the majority of cases, serial hCG monitoring and high-quality vaginal echography make suction curettage obsolete, by providing a highly probable diagnosis of extrauterine pregnancy. The risk of intrauterine synechiae (Figure 1), due to unnecessary suction curettage, has to be considered and compared with the administration of a chemotherapeutic agent that has no benefit in this instance and is potentially toxic.

METHOTREXATE AS SECOND-LINE THERAPY

MTX can be given as second-line therapy in cases of failure of laparoscopic linear salpingotomy.

Diagnosis of persistent trophoblast

The diagnosis of persistent trophoblast after laparoscopic salpingotomy is made by measuring hCG levels postoperatively. It has been shown and proved in one of our studies[27] that, 2 days postoperatively, the hCG level should be less than 50% of the preoperative level, and after 4 days, less than 25% of the preoperative level. Figure 2 illustrates the postoperative decrease in hCG: if the postoperative hCG level is within the purple area, the laparoscopic treatment is considered to have been successful. If the postoperative hCG level is within the dark blue area, the diagnosis of persistent ectopic tissue is made. Indeed, an absence of any decrease proves the active secretion of hCG by persistent and well-vascularized trophoblastic tissue. However, if the hCG level falls within the light blue intermediate area (between the purple and dark blue), then a follow-up evaluation must be made by repeated hCG level monitoring 2 days later in order to evaluate the presence or absence of any significant decrease.

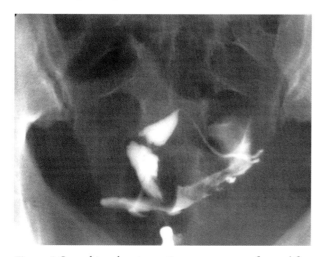

Figure 1 Synechiae due to suction curettage performed for diagnosis of extrauterine pregnancy

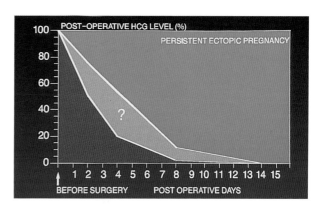

Figure 2 Graph illustrating the postoperative decrease in the human chorionic gonadotropin (hCG) level: the purple area is the successful area; the blue area is the failed area; the intermediate light purple area is the repeated monitoring area

In our department, if the 2-day postoperative hCG level remained higher than 50% of the initial (before laparoscopy) value, MTX (40 mg, intramuscularly) was administered. The hCG level was evaluated 4 days postoperatively and, if necessary, MTX was again given intramuscularly if hCG levels were > 25% of the initial value.

Prevalence and management

In a first series of 300 patients[27] treated conservatively by laparoscopic salpingotomy (Table 2), two cases in 1982 required a second-look laparotomy for recurrent bleeding due to persistent trophoblast. In 15 other cases, persistent trophoblast was also observed. All were treated successfully with methotrexate (Figure 3). The incidence of persistent ectopic gestation following conservative surgery was 5%. This incidence was similar to that observed in the literature review by Morlock and co-workers[11], who estimated the average failure rate to be 10%.

In a second series of 320 patients who underwent conservative laparoscopic treatment, persistent trophoblastic tissue was observed in 41 cases (13%) (Table 2). Again, all patients were treated with intramuscular MTX. However, in this second series, eight failures were encountered despite MTX administration.

Thus, two important questions remained to be answered, namely: why was there an increased persistent EP rate in the second series and why, in this series, did the administration of MTX fail in eight cases?

Concerning the increased use of MTX, a distinction must be made between true and false failures. True failures can be explained by the fact that, in a university teaching hospital, residents are in the process of learning, when performing laparoscopic procedures. The rate of such failures in our series was 8.5%, higher than the rate observed in the first series of 300 patients treated by the same surgeons (i.e. J.D. and M.N.). In these cases, MTX was required because of the abnormal decrease in the hCG level. After an initial decrease, the hCG level increased into the dark blue area. The diagnosis of persistent trophoblast was made and MTX was administered intramuscularly twice or three times, if needed (Figure 4). False failures can be accounted for by the inadequate use of MTX (4.5%). Indeed, in a few cases, MTX was given when it was not required, when the hCG level decrease was normal.

In conclusion, the failure rate of 8.5% observed in the second series was higher than that noted in the first series, as a result of necessary 'internship' in the department.

The second question to be addressed was why the administration of MTX failed in eight cases of the second series published in 1994[36] (Table 3). In patients receiving medication for ovulation, EP risk may be double. In one case, we observed a heterotubal pregnancy and another patient presented with a double tubal implantation site. Both patients had received clomiphene citrate and both underwent a second-look laparoscopy. In the case of the heterotubal pregnancy, a salpingotomy was carried out and was successful. The second patient underwent a third laparoscopy because of recurrent bleeding after the second salpingotomy. Laparoscopic salpingectomy was then carried out. There was one implantation site in the ampulla and another in the isthmus. In this case, the first procedure (ampullary salpingotomy) was well chosen, as proved by the anatomical aspect observed at the time of the third laparoscopy. The recurrent bleeding was provoked by persistent trophoblast in the isthmic tubal portion.

Table 2 Tubal pregnancy: laparoscopic procedures

	1980–1986 (n = 300)	1987–1990 (n = 320)
Persistent ectopic pregnancy	n = 15 (5%)	n = 41 (13%)
Therapy	methotrexate	methotrexate
Failure	0	8

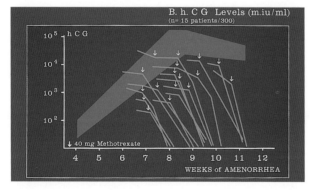

Figure 3 Levels of human chorionic gonadotropin (hCG) before and after administration of 40 mg of methotrexate intramuscularly in 15 cases of persistent trophoblast (first series)

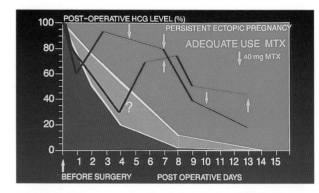

Figure 4 Adequate use of methotrexate: 4–5 days postoperatively, the human chorionic gonadotropin (hCG) level was abnormal (blue area) and methotrexate was required

In two cases, the laparoscopy was performed too early (< 6 weeks of amenorrhea) and the EP was not visible (too small); no surgical therapy was administered. A salpingotomy was performed 2 weeks later in one case. In the second case, an echo-guided MTX injection was given: the hCG level decreased, but the hysterosalpingography performed 3 months later showed ampullary dilatation and occlusion at the EP site.

In four cases, the laparoscopic procedure itself was at fault. The salpingotomy site was incorrect in three cases, requiring a second salpingotomy. In one case, the trophoblastic aspiration was insufficient and a salpingotomy and injection of MTX into the broad ligament were required.

In a series of 321 patients who had undergone conservative laparoscopic surgery, Pouly and colleagues[24]

reported 15 cases with residual trophoblast. Of these patients, seven underwent a second laparoscopic procedure, and six required a salpingectomy via laparotomy[25] (Table 4).

Rivlin and co-workers[41,42] reviewed five case reports of persistent ectopic gestation, and recommended that salpingectomy be the standard procedure undertaken.

In 1987, Di Marchi and colleagues[43] reported four cases (4.8%) of EP, out of 84 patients who had undergone a salpingotomy or fimbrial expression. Three patients required a repeat laparotomy and salpingectomy, and one was managed expectantly.

Table 4, showing more recent results, demonstrates that MTX is the therapy of choice to manage persistent ectopic trophoblast.

Table 3 Failures of methotrexate (MTX) used as therapy for persistent ectopic pregnancy ($n = 8$) (series published by Donnez and Nisolle in 1994[36])

Problem	n	Post-methotrexate procedure
Heterotubal pregnancy (clomiphene citrate)	1	salpingotomy (second-look)
Double implantation site (clomiphene citrate)	1	salpingotomy (second-look) salpingotomy (third-look)
(Too) early laparoscopic procedure	2	salpingotomy (second-look) echo-guided MTX injection
Imperfect laparoscopic procedure incorrect salpingotomy site	3	salpingotomy (second-look)
insufficient trophoblastic aspiration	1	salpingotomy and injection of MTX into the broad ligament (second-look)

Table 4 Management of persistent ectopic pregnancy after laparoscopic treatment

	Number of patients	Primary procedure	Management
Donnez[26]	2	salpingotomy	salpingotomy and coagulation
Rivlin et al.[41,42]	1	salpingotomy	salpingectomy
Cartwright et al.[44]	2	salpingotomy	expectant
Pouly et al.[24]	11	salpingotomy	salpingotomy
	4	fimbrial expression	salpingectomy
DiMarchi et al.[43]	3	salpingotomy	salpingectomy
	1	fimbrial expression	expectant
Donnez and Nisolle[27]	13	salpingotomy	methotrexate
Donnez and Nisolle[36]	56	salpingotomy	methotrexate
Seifer et al.[46]	50	salpingotomy	repeat salpingotomy ($n = 16$) or salpingectomy ($n = 18$)
Hoppe et al.[18]	19	salpingotomy	methotrexate

In a series of 20 patients undergoing linear salpingectomy[44,45], two patients demonstrated a postoperative rise in serum β-hCG levels, suggesting the persistence of trophoblastic tissue. Both patients were asymptomatic and were managed expectantly.

Discussion

After conservative surgical treatment of EP, a decrease in hCG levels must ensue until non-pregnant levels are achieved, because persistent EP may cause delayed intraabdominal hemorrhage.

The risk of persistent tubal pregnancy must be considered if the hCG level falls by less than 50% on day 2, according to Donnez and Nisolle[36].

Spandorfer and colleagues[47] were even stricter in their criteria in 1997, claiming that the hCG level must fall by more than 50% on day 1. Hagstrom[48] and Kemmann[49] and their groups found that the risk of persistent tubal pregnancy could be predicted by progesterone and hCG levels observed 24 h preoperatively. In our opinion, a decrease in the hCG level to less than 50% of the initial value on day 2 is the main criterion.

Persistent ectopic pregnancy can appear as increasing hCG titer or as 'slow-falling hCG' after conservative surgery. If a stable clinical condition is present, intramuscular MTX injection can be proposed as second-line therapy; otherwise, surgical treatment must be repeated. We do not consider the proposal of Graczykowski and colleagues[50], to administer prophylactic MTX (1 mg/kg) to reduce the incidence of persistent EP, to be ethically acceptable. Indeed, this would constitute unnecessary treatment in more than 90% of cases.

Administration of MTX is definitely the therapy of choice for persistent EP diagnosed by an insufficient decrease in hCG after salpingotomy.

PROGNOSIS FOR FUTURE FERTILITY

Postoperative fertility after linear salpingotomy

In a review in 1994[36], Donnez and Nisolle observed an intrauterine pregnancy rate of 57% and a recurrent EP rate of 16% after linear salpingotomy (Table 5).

In a series of 120 patients without any history of infertility who wished to become pregnant, an intrauterine pregnancy rate of 54% was achieved (Table 6). The recurrent tubal pregnancy rate after laparoscopy was similar to that obtained in another series of 148 patients who

Table 5 Pregnancy rates following linear salpingotomy for ectopic pregnancy in women desiring to become pregnant (from Donnez and Nisolle[36])

Laparoscopy	Number of patients	Intrauterine pregnancy n (%)	Ectopic pregnancy n (%)
Pouly et al.[24]	118	75 (64)	26 (22)
Donnez and Nisolle[27]	138	70 (51)	14 (10)
Total	256	145 (57)	40 (16)

Table 6 Postoperative fertility after conservative management of ectopic pregnancy. Comparison of laparotomy vs. laparoscopy (from Donnez and Nisolle 1989[27], 1994[36])

	Number of patients	Intrauterine pregnancy n (%)	Ectopic pregnancy n (%)
Laparotomy			
No history of infertility	148	92 (62)	12 (8)
After microsurgical tuboplasty	64	19 (30)	13 (20)
Total	212	111 (52)	25 (12)
Laparoscopy			
No history of infertility	120	65 (54)	10 (8)
After microsurgical tuboplasty	18	5 (27)*	4 (22)*
Total	138	70 (51)	14 (10)

* *p* < 0.005; significantly different from the group of women without any history of infertility

underwent conservative surgery (linear salpingotomy) by laparotomy (8% in both groups).

Among patients with a history of microsurgical tuboplasty, the postoperative intrauterine pregnancy rate was significantly lower ($p < 0.005$) than that obtained in the group of patients without a history of infertility (27% vs. 54%). The recurrent tubal pregnancy rates were also significantly different ($p < 0.005$; 22% vs. 8%). Similar data were obtained from the group of patients who underwent a conservative approach by laparotomy.

Among patients with a single tube in a review by Donnez and Nisolle in 1994[36], the intrauterine pregnancy rate was 51% and the recurrent tubal pregnancy rate was 22%. In a review by Yao and Tulandi[51] of a series of 1514 women, the intrauterine pregnancy rate was 61.4%, with a 15.4% risk of recurrent EP. Linear salpingotomy seems to result in a higher rate of subsequent intrauterine pregnancy than either total or partial salpingectomy. However, the more favorable reproductive outcome may, in part, reflect a selection bias, since linear salpingotomy was performed in cases of unruptured gestations, whereas salpingectomy was usually performed in cases of ruptured ectopic gestations. The advantage of conservative surgery over radical surgery is clear when treating ectopic gestations, when there is only one tube. In these cases, a conservative approach is the only one that preserves reproductive potential.

Although tubal rupture seriously affects the immediate health of the women concerned, it seems to have no independent effect on subsequent fertility[51].

Is medical or surgical treatment better for subsequent fertility?

In 1998, Fernandez and colleagues[9] published a study comparing MTX injected transvaginally, or administered intramuscularly, with laparoscopic salpingotomy and concluded: 'Spontaneous reproductive performance was similar in both groups, but overall intrauterine pregnancy was higher, and repeat EP lower, after methotrexate treatment' (but it was not statistically significant).

Do ruptured EPs have an adverse effect on subsequent pregnancies?

Job-Spira and colleagues[52] concluded, in their study in 1999, that there was no decrease in the rate of intrauterine pregnancy in the year following treatment, except if the woman was over 35 years of age, had a previous history of infertility or previous tubal damage (all factors that were present before the rupture).

In conclusion

'Fertility after ectopic pregnancy is affected much more by the status of the contralateral tube than by the procedure performed, with fertility rates exceeding 80% after salpingectomy when the opposite tube is normal'[53].

REFERENCES

1. Stovall TG, Ling FW, Buster JE. Outpatient chemotherapy of unruptured ectopic pregnancy. *Fertil Steril* 1989;51:535–8
2. Stovall TG, Ling FW, Gray LA, *et al*. Methotrexate treatment of unruptured ectopic pregnancy: a report of 100 cases. *Obstet Gynecol* 1991;77:749–53
3. Hitara AJ, Soper DE, Bump RC, *et al*. Ectopic pregnancy in an urban teaching hospital: can tubal rupture be predicted? *South Med J* 1991;84:1467
4. Mol BWJ, Hajenius PJ, Engelsbel S, *et al*. Can noninvasive diagnosis tools predict tubal rupture or active bleeding in patients with tubal pregnancy? *Fertil Steril* 1999;71:167
5. Fernandez H, Lelaidier C, Thouvenez V, *et al*. The use of a pretherapeutic predictive score to determine inclusion criteria for the non-surgical treatment of ectopic pregnancy. *Hum Reprod* 1991;6:995–8
6. Fernandez H, Lelaidier C, Baton C, *et al*. Return of reproductive performance after expectant management and local treatment for ectopic pregnancy. *Hum Reprod* 1991;6:1474–7
7. Fernandez H, Benifla JL, Lelaidier C, *et al*. Methotrexate treatment of ectopic pregnancy: 100 cases treated by primary transvaginal injection under sonographic control. *Fertil Steril* 1993;59:773–7
8. Fernandez H, Bourget P, Ville Y, *et al*. Treatment of unruptured tubal pregnancy with methotrexate: pharmacokinetic analysis of local versus intramuscular administration. *Fertil Steril* 1994;62:943
9. Fernandez H, Cappella-Allouc S, Vincent Y, *et al*. Randomized trial of conservative laparoscopic treatment and methotrexate administration in ectopic pregnancy and subsequent fertility. *Hum Reprod* 1998;13:3239
10. Pansky M, Bukovsky J, Golan A, *et al*. Reproductive outcome after laparoscopic local methotrexate injection for tubal pregnancy. *Fertil Steril* 1993;60:85–7
11. Morlock RJ, Lafata JE, Eisenstein D. Cost-effectiveness of single-dose methotrexate compared with laparoscopic treatment of ectopic pregnancy. *Obstet Gynecol* 2000;95:407
12. Vermesh M, Silva PD, Rosen GF, *et al*. Management of unruptured ectopic gestation by linear salpingostomy: a prospective randomized clinical trial of laparoscopy versus laparotomy. *Obstet Gynecol* 1989;73:400–4
13. Lecuru F, Robin F, Bernard JP, *et al*. Single-dose Methotrexate for unruptured ectopic pregnancy. *Int J Gynaecol Obstet* 1998;61:253–9
14. Yao M, Tulandi T, Falcone T. Treatment of ectopic pregnancy by systemic methotrexate, transvaginal

methotrexate, and operative laparoscopy. *Int J Fertil* 1996;41:470–5

15. Hajenius P, Engelsbel S, Mol B, *et al.* Randomised trial of systemic methotrexate versus laparoscopic salpingostomy in tubal pregnancy. *Lancet* 1997;350:774–9

16. Tan H, Tay S. Laparoscopic treatment of ectopic pregnancies – a study of 100 cases. *Ann Acad Med Singapore* 1996;25:665–7

17. Shalev E, Peleg D, Bustan M, *et al.* Limited role for intratubal methotrexate treatment of ectopic pregnancy. *Fertil Steril* 1995;63:20–4

18. Hoppe DE, Bekkar BE, Nager CW. Single-dose systemic methotrexate for the treatment of persistent ectopic pregnancy after conservative surgery. *Obstet Gynecol* 1994;83:51–4

19. Seifer DB, Gutmann JN, Grant WD, *et al.* Comparison of persistent ectopic pregnancy after laparoscopic salpingostomy versus salpingostomy at laparotomy for ectopic pregnancy. *Obstet Gynecol* 1993;81:378–82

20. Lundorff P, Hahlin M, Sjoblom P, *et al.* Persistent trophoblast after conservative treatment of tubal pregnancy: prediction and detection. *Obstet Gynecol* 1991;77:129–33

21. Letterie GS, Fasolak WS, Miyazowa K. Laparoscopy and minilaparotomy as operative management of ectopic pregnancy. *Mil Med* 1990;155:305–7

22. Mecke H, Semm K, Lehmann-Willenbrock E. Results of operative pelviscopy in 202 cases of ectopic pregnancy. *Int J Fertil* 1989;34:93–100

23. DeCherney AH, Diamond MP. Laparoscopic salpingostomy for ectopic pregnancy. *Obstet Gynecol* 1987;70:948–50

24. Pouly JL, Manhes H, Mage G, *et al.* Conservative laparoscopic treatment of 321 ectopic pregnancies. *Fertil Steril* 1986;46:1093–7

25. Bruhat MA, Manhes H, Mage G, *et al.* Treatment of ectopic pregnancy by means of laparoscopy. *Fertil Steril* 1980;33:411–44

26. Donnez J. Conservative treatment of ectopic pregnancy. A first series of 50 cases. *Acta Endosc* 1982;4:62

27. Donnez J, Nisolle M. Laparoscopic treatment of ampullary tubal pregnancy. *J Gynecol Surg* 1989;5:19

28. Jimenez-Caraballo A, Rodriguez-Donoso G. A 6-year clinical trial of methotrexate therapy in the treatment of ectopic pregnancy. *Eur J Obstet Gynecol* 1998;79:167–71

29. Lipscomb GH, Bran D, McCord ML, *et al.* Analysis of three hundred and fifteen ectopic pregnancies treated with single-dose methotrexate. *Am J Obstet Gynecol* 1998;178:1354–8

30. Thoen LD, Creinin MD. Medical treatment of ectopic pregnancy with methotrexate. *Fertil Steril* 1997;68:727–30

31. Stika CS, Anderson L, Frederiksen MC. Single-dose methotrexate for the treatment of ectopic pregnancy: Northwestern Memorial Hospital three-year experience. *Am J Obstet Gynecol* 1996;174:1840–8

32. Corsan GH, Karacan M, Qasim S, *et al.* Identification of hormonal parameters for successful systemic single-dose methotrexate therapy in ectopic pregnancy. *Hum Reprod* 1995;10:2719–22

33. Glock JL, Johnson JV, Brumsted JR. Efficacy and safety of single-dose systemic methotrexate in the treatment of ectopic pregnancy. *Fertil Steril* 1994;62:716–21

34. Henry MA, Gentry WL. Single-injection of methotrexate for treatment of ectopic pregnancies. *Am J Obstet Gynecol* 1994;171:1584–7

35. Stovall TG, Ling FW. Single-dose methotrexate: an expanded clinical trial. *Am J Obstet Gynecol* 1993;168:1759–65

36. Donnez J, Nisolle M. Postoperative management and reproductive outcome after conservative laparoscopic procedures. In Donnez J, Nisolle M, eds. *An Atlas of Laser Operative Laparoscopy and Hysteroscopy.* Carnforth, UK: Parthenon Publishing, 1994:131–44

37. Saraj AJ, Wilcox JG, Najmabadi S, *et al.* Resolution of hormonal markers of ectopic gestation: a randomized trial comparing single-dose intramuscular methotrexate with salpingostomy. *Obstet Gynecol* 1998;92:989–94

38. Lipscomb GH, McCord ML, Stovall TG, *et al.* Predictors of success of methotrexate treatment in women with tubal ectopic pregnancy. *N Engl J Med* 1999;341:1974

39. Schafer D, Kryss J, Pfuhl J, *et al.* Systemic treatment of ectopic pregnancies with single-dose methotrexate. *J Am Assoc Gynecol Laparosc* 1994;1:213–18

40. Lipscomb GH, Stovall TG, Ling FW. Nonsurgical treatment of ectopic pregnancy. *N Engl J Med* 2000;343:1325–9

41. Rivlin ME, Meeks GR, Cowan BD, *et al.* Persistent trophoblastic tissue following salpingostomy for unruptured ectopic pregnancy. *Fertil Steril* 1985;43:323

42. Rivlin, ME. Persistent ectopic pregnancy: complication of conservative surgery. *Int J Fertil* 1985;30:10

43. DiMarchi JM, Losasa TS, Kobara TY, *et al.* Persistent ectopic pregnancy. *Obstet Gynecol* 1987;70:555

44. Cartwright PS, Herbert CM, Mawson WS. Operative laparoscopy for the management of tubal pregnancy. *J Reprod Med* 1986;31:589

45. Cartwright PS, Etmann SS. Repeat ipsilateral tubal pregnancy following partial salpingectomy: a case report. *Fertil Steril* 1984;42:647

46. Seifer DB, Silva PD, Grainger DA, *et al.* Reproductive potential after treatment for persistent ectopic pregnancy. *Fertil Steril* 1994;62:194-6

47. Spandorfer SD, Sawin SW, Benjamin I, *et al.* Postoperative day 1 serum human chorionic gonadotropin level as a predictor of persistent ectopic pregnancy after conservative surgical management. *Fertil Steril* 1997;63:430–4

48. Hagstrom HG, Hahlin M, Bennegard-Eden B, *et al.* Prediction of persistent ectopic pregnancy after laparoscopic salpingostomy. *Obstet Gynecol* 1994;84:798–802

49. Kemmann E, Trout S, Garcia A. Can we predict patients at risk for persistent ectopic pregnancy after laparoscopic salpingotomy? *J Am Assoc Gynecol Laparosc* 1994;1:122–6

50. Graczykowski JW, Mishell DR Jr. Methotrexate prophylaxis for persistent ectopic pregnancy after conservative treatment by salpingostomy. *Obstet Gynecol* 1997;89:118–22

51. Yao M, Tulandi T. Current status of surgical and nonsurgical management of ectopic pregnancy. *Fertil Steril* 1997;67:421–33

52. Job-Spira N, Fernandez H, Bouyer J, *et al.* Ruptured tubal ectopic pregnancy: risk factors and reproductive outcome: results of a population-based study in France. *Am J Obstet Gynecol* 1999;180:938–44

53. Rulin MC. Is salpingostomy the surgical treatment of choice for unruptured tubal pregnancy? *Obstet Gynecol* 1995;86:1010

Laparoscopic management of ectopic pregnancy: a 500-case evaluation

17

G. Mage, J.L. Pouly, M. Canis, A. Wattiez, C. Chapron and M.A. Bruhat

The combination of sensitive human chorionic gonadotropin (hCG) assays and ultrasonography makes an early diagnosis of ectopic pregnancy possible. Progress in operative laparoscopy allows an endoscopic management of ectopic pregnancy[1-3]. From 1974 to 1987, 500 cases of ectopic pregnancy were treated by laparoscopic procedures by our team.

MATERIALS AND METHODS

Patients

A total of 500 cases were managed by a laparoscopic approach: 427 were treated conservatively and 73 were treated by salpingectomy. The average age of the patients was 25.4 ± 4.9 years (in the first 321 cases). The absolute and relative contraindications to the laparoscopic treatment of ectopic pregnancy, reported in Table 1, were respected.

Table I Contraindications to the laparoscopic treatment of ectopic pregnancy

Absolute contraindications
Interstitial pregnancy
Retrouterine hematocela
Shock
Relative contraindications
Hemoperitoneum over 1500 ml
Obesity
Large adhesions

Laparoscopic treatment

The laparoscopic management of ectopic pregnancy requires the following equipment:

(1) An 11-mm laparoscope with its trocar (Storz France, Paris, France) introduced through the umbilicus;

(2) Two operating trocars (5 and 7 mm) inserted by means of two small lateral suprapubic incisions;

(3) A 5-mm atraumatic forceps (Microfrance, Bourbon l'Archambault, France);

(4) The 7-mm Triton (Microfrance), an instrument with three functions: potential aspiration through a 6-mm diameter channel, injection of saline solution under pressure and electrocoagulation with a retractable monopolar needle electrode;

(5) A 19-gauge needle;

(6) 5 IU of Vasopressin (POR 8, Sandoz Laboratories, Basel, Switzerland);

(7) In cases of radical treatment, bipolar cautery forceps and laparoscopic scissors;

(8) Since 1984, we have been using a video system, which gives us more precision and comfort and allows better teaching.

Methods

After diagnosis of ectopic pregnancy, two suprapubic operative trocars are inserted: a 5-mm trocar at the end of an imaginary Pfannenstiel at the site of ectopic pregnancy and a 7-mm one on the opposite side. The first stages of conservative or radical laparoscopic management are the same:

(1) Aspiration of the hemoperitoneum with the Triton;

(2) Washing of the pelvis with saline solution under pressure;

(3) Evaluation of the ectopic pregnancy for location and operability.

The factors reported in Table 2 determine the choice between conservative and radical treatment.

Conservative treatment

In the case of conservative treatment, the different stages of the treatment are:

(1) Preventive hemostasis: vasopressin is diluted in 20 ml of serum saline and injected into the mesosalpinx through a 19-gauge needle (Figure 1). Blanching of the tube and temporary ischemia provides a virtually bloodless operating field. The use of this drug must be carefully controlled due to the dramatic arterial hypertension in cases of intravascular injection. Extravascular injection induces a moderate increase in arterial pressure and a moderate bradycardia in some cases. The temporary ischemia does not affect tubal patency, as was verified by a second-look laparoscopy (15 cases), and provides a similar

Table 2 Choosing between conservative and radical treatment of ectopic pregnancy: scoring system

History of the patient		
Infertility	2	
Ectopic pregnancy	2	(+ for following ectopic pregnancies)
Tubal plasty	2	
Location		
Isthmus	1	
Ampulla	0	
Fimbria	–1	
In case of solitary tube		
Salpingectomy	2	
Obstructed tube	1	
Bilateral ectopic pregnancy	2	
In case of rupture	1	
Score 1–4	conservative treatment	
Score 6 or more	radical treatment	
Score = 5	?	

Table 3 Postoperative fertility and ectopic pregnancy in relation to the status of the tubal wall, the location of ectopic pregnancy and the use of vasopressin

	n	Intrauterine pregnancy *n* (%)	Extrauterine pregnancy *n* (%)
Use of vasopressin			
no	54	33 (61.1)	12 (22.2)
yes	95	64 (67.4)	13 (13.7)
Tubal wall			
ruptured	55	35 (63.6)	8 (14.5)
unruptured	94	62 (66)	17 (18.1)
Location			
isthmus	27	16 (59.3)	8 (29.6)
ampulla	101	63 (62.4)	16 (15.8)
fimbria	21	18 (85.7)	1 (4.8)

intrauterine pregnancy rate in groups with or without vasopressin (Table 3).

(2) Salpingotomy: a 10–15-mm incision is made in the antimesenteric proximal portion of the hematosalpinx with the needle electrode of the Triton (Figures 2 and 3). Salpingotomy must be the systematic approach whenever there is a hematosalpinx. The high incidence of residual trophoblastic tissue in women treated without salpingotomy led us to perform tubal abortion only in cases of fimbrial ectopic pregnancies. The salpingotomy must be performed in the proximal portion of the hematosalpinx, which is the usual location of the trophoblast (Figure 2).

(3) Extraction of the trophoblast (Figure 4): the Triton is introduced through the salpingotomy incision; clots and trophoblast are aspirated. In most cases, aspiration removes the product of conception entirely. In some cases, saline solution injected under pressure by the Triton or grasping forceps, is used to separate the trophoblast from the tubal wall. In all cases, the salpingotomy is left open (Figure 5).

At the end of the procedure, it is necessary to:

(1) Check the tube vacuity;

(2) Wash the pelvis with saline solution under pressure (Figure 6);

(3) Remove all clots and products of conception with the Triton;

(4) Assess the contralateral Fallopian tube.

It is not necessary to insert an intraperitoneal drain through the pouch of Douglas.

The postoperative follow-up includes weekly hCG assays from the 2nd day after the operation until the level is undetectable (less than 5 mIU/ml)[4].

Radical treatment

In the case of radical treatment[5], a salpingotomy is performed by bipolar coagulation and scissors after aspiration of the ectopic pregnancy from the tube, as in conservative treatment. The proximal part of the isthmus is coagulated and sectioned. Then the mesosalpinx is progressively coagulated and sectioned until the tube can be removed with grasping forceps and extracted from the abdomen.

RESULTS

A total of 427 cases of ectopic pregnancy treated conservatively between 1974 and 1986 were studied. Failures occurred in 22 cases (5.15%) because of an incomplete removal of the trophoblast, requiring a second laparoscopic procedure in ten cases and laparotomy in 12 cases. Of the 73 patients treated by salpingectomy, we had only one postsurgical complication (1.36%): a 10th postoperative day hemorrhage which was successfully resolved by laparotomy. Postectopic fertility was evaluated in 149

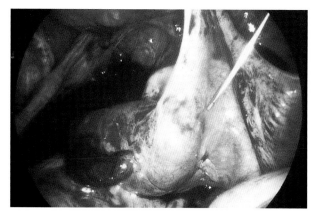

Figure 1 Injection of vasopressin into the mesosalpinx

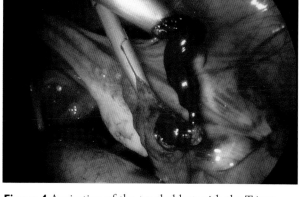

Figure 4 Aspiration of the trophoblast with the Triton

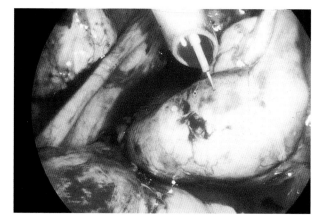

Figure 2 Salpingotomy in the antimesenteric proximal portion of the hematosalpinx with the needle electrode of the Triton

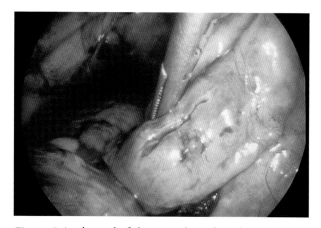

Figure 5 At the end of the procedure, the salpingotomy is left open

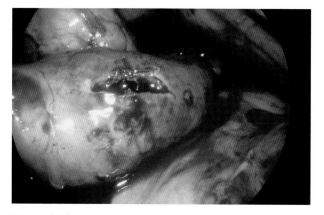

Figure 3 The incision

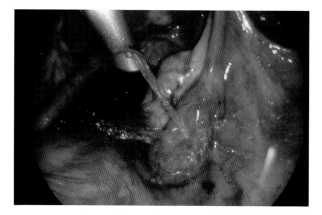

Figure 6 Washing of the pelvis

patients who wished to become pregnant, with a minimum follow-up of 1 year.

Fertility results are summarized in Table 4. Of the 149 women who desired fertility, 97 (65.1%) had a subsequent intrauterine pregnancy. Five intrauterine pregnancies occurred after a second ectopic pregnancy which was also treated using a conservative laparoscopic procedure. The ectopic pregnancy rate was 16.8% (25 patients) and 49

patients (32.9%) suffered subsequent infertility (recurrent ectopic pregnancy + failure to conceive). (As can be seen in Table 6, our results compare favorably with those of other studies.)

According to their history, the 149 patients were divided into two groups: group I, 80 patients without any history of infertility or ectopic pregnancy; and group II, the other 69 patients. The results are summarized in Table 5.

Statistical differences exist between the subsequent fertility rates of these two groups. An intrauterine pregnancy occurred in 68 patients in group I (85%) and in 29 patients (42%) in group II ($p < 0.001$). An ectopic pregnancy occurred in 12% of cases (ten patients) in group I and 22% of cases (15 patients) in group II. The postectopic infertility rate was 12% (ten cases) in group I and 56% (39 cases) in group II ($p < 0.001$).

Group III included 21 patients who had an ectopic pregnancy after microsurgical tuboplasty: four subsequently had an intrauterine pregnancy (19%), 17 remained sterile (81%) and six (29%) had a recurrence.

The 'solitary tube' group included patients who had undergone a previous salpingectomy, patients with a previously obstructed contralateral tube and patients who presented an ectopic pregnancy in each tube successively, both treated by laparoscopy.

Postoperative fertility and recurrence of ectopic pregnancy were studied in relation to the rupture of the tubal wall and location of the ectopic pregnancy (Table 3). The tube was ruptured in 55 patients. Among these women, there were 35 intrauterine pregnancies (63.6%) and eight had a recurrence of ectopic pregnancy (14.5%). Of the 94 with an unruptured ectopic pregnancy, 62 developed an intrauterine pregnancy (66%) and 17 a recurrence of ectopic pregnancy (18.1%).

Table 4 Fertility results

Number of cases	Intrauterine pregnancy n (%)	Ectopic pregnancy n (%)	Sterility n (%)
149	97* (65.1)	25 (16.8)	49† (32.9)

*, five after a second ectopic pregnancy; †, 17 after a second ectopic pregnancy

The first ectopic pregnancy was located in the ampulla in 101 cases (67.8%), in the fimbria in 21 cases (44%) and in the isthmus in 27 cases (18.2%). The intrauterine pregnancy rates in these groups were 62.4%, 85.7% and 59.3%, respectively. The recurrence rates in these groups were 15.8%, 4.8% and 29.6%, respectively.

A simple scoring system (Table 2) allows the categorization of patients into two groups according to a high or poor chance of subsequent intrauterine pregnancy. This scoring system has been used by our team for 2 years now to choose between radical and conservative treatment.

CONCLUSION

Conservative laparoscopic treatment of ectopic pregnancy is a safe and effective laparoscopic procedure. In cases with contraindications to conservative management, a salpingectomy can be performed with a laparoscopic procedure. Failure due to residual trophoblastic tissue can occur. The failure necessitates a careful follow-up by monitoring of hCG levels.

Comparisons of postectopic pregnancy fertility results must be made critically. However, our postoperative rate of 65.1% intrauterine pregnancies compares favorably with previous studies (Table 6). The incidence of a previous history in relation to the success rate of the patient is emphasized in our series and must be taken into account when making the choice between radical and conservative treatment. Broad experience in operative laparoscopy is, however, required before management of ectopic pregnancy by laparoscopy is undertaken. Our techniques are, by and large, simple and easily feasible for most laparoscopic surgeons after adequate training. The advantages of laparoscopic procedures compared to laparotomy are evident in the reduction of hospital stay and patient trauma.

Table 5 Fertility according to history

	Number of patients	Intrauterine pregnancy n (%)	Ectopic pregnancy n (%)	Sterility n (%)
Group I: without history†	80	68* (85)	10** (12)	10* (12)
Group II: with history†	69	29* (42)	15** (22)	39* (56)
Group III: post-plasty	21	4 (19)	6 (29)	17 (81)
Solitary tube	27	11 (41)	6 (22)	15 (55)
Postectopic	38	7 (18)	15 (39)	29 (76)
Non-tubal infertility	38	23 (60)	6 (16)	15 (39)

*, $p < 0.001$; **, not significant; †, refers to history of infertility or ectopic pregnancy

Table 6 Comparison of our postectopic pregnancy fertility results with other principal series

Author	Year	Number of patients	Intrauterine pregnancy n (%)	Ectopic pregnancy n (%)
Conservative treatment				
Ploman	(1960)[6]	31	16 (52)	1 (3)
Skjul	(1964)[7]	92	23 (25)	1 (1)
Timonen	(1967)[8]	185	46 (25)	21 (11)
Palmer	(1972)[9]	55	11 (20)	9 (16)
Swollin	(1972)[10]	40	10 (25)	7 (17)
Jarvinen	(1972)[11]	43	22 (51)	4 (9)
Stromme	(1973)[12]	37	20 (54)	7 (19)
Bukovsky	(1979)[13]	20	14 (70)	1 (5)
DeCherney	(1979)[14]	48	19 (39)	4 (8)
Giana	(1979)[15]	51	17 (33)	4 (8)
Henri-Suchet	(1979)[16]	52	22 (42)	10 (19)
Sherman	(1982)[17]	47	39 (83)	7 (15)
Lalau	(1985)[18]	118	35 (30)	29 (25)
Microsurgery				
DeCherney	(1980)[19]	9	5 (55)	0 (0)
Janecek	(1980)[20]	10	6 (60)	2 (20)
Laparoscopic treatment				
Our results	(1987)	149	97 (65)	25 (17)

REFERENCES

1. Bruhat MA, Manhes H, Mage G, *et al.* Treatment of ectopic pregnancy by means of laparoscopy. *Fertil Steril* 1980;33:411

2. Manhes H, Mage G, Pouly JL, *et al.* Traitement coelioscopique de la grossesse extra utérine non rompue: améliorations techniques. *Nelle Presse Med* 1983;12:1431

3. Pouly JL, Manhes H, Mage G, *et al.* Conservative laparoscopic treatment of 321 ectopic pregnancies. *Fertil Steril* 1986;46:1093

4. Pouly JL, Gachon M, Gaillard G, *et al.* La décroissance de l'HCG après traitement coelioscopique conservateur de la grossesse extra-utérine. *J Gynecol Obstet Biol Reprod* 1987;16:195

5. Dubuisson JB, Aubriot FX, Cardone V. Laparoscopic salpingectomy for tubal pregnancy. *Fertil Steril* 1987;47:225

6. Ploman L, Wicksell F. Fertility after conservative surgery in tubal pregnancy. *Acta Obstet Gynecol Scand* 1960;39:143

7. Skjul V, Palvic Z, Stoiljkovic C, *et al.* Conservative operative treatment of tubal pregnancy. *Fertil Steril* 1964;15:634

8. Timonen S, Nieminen U. Tubal pregnancy, choice of operative method of treatment. *Acta Obstet Gynecol Scand* 1967;46:327

9. Palmer R. Résultats et indications de la chirurgie conservatrice au cours de la grossesse extra-utérine. *C R Soc Fr Gynecol* 1972;42:317

10. Swollin K, Fall M. Ectopic pregnancy. *Acta Eur Fertil* 1972;3:147

11. Jarvinen PA. Conservative operative treatment of tubal pregnancy with post-operative daily hydrotubation. *Acta Obstet Gynecol Scand* 1972;51:169

12. Stromme WB. Conservative surgery for ectopic pregnancy. *Obstet Gynecol* 1973;41:251

13. Bukovsky J, Langer R, Herman A, *et al.* Conservative surgery for ectopic pregnancy. *Obstet Gynecol* 1979;53:709

14. DeCherney A, Kase N. The conservative surgical management of unruptured ectopic pregnancy. *Obstet Gynecol* 1979;54:541

15. Giana M. Tratamento chirurgico conservativo in 51 caza digravidenza tubarica. *Minera Ginecol* 1979;30:99

16. Henri-Suchet J. Chirurgie conservatrice de la grossesse extra-utérine. In *Oviducte et Fertilité*. Paris: Masson, 1979:393

17. Sherman D, Langer R, Sadovsky G, *et al.* Improved fertility following ectopic pregnancy. *Fertil Steril* 1982;37:497

18. Lalau Keraly M. Récidives de grossesse extra-utérine. A propos d'une étude multicentrique de 470 cas de GEU. Thèse Paris 1985

19. DeCherney AH, Polan ML, Kort H, *et al.* Microsurgical technique in the management of tubal ectopic pregnancy. *Fertil Steril* 1980;34:324

20. Janecek J. Resultats de la chirurgie reconstructrice dans les grossesses extra-utérines non rompues. *Rev Méd Suisse Romande* 1979;99:603

Laparoscopic microsurgical tubal anastomosis

18

C.H. Koh

LAPAROSCOPIC MICROSURGERY: A NEW TOOL FOR CONTINUOUS MICROSURGERY

Laparoscopic microsurgery is a new discipline that synergizes the potential of classical microsurgery and laparoscopy. It can overcome the deficits inherent in each. With classical microsurgery, the delicate and precise surgery can only happen after laparotomy, retraction, packing and crude macro-adhesiolysis to bring the adnexae under the operating microscope, a situation responsible for *de novo* adhesions. On the other hand, the superior and atraumatic exposure obtainable by laparoscopy has often not been matched by delicate surgery, causing concern for irreparable tissue damage[1]. These problems are well addressed by this new tool. In fact, as our experience and technique of laparoscopic microsurgery have evolved and improved, it is becoming evident that we are exceeding our surgical expectations, moving beyond 'new access, old technique'[1] into the era of what we would call 'new access, new technique'.

This is the technique of *continuous microsurgery*, only achievable via laparoscopy. Reproductive surgery can now be performed in ways that were not possible for either operative laparoscopy or classical microsurgery. In the performance of tubal anastomosis, one can be truly minimally interventionist, by omitting the use of retractors and packing, while the treatment of severe adhesions, endometriosis of the cul-de-sac and microsurgical repair of the ureters, for example, were not previously achievable under conditions of continuous microsurgery and minimal collateral trauma. With the further evolution of technology, this tool is poised for applications as yet unimagined.

INDICATIONS FOR LAPAROSCOPIC TUBAL ANASTOMOSIS

(1) Reversal of sterilization;

(2) Mid-tubal block secondary to various pathology;

(3) Tubal occlusion secondary to ectopic pregnancy treatment;

(4) Salpingitis isthmica nodosa;

(5) Failed tubal cannulation for proximal block;

(6) Failed previous macrosurgical sterilization reversal.

EQUIPMENT AND INSTRUMENT REQUISITES FOR LAPAROSCOPIC MICROSURGERY

Magnification, resolution and digital enhancement

Magnification of 25–40 times is essential to identify healthy mucosa and muscularis before anastomosis can be performed. For microsuturing, magnification at 10–15 times is adequate. We measure laparoscopic magnification by using a 20-inch (50-cm) monitor and determining the ratio of the size of the image on the monitor to actual life size. We call this the 'magnification factor of video laparoscopy'. With the current three-chip cameras available with zoom capability, magnification up to 40 times is achievable.

Magnification requires a correspondingly high resolution for it to be usable, and this is achieved by cameras and monitors capable of at least 800 lines of resolution. The three-chip camera is also indispensable for accurate color resolution. An 8-0 suture, which is 45 μm in diameter, is easily seen using such a video system.

To enhance contrast further, some companies have built digital enhancement into their cameras or as an add-on unit. This enhances small vessels and edge detail, thus improving discrimination. An extremely sensitive auto-iris built into the camera provides rapid control of illumination, avoiding the dreaded 'white-out' when the telescope is brought close to tissue. This is particularly important in microsuturing, as the telescope has to be panned in and out frequently during the case. We use the Storz three-chip camera which incorporates all the above features as standard.

Micro-instrumentation

Micro-instrumentation has been designed that allows laparoscopic microsuturing to be performed with precision and ease (Storz 'Koh Ultramicro Series'™). This avoids the inefficiency and frustration caused by suture fraying and breakage and poor needle stability.

Special design elements include sand-blasted tips to reduce glare, atraumatic terminal serrations, jaw apposition without slippage of 8-0 suture, with a responsive and sensitive handle design.

Sutures and needles

A more rigid needle is necessary for laparoscopic micro-suturing than for classical microsurgery. Furthermore, it is often easier to insert the needle directly into tissue without the use of a counter-pressing grasper. To achieve this, the needle needs low-force penetration characteristics and superior rigidity. Suitable examples include the BV 175-6 needle swaged to 7-0 and 8-0 Prolene™ or a BV 130-5 needle swaged to 8-0 polypropylene (Ethalloy TruTaper needle, Ethicon). Another excellent needle we have used recently is the Surgipro™ 135-5 needle swaged to 8-0 polypropylene (US Surgical Corporation). Although black nylon would give better discrimination laparoscopically, the needle is not ideal. Plain Vicryl is the most difficult to see laparoscopically and becomes limp when wet. Monofilament sutures tend not to fray and allow easier intracorporeal suturing.

Other equipment

Trocars

Reusable 3-mm trocars are available with the Ultramicro Series, or 5-mm trocars with rubber valves that allow 3-mm instruments to be used without reducers. Three-millimeter suction irrigators are available and provide a more suitable jet for microsurgery than the 5-mm counterparts.

Stents

These are not used as it can be traumatic to cannulate the distal Fallopian tube.

Uterine manipulator

The Rumi™ uterine manipulator (Cooper Surgical, USA), with its superior anteversion mechanism, is indispensable for tubal anastomosis as multiple permutations of uterine position can be obtained, thereby presenting the proximal tube at a favorable angle for microsuturing. The lateral openings of the Rumi intrauterine tip facilitate retrograde chromopertubation. Uterine manipulators having a terminal opening tend to be lodged in the endometrium and cause intravasation of dye and a false diagnosis of a proximal block.

Energy

A 150-μm microneedle unipolar electrode (Storz 'Koh Ultramicro Series'™) is used for incision and dissection, powered from a low-voltage generator. Power settings of 15–20 W for cutting and 15 W for fulguration are adequate. When the mesenteric vasculature is inadvertently cut, causing more vigorous bleeding, a microbipolar electrode of 1-mm diameter is used.

PREREQUISITES OF THE SURGEON

The aspiring laparoscopic microsurgeon should be highly experienced in classical microsurgery and have highly developed two-handed laparoscopic skills for intracorporeal knotting. Extracorporeal techniques for 7-0 and 8-0 sutures are impractical and crude and cause 'cutting through', or disruption, of tissue.

TYPES OF ANASTOMOSIS

Isthmic–isthmic anastomosis

Although the lumen may be as small as 500 μm to 1 mm, equivalent luminal size and a thick muscularis allow a technically easier anastomosis, particularly if 8-0 suture is used.

Isthmic–ampullary anastomosis

Luminal disparity is a potential problem. Preliminary dissection of the serosa and visualization of the proximal stump make it possible to create a lumen only slightly larger than the proximal ostium.

Ampullary–ampullary anastomosis

The awkwardness in these cases is due to the thin muscularis and the tendency for prolapse or extrusion of the mucosal folds. The angled probe can be used to delineate the muscularis as well as push the redundant mucosa back into the lumen after tying the muscularis sutures.

Tubo–cornual anastomosis

A linear slit at 12 o'clock is made in the cornual muscularis, using the microneedle electrode after pitressin injection. This allows some mobility of the interstitial tube so that it can be aligned to the needle and needleholder to effect suturing.

Selection of cases for the learning curve

The easiest cases for laparoscopic microsurgical anastomosis are mechanical sterilizations. The tissue damage is predictable and there is enough proximal and distal tube available with equivalent luminal sizes. In particular, the availability of proximal tube allows its mobilization to conform with the needle position whereas, with cornual anastomosis, extra steps are needed to mobilize the intramural tube and the suture placement may be inaccurate without a considerable amount of experience. Therefore, cases of electrosurgical sterilization, salpingitis isthmica nodosa and failed tubal cannulation are not suitable for anastomosis until the operator has performed more than 50 cases of isthmic anastomosis with good outcome. In this

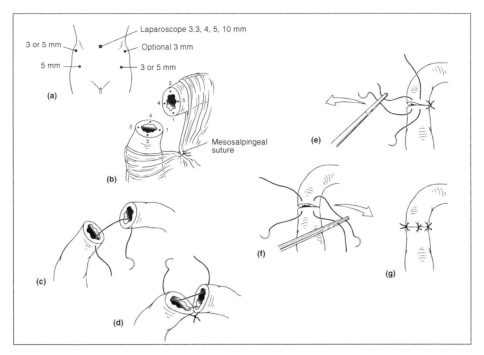

Figure 1 Surgical technique for anastomosis. (a) Placement of secondary ports; (b) suturing of the mesosalpinx; (c)–(g) suturing of the proximal tube to the distal tube

regard, a preoperative hysterosalpingogram may provide good prescreening.

SURGICAL TECHNIQUE

After insertion of a Foley catheter, the Rumi uterine manipulator with diagnostic tip is inserted into the uterus for mobilization. The intrauterine balloon is inflated with 3 ml saline. Dilute methylene blue is attached via a syringe to the chromopertubation port. After sterile preparation and draping, the trocars are inserted.

We employ the direct puncture technique using a 10-mm disposable trocar through the umbilical incision. After pneumoperitoneum has been created under direct visualization, the 3- or 5-mm secondary ports are then placed according to the position in the diagram (Figure 1a). The surgeon stands on the patient's right side.

Following this, the uterus is mobilized and anteverted and retroverted to inspect the pelvis. The lengths of the proximal and distal tubes are examined, as well as the condition of the fimbria. Any paratubal and periovarian adhesions are treated at this point, using the microelectrode. If all conditions are satisfactory for anastomosis, the operation proceeds.

The instruments described are all part of the complete Storz 'Koh Ultramicro Series'™ set.

The pitressin injector is inserted through the right lower port and 1 : 30 dilute pitressin is injected into the terminal serosa of the proximal tube, just enough to bulge the serosa. Next, using the Ultramicro I grasper with his

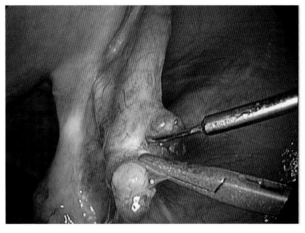

Figure 2 A grasper stabilizes the proximal tip of the tube. The surgeon circumscribes the serosa of the proximal tube

left hand to stabilize the tip of the tube, the operator introduces the microneedle electrode through the right lower port, to circumscribe the serosa of the proximal tube about 5 mm away from the tip (Figure 2). If the tubal length is generous and there is obvious bulbous dilatation of the tip, more tube can be sacrificed and the serosal cut would be 1 cm away from the tip. Following this, the microneedle is used to divide the tubal mesentery up to the chosen point for transection. By keeping this incision close to the tube, the mesosalpingeal vessels are not damaged and, therefore, do not require cautery, which may compromise the blood supply to the Fallopian tube (Figure 3).

The guillotine is inserted into the right lower port and a right-angled cut is made of the proximal tube (Figure 4). Chromopertubation is performed retrogradely by means of the syringe attached to the Rumi uterine manipulator. When dye emerges freely from the proximal tube, the laparoscope is brought to within 1 cm of the tissue to examine the muscularis and the mucosa at 40 times magnification (Figure 5). Normal isthmic mucosa stains blue and exhibits three to four folds. The muscularis is found to be circular and non-fibrotic.

The proximal end of the distal tube is now held up and pitressin is injected, via the right lower port, subserosally. Following this, the microelectrode is used to dissect and expose the proximal stump of the distal tube, which is regrasped using the Ultramicro II grasper at the very tip (Figure 6). At this point, the tubal lumen is compared to that of the proximal tube by using the straight chromo-pertubator, which has 1-mm markings along its tip. The aim is to obtain a distal lumen that is no more than 1 mm larger than the proximal stump (Figure 7).

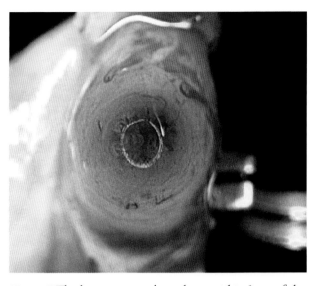

Figure 5 The laparoscope is brought to within 1 cm of the tissue to examine the muscularis and the mucosa at 40 times magnification

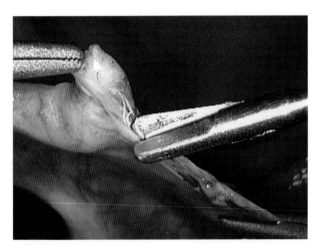

Figure 3 During dissection, care is taken to avoid damage to mesosalpingeal vessels

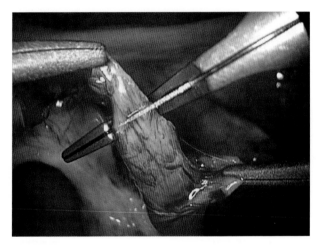

Figure 6 Dissection of the proximal end of the distal tube. The guillotine is also used to make a right-angled cut

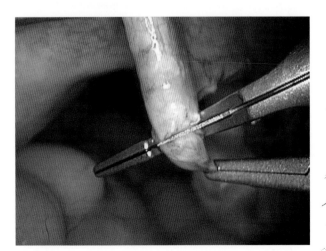

Figure 4 By using a guillotine, a right-angled cut is made of the proximal tube

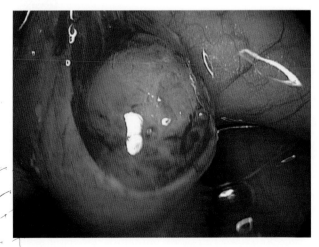

Figure 7 The aim is to obtain a distal lumen that is no more than 1 mm larger than the proximal stump

The guillotine is then reintroduced to cut the distal stump. The curved chromopertubator is introduced to inject methylene blue dye through the proximal lumen, gently, to see that it emerges through the fimbria. When this has been achieved, it confirms patency of the distal tube without the need for cannulation, which is traumatic and difficult to achieve laparoscopically. The lumen is inspected to ensure that the size is adequate and, if not, further cuts are made with the guillotine. Pinpoint hemostasis is performed as necessary. Any redundant segment of Fallopian tube with attached loop or clip may now be removed using the unipolar electrode.

An 8-cm length of 6-0 PDS or Prolene is now introduced by holding the suture 2 cm from the needle with the Ultramicro needleholder through the right lower 5-mm port. A grasper (Ultramicro I) is introduced through the right upper quadrant with the operator's left hand. The needle is grasped by the grasper, oriented and then grasped by the needleholder. The mesosalpinx is sutured together using an intracorporeal knot, tying about 5 mm away from the Fallopian tube (Figure 8). Care should be taken not to approximate the mesosalpinx too near the tube as it will hinder subsequent anastomosis (Figure 1b).

A 6-cm length of 7-0 or 8-0 suture is now introduced in the same way as previously and the needle is positioned on the needleholder similarly. The Ultramicro II grasper is used in the left hand for this suture. Using clockwise rotation of the wrist, the muscularis at 6 o'clock on the distal tube is pierced, including the mucosa (Figure 9). The needle is then inserted at 6 o'clock of the proximal tube from mucosa through muscularis, again maintaining the clockwise motion of the wrist (Figure 1c). Intracorporeal knot-tying is performed, with three knots thrown (Figure 10). Facilitation with intracorporeal knotting can be achieved using a curved Ultramicro II grasper. The suture is then cut precisely using the Ultramicro suture scissors. Another 7-0 or 8-0 suture (Figure 11) is placed at

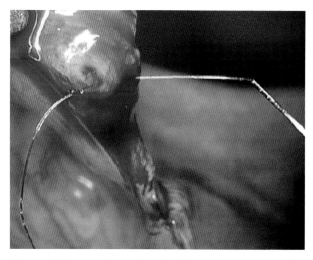

Figure 9 Using a 6-cm length of 7-0 or 8-0 suture, the muscularis at 6 o'clock on the distal tube is pierced, including the mucosa

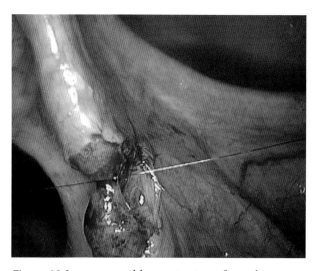

Figure 10 Intracorporeal knot-tying is performed

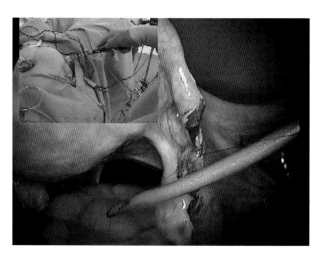

Figure 8 The mesosalpinx is sutured together using intracorporeal knot-tying about 5 mm away from the Fallopian tube

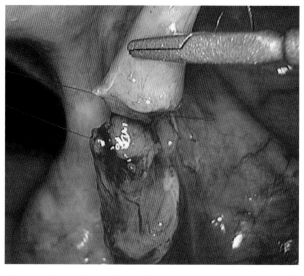

Figure 11 Another 7-0 or 8-0 suture is placed at 12 o'clock

12 o'clock of the proximal tube from muscularis to submucosa or mucosa and then to the 12 o'clock position of the distal tube with the needle entering from mucosa/submucosa through muscularis (Figure 1d). This suture is now held by the assistant using the Ultramicro II grasper and, together with the use of the uterine manipulator, one is able to rotate the tube so that both the 3 and 9 o'clock positions become available for accurate suture placement (Figures 1e and f, 12 and 13). These are placed next and tied and, finally, the 12 o'clock suture is tied (Figure 14). Chromopertubation is performed via the uterine manipulator and the patency of the tube can now be demonstrated. Slight leakage at the anastomotic site is no cause for concern as long as dye emerges from the distal fimbria. The 6-0 or 7-0 Prolene or PDS is then used to place one or two interrupted serosal sutures (Figure 15).

These sutures may incorporate the outer muscularis to maintain support of the anastomosis (Figure 1g). Any gaps evident in the mesosalpinx are similarly closed using 6-0 nylon. The opposite tube is then treated in the same manner (Figure 16).

CONCLUSIONS

Laparoscopic microsurgery is an exciting new tool with great promise, like classical microsurgery before it. However, the learning curve is steep, and skill development very intensive. It requires at least 20 mid-tubal cases before operators begin to develop a fluid rhythm. After 50 cases, one can perform bilateral midtubal anastomosis in 90 min, making it a very efficient procedure.

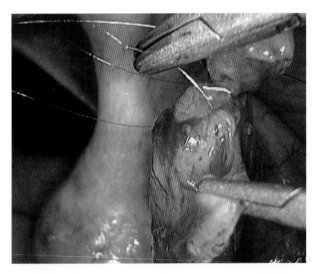

Figure 12 Using the UltraMicro II grasper, one is able to rotate the tube so that both the 3 and 9 o'clock positions become available for accurate suture placement

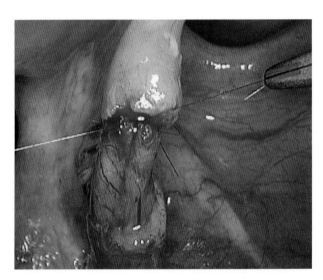

Figure 14 Finally, the 12 o'clock suture is tied

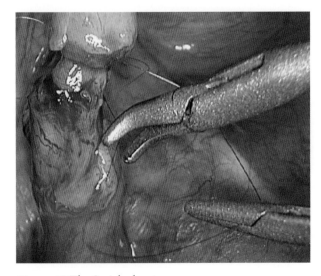

Figure 13 The 3 o'clock suture

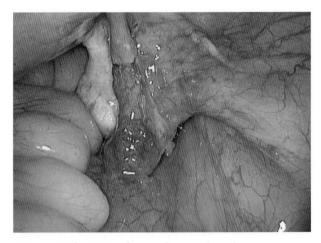

Figure 15 The 6-0 Prolene is then used to place one or two interrupted serosal sutures which may incorporate the outer muscularis to maintain support of the anastomosis

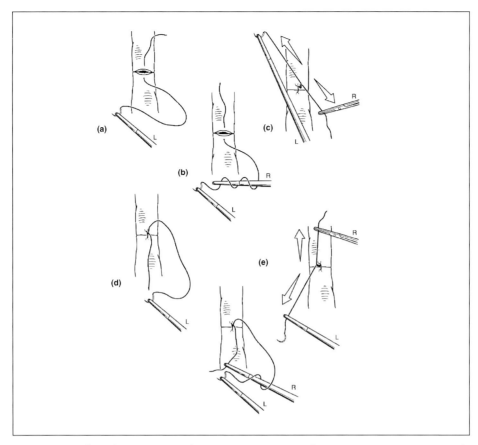

Figure 16 Ipsilateral intracorporeal microsuturing using Ultramicro instrumentation with 7-0 and 8-0 Prolene

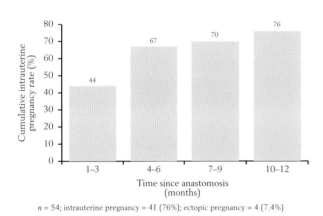

n = 54; intrauterine pregnancy = 41 (76%); ectopic pregnancy = 4 (7.4%)

Figure 17 Cumulative intrauterine pregnancy rate (%) 1992–1997 (follow-up 6–12 months). Reproductive Specialty Center, Milwaukee, USA

Laparoscopic microsurgery will introduce a new dimension to reproductive surgery and over time will replace laparotomy for microsurgery (Figure 17). It is important to realize, however, that the learning curve is considerable and the technique may not be attainable by all, despite their best efforts. The reproductive surgeon of tomorrow will be an expert in microendoscopy and laparoscopic microsurgery, with sufficient numbers of cases to maintain and develop his expertise.

REFERENCE

1. Brosens IA. Risks and benefits of endoscopic surgery in reproductive medicine. In *Proceedings of the 15th World Congress on Fertility and Sterility*. ASRM 1995;47:339–43

Laparoscopic management of ovarian cysts

19

M. Nisolle, J. Squifflet, M. Smets and J. Donnez

In most clinical circumstances, a unilocular ovarian cyst does not require aspiration, but does require medical therapy (such as oral contraceptives) for 3 months. If the cyst does not disappear after a 3-month course of therapy, it requires careful evaluation (echography, CA-125 level and, in some instances, computerized tomography (CT) and magnetic resonance imaging (MRI)), and, finally, laparoscopic diagnosis and management. The most frequent types of cysts found in young women are:

(1) The unilocular clear fluid cyst (mucous or serous);

(2) The dermoid cyst;

(3) The endometrial cyst (endometrioma).

Laparoscopic removal of benign ovarian cysts is an effective technique, involving little risk of complications[1,2]. Nevertheless, several criteria must be taken into account before performing this procedure. Various diagnostic methods have been used to discriminate between benign and malignant ovarian tumors: physical examination, transvaginal ultrasound color flow imaging and tumor markers such as CA-125.

PREOPERATIVE EVALUATION

Ultrasound examination

Using high-frequency transvaginal sonography, it is possible to detect malignant ovarian tumors more efficiently than by transabdominal echography[3]. The vaginal approach produces greater image resolution than the abdominal, thus allowing a more detailed morphological assessment of ovarian masses (Figure 1a and b).

The following criteria must be assessed: size and location, borders of the mass and free pelvic fluid (ascites). The internal structure of a mass is considered to be the most important sonographic criterion for distinguishing benign from malignant disorders. The tumor can be purely cystic, complex (mainly cystic, or mainly solid) or purely solid. Loculations, thick septa, irregular solid parts within a mass, undefined margins, and the presence of ascites are considered as malignant patterns (Figure 1c). Such cases certainly require conventional surgery by laparotomy. A sonographic diagnosis of benign disease is generally accurate; indeed, a predictive non-malignant rate of 95.6% was found by Herrmann and colleagues[4].

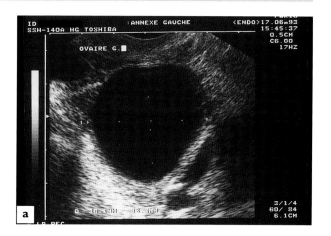

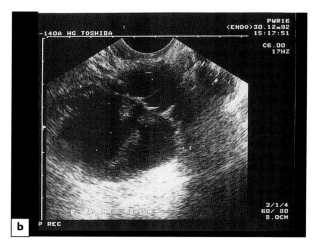

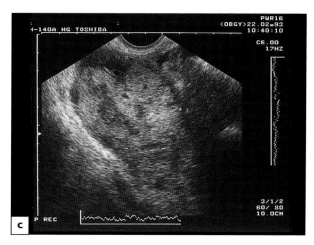

Figure 1 Transvaginal sonography: (a) unilocular cyst, without solid structures; (b) multilocular cyst; (c) cyst with thick septa and irregular solid parts suspected to be malignant

Transvaginal Doppler ultrasound with color flow imaging

Transvaginal Doppler ultrasound with color flow imaging is a new technique for the evaluation of ovarian masses[5–7]. It allows the positioning of the probe closer to the tumor and visually reflects the state of blood flow of the ovarian tumor (Figure 2a and b); it permits the detection of low-resistance intratumoral blood vessels, characteristic of malignant tumors (Figure 2c).

The pulsatility index (PI), defined as the difference between the peak systolic and the end-diastolic flow velocity divided by the mean flow velocity, is calculated. Bourne and co-workers[5] reported that this method can be used to differentiate between primary ovarian cancer and other forms of benign pelvic masses. In their study, low impedance to ovarian blood flow was associated with malignant ovarian tumors (PI < 1).

Weiner and associates[8] made an attempt to compare transvaginal color flow imaging with conventional sonographic findings and other screening procedures to predict ovarian malignancy. They found that suspicious sonographic findings had low specificity and were inadequate in distinguishing between benign and malignant ovarian tumors. They concluded that transvaginal color flow imaging provided high sensitivity and specificity and was superior to the other methods used for preoperative evaluation of ovarian masses.

A simple measurement of the PI in the newly formed intratumoral blood vessels can discriminate accurately between malignant and non-malignant ovarian tumors. Moreover, because early development of neovascularity may precede tumor growth, screening for ovarian malignancy with transvaginal color flow imaging may detect early ovarian neoplasms before sonography. According to the results of Bourne and colleagues[5], Fleischer and co-workers[9], and Kurjak and associates[6], transvaginal color Doppler is a valuable method of differentiating benign from malignant ovarian tumors. However, others[10] have recently been unable to reproduce their results.

CA-125

The preoperative evaluation of serum CA-125 levels must be made before endoscopic surgery, especially in premenopausal and postmenopausal patients, in order to suspect malignant disease preoperatively. Values of CA-125 in excess of 65 IU/ml distinguished malignant from benign disease with a specificity of 92% and a sensitivity of 75% when both premenopausal and postmenopausal patients were studied together[11]. Greater specificity and sensitivity were observed in postmenopausal subjects, in whom the specificity of the assay was 97% and the sensitivity 78%[11].

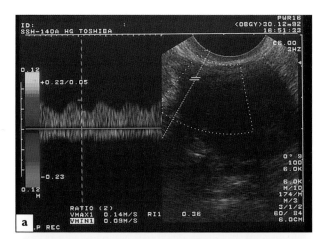

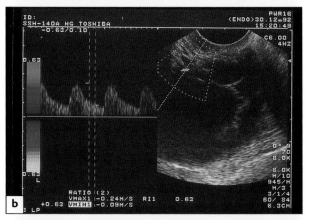

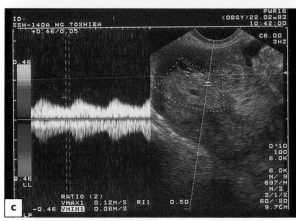

Figure 2 Transvaginal Doppler ultrasound with color flow imaging (corresponding to the cysts shown in Figure 1): (a) unilocular cyst: normal pulsatility index; (b) multilocular cyst: normal pulsatility index; (c) multilocular cyst with hyperechogenic areas. Low-resistant intratumoral blood vessels, suggesting malignancy

CT and MRI

CT provides high quality images of the ovaries but does not give more information than ultrasound, except in cases of dermoid cysts (Figure 3). In our experience, CT is less sensitive and less specific than transvaginal echography in the detection of intracystic structures or septa (Figure 3).

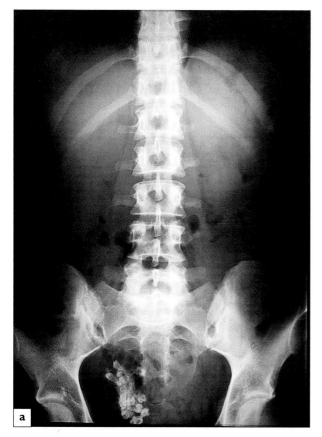

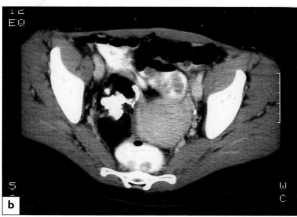

Figure 3 (a) and (b) Computerized tomography; in the case of dermoid cyst, high-quality images are obtained

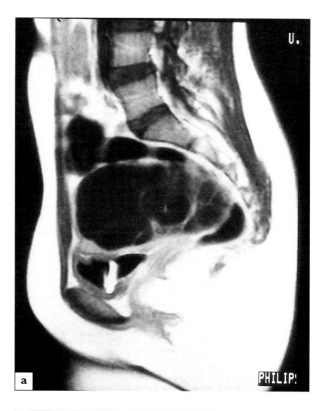

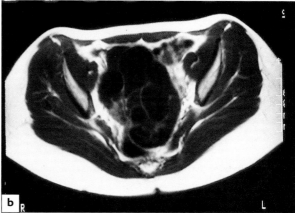

Figure 4 (a) and (b) Magnetic resonance imaging provides soft tissue contrast and clear pictures of pelvic organs. Multilocular cyst (histology: mucinous cyst)

MRI provides soft tissue contrast and clear pictures of pelvic organs (Figure 4). This modality is biologically safe and more sensitive than CT in the diagnosis of intracystic structures, and more sensitive and specific than either CT or ultrasound in the evaluation of an ovarian mass.

As a result of the accuracy, convenience, relatively low cost and availability of high-resolution ultrasound equipment, this technique has remained the principal imaging modality in assessing pelvic pathology. In our department, CT and MRI are indicated in cases of suspected malignant lesions.

INDICATIONS

Indications for laparoscopic cystectomy include serous, mucous, dermoid and endometriotic cysts. The internal wall of the endometriotic cyst, whose complete dissection from the ovarian cortex could be difficult, can also be vaporized with the CO_2 laser, as previously described[12,13].

The indications for laparoscopic oophorectomy usually include large endometriotic cysts and benign ovarian cysts in patients aged over 40 years.

The laparoscopic aspiration of unilocular, smooth-walled, translucent ovarian cysts remains controversial. The main concern is spillage of malignancy. Thorough preoperative evaluation of the patient, combining ultrasonography of ovarian tumors with the measurement of tumor markers, may greatly improve the accuracy of diagnosis of ovarian malignancy. Moreover, laparoscopy is, in the first place, used as a diagnostic tool whereby the pelvis and the abdominal cavity are thoroughly evaluated.

The ovaries are inspected carefully to ensure that the cyst wall is smooth and that there is no vegetation (Figure 5). The interior wall of the cyst can also be carefully examined (Figure 6) and a biopsy with frozen histological evaluation can be carried out.

In a retrospective study of 226 patients, Mage and colleagues[14] reported that the diagnosis of malignant tumors by laparoscopy was 100% accurate. The anatomopathological examination of specimens in benign conditions was never wrong. They concluded that laparoscopy is a reliable way of diagnosing the type of ovarian cyst.

According to these data, we have proposed the scheme outlined in Figure 7 for the laparoscopic management of ovarian cysts. In patients aged under 35 years, hormonal therapy is first attempted for 3 months if the echography reveals a unilocular, smooth-walled cyst without septa or intracystic structures. If the cyst persists, an ultrasound examination is carried out and the CA-125 level is measured, in order to exclude a malignant lesion. In patients under 40 years of age, a cystectomy is usually performed. In patients aged over 40 years, the preoperative evaluation (echography and CA-125) is made directly. If data suggest malignancy, a laparotomy is performed after computerized tomography and/or magnetic resonance imaging have been performed. Only when a malignant lesion can be excluded is a laparoscopy performed. If at all possible, the cyst is removed intact. Otherwise, the interior wall of the cyst is examined to exclude the presence of any suspect vegetation, which would require a biopsy and a frozen histological examination.

In patients over age 40 years, a cystectomy is rarely performed and a unilateral oophorectomy is the preferred procedure. If the frozen histological examination reveals the presence of malignant cells, a laparotomy and total abdominal hysterectomy are mandatory.

In patients aged over 50 years, after all the same precautions have been taken, a bilateral oophorectomy is carried out, even if the contralateral ovary is normal.

SURGICAL PROCEDURES

The procedure is performed under general anesthesia. After induction of a pneumoperitoneum, a 12-mm trocar is inserted subumbilically. The laparoscope is connected to a video camera. Three 5-mm trocars are systematically inserted suprapubically: one in the midline approximately 3 cm above the symphysis pubis, and the other two a few centimeters on either side, taking care to avoid the epigastric vessels.

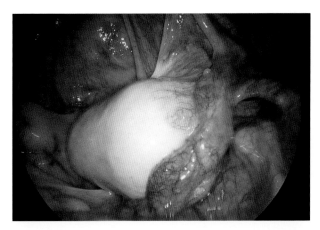

Figure 5 Laparoscopic examination of the external cyst wall which must have a smooth appearance

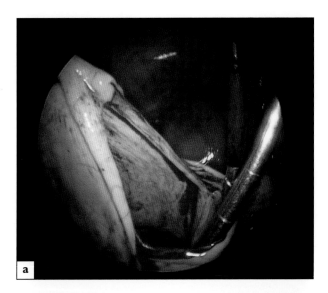

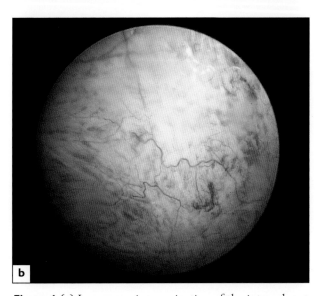

Figure 6 (a) Laparoscopic examination of the internal cyst wall; (b) internal view of the cyst. Note the absence of intracystic vegetations (no biopsy required)

The initial phase of the laparoscopy is purely diagnostic. First, the abdominal cavity is inspected thoroughly and a peritoneal sampling is sent for cytology. The ovaries are examined carefully in order to exclude the presence of excrescences or other evidence suggesting malignancy.

It is important to differentiate between organic and functional cysts during laparoscopy; 10–20% of functional cysts do not disappear after 3 months of treatment with combination oral contraceptive pills containing 50 µg of ethinylestradiol. According to Mage and associates[14], there are five laparoscopic criteria which allow us to distinguish between functional and organic cysts (Table 1).

Intraperitoneal cystectomy

The utero-ovarian ligament is grasped with an atraumatic forceps introduced on the side of the tumor, in order to completely expose the ovary (Figure 8).

The first step consists of making an incision in the ovarian cortex with the scissors or with the CO_2 laser

(Figure 9). The incision must be made in the ovarian cortex overlying the cyst and it must be long enough to permit a straightforward cystectomy. In some cases, the cyst is first aspirated and the liquid examined (Figure 10).

The interior wall of the cyst can be checked by introducing the laparoscope into the ovarian cyst (Figure 11). If there is any intracystic vegetation, a biopsy with frozen histological evaluation can be carried out before a decision is made whether to perform a cystectomy or oophorectomy. In fact, ideally, the cyst should be removed intact from the ovary, without aspirating any of the contents.

The second step is the separation of the ovarian cyst capsule from the surrounding ovarian cortex. The ovarian cyst is held using an atraumatic forceps and the ovarian cortex is grasped with another forceps placed close to the ovarian cyst (Figure 12). By traction and counter-traction, the dissection is easily carried out and the cyst is removed.

Nezhat and colleagues[15] inject 3–5 ml of dilute vasopressin between the capsule and ovarian cortex, to create a tissue plane (hydrodissection) and to reduce oozing from

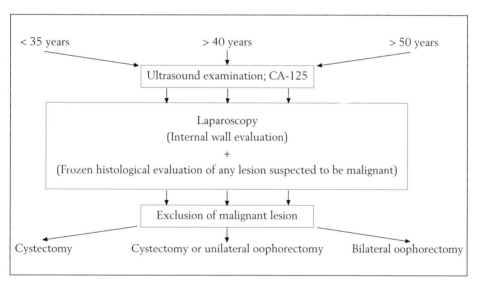

Figure 7 Laparoscopic management of ovarian cysts

Table 1 Laparoscopic criteria for differentiation between functional and organic ovarian cysts (from reference 14)

Criterion	Organic cysts	Functional cysts
Utero-ovarian ligament	lengthened	normal
Cyst wall	thick	thin
Ovarian vessels	numerous and regular starting from the mesovarium	more scanty, coral-like
Cyst fluid	clear, dark, brown, or dermoid	saffron yellow
Internal cyst wall appearance	smooth or fibrotic with areas of hypervascularization	retina-like aspect

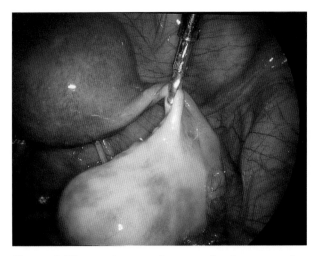

Figure 8 The ovarian cyst is exposed using a grasping forceps

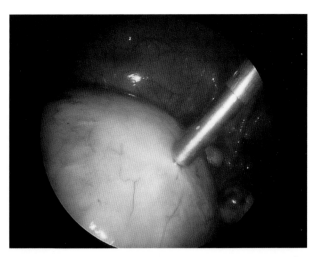

Figure 10 In order to perform an ovarian cystoscopy, the aspiration of the intracystic contents can be carried out in some instances

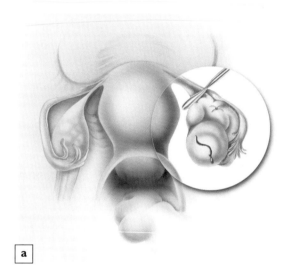

a

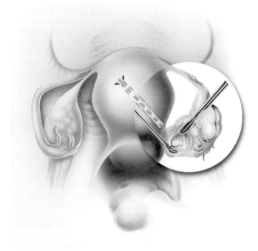

Figure 11 Ovarian cystoscopy by the introduction of the laparoscope into the cyst

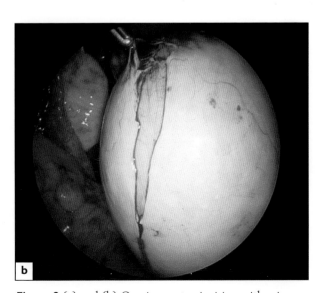

b

Figure 9 (a) and (b) Ovarian cortex incision with scissors

the ovarian bed. We do not consider this procedure to be useful and it is not used in our department.

The surgeon must constantly observe the tissue tension, and the grasping forceps must be moved often in order to apply the traction in just the right place to avoid tearing the ovary.

At the ovarian hilus, the dissection is often more difficult, but nevertheless, the dissection should continue until the cyst is completely removed from the ovary (Figure 13).

Thereafter, the interior ovarian surface is examined and rinsed. Hemostasis is usually achieved spontaneously but, if necessary, bipolar coagulation can be used. However, aggressive electrocoagulation can be the cause of ovarian destruction and premature ovarian failure.

Generally, there is no bleeding and the ovary is left to heal without suturing (Figure 14). Indeed, the ovarian edges approximate spontaneously. In cases of large cysts

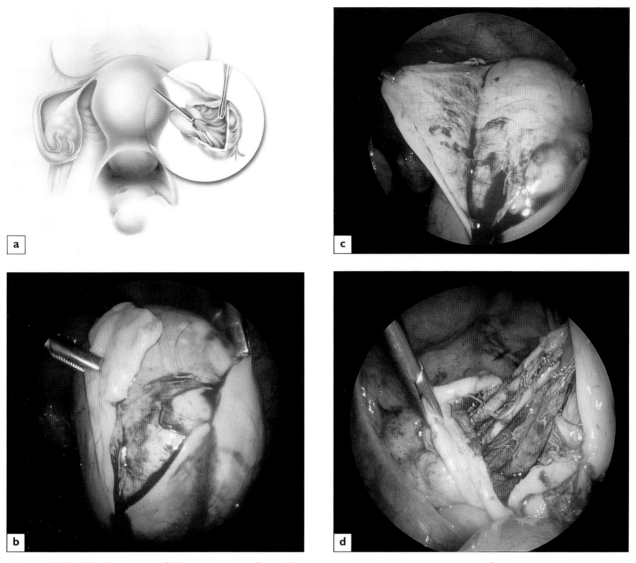

Figure 12 (a)–(d) Separation of the ovarian cyst from the ovarian cortex using two atraumatic forceps

where approximation does not occur spontaneously, closure can be undertaken using the following techniques.

Suturing

The ability to suture during laparoscopy was initially developed by Semm[16]. Loop ligation using the endoloop or Roeder loop is most often used as an adjuvant to hemostasis, and as a classic ligature in the case of salpingo-oophorectomy or oophorectomy.

With the advent of endoligature and the intra- and extracorporeal operative knotting techniques, classic methods used at laparotomy were introduced in endoscopic surgery and have become a mainstay. The intracorporeal knotting technique has been recommended by Semm[16] for fine ovarian sutures. Two lower abdominal puncture sites are necessary, and, through these, laparoscopic needle holders are introduced to manipulate the suture, needle and involved tissue. The suture material

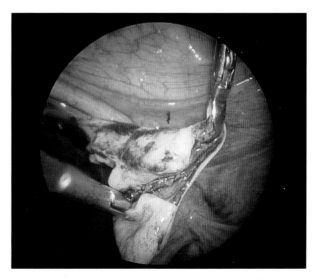

Figure 13 Complete removal of the cyst. The remaining ovarian cortex is grasped with the help of two atraumatic forceps

suture, needle and involved tissue. The suture material used is 4/0 or 6/0 polydioxanone.

Clips

Clips can also be used for closing the ovarian cortex after cystectomy. The clip is of medium to large size and is made of titanium, an inert, non-reactive metal (Autosuture (Eudohernia®); Ethicon). Three to four clips are applied using the 10-mm clip applicator; this is usually sufficient to achieve ovarian closure (Figure 15). For ovarian surgery, a titanium clip is preferred to one made of polydioxanone material.

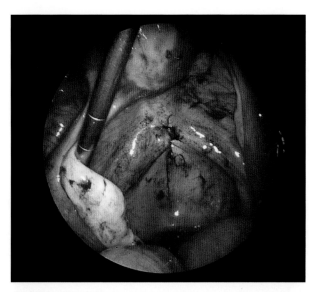

Figure 14 Final aspect of the ovarian cortex. The dermoid cyst was removed through a colpotomy incision whose closure is clearly visible between the uterosacral ligaments

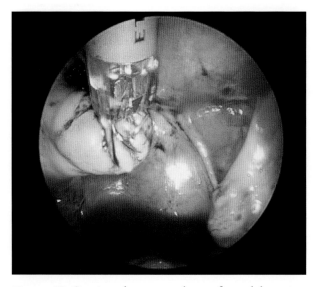

Figure 15 Ovarian closure can be performed by using titanium clips, but usually the ovary is left open

Fibrin sealant

Fibrin sealant[13] is useful in controlling microvascular or capillary bleeding from ruptured or surgically dissected tissue. It is particularly beneficial during surgery on patients with increased bleeding tendencies. It might also be used to seal tissue with different kinds of biomaterials. Thus, fibrin sealant has a place in all surgical disciplines for the purposes of tissue sealing, hemostasis and support of wound healing. There seem to be a few drawbacks, such as the risk of viral transmission; however, the benefits of combining fibrin sealing with modern-day surgery far outweigh any known risks.

For the optimal use of fibrin sealant, the application technique should meet the following requirements:

(1)   The sealant components should be fully dissolved and kept at a temperature of 37°C (which is easy with the Fibrinotherm system);

(2)   The wound surfaces should be as dry as possible (though application to wet surfaces is feasible);

(3)   The components should be mixed thoroughly on application;

(4)   The thrombin and aprotinin concentrations may be adjusted to the purpose of application;

(5)   The sealant should be applied as a thin film through a catheter introduced into one of the trocars;

(6)   After clotting has occurred, further mechanical stresses should be avoided for about 3–5 min. The edges of the ovarian cortex are approximated with atraumatic forceps (Figure 16).

Laparoscopic oophorectomy

In most cases, the tube is removed with the ovary intact unless a previous salpingectomy has been performed. Different methods of laparoscopic oophorectomy have been described. The initial technique described the placement of pre-tied loop ligatures[16]; three chromic endoloop sutures were placed around the ovary and the tube and pulled tight. The ovary was then cut away from its pedicle, cut into strips, and removed laparoscopically.

The second method of laparoscopic oophorectomy was bipolar coagulation with excision (Figure 17a). This technique involved four punctures, with traction (Figure 17b) on the adnexum. A bipolar coagulation forceps was then used to coagulate the ovarian pedicle (Figure 17c and d). After total desiccation of the tissue, 5-mm scissors or the CO_2 laser were used to cut (Figure 17e and f). Successive portions of the meso-ovarium and mesosalpinx were treated in a similar fashion (Figure 17g), and the proximal tube and ovarian ligament were also coagulated (Figure 17h) and cut (Figure 17i). Once the tube and ovary had been separated, they were removed laparoscopically using a LapSac® (Figure 17j–l). Recent studies have shown

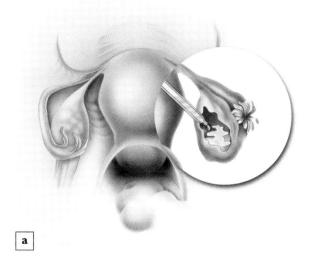

a

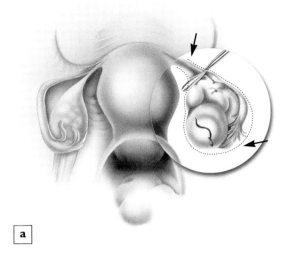

a

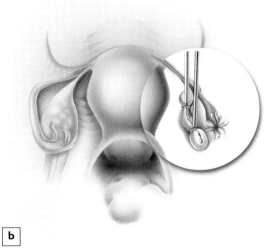

b

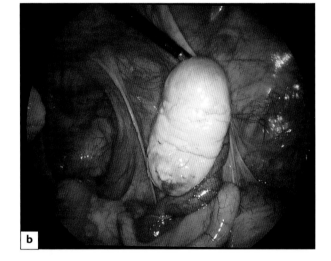

b

Figure 16 (a) Ovarian closure by using fibrin sealant; (b) approximation of the ovarian cortex with two atraumatic forceps

equally good results using tissue desiccation with bipolar coagulation followed by excision without ligatures.

The most recent technique for laparoscopic oophorectomy is the automatic laparoscopic stapling device. Disposable stapling instruments for laparoscopic surgery are now available. The Multifire GIA surgical stapler (United States Surgical Corporation, Newark, NJ, USA) is readily available and is proving to be effective for appendicectomy, hysterectomy and adnexectomy (Figure 18).

A staple cartridge 3 cm in length is fired across the infundibulopelvic vessels. Two triple-staggered lines of titanium staples are automatically placed, with a knife cutting between them (Figure 18). In most cases, two firings of the automatic stapling device are necessary to accomplish removal of the tube and ovary. They are then extracted in a similar way to that used in other laparoscopic techniques. The automatic stapling device reduces operating time but is nevertheless more expensive than bipolar coagulation.

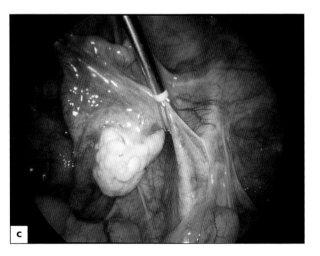

c

Figure 17 Laparoscopic adnexectomy: (a) illustration of the technique – coagulation of the ovarian pedicle, the ligament, the Fallopian tube and the utero-ovarian ligament; (b) laparoscopic view of a 3-cm multilocular cyst in a perimenopausal woman; (c) the ovarian pedicle is grasped and elevated. *Continued on next page*

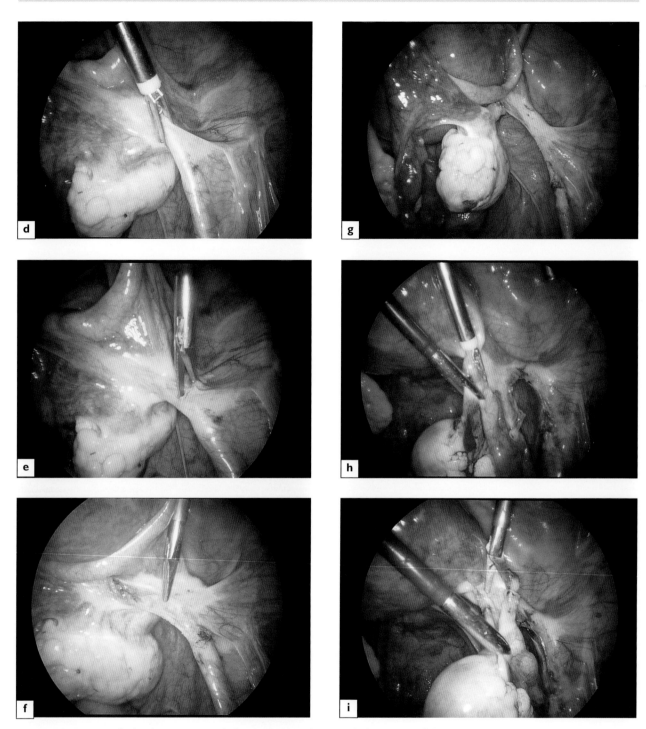

Figure 17 *Continued* (d) The ovarian pedicle is coagulated; (e) and (f) section of the ovarian pedicle with scissors; (g) the broad ligament is cut up to the round ligament; (h) coagulation of the proximal part of the annexa; (i) section of the proximal part of the adnexa. *Continued on next page*

In certain cases, it is impossible to use pre-tied ligatures as the primary method because the ovary adheres too strongly to the side-wall to allow the placement of the ligature around the adnexa. In such cases, dissection and bipolar coagulation are necessary before beginning the oophorectomy. Similarly, the automatic stapling device, which is 12 mm in diameter, cannot be placed around the whole adnexa; it must be mobile and free before the auto-

matic stapling device can be used[17]. Aquadissection, blunt probing, scissors and judicious use of bipolar coagulation are necessary in certain cases to mobilize the ovary for laparoscopic removal using any of the three techniques described. Aggressive ovariolysis increases the risk of ureteral or bowel injury, or severe bleeding.

The absence of ovarian adhesiolysis before oophorectomy can lead to the incomplete removal of all functional

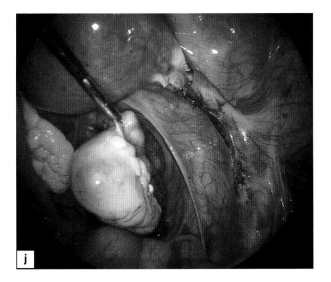

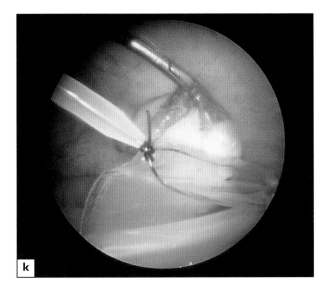

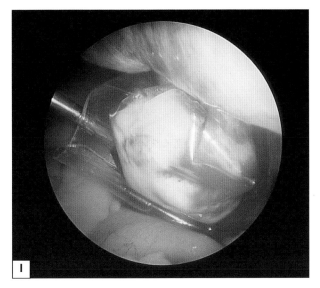

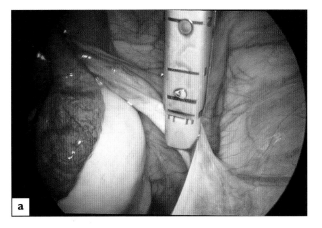

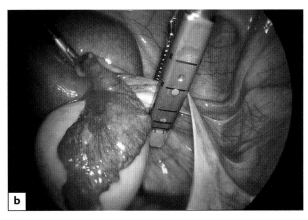

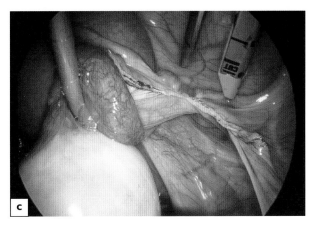

Figure 18 (a)–(c) Multifire GIA surgical stapler: application on the ovarian vessels

ovarian tissue. The endoloop sutures must be placed below the ovary, to avoid trapping ovarian tissue in the pedicle. Persistent ovarian remnant syndrome after laparoscopic oophorectomy has been described by several authors[15].

Cyst at adnexa removal

There are several techniques used for the removal of a cyst or of the adnexa:

(1)   After enucleation from the ovaries or after oophorectomy, the tissue is grasped with the grasping

Figure 17 *Continued*. (j) The adnexa is dissected free; (k) to avoid spillage, the ovary, with intact cyst, is placed in the bag; (l) the bag is closed by pulling its drawstrings

forceps introduced through the operating channel of the laparoscope and removed from the abdominal cavity. Such removal can be performed only in cases of small ovarian cysts or after aspiration of the cyst.

However, in cases where spillage should be avoided at all costs (separate cysts or CA-125 > 35 IU/ml), an impermeable bag can be used (LapSac, Ethicon or Cook) (Figure 17k and l). The bag is introduced through a second puncture trocar. The cyst or the ovary with the intact cyst is placed in the bag, which is closed by pulling its drawstring. The bag is raised to just beneath the abdominal wall and a needle is introduced into the bag in order to aspirate the cyst and decompress it. Then the bag is removed without spillage from the abdominal cavity through a 2-cm suprapubic incision. Reich[18] describes a different technique: the bag is inserted intraperitoneally through the colpotomy incision and it is removed by pulling the drawstring through the posterior vaginal incision. The bag is opened and the intact specimen visually identified, decompressed and removed.

(2) In some cases, the tissue is grasped directly with an instrument introduced through a suprapubic incision without using a bag. Theoretically, removing the cyst through a puncture site could lead to a surviving ovarian remnant in the abdominal wall. Nezhat and co-workers[15] have not observed this phenomenon in their 1–3-year follow-up in the patients who underwent this technique of cyst wall removal. However, Canis (personal communication) has recently reported induced endometriosis at the trocar site after removal of an endometriotic cyst through the abdominal wall. A metastatic tumor has been reported in three cases on the anterior abdominal wall at the trocar site, following biopsy of ovarian cancer[19]. It is suggested that any suspicious ovarian tissue must be removed from the abdomen while avoiding direct contact with the abdominal incision.

(3) In cases of large dermoid cysts, the cyst can be placed in the cul-de-sac of Douglas using a grasping forceps. A colpotomy incision is made and the cyst is then removed intact or aspirated through the vagina[20]: a needle is directed through the vagina for cyst decompression. The thick cyst contents can be evacuated by introducing the suction cannula into the cyst after making an incision of 5–6 mm. When the mass is small enough, it can be pulled through the vaginal incision. Copious vaginal and intraperitoneal irrigation with antiseptic solution is performed after cyst removal.

In our department, a colpotomy incision is made through the vagina and the overlying peritoneum using scissors. We have never encountered any complications – no bleeding, rectal injuries or infections – using this technique.

However, Reich[18] suggests that a posterior colpotomy incision using the CO_2 laser or electrosurgery through the cul-de-sac of Douglas into the vagina is preferable to a vaginal incision because complete hemostasis is obtained while making the colpotomy incision. The anatomical relationship between the rectum and the posterior vagina must be confirmed before making the laparoscopic colpotomy incision to avoid cutting the rectum. Reich[18,21,22] uses an instrument placed in the uterus for elevation and anteversion. The posterior vaginal fornix is identified by placing a wet sponge in a ring forceps just behind the cervix. A rectal probe can also be used in order to ensure that the rectum is out of the way.

DISCUSSION

Risk of borderline tumor

The advantages of the laparoscopic treatment of ovarian cysts have been described for women under the age of 35 years with simple ovarian cysts, for whom the overall risk of malignancy is only 4.5 per 100 000 cases[14].

The risk is much higher in postmenopausal women. Indeed, a 10-year study[23] suggested that, when a postmenopausal woman undergoes surgery for an ovarian neoplasm, the rate of malignancy may be as high as 45%. Very often, a malignant tumor is diagnosed or suspected by means of echography, CA-125, CT or MRI. We have tried to evaluate the 'true' risk of underdiagnosing an ovarian tumor preoperatively.

In a series of 114 postmenopausal women who underwent bilateral adnexectomy, 78 were found to have a serous or mucinous cystadenoma, ten an endometrial cyst, eight a paraovarian cyst, 14 a dermoid cyst and four (< 4%) a borderline tumor (Table 2). In this series, all patients had a preoperative check-up including the measurement of the CA-125 level and an ultrasound examination. Three of the four borderline tumor cases presented abnormalities at the preoperative check-up (Table 3). Indeed, in two cases, in spite of a normal CA-125 level, the echography showed a multilocular cyst. In one case, the cyst was unilocular but

Table 2 Bilateral adnexectomy (n = 114 postmenopausal women)

Pathology	Number
Serous or mucinous cystadenoma	78
Endometrial cyst	10
'Paraovarian' cyst (Wolffian)	8
Dermoid	14
Borderline tumor	4

the CA-125 level was elevated. In the last case, however, there were no evident abnormalities (unilocular cyst, normal CA-125 level); therefore, an accurate preoperative diagnosis was impossible (0.9%) (Figure 19). In these four borderline cases, the abnormal cells could not be detected on frozen pathology. These four patients underwent hysterectomy 2 weeks later. Peritoneal sampling for cytology did not reveal any abnormal cells, and the histology did not show any residual malignant tissue; to date, no sign of recurrence has been demonstrated.

The preoperative check-up of a mass diagnosed in postmenopausal women is, in most cases, accurate. Indeed, in our series, only one case (< 1%) went undetected preoperatively. However, when an abnormality is observed

(Figure 20), certain peri-operative precautions must be taken to avoid spillage of the intracystic contents.

Risk of spillage

Spillage of benign material in cases of benign cystic teratomas or endometriomas can theoretically produce chemical peritonitis. Intraoperative spillage of a mucinous cystadenoma may theoretically initiate pseudomyxoma peritonei. The risk appears to be very low, since pseudomyxoma peritonei, when reported, is usually present at the time of initial surgery[24]. According to several authors, pseudomyxoma peritonei is almost always associated with mucinous cystadenocarcinoma[25]. Furthermore,

Table 3 Borderline tumors (n = 4); preoperative check-up

Case	Echography	CA-125 (IU/ml)	Frozen pathology
1	multilocular	< 35	negative
2	multilocular	< 35	negative
3	unilocular	56	negative
4	unilocular	< 35	negative

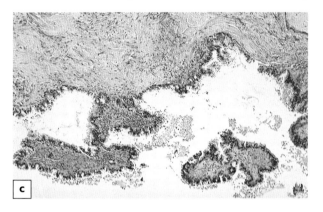
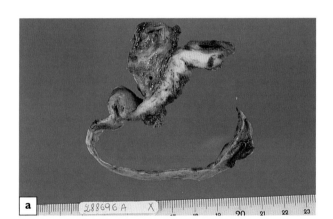
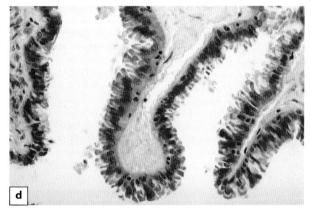
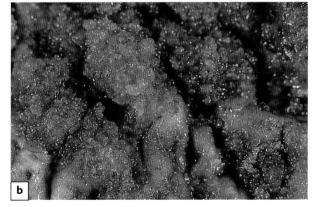
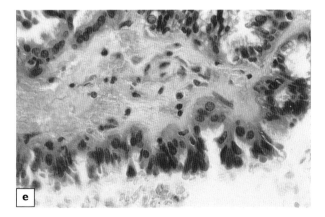

Figure 19 Borderline ovarian tumor: (a) unilocular cyst with a normal CA-125 level; (b) small (< 1 mm) papillary lesions were visible over an area of 1 cm²; (c)–(e) histology reveals the presence of an ovarian borderline tumor

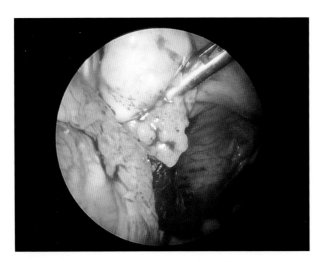

Figure 20 Laparoscopic diagnosis of small vegetations on the surface of the ovary. These were not suspected by echography. Frozen histology revealed a 'borderline' tumor. Ovariectomy was carried out. The ovary was removed by using a LapSac

pseudomyxoma peritonei does not appear to be a frequent complication of mucinous carcinoma, even when ruptured at laparotomy. To date, Mage and co-workers[1,14] have observed no cases of pseudomyxoma peritonei after laparoscopic treatment of mucinous cystadenoma. Similar results have been reported after laparotomy with cyst rupture. The treatment of the cyst must include careful and copious peritoneal lavage performed immediately, using several liters of Ringer's lactate, with the patient in a reverse Trendelenburg position. Operative spillage should be avoided as much as possible by using 5-mm aspiration systems or a LapSac. In cases of large cysts, the cyst can be punctured before it is placed in the LapSac, which is positioned directly beneath the cyst in order to catch any possible spillage. Moreover, peritoneal lavage and the appropriate surgical treatment, carried out immediately after diagnosis, seem to make the risks of spillage negligible[1,26] (also Donnez and Nisolle, present study). A recent re-evaluation of intraoperative spillage at laparotomy has demonstrated no adverse effect on the prognosis of stage I ovarian cancer[27]. According to this study, the survival term depends primarily on three factors:

(1) The tumor grading;

(2) The density of adhesions;

(3) Ascites > 250 ml.

However, the capsule penetration, the tumor size, the histological type, the age of the patient and the rupture of the tumor were found to have no influence on the prognosis.

It is generally agreed that ovarian cancer should not be managed laparoscopically. One of the drawbacks of operative laparoscopy may be that, in certain cases, malignant cysts cannot be detected.

Risk of postoperative adhesions

What is the risk of postoperative adhesion formation following closure versus non-closure of ovarian defects? It is well known that the ovary is particularly sensitive to surgical trauma, as demonstrated by the high incidence of adhesions after ovarian wedge resection. Buttram and Vaquero[28] performed bilateral ovarian wedge resection for polycystic ovarian disease in 173 patients. Of these, 34% underwent endoscopy or laparotomy at some time after bilateral wedge resection. Although the degree of severity varied, all 59 women were found to have adhesions.

Of nine women of reproductive age who underwent removal of dermoid cysts via laparoscopy without an ovarian suture, Nezhat and associates[15] performed a repeat laparoscopy in four for the evaluation of possible pelvic adhesion formation. Only one had mild periovarian adhesions and she had experienced no previous spillage of cyst contents; in the other three women without adhesions at the time of their second laparoscopy, spillage had previously occurred during the cystectomy. Because there is little adhesion formation after intraperitoneal cystectomy, most authors consider that no suture is required and that the ovary can be left open. In our department, ovarian closure is performed only in cases of large endometriotic cysts. Indeed, such cysts are vaporized using the CO_2 laser instead of dissection. Following this type of procedure, the ovarian edges do not approximate spontaneously, and adhesion formation can occur between the vaporized area and the fimbria[12,13]. For this reason, Tissucol® or clips can be used for the ovarian closure[13].

CONCLUSION: THE RIGHT WAY IS THE SELECTION OF PATIENTS

Selection of patients for laparoscopic treatment can be accomplished successfully by excluding those with elevated CA-125 levels, suspect ultrasound appearances of cysts containing > 3-mm thick septations, solid components within a cyst, matted loops of bowel, or ascites. Large series have demonstrated a reassuringly low incidence of inadvertently encountered malignancy at laparoscopy (0.4%[29,30], 0.9% (Nisolle and Donnez, present study), 1.1%[24], 1.2%[1]), but intraoperative surveillance and numerous biopsies are necessary if unsuspected cancer is to be correctly diagnosed.

We are of the opinion that careful preoperative and peri-operative examination will eliminate the high rate of mistakes published in 1991 by Maiman and colleagues[31]. For us, this manuscript reveals a lack of experience or the absence of strict guidelines by the 29 respondents who took part in a survey concerning the 'laparoscopic management of ovarian neoplasms subsequently found to be malignant'.

REFERENCES

1. Mage G, Canis M, Manhes H, *et al*. Laparoscopic management of adnexal cystic masses. *J Gynecol Surg* 1990;6:71–9
2. Bruhat MA, Mage G, Chapron C, *et al*. Present day endoscopic surgery in gynecology. *Eur J Obstet Gynecol Reprod Biol* 1991;41:4–13
3. Campbell S, Bhan V, Royston P, *et al*. Transabdominal ultrasound screening for early ovarian cancer. *Br Med J* 1989;299:1363–7
4. Hermann UJ, Locher GW, Goldhirsch A. Sonographic patterns of ovarian tumors: prediction of malignancy. *Obstet Gynecol* 1987;69:777–81
5. Bourne T, Campbell S, Steer C, *et al*. Transvaginal colour flow imaging: a possible new screening technique for ovarian cancer. *Br Med J* 1989;299:1367–70
6. Kurjak A, Schulman H, Sosic A, *et al*. Transvaginal ultrasound, color flow, and Doppler waveform of the postmenopausal adnexal mass. *Obstet Gynecol* 1992;80:917–21
7. Kawai M, Kano T, Kikkawa F, *et al*. Transvaginal Doppler ultrasound with color flow imaging in the diagnosis of ovarian cancer. *Obstet Gynecol* 1992;79:163–7
8. Weiner Z, Thaler I, Beck D, *et al*. Differentiating malignant from benign ovarian tumors with transvaginal color flow imaging. *Obstet Gynecol* 1992;79:159–62
9. Fleischer AC, McKee MS, Gordon AN, *et al*. Transvaginal sonography of postmenopausal ovaries with pathologic correlation. *J Ultrasound Med* 1990;9:637–44
10. Hata K, Hata T, Manabe A, *et al*. A critical evaluation of transvaginal Doppler studies, transvaginal sonography, magnetic resonance imaging, and CA-125 in detecting ovarian cancer. *Obstet Gynecol* 1992;00:922–6
11. Malkasian GD, Knapp RC, Lavin PT, *et al*. Preoperative evaluation of serum CA-125 levels in premenopausal and postmenopausal patients with pelvic masses: discrimination of benign from malignant disease. *Am J Obstet Gynecol* 1988;159:341–6
12. Donnez J, Nisolle M, Karaman Y, *et al*. CO_2 laser laparoscopy in peritoneal endometriosis and in ovarian cyst. *J Gynecol Surg* 1990;5:391
13. Donnez J, Nisolle M. Laparoscopic management of large ovarian endometrial cysts: use of fibrin sealant. *J Gynecol Surg* 1991;7:163–7
14. Mage G, Canis M, Manhes G, *et al*. Kystes ovariens et coelioscopie. A propos de 226 observations. *J Gynecol Obstet Biol Reprod* 1987;16:1053–61
15. Nezhat C, Winer WK, Nezhat F. Laparoscopic removal of dermoid cyst. *Obstet Gynecol* 1989;73:278–80
16. Semm K, Mettler L. Technical progress in pelvic surgery via operative laparoscopy. *Am J Obstet Gynecol* 1980;138:121–7
17. Daniell JF, Kurts BR, Lee J. Laparoscopic oophorectomy: comparative study of ligatures, bipolar coagulation, and automatic stapling devices. *Obstet Gynecol* 1992;80:325–8
18. Reich H. Difficulties in removing large masses from the abdomen. In Corfman RS, Diamond MP, DeCherney A, eds. *Complications of Laparoscopy and Hysteroscopy*. New York: Blackwell Scientific Publications, 1993:103–7
19. Hsiu JG, Given FT, Kemp GM. Tumor implantation after diagnostic laparoscopic biopsy of serous ovarian tumors of low malignant potential. *Obstet Gynecol* 1986;68:91–3
20. Nisolle M, Donnez J. Laparoscopic ovarian cystectomy. Presented at the *Seventh International Symposium on Laser Endoscopic Surgery*, Brussels, 1992
21. Reich H. Laparoscopic oophorectomy and salpingo-oophorectomy in the treatment of benign tubo-ovarian disease. *Int J Fertil* 1987;32:233–6
22. Reich H. New techniques in advanced laparoscopic surgery. In Sutton CJG, ed. *Baillière's Clinical Obstetrics and Gynaecology, Laparoscopic Surgery*. 1989;3:655–82
23. Koonings RP, Campbell K, Mishell DR, *et al*. Relative frequency of primary ovarian neoplasms: a 10-year review. *Obstet Gynecol* 1989;74:921–6
24. Tasker M, Langley FA. The outlook for women with borderline epithelial tumours of the ovary. *Br J Obstet Gynaecol* 1985;92:969
25. Fernandez RN, Daly JM. Pseudomyxoma peritonei. *Arch Surg* 1980;115:409
26. Lueken RP. Laparoscopic-ovarian surgery. In Lueken RP, Gallinat A, eds. *Endoscopic Surgery in Gynecology*. Berlin: Demeter Verlag GMBH, 1993:43–7
27. Dembo AJ, Davy M, Stenwig AE, *et al*. Prognostic factors in patients with stage I epithelial ovarian cancer. *Obstet Gynecol* 1990;75:263–73
28. Buttram VC, Vaquero C. Post-ovarian wedge resection adhesive disease. *Fertil Steril* 1975;26:874
29. Nezhat C, Nezhat F. Complications of laparoscopic ovarian cystectomy. In Corfman RS, Diamond MP, DeCherney A, eds. *Complications of Laparoscopy and Hysteroscopy*. New York: Blackwell Scientific Publications, 1993:108–12
30. Nezhat F, Nezhat C, Welander CE, *et al*. Four ovarian cancers diagnosed during laparoscopic management of 1011 women with adnexal masses. *Am J Obstet Gynecol* 1992;167:790–6
31. Maiman M, Seltzer V, Boyce J. Laparoscopic excision of ovarian neoplasms subsequently found to be malignant. *Obstet Gynecol* 1991;77:563–5

Laparoscopic management of adnexal torsion

20

M. Canis, G. Mage, A. Wattiez, H. Manhes, J.L. Pouly and M.A. Bruhat

Laparoscopy is useful for the accurate diagnosis of adnexal torsion. Early diagnosis prevents adnexal necrosis[1,2] and allows conservative treatment of this rare condition[3,4]. We assumed it would be possible to perform complete conservative treatment by laparoscopy in most cases. Here we present our experience of 33 cases treated by laparoscopy from a series of 41 cases.

MATERIAL AND METHODS

Patients

A total of 41 cases of adnexal torsion were diagnosed between June 1978 and June 1988. Only cases with at least a 360° rotation of the ovarian pedicle or the tube were included in this study. Malignant tumors, always treated by laparotomy, were excluded. According to their clinical data, patients were divided into two groups.

Group 1

This group consisted of 30 patients (73.2% of the total) with acute pelvic pain; the interval between the onset of pain and laparoscopy ranged from 6 h to 4 days. The preoperative diagnosis was correct in about 70% of cases.

Group 2

In this group of 11 cases (26.8%), laparoscopy was performed for the surgical evaluation of adnexal cystic tumors. The time lapse between the first visit to our department and laparoscopy ranged from 1 to 3 months. Torsion was never suspected before laparoscopy.

Method

Laparoscopy was performed under general anesthesia with endotracheal intubation. The technique and the instrumentation used have been described previously[5-7]. After diagnosis, the laparoscopic management included two stages: management of ischemic lesions and treatment of the etiology (Figures 1 and 2).

Management of ischemic lesions

As recommended by Way[4], the organs involved were always untwisted to assess ischemic lesions. This procedure was performed slowly with an atraumatic forceps to avoid

additional adnexal damage. Treatment was chosen according to the initial lesions and the speed of recovery. The women were assigned to one of the following groups:

(1)   Group A: no evidence of ischemia, or mild lesions with immediate and complete recovery;

(2)   Group B: severe ischemia (tube and ovary were dark red or black at the time of diagnosis) with partial recovery 10 min after the pedicle was untwisted;

(3)   Group C: gangrenous adnexa without recovery.

In groups A and B, conservative management was chosen whenever it was possible to treat the etiology in this way. In group B, a second-look laparoscopy was performed 6–8 weeks after the initial procedure to assess definitive

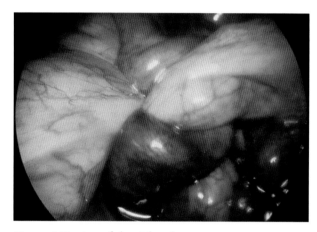

Figure 1 Torsion of the right adnexa

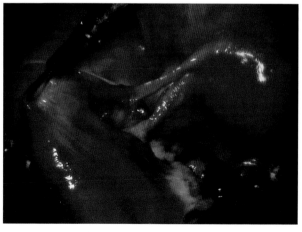

Figure 2 Partial ovarian recovery at the end of the laparoscopy

recovery. In group C, gangrenous adnexa were removed either by laparotomy or by laparoscopy.

Treatment of the etiology

Various laparoscopic procedures, such as the treatment of ectopic pregnancy[6], adhesiolysis[8] or ovarian cystectomy[5], were used for the treatment of the etiology. All patients were closely followed clinically, looking for any recurrence of torsion after conservative management.

RESULTS

Laparoscopy permitted a diagnosis in all cases. The whole adnexa was involved in 31 cases, the tube in nine cases and the ovary in one case.

Detorsion

The laparoscopic unwinding of torsion was possible in 38 cases. In the three remaining cases, the manipulation of gangrenous tubes resulted in a salpingectomy without any bleeding. Ischemic lesions were mild in 25 cases (group A), severe in nine cases (group B), and beyond recovery in seven cases. All patients with chronic pelvic pain were included in group A.

Etiology

Pathological findings are listed in Table 1. Paroophoritic and ovarian cysts were the most common etiologies. In two cases, the etiology was thought to be congenital; we found a rather short mesovarium (4 mm in length) in one case and a utero-ovarian ligament which was too long in the other case. Normal-size adnexa underwent spontaneous torsion; in such cases, several ovarian punctures were performed to rule out the presence of a small ovarian cyst.

Management

Management is shown in Table 2. Laparoscopic treatment was achieved in 33 cases (80.5%). Indications for laparotomy are listed in Table 3. Conservative management was possible in 32 cases and was performed by laparoscopy in 27 cases (Table 4) and by laparotomy in five cases.

There were no significant postoperative problems. Although heparin therapy was never used, we observed no thromboembolic complications. Patients were discharged 2–3 days after a laparoscopic procedure and 6 days after laparotomy.

In group B, six patients had a second-look laparoscopy which showed a complete and even surprising recovery of ischemic lesions (Figure 3). Ovarian biopsy was performed

Table 1 Adnexal torsions

Pathological findings	Tube (n = 9)	Ovary (n = 1)	Adnexa (n = 31)	Total (n = 41)
Paroophoritic cysts	6	–	7	13
Functional ovarian cysts	–	–	5*	5
Organic ovarian cysts	–	–	12	12
Ectopic pregnancy	2	–	–	2
Adhesions	1	–	1*	2
Congenital malformation	–	1	1	2
Normal adnexa	–	–	6	6

* One case with adhesions associated with a functional cyst

Table 2 Management of adnexal torsions according to laparoscopic findings

	Radical treatment		Conservative treatment	
Laparoscopic findings	Laparoscopy	Laparotomy	Laparoscopy	Laparotomy
Mild (n = 25)	1	1	19	4
Severe (n = 9)	0	0	8	1
Gangrenous (n = 7)	5	2	0	0

Table 3 Treatment of adnexal torsions; indications are given for cases in which laparotomy was performed

Treatment	Number of cases (%)
Laparoscopic	33 (80.5)
Laparotomy	8 (19.5)
gangrenous organs	2
ovarian cystectomy	4
ovariopexis	1
oophorectomy for large dermoid cyst	1

Table 4 Adnexal torsions: secondary laparoscopic procedures

Procedure	Number
Adhesiolysis	2
Puncture biopsy of functional cysts	5
Conservative treatment of ectopic pregnancy	1
Paroophoritic cystectomy	10
Ovarian cystectomy	4
Oophorectomy	2
Salpingectomy	4
Ovariopexis with Fallopian ring	3

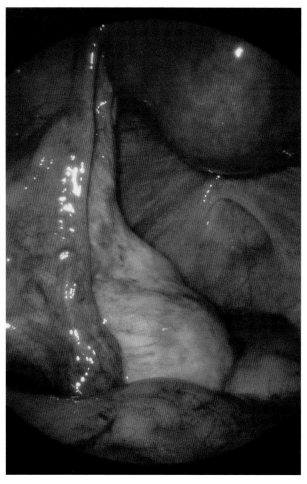

Figure 3 The same ovary at the second-look laparoscopy 3 months later

in only one case and histological examination showed a thickened ovarian capsule with a normal follicular population.

Follow-up

The duration of follow-up ranged from 9 months to 6 years. Ten patients were lost to follow-up 1 month after the treatment. Two recurrences were observed:

(1) One recurrence involved the same adnexa: 12 months after a laparoscopic ovariopexis using a Fallopian ring to treat an over-long utero-ovarian ligament, a second laparoscopy was performed to evaluate an ovary which was 6 cm in diameter; a recurrence of torsion was found with four twists without any evidence of ischemia. A bilateral surgical ovariopexis was then performed by laparotomy.

(2) The second recurrence involved the contralateral adnexa and was diagnosed 12 months after the initial procedure (which included a right ovariopexis and a right ovarian cystectomy); the recurrence was explained only by an over-long utero-ovarian ligament. This recurrence was treated conservatively; a

laparoscopic ovariopexis was performed using non-absorbable suture and fibrin glue.

DISCUSSION

In our experience, laparoscopy always permits an accurate diagnosis of adnexal torsion, an infrequent condition[9,10]. As the clinical symptoms can be associated with more common diseases such as ectopic pregnancy, salpingitis or corpus luteum hemorrhage that can be managed by laparoscopy, we and others[9,10] believe that surgical exploration should be carried out in this way.

In group C (gangrenous adnexa), laparoscopy was performed more than 72 h after the onset of pain in five cases, emphasizing the need for an early diagnosis of torsion. Indeed a delayed exploration will find a gangrenous adnexa which must be removed; spontaneous evolution probably results in spontaneous tubo-ovarian auto-amputation[11,12].

Conservative management was possible in 78% of our patients and appeared necessary as many patients were under 30 years of age. Conservative management requires, first, the unwinding of the torsion, a procedure which was previously condemned for fear of freeing a potentially fatal embolus[13,14]. In a recent report, fear of this complication appeared to be one of the main indications for radical management of adnexal torsion[10]. We and other authors[3,4] have never observed any embolic complications; prompt diagnosis and treatment probably account for this. Embolic complications could have been encountered when adnexal torsion was managed in a phlegmatic manner and twisted organs were found to be obviously gangrenous at laparotomy. Furthermore, in many cases of gangrenous adnexa, an unwinding of the torsion appears to be impossible; indeed, in three of our patients, gentle exploration of the adnexa with a probe resulted in spontaneous salpingectomy. As we observed no bleeding in these cases, we feel that no embolus is likely to be freed during this procedure. Conservative management remains questionable in cases of mild ischemia (group A). Indeed, Azoury and colleagues[2] reported that histological examination of a tube removed in spite of a complete recovery from mild ischemia showed definite mucosal damage. They concluded that conservative management should be attempted only in young women with bilateral adnexal torsion. Our experience differs from this since one of our patients had an intrauterine pregnancy following conservative treatment of a solitary twisted adnexa with severe ischemic damage. Furthermore, tubal patency was previously confirmed by hysterosalpingography[4]. Therefore, conservative management of mild and severe ischemic lesions appears to be safe and effective even if further studies are required to assess fertility after this procedure.

A complete laparoscopic treatment was achieved in 33 cases (80.5%). Physical stress, postoperative recovery and economic cost are reduced with such treatment, making it more acceptable and more desirable than conventional surgical management. This method should, however, be restricted to physicians trained in operative laparoscopy with a complete set of instruments available.

Many etiological factors have been discussed previously in the literature. The main problem is the correct and safe management of ovarian cysts. When an organic cyst is diagnosed or even suspected, a complete cystectomy must be performed for histological examination, either by laparoscopy or by laparotomy[5]. Infarction makes accurate pathological diagnosis quite difficult and Lomano[15] reported 26 non-specific ovarian cysts among 44 cases of twisted ovarian cysts. We encountered this problem in only one case.

When ischemic lesions are severe, laparoscopic differentiation between torsion of a normal tube and torsion of a tubal pregnancy is quite difficult. We believe that, if a hematosalpinx is diagnosed in women of reproductive age, a salpingotomy with tubal aspiration must be performed in every case[6]. In our series, two cases of adnexal torsion were attributed to congenitally unusual ovarian attachment. In one of these patients, a laparoscopic ovariopexis, using a Fallopian ring, resulted 12 months later in a recurrence of

torsion with the disappearance of the utero-ovarian ligament. Although we observed no complication when the utero-ovarian ligament was shortened after the treatment of a paroophoritic cyst, we believe that this procedure should not be used to prevent recurrence of torsion. Laparoscopic ovariopexis should use non-absorbable sutures. Several authors report that a routine ovariopexis is required during every conservative treatment of adnexal torsion[9,14]. In our study and in other reports[1,3,4], a recurrence of torsion seems to be quite rare, so we believe that, once an etiology has been found and correctly treated, the risk of recurrence is quite low. In our opinion, ovariopexis should be performed in cases of unusual ovarian attachment and/or immediate recurrence of torsion but it is questionable in cases of normal adnexa.

REFERENCES

1. Lee RA, Welch JS. Torsion of the uterine adnexa. *Am J Obstet Gynecol* 1967;97:974
2. Azoury RS, Chemab RM, Muffarrij IK. The twisted adnexa: a clinical pathological review. *Diagn Gynecol Obstet* 1980;2:185
3. MacGowan L. Torsion of cystic or diseased tissue. *Am J Obstet Gynecol* 1964;88:135
4. Way S. Ovarian cystectomy of twisted cysts. *Lancet* 1946;2:47
5. Mage G, Canis M, Manhes H, *et al.* Kystes ovariens et coelioscopie. *J Gynecol Obstet Biol Reprod* 1987;16:1053–61
6. Pouly JL, Manhes H, Mage G, *et al.* Conservative laparoscopic treatment of 321 ectopic pregnancies. *Fertil Steril* 1986;46:1093
7. Bruhat MA, Mage G, Pouly JL, *et al.* Coelioscopie Opératoire. Editions Medsi, Juin. Paris: McGraw Hill, 1989
8. Bruhat MA, Mage G, Manhes H, *et al.* Laparoscopic procedures to promote fertility: result of 93 selected cases. *Acta Eur Fertil* 1983;14:113
9. Nicols DH, Julian PJ. Torsion of the adnexa. *Clin Obstet Gynecol* 1985;28:375–80
10. Hibbart LT. Adnexal torsion. *Am J Obstet Gynecol* 1985;152:456
11. Sebastian JA, Baker RL, Cordray F. Asymptomatic infarction and separation of ovary and distal uterine tube. *Obstet Gynecol* 1973;41:531–5
12. Beyth Y, Barin E. Tubo-ovarian autoamputation and infertility. *Fertil Steril* 1984;42:932
13. James DF, Barber HRK, Graber EA. Torsion of uterine adnexa in children. Report of 3 cases. *Obstet Gynecol* 1970;365:226
14. Powell JL, Foley FP, Llorens AS. Torsion of the Fallopian tube in post menopausal women. *Am J Obstet Gynecol* 1972;111:113–15
15. Lomano JM, Trelford JD, Ullery JC. Torsion of the uterine adnexa causing an acute abdomen. *Obstet Gynecol* 1970;35:221

Part 3
Uterine and pelvic floor pathology

21

Laparoscopic myomectomy

J.B. Dubuisson, A. Fauconnier and C. Chapron

The indications for operative laparoscopy have expanded greatly over the past decades as its many advantages over laparotomy have been recognized. Myomectomy may be performed by laparoscopy in selected cases, particularly in subserous and interstitial myomas[1–4]. At present, a large number of teams use laparoscopic myomectomy, proving that this technique is feasible and reproducible; it is nevertheless a difficult operation.

PREOPERATIVE EVALUATION

Preoperative detection and evaluation of the myomas should be particularly meticulous, because, with the laparoscopic approach, it is impossible to palpate the myometrium thoroughly. This preoperative work-up must include abdominal and transvaginal ultrasonography, examination of the uterine cavity, either by diagnostic hysteroscopy or by hysterosalpingography, and measurement of preoperative hemoglobin levels.

Abdominal and transvaginal ultrasound examination must include the measurement of the diameter of the entire uterus (length, thickness and width), the number of myomas and characteristics of the dominant myomas, i.e. their type (intramural, subserous or pedunculated), size, and location (anterior, posterior or fundus). The examination includes the measurement of the distance between the endometrium and the myoma[5]. It is also important to include a systematic search for adenomyosis, because adenomyoma have a different pathology. Adenomyoma is very difficult to cleave and the best access is certainly not by laparoscopy. Ultrasound criteria for the diagnosis of adenomyosis are available[6,7].

Diagnostic hysteroscopy must be performed in patients with menometrorrhagia, in cases of multiple myomas, in cases of suspected intrauterine abnormalities at ultrasound and in infertile patients. Hysteroscopy allows the surgeon to differentiate between a deep interstitial myoma and a submucous myoma or a polyp. Comparison of the results of the ultrasound examination and the hysteroscopy is important to determine the operative strategy. In case of discrepancy, hysterosonography might be useful for evaluating relationships between the myomas and the uterine cavity[8].

Hysterosalpingography should be performed in cases of infertility or if adenomyosis is suspected by hysteroscopy or ultrasound examination. It permits an evaluation of the distortion of the uterine cavity and of the tubal status. In the case of infertility, the investigation should be completed by including a study of ovarian function (monthly temperature curve, levels of follicle stimulating hormone, luteinizing hormone and estradiol) and the partner's semen analysis. Since, in the presence of an associated male, or ovulatory factor, the postoperative fertility results are poor[9], in these cases the perioperative and postoperative strategy should be carefully discussed.

The blood count and serum ferritin provide information as to whether to give oral iron (see preoperative treatment), particularly in patients with menometrorrhagia.

PREOPERATIVE TREATMENT

Correction of sideropenic anemia by giving oral iron is essential in order to reduce the risk of blood transfusion. In some cases it is necessary to postpone laparoscopic myomectomy until the blood count has been normalized.

Gonadotropin releasing hormone (GnRH) agonists cause myoma shrinkage by reducing the circulating estrogen levels[10]. Maximal reduction of myoma size is achieved by 12 weeks of therapy, with no further change observed after 24 weeks of treatment[11]. Matta and colleagues[12] observed that GnRH agonists reduce uterine blood flow.

In patients undergoing laparoscopic myomectomy, preoperative treatment with GnRH agonists may have controversial effects. A marked reduction in blood loss during laparotomic myomectomy has been demonstrated[13]. During laparoscopic myomectomy, preoperative use of GnRH agonists also has the advantage of reducing blood loss[14,15]. However, in our experience, we have found that preoperative treatment with GnRH agonists (whatever the duration of treatment) increased the risk of conversion[5]. We consider, with others[16–18], that preoperative treatment with GnRH agonists may increase the difficulties in identifying and dissecting the cleavage plane between the myoma and its pseudocapsule. In addition, their use could increase the risk of recurrence of myoma[19] by making it more difficult to detect small intramural nuclei perioperatively. In our opinion, preoperative use of GnRH agonists should only be made in a case of sideropenic anemia in a bleeding patient[20] or in cases of myomas with highly developed perimyomatous vascularization. Doppler ultrasonography may be useful for selecting the cases that will most benefit from preoperative use of GnRH agonists[21].

INDICATIONS FOR OPERATIVE LAPAROSCOPY

The indications depend on the number, size, type and localization of myomas. Analysis of the main published series of laparoscopic myomectomy shows that the operation is used for medium-sized myomas (about 5 cm) which are relatively few in number (one to two per patient)[22].

The number of myomas may be a problem during operative laparoscopy. In our opinion, this procedure should not be attempted when more than two or three myomas are present at ultrasound investigation for several reasons. First, the conversion rate increases with the number of myomas[23]. Second, in our experience, operative time and difficulties increase with the number of myomas, leading to strain on the surgeon. Third, when myomas are numerous, ultrasound investigation might underestimate the true number of myomas.

We recommend that laparoscopic myomectomy should only be performed for myomas not exceeding 8–10 cm[22,24], although other teams have far higher limits, indeed up to 15 cm[25,26]. Difficulties increase with the myoma size for many reasons: the biggest myomas will have a highly distended perimyomatous vascularization due to compression by the myoma[16,27,28]; growth of certain myomas results in reorganization of the myomatous tissues and neighboring myometrium, making the attachments of the myomas difficult to cleave; the time required for laparoscopic myomectomy increases with the size of the myoma[22]; and, finally, the large dimensions of the myoma can cause a lack of operating space. In fact the upper limit that should be proposed mostly depends on other characteristics (i.e. location, depth of penetration) of the myoma[5].

Subserous and interstitial myomas are an indication for elective operative laparoscopy. Although the ablation of a entirely submucous myoma must be performed by operative hysteroscopy when its diameter is less than 4–5 cm, cases with deep intramural myoma with a submucosal component are difficult to treat by this method and usually require repeat procedures[29,30]. Cases of medium-sized (4–7 cm) myomas involving the uterine cavity appear to be easy to treat by the laparoscopic approach[5], thus providing an interesting alternative to hysteroscopic resection. On the other hand, in cases where an entirely submucous myoma of small diameter (2 or 3 cm) is associated with other subserous or interstitial myomas, the submucous myoma is treated first by operative hysteroscopy. The laparoscopic treatment of the other myomas will be discussed later, depending on the efficacy of operative hysteroscopy to treat the symptoms (i.e. menorrhagia, infertility). We rarely associate operative hysteroscopy with operative laparoscopy because operative hysteroscopy provokes a distension of the uterus which may cause bleeding when performing hysterotomy and enucleation.

An anterior location of the dominant myoma increases the difficulties and conversion rate[5,24]. This may be explained by the fact that the anterior wall of the uterus is less accessible to the operating trocars when the myoma is large. This is particularly true for the step of hemostasis and suturing. It is difficult to close an anterior hysterotomy. Indeed, the curved needles have to penetrate through the myometrium perpendicularly to ensure a good approximation and hemostasis. Myomas situated in the broad ligament or at the uterine isthmus can also be treated by operative laparoscopy, taking care not to damage the ureter and the uterine vessels.

OPERATIVE TECHNIQUE

Technical principles

The main complications with this operation, as with myomectomy by laparotomy, are the risk of perioperative hemorrhage and the risk of postoperative adhesions. The use of the laparoscopic access for the myomectomy also raises certain particular problems: bloodless enucleation of the myomas is absolutely essential for a clear view and to continue the procedure. As with laparotomy, a perfect suture must be achieved to obtain a good-quality scar. So the use of the technique of laparoscopic myomectomy is based on several basic principles:

(1) The principles of microsurgery must be applied to laparoscopic myomectomy: avoidance of intraperitoneal contamination, use of fine and atraumatic instruments, gentle and atraumatic manipulation of the uterus without grasping the pelvic organs (except the myoma itself);

(2) With laparoscopic myomectomy, each myoma must be excised via its own hysterotomy; it is not possible to use the same incision to remove all the myomas as with laparotomy[31,32]. Indeed, a long anterior sagittal hysterotomy is too hemorrhagic and takes too long a time for suturing by laparoscopy;

(3) Dissection must take place in every case along the cleavage plane separating the myoma from the adjacent myometrium. This cleavage plane is bounded by a pseudocapsule made up of compressed muscular fibers and diverted uterine vessels[16,28]. This allows healthy adjacent myometrium to be preserved and damage is avoided to the perimyomatous vessels, which are often distended due to compression by the myoma[27] and could be the origin of considerable hemorrhage;

(4) Electrocoagulation must be used as sparingly as possible to achieve hemostasis of the edges after myomectomy. Certain cases of uterine rupture during pregnancy reported after laparoscopic myomectomy[33–35] and after myolysis[36] suggest that

the use of electrocoagulation may induce necrosis of the myometrium resulting in a postoperative fistula;

(5) Suture of the hysterotomy must always respect a certain number of principles. Indeed, any technical deficiency when carrying it out may result in uterine rupture during a subsequent pregnancy[33]. Apart from pedunculated myomas or subserosal myoma with a small implantation surface (i.e. < 1 cm^2), the myomectomy sites must always be sutured. In the experience of certain teams at the beginning, when no suture was carried out, the resulting scars were fine or dehiscent[4,26]. The uterine suture does not necessarily have to use several planes but must always take up the full depth of the edges of the hysterotomy and result in total contact over the whole of the myomectomy defect, in order to avoid secondary constitution of a hematoma. This kind of hematoma can cause weakness in the scar tissues and the constitution of a secondary fistula[26,37]. When the uterine cavity has been opened or when the myomectomy defect is deep, it is necessary to make a suture in two planes. It is possible to make this type of suture in several planes by laparoscopy[37–39]. However, if it is difficult, there should be no hesitation in using laparoscopic-assisted myomectomy (LAM) to complete it successfully. This procedure is an alternative procedure between laparotomy and laparoscopic myomectomy: laparoscopy is used to perform the myoma(s) exposure and to begin or achieve enucleation; the uterine suture is then carried out by minilaparotomy in a traditional fashion[40,41]. The myoma is then removed by mini-laparotomy.

Instrumentation

In addition to the standard instrumentation for any operative laparoscopy, certain specific instruments are useful when carrying out laparoscopic myomectomy. Short curved monopolar scissors enable incision of the myometrium and section of the tracti between the myoma and myometrium. Other instruments are useful when making the intra- or extracorporeal sutures: needleholders, atraumatic forceps with no slot nor claws, suture pusher. A strong grasping 10-mm forceps (tenaculum or claw forceps) is useful to perform an efficient traction during enucleation. High-frequency electrosurgical generators are employed.

Ideally, an electric morcellation device such as the Steiner (Karl Storz, Germany) or SEMM (Wisap/AMSA) allows large myomas to be extracted by a 12-, 15- or 20-mm suprapubic port. This device has proved easy to use after a certain learning phase and reduces the operative times[42]. This morcellation device also exists as a disposable instrument (Gynecare). The C.C.L. Vaginal Extractor

(Karl Storz, Germany) enables removal of myomas by posterior colpotomy without leakage of gas.

Installation

The patient lies with thighs spread with abduction, providing access to the vagina, and buttocks protruding generously over the edge of the table in order to be able to manipulate the uterus with an intrauterine cannula. The main surgeon stands to the patient's left with the first assistant opposite, and the second assistant between the patient's legs.

Injection of undiluted methylene blue into the uterine cavity is useful to confirm the tubal patency and to enable the endometrium to be identified during surgery. The uterus is then cannulated, enabling it to be manipulated during the operation. Laparoscopy can be performed transumbilically or 2 cm supraumbilically depending on the uterine size. Two 5-mm lateral trocars and one 12-mm midline trocar are inserted in the suprapubic position. The positions of the trocars should be adapted whenever possible to the size and location of the myomas. Generally speaking, the two lateral trocars should be placed high and outside the epigastric vessels so that good access is provided for myomas in various locations and to ensure that the surgeon has sufficient operating space for movement when performing enucleation or carrying out the sutures.

Description of the operative technique

The technique of laparoscopic myomectomy that we use in our institution[43] comprises four main phases schematically speaking: hysterotomy and revelation of the myoma, enucleation, suture of the myomectomy site, and extraction of the myoma.

Incision of the myometrium and exposure of the myoma

The hysterotomy is direct, in line with the myoma. In the case of a posterior myoma, we use sagittal hysterotomies. In the case of an anterior myoma, we tend to use oblique hysterotomies because they are easier to suture. The myometrium is incised using low-voltage monopolar current in section mode in order to safeguard the myometrium as far as possible (Figure 1). Hemostasis of the intramyometrial vessels is carried out progressively using mono- or bipolar current. The myoma is easy to recognize by its smooth appearance and pearly white color which contrasts with the adjacent myometrium.

Enucleation (Figure 2)

Dissection of the myoma should run inside the avascular plane surrounding the myoma, leaving the pseudocapsule around the outside and with the uterine vessels pushed back. Identification of this avascular plane is assisted by the magnifying effect of the laparoscopic images (Figure 3). The myoma is grasped with a strong grasping forceps designed specifically for myomas (with claw or tenaculum) and pulled hard towards the anterior abdominal wall or upwards; at the same time, the surgeon or his assistant exert traction in the opposite direction, using the endouterine cannula or by pushing on the edges of the hysterotomy with an instrument. This dissection proceeds from the superficial areas inwards, and always under visual control in order to identify the fine tracti adhering to the myoma. The tip of a blunt instrument is used to press against the myoma. The tracti adhering to the myoma are coagulated, then sectioned. The bed of the myomectomy is most often free from hemorrhage at the end of dissection if care has been taken to follow the avascular cleavage plane, and there is no need to take further steps for hemostasis.

Hysterotomy suture (Figures 4 and 5)

We use fine resorbable suture, diameter 00 or 0 gauge, mounted on a curved needle with atraumatic tip (Vicryl, Polyglactine 910, Ethicon, Neuilly, France). The suture is usually carried out in a single plane. We use single, separate intra- or extracorporeal knots. The stitches go through the whole thickness of the edges of the hysterotomy, and through the uterine serosa. They are placed sufficiently close for the edges to be approximated completely yet far enough apart to avoid making the myometrium too fragile (Figure 6). When the myomectomy is located deeply, or the uterine cavity has been opened, we suture along a deep plane with a few single stitches deep in the myometrium, and along a superficial plane taking in the serosa and the superficial part of the myometrium. The superficial plane can be dealt with using a running suture or with individual stitches. When suturing the deep plane, it can sometimes be difficult to take the needle through the thickness of the defect. In this case, it can be an advantage to use Vicryl-1 with a large curved needle and to perform a U-shaped transfixing stitch[26], running through the uterine serosa and taking in the whole thickness of the edges of the myomectomy. One or two of these stitches are sufficient to ensure that all the deep part of the hysterotomy is brought into contact. When the uterine suture proves difficult to carry out, it is essential to know when to stop and use a

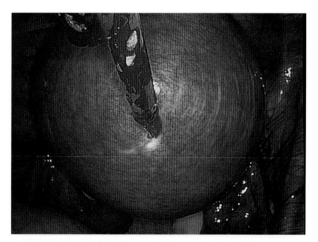

Figure 1 Hysterotomy of a posterior intramural myoma

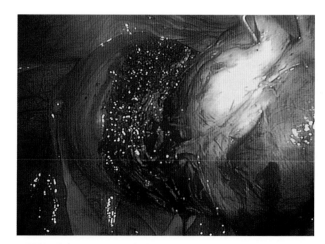

Figure 3 End of the myomectomy

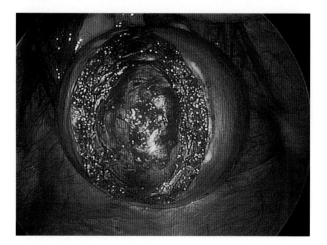

Figure 2 Enucleation of the myoma

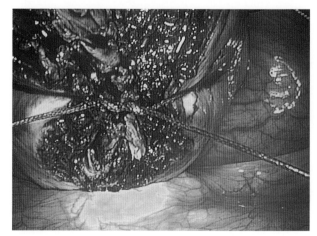

Figure 4 Uterine suture

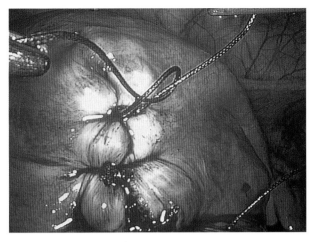

Figure 5 Intracorporeal separate sutures

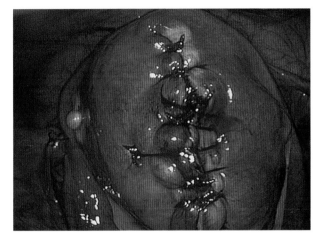

Figure 6 Final result

minilaparotomy for the suture. We recommend, in particular, its use for large anterior or deep intramural myomas.

Extraction of the myomas

There are various methods for extraction: direct suprapubic extraction, electric morcellation or extraction via posterior colpotomy.

(1) Direct suprapubic extraction is appropriate only for small myomas. Extraction takes place through the midline suprapubic incision which may be enlarged (2 cm). If needed, a manual morcellation is carried out: with one or two single-tooth tenaculums, the myoma is brought up to the suprapubic incision and held against the peritoneum to prevent loss of CO_2 and then fragmented under laparoscopic control, using a small blade passed through the incision.

(2) Electric morcellation is carried out with the use of an electrical morcellator (see Instrumentation). This device is an external rotating cylindrical blade that is introduced via a 12-, 15- or 20-mm suprapubic

trocar. A forceps with 10-mm jaws is inserted through the morcellator channel to grasp the fibroid and cut it progressively, like peeling an orange. The position of the rotating blade must be carefully controlled in order to avoid any risk of damaging any neighboring organs.

(3) Posterior colpotomy also allows large myomas to be extracted[44]. The colpotomy may be performed by laparoscopy, using the monopolar hook, or conventionally through the vagina. The myoma is then grasped with a forceps with 10-mm jaws inserted through the colpotomy under laparoscopic control. The myoma is extracted vaginally, either directly or after morcellation. In the case of large or numerous myomas, the C.C.L. Vaginal Extractor (Karl Storz, Germany) is useful to prevent leakage of gas.

Second-look laparoscopy

A second-look laparoscopy should be proposed to those patients who desire pregnancy and who have sutured uterine scars, in order to eliminate adhesions after myomectomy and to assess the strength of the uterine scar[45,46]. Systematic use of second-look laparoscopy could reduce adhesions after myomectomy and consequently enhance fertility[47,48]. The thickness and quality of the hysterotomy scar is assessed on this occasion, using a methylene blue test. It is a useful guide for management of future obstetric practice[49]. This procedure should take place 2 or 3 months after laparoscopic myomectomy to evaluate the uterine scar well.

RESULTS

Conversion rate and operative time

The percentage of conversions to laparotomy reported in retrospective studies varies from 0 to 41%[22]. In our experience with 426 laparoscopic myomectomies, the rate of conversion to an open procedure (either laparotomy or LAM) was 11.3%. Several independent factors were found to increase the risk of conversion: size of the dominant myoma at ultrasound, anterior location, intramural type or preoperative use of GnRH agonists[5]. Because of the difficulties of identifying the cleavage plane, the presence of an adenomyoma or associated adenomyosis make laparoscopic myomectomy very difficult[24]. In one study, where the use of laparoscopic myomectomy was not restricted to cases with a low number of myomas, the conversion rate was found to increase with the number of myomas[23].

The mean operative time is about 2 h for the main series published[22]. This could be considered to be rather long. Indeed, two controlled studies comparing laparoscopic myomectomy with myomectomy by laparotomy[50,51] found an increase in the operative time when it was carried out by the laparoscopic route. The size and depth of penetration in the myometrium of the dominant myoma are the most important parameters to consider. In the case of large and deeply infiltrating myomas, the time will increase with enucleation, suturing and morcellation. The surgeon must also take into account his/her own experience.

Risk of hemorrhage

Myomectomy itself has the reputation of being a hemorrhagic operation. However, the use of the laparoscopic approach reduces the hemorrhagic risk connected with myomectomy. Indeed, in three controlled studies[50–52] there was a significant reduction of the hemoglobin decrease connected with the use of laparoscopic myomectomy. The laparoscopic route presents two advantages over laparotomy in terms of limiting the hemorrhagic risk during myomectomy: the pressure of the pneumoperitoneum prevents blood extravasation from the intramyometrial capillaries and veins, and the magnification provided by the laparoscope lens helps to identify the cleavage plane more precisely and enables selective coagulation of the small vessels feeding the myoma.

It can be useful to take certain steps to reduce perioperative bleeding. Meticulous preventive coagulation of the tracti connecting the myoma to the adjacent myometrium must be carried out[24]. Preoperative use of GnRH agonists is efficient in reducing perioperative bleeding[14,15], but problems with their use have already been discussed (see Preoperative treatment). One author[39] has proposed a technique for temporary hemostasis which can be used with laparoscopy (compression of the uterine pedicles at the isthmus, using a broad, single-strand suture), but we ourselves have no experience of this technique. Infiltration of the adjacent myometrium with vasoconstrictive agents is very useful for limiting the bleeding. However, in France, the use of powerful vasoconstrictors like vasopressin derivatives (POR-8) is not allowed. We sometimes use lidocaïne + epinephrine (Xylocaïne adrénaliné 1%) but it is far less efficient.

Postoperative course

Two randomized clinical trials have demonstrated that laparoscopic myomectomy has proven advantages compared to the laparotomic approach in terms of the postoperative course. The laparoscopic approach may offer the benefits of lower postoperative pain and shorter recovery time in comparison with laparotomy[52]. It also reduces the length of the hospital stay and transient episodes of febrile morbidity[50].

Postoperative adhesions

There are several arguments suggesting that the laparoscopic approach reduces the risk of postoperative adhesions after myomectomy. In a non-randomized comparative study, Bulletti and colleagues[53] found a statistically significant decrease in the degree of postoperative adhesions and the proportion of patients with adhesions associated with the use of the laparoscopic route. In this study, the potential factors for confusion are taken into account, because a match is made for size, location and the type of myoma. Furthermore, in the retrospective studies with a systematic laparoscopic second-look after myomectomy, the percentages of patients presenting adhesions (wherever these are located) after laparoscopic myomectomy are 51.1% (95% confidence interval (CI): 42.6–59.6) and 89.6% (95% CI: 84.5–94.8) after laparotomy. The proportions of patients presenting adnexal adhesions connected to the myomectomy scar are 30.5% (95% CI: 21.3–39.8) after laparoscopic myomectomy and 68.9% (95% CI: 58.4–79.5) after laparotomy[22]. Laparoscopic surgery offers the advantage of respecting the principles of microsurgery by its very nature (atraumatic manipulation, fine instruments, thorough washing). In addition, it avoids intraperitoneal contamination and has less effect on the equilibrium of the peritoneum.

Obstetric quality of laparoscopic myomectomy scars

There is considerable debate concerning the strength of hysterotomy scars after laparoscopic myomectomy[54] because of the possibility of uterine rupture during pregnancy after laparoscopic myomectomy. To date, five cases have been reported over a short period[33–35,55,56]. All these cases of rupture occurred after small (3–5 cm), single myomas were removed, and quite remarkably they took place before labor actually began. However, it is difficult to draw any definite conclusions from these cases because it is not known how frequently this accident occurs: the cases are reported in isolation, without any indication of the number of pregnancies occurring after laparoscopic myomectomy.

The incidence of uterine rupture after laparoscopic myomectomy is probably low. Between 1989 and 1996 in our institution, the risk of uterine rupture specifically due to laparoscopic myomectomy was 1.0% (95% CI: 0.0–5.5) in 100 deliveries after laparoscopic myomectomy[49]. To date, apart from our study, seven teams have reported on pregnancies after laparoscopic myomectomy and none has observed any uterine rupture[3,37,57–61]. It is difficult to say whether this risk is greater than after myomectomy by laparotomy. The good reputation that scars after myomectomy by laparotomy have in obstetrics is based on the fact that many pregnancies have been reported after this operation without any case of rupture[16,62–72]. However, the largest series are old and the rate of cases lost to follow-up is not specified. Furthermore, observations of uterine ruptures after laparotomy have been reported regularly in the literature[73–78]. Finally, in a retrospective study made in the Trinidad maternity hospital, the rate of rupture observed during labor after myomectomy by laparotomy was 4.4% (95% CI 0.5–14.8)[79]. All these elements suggest, in fact, that the risk of rupture after myomectomy by laparotomy is underestimated. In the randomized clinical trial by Seracchioli and colleagues[50], 27 women in the laparotomic group and 20 women in the laparoscopic myomectomy group had deliveries after myomectomy. There was no uterine rupture in either group. However, comparative studies covering a larger number of cases are still needed to see if the risk of rupture differs according to the approach.

At present, we consider that this risk is acceptable and that it should not prevent the laparoscopic approach being used when the myomectomy is needed. However, when performing laparoscopic myomectomy, particular care must be given to the uterine closure (see Operative technique). Indeed, intraperitoneal sutures need surgeons who are well experienced in laparoscopic surgery.

Fertility after laparoscopic myomectomy

In our series of 91 infertile women treated with laparoscopic myomectomy, the 2-year cumulative rate of spontaneous intrauterine pregnancy was 44% after laparoscopic myomectomy. This rate was 70% when no infertility factor associated with myoma was found and 32% when one or more infertility factors were associated with myoma[46]. The fertility results in our population are comparable to those observed in the series of infertile women treated by laparotomy[80]. In particular, if we only take into account those patients who present no associated infertility factor, the conception rate observed in our series is at least equivalent to that of the series of women treated by laparotomy[46]. In the randomized clinical trial of Seracchioli and colleagues[50], including patients with infertility and at least one myoma of more than 4 cm, the fertility rate did not differ between the laparotomic and laparoscopic approaches.

Recurrence after laparoscopic myomectomy

Only one study has been devoted specifically to the risk of recurrence after laparoscopic myomectomy[81]. The cumulative rate at 5 years (51%) is distinctly higher than those observed in the series of myomectomy by laparotomy[16,67,82], and the time lapse before recurrence is shorter. With the laparoscopic route, it is impossible to palpate the myometrium thoroughly and small intramural nuclei which do not deform the uterine serosa can be overlooked, resulting in incomplete exeresis more often than when the myomectomy uses laparotomy. If these results are confirmed, then considerable caution should be exercised before using the laparoscopic route for multiple myomas.

CONCLUSIONS

Laparoscopic myomectomy is a safe technique which has several advantages, including lower postoperative pain, shorter recovery time and reduction of postmyomectomy adhesion formation in comparison with the laparotomic approach. However, it is a difficult operation and the surgeon needs to be well experienced in laparoscopic surgery. Because of increasing difficulties during laparoscopic myomectomy, it is essential to respect the limits. We recommend the following:

(1) Preoperative evaluation of the myomas should be meticulous, in particular concerning ultrasound and hysteroscopic examination;

(2) The preoperative blood count should be controlled and sideropenic anemia should be corrected;

(3) High-frequency electrosurgical generators and monopolar scissors or hook should be used;

(4) Particular care must be paid when suturing the uterus to prevent bleeding and weakening of the myometrium;

(5) An electric morcellator or posterior colpotomy should be employed for the extraction of large myomas.

REFERENCES

1. Daniell JF, Gurley LD. Laparoscopic treatment of clinically significant symptomatic uterine fibroids. *J Gynecol Surg* 1991;7:37–9

2. Dubuisson JB, Lecuru F, Foulot H, *et al.* Myomectomy by laparoscopy: a preliminary report of 43 cases. *Fertil Steril* 1991;56:827–30

3. Hasson HM, Rotman C, Rana N, *et al.* Laparoscopic myomectomy. *Obstet Gynecol* 1992;80:884–8

4. Nezhat C, Nezhat F, Silfen SL, *et al.* Laparoscopic myomectomy. *Int J Fertil* 1991;36:275–80

5. Dubuisson J-B, Fauconnier A, Fourchotte, V, *et al.* Laparoscopic myomectomy: predicting the risk of conversion to an open procedure. *Hum Reprod* 2001:in press

6. Atri M, Reinhold C, Mehio AR, *et al.* Adenomyosis: US features with histologic correlation in an *in-vitro* study. *Radiology* 2000;215:783–90

7. Chiang CH, Chang MY, Hsu JJ, *et al.* Tumor vascular pattern and blood flow impedance in the differential diagnosis of leiomyoma and adenomyosis by color Doppler sonography. *J Assist Reprod Genet* 1999;16:268–75

8. Cohen LS, Valle RF. Role of vaginal sonography and hysterosonography in the endoscopic treatment of uterine myomas. *Fertil Steril* 2000;73:197–204

9. Fauconnier A, Dubuisson J-B, Ancel P-Y, *et al.* Prognostic factors of reproductive outcome after myomectomy in infertile patients. *Hum Reprod* 2000;15:1751–7

10. Friedman AJ, Harrison-Atlas D, Barbieri RL, *et al.* A randomized, placebo-controlled, double-blind study evaluating the efficacy of leuprolide acetate depot in the treatment of uterine leiomyomata. *Fertil Steril* 1989;51:251–6

11. Lumsden MA, West CP, Baird DT. Goserelin therapy before surgery for uterine fibroids. *Lancet* 1987;1:36–7

12. Matta WH, Stabile I, Shaw RW, *et al.* Doppler assessment of uterine blood flow changes in patients with fibroids receiving the gonadotropin-releasing hormone agonist buserelin. *Fertil Steril* 1988;49:1083–5

13. Friedman AJ, Rein MS, Harrison-Atlas D, *et al.* A randomized, placebo-controlled, double-blind study evaluating leuprolide acetate depot treatment before myomectomy. *Fertil Steril* 1989;52:728–33

14. Campo S, Garcea N. Laparoscopic myomectomy in premenopausal women with and without preoperative treatment using gonadotrophin-releasing hormone analogues. *Hum Reprod* 1999;14:44–8

15. Zullo F, Pellicano M, De Stefano R, *et al.* A prospective randomized study to evaluate leuprolide acetate treatment before laparoscopic myomectomy: efficacy and ultrasonographic predictors. *Am J Obstet Gynecol* 1998;178:108–12

16. Acien P, Quereda F. Abdominal myomectomy: results of a simple operative technique. *Fertil Steril* 1996;65:41–51

17. Beyth Y. Gonadotropin-releasing hormone analog treatment should not precede conservative myomectomy [Letter]. *Fertil Steril* 1990;53:187–8

18. Reich H, Thompson KA, Nataupsky LG, *et al.* Laparoscopic myomectomy: an alternative to laparotomy or hysterectomy? *Gynaecol Endosc* 1997;6:7–12

19. Fedele L, Vercellini P, Bianchi S, *et al.* Treatment with GnRH agonists before myomectomy and the risk of short-term myoma recurrence. *Br J Obstet Gynaecol* 1990;97:393–6

20. Crosignani PG, Vercellini P, Meschia M, *et al.* GnRH agonists before surgery for uterine leiomyomas. A review [see comments]. *J Reprod Med* 1996;41:415–21

21. Zullo F, Pellicano M, Di Carlo C, *et al.* Ultrasonographic prediction of the efficacy of GnRH agonist therapy before laparoscopic myomectomy. *J Am Assoc Gynecol Laparosc* 1998;5:361–6

22. Dubuisson J-B, Fauconnier A, Babaki-Fard K, *et al.* Laparoscopic myomectomy: a current view. *Hum Reprod Update* 2000;6:558–94

23. Daraï E, Deval B, Darles C, *et al.* Myomectomie: coelioscopie ou laparotomie. *Contracept Fertil Sex* 1996;24:751–6

24. Dubuisson JB, Chapron C, Lévy L. Difficulties and complications of laparoscopic myomectomy. *J Gynecol Surg* 1996;12:159–65

25. Adamian LV, Kulakov VI, Kiselev SI, *et al.* Laparoscopic myomectomy in treatment of large myomas. *J Am Assoc Gynecol Laparosc* 1996;3:S1

26. Hasson HM. Laparoscopic myomectomy. *Infertil Reprod Med Clin N Am* 1996;7:143–59

27. Farrer-Brown G, Beilby J, Tarbit MH. Venous changes in the endometrium of myomatous uteri. *Obstet Gynecol* 1971;38:743–51

28. Vollenhoven BJ, Lawrence AS, Healy DL. Uterine fibroids: a clinical review. *Br J Obstet Gynaecol* 1990;97:285–98

29. Donnez J, Polet R, Smets M, *et al.* Hysteroscopic myomectomy. *Curr Opin Obstet Gynecol* 1995;7:311–16

30. Wamsteker K, Emanuel MH, de Kruif JH. Transcervical hysteroscopic resection of submucous fibroids for abnormal uterine bleeding: results regarding the degree of intramural extension. *Obstet Gynecol* 1993;82:736–40

31. Bonney V. The technique and results of myomectomy. *Lancet* 1931;220:171–3

32. Buttram VC, Reiter R. Uterine leiomyomata: etiology, symptomatology and management. *Fertil Steril* 1981;36:433–45

33. Dubuisson JB, Chavet X, Chapron C, *et al.* Uterine rupture during pregnancy after laparoscopic myomectomy. *Hum Reprod* 1995;10:1475–7

34. Harris WJ. Uterine dehiscence following laparoscopic myomectomy. *Obstet Gynecol* 1992;80:545–6

35. Pelosi M, Pelosi MA. Spontaneous uterine rupture at thirty-three weeks subsequent to previous superficial laparoscopic myomectomy. *Am J Obstet Gynecol* 1997;177:1547–9

36. Vilos GA, Daly LJ, Tse BM. Pregnancy outcome after laparoscopic electromyolysis. *J Am Assoc Gynecol Laparosc* 1998;5:289–92

37. Miller CE, Johnston M, Rundell M. Laparoscopic myomectomy in the infertile woman. *J Am Assoc Gynecol Laparosc* 1996;3:525–32

38. Dubuisson JB, Chapron C, Chavet X, *et al.* Traitement coeliochirurgical des volumineux fibromes utérins. Technique opératoire et résultats. *J Gynecol Obstet Biol Reprod* 1995;24:705–10

39. Ostrzenski A. A new laparoscopic myomectomy technique for intramural fibroids penetrating the uterine cavity. *Eur J Obstet Gynecol Reprod Biol* 1997;74:189–93

40. Nezhat C, Nezhat F, Bess O, *et al.* Laparoscopically assisted myomectomy: a report of a new technique in 57 cases. *Int J Fertil Menopausal Stud* 1994;39:39–44

41. Tulandi T, Youseff H. Laparoscopy assisted myomectomy of large uterine myomas. *Gynaecol Endosc* 1997;6:105–8

42. Carter JE, McCarus SD. Laparoscopic myomectomy. Time and cost analysis of power vs. manual morcellation. *J Reprod Med* 1997;42:383–8

43. Dubuisson JB, Chapron C, Fauconnier A, *et al.* Laparoscopic myomectomy and myolysis. *Curr Opin Obstet Gynecol* 1997;9:233–8

44. Mangeshikar PR. New instrumentation and technique for laparoscopic myomectomy. *J Am Assoc Gynecol Laparosc* 1995;2:S29

45. Dubuisson JB, Fauconnier A, Chapron C, *et al.* Second look after laparoscopic myomectomy. *Hum Reprod* 1998;13:2102–6

46. Dubuisson JB, Fauconnier A, Chapron C, *et al.* Reproductive outcome after laparoscopic myomectomy in infertile women. *J Reprod Med* 2000;45:23–31

47. Tulandi T, Murray C, Guralnick M. Adhesion formation and reproductive outcome after myomectomy and second look laparoscopy. *Obstet Gynecol* 1993;82:213–15

48. Ugur M, Turan C, Mungan T, *et al.* Laparoscopy for adhesion prevention following myomectomy. *Int J Gynecol Obstet* 1996;53:145–9

49. Dubuisson JB, Fauconnier A, Deffarges J-V, *et al.* Pregnancy outcome and deliveries following laparoscopic myomectomy. *Hum Reprod* 2000;15:869–73

50. Seracchioli R, Rossi S, Govoni F, *et al.* Fertility and obstetric outcome after laparoscopic myomectomy of large myomata: a randomized comparison with abdominal myomectomy. *Hum Reprod* 2000;15:2663–8

51. Stringer NH, Walker JC, Meyer PM. Comparison of 49 laparoscopic myomectomies with 49 open myomectomies. *J Am Assoc Gynecol Laparosc* 1997;4:457–64

52. Mais V, Ajossa S, Guerriero S, *et al.* Laparoscopic versus abdominal myomectomy: a prospective, randomized trial to evaluate benefits in early outcome. *Am J Obstet Gynecol* 1996;174:654–8

53. Bulletti C, Polli V, Negrini V, *et al.* Adhesion formation after laparoscopic myomectomy. *J Am Assoc Gynecol Laparosc* 1996;3:533–6

54. Nezhat C. The 'cons' of laparoscopic myomectomy in women who may reproduce in the future. *Int J Fertil Menopausal Stud* 1996;41:280–3

55. Friedmann W, Maier RF, Luttkus A, *et al.* Uterine rupture after laparoscopic myomectomy. *Acta Obstet Gynecol Scand* 1996;75:683–4

56. Mecke H, Wallas F, Brocker A, *et al.* Pelviskopische Myomenukleation: Technik, Grenzen, Komplicationen. *Geburtsh Frauenheilk* 1995;55:374–9

57. Daraï E, Dechaud H, Benifla JL, *et al.* Fertility after laparoscopic myomectomy: preliminary results. *Hum Reprod* 1997;12:1931–4

58. Nezhat CH, Nezhat F, Roemisch M, *et al.* Pregnancy following laparoscopic myomectomy: preliminary results. *Hum Reprod* 1999;14:1219–21

59. Reich H. Laparoscopic myomectomy. *Obstet Gynecol Clin North Am* 1995;22:757–80

60. Ribeiro SC, Reich H, Rosenberg J, *et al.* Laparoscopic myomectomy and pregnancy outcome in infertile patients. *Fertil Steril* 1999;71:571–4

61. Seinera P, Arisio R, Decko A, *et al.* Laparoscopic myomectomy: indications, surgical technique and complications. *Hum Reprod* 1997;12:1927–30

62. Berkeley AS, DeCherney AH, Polan ML. Abdominal myomectomy and subsequent fertility. *Surg Gynecol Obstet* 1983;156:319–22

63. Brown AB, Chamberlain R, Te Linde RW. Myomectomy. *Am J Obstet Gynecol* 1956;71:759–63

64. Brown JM, Malkasian GD, Symmonds RE. Abdominal myomectomy. *Am J Obstet Gynecol* 1967;90:126–8

65. Davids A. Myomectomy: surgical technique and results in series of 1150 cases. *Am J Obstet Gynecol* 1952;63:592–604

66. Egwuatu VE. Fertility and fetal salvage among women with uterine leiomyomas in a Nigerian Teaching Hospital. *Int J Fertil* 1989;34:341–6

67. Finn WF, Muller PF. Abdominal myomectomy: special reference to subsequent pregnancy and to the reappearance of fibromyomas of the uterus. *Am J Obstet Gynecol* 1950;60:109–14

68. Loeffler FE, Noble AD. Myomectomy at the Chelsea Hospital for Women. *J Obstet Gynaecol Br Commonw* 1970;77:167–70

69. Mussey RD, Randall LM, Doyle LW. Pregnancy following myomectomy. *Am J Obstet Gynecol* 1945;49:508–12

70. Sirjusingh A, Bassaw B, Roopnarinesingh S. The results of abdominal myomectomy. *West Ind Med J* 1994;43:138–9

71. Smith DC, Uhlir JK. Myomectomy as a reproductive procedure. *Am J Obstet Gynecol* 1990;162:1476–9

72. Sudik R, Husch K, Steller J, *et al.* Fertility and pregnancy outcome after myomectomy in sterility patients. *Eur J Obstet Gynecol Reprod Biol* 1996;65:209–14

73. Garnet JD. Uterine rupture during pregnancy. *Obstet Gynecol* 1964;23:898–902

74. Georgakopoulos PA, Bersis G. Sigmoido-uterine rupture in pregnancy after multiple myomectomy. *Int Surg* 1981;66:367–8

75. Golan D, Aharoni A, Gonon R, *et al.* Early spontaneous rupture of the post myomectomy gravid uterus. *Int J Gynecol Obstet* 1990;31:167–70

76. Ozeren M, Ulusoy M, Uyanik, E. First-trimester spontaneous uterine rupture after traditional myomectomy: case report. *Isr J Med Sci* 1997;33:752–3

77. Palerme GR, Friedman EA. Rupture of the gravid uterus in the third trimester. *Am J Obstet Gynecol* 1966;94:571–6

78. Quakernack K, Bordt J, Nienhaus H. [Placenta percreta and rupture of the uterus]. *Geburtsh Frauenheilk* 1980;40:520–3

79. Roopnarinesingh S, Suratsingh J, Roopnarinesingh A. The obstetric outcome of patients with previous myomectomy or hysterotomy. *West Ind Med J* 1985;34:59–62

80. Vercellini P, Maddalena S, De Giorgi O, *et al.* Determinants of reproductive outcome after abdominal myomectomy for infertility. *Fertil Steril* 1999;72:109–14

81. Nezhat FR, Roemisch M, Nezhat CH, *et al.* Recurrence rate after laparoscopic myomectomy. *J Am Assoc Gynecol Laparosc* 1998;5:237–40

82. Candiani GB, Fedele L, Parazzini F, *et al.* Risk of recurrence after myomectomy. *Br J Obstet Gynaecol* 1991;98:385–9

22

Laparoscopic myolysis

J. Donnez, M. Nisolle, R. Polet and J. Squifflet

Uterine fibroids are common, benign, solid tumors of the genital tract and, depending on their size and location, can lead to hysterectomy. In the early 1990s, advanced operative laparoscopy techniques were developed and large uterine fibroids can now be removed laparoscopically in patients wishing to avoid hysterectomy[1,2]. On the other hand, laparoscopic myolysis has been proposed in cases of subserous or intramural myomas as an alternative to myomectomy or hysterectomy. This technique was first performed in the late 1980s in Europe. In fact, the concept of myolysis was first proposed by Donnez and colleagues[3,4] for hysteroscopic myolysis and then applied to laparoscopic myolysis[5]. Initially, myoma coagulation was viewed as an alternative to myomectomy for women interested in preserving fertility. Using the energy of the neodymium : yttrium–aluminum–garnet (Nd : YAG) laser, leiomyomas were coagulated around the point of laser penetration, necrosing the myometrium, denaturing protein and destroying vascularity. No reports on the procedure appeared in the United States until Goldfarb reported his first series[6]. As an alternative to myomectomy and hysterectomy, the author performed myoma coagulation on leiomyomas up to 10 cm in diameter, but limited the procedure to post-reproductive and perimenopausal women.

In this chapter, we have evaluated the different techniques, and the long-term effects on myoma growth, of the technique called myolysis.

INDICATIONS

According to Nisolle and colleagues[5], indications for myolysis were pelvic pain, compression symptoms and a global uterine volume between 9 and 12 weeks (in order to avoid hysterectomy).

Myolysis was also considered as an alternative to laparoscopic myomectomy if myomectomy was judged to be too difficult or not mandatory, or in cases of multiple intramural myomas, to avoid a time-consuming laparoscopic myomectomy.

THE FIRST SERIES OF MYOLYSIS WITH Nd : YAG LASER

In the late 1980s, myolysis was proposed to 48 women over 35 years of age with intramural myomas up to 8 cm in diameter who did not wish to bear any more children[5,7].

The mean age was 42 years (ranging from 35 to 48 years). Myomas were diagnosed by pelvic examination. Their size and location were confirmed by ultrasonography (Figure 1). The vascularization was evaluated by means of Doppler ultrasound with color flow imaging (Figure 2). No previous laparoscopy had been performed in these women.

Technique

Laparoscopy was performed transumbilically using a 10-mm endoscope adapted to a video camera. The instruments were introduced through three suprapubic puncture sites (5 mm in diameter).

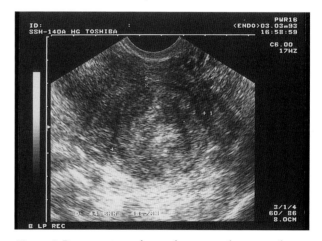

Figure 1 Preoperative echography: size is determined

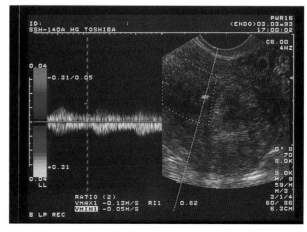

Figure 2 Myoma: the vascularization is evaluated by means of Doppler ultrasound with color flow imaging

225

The bare laser fiber was introduced as close to perpendicular as possible into the fibroid through a second puncture trocar to a depth depending on the myoma diameter (Figure 3). During the application of laser energy, the fiber was introduced, reaching the central part of the fibroid, and was then removed slowly in order to provoke a 'strong coagulation'. The power used was 80 W. The procedure was repeated on the entire surface of the myoma in order to coagulate most of the myoma volume. The surface of the myoma was rinsed with 0.9% saline solution during the laser application to reduce thermal conduction through the uterine wall. The distance between the holes was about 5–7 mm (Figure 4).

Vasopressin (POR8, Sandoz, Brussels, Belgium) was never used to infiltrate the myometrium adjacent to the fibroid to induce temporary myometrial ischemia, reducing blood loss. However, in one case, diluted vasopressin was required to obtain complete uterine hemostasis: 5 U of vasopressin in 20 ml of saline solution was injected just around the hemorrhagic site at the end of the procedure.

Immediately following myolysis, many laser scars can be seen on the myoma, which appears paler than normal (Figure 5a). In the last ten cases, an Interceed® graft (Johnson and Johnson, New Brunswick, NJ) was used to cover the coagulated area after hemostatic control was obtained, in order to decrease the risk of adhesions (Figure

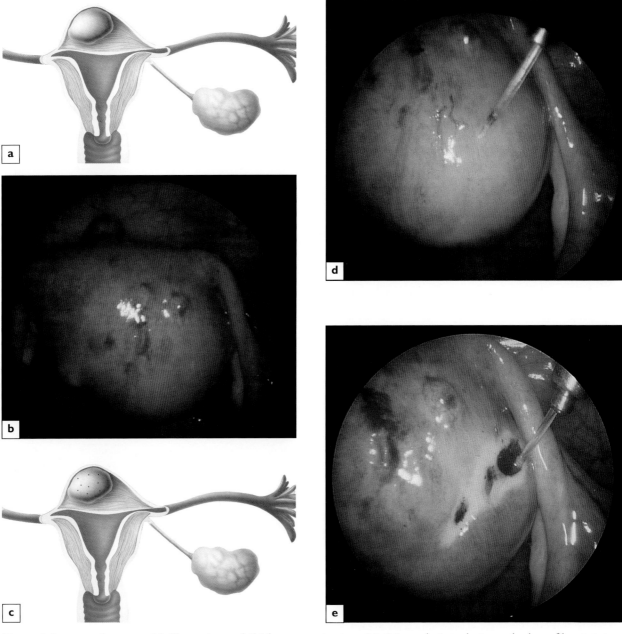

Figure 3 Intramural myoma: (a) illustration and (b) laparoscopic view; (c)–(e) myolysis technique: the laser fiber is introduced at an angle perpendicular to the fibroid and removed during the application of laser energy

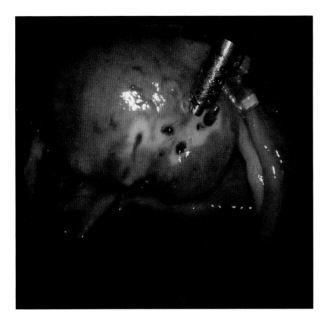

Figure 4 Laparoscopic view: the distance between holes is about 5–7 mm

5b and c). Careful aspiration of peritoneal fluid was then carried out and a suction catheter was left in the pouch of Douglas.

In the first series of 48 patients, none required laparotomy for bleeding, and no bladder or bowel injury was reported. During surgery, some problems arose because of difficult access to posterior myomas by the laser fiber, introduced through a second puncture. In such cases, the laser fiber can be introduced directly through the laparoscope to achieve better access. The estimated blood loss was minimal (< 50 ml) in all cases but one. The operating time varied from 20 to 45 min, depending on the diameter and number of myomas. All patients were released in good physical condition the following day; none experienced any postoperative infection or hemorrhage.

Evaluation of myoma size

The number, size and location of the myomas were evaluated by vaginal echography before laparoscopic myolysis (Figures 1 and 2). The size of the myomas, measured by ultrasound, ranged from 3 to 8 cm in diameter. Postoperatively, myoma evaluation was echographically performed at weeks 3, 6 and 12, after 6 months and after 1 year; 15 patients were evaluated after 3 years. Changes in the myoma structure and size were analyzed by echography (Figures 6 and 7). In the first 3 weeks, areas of necrosis were suspected by the presence of numerous anechogenic areas in the myoma. Subsequently, a more echogenic structure appeared.

Fibroids treated by myolysis ranged from 3 to 8 cm in diameter. The mean decrease in the myoma diameter after myolysis was 4% (range 0–6%) at week 6, 12% (range 2–18%) at week 12 and 41% (range 18–62%) after 6

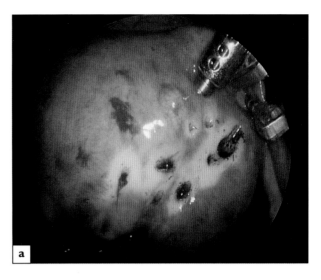

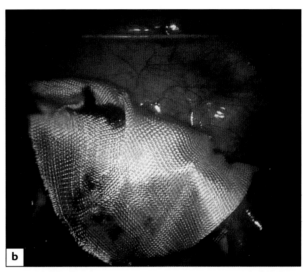

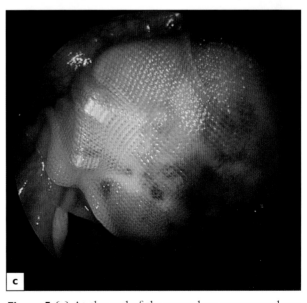

Figure 5 (a) At the end of the procedure, numerous laser scars are seen; the paler color of the myoma is due to the coagulation; (b) and (c) to avoid adhesions, Interceed® is used to cover the laser scars

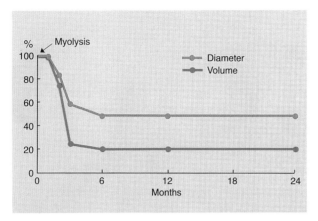

Figure 6 Decrease in the myoma diameter and volume after myolysis

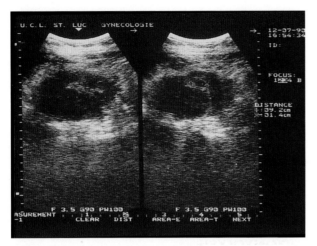

Figure 7 Ultrasound evaluation of the myoma 3 weeks after myolysis: areas of necrosis, characterized by anechogenic structures, are observed

months. The echostructure of the coagulated myoma was such that only experienced echographists could really distinguish the limits of the myoma.

The results observed after 1 year were similar to those seen after 6 months; there was neither any further decrease in size nor a regrowth of the myoma.

After 3 years, 15 patients were evaluated by echography. In ten of them who had two to three myomas (between 3 and 5 cm in diameter), echography revealed only small areas (< 1 cm in diameter) whose echographic structure was slightly different from the normal myometrium. Among the five remaining patients, three were stable and two showed a reappearance of myomas in other sites. The last two patients underwent laparoscopic subtotal hysterectomy. Only a few adhesions were present.

Failure of treatment, indicated by an absence of any significant decrease in the myoma diameter, was never observed.

Complications: adhesions confirmed by second-look laparoscopy

In 15 patients, a second-look laparoscopy was carried out more than 6 months after myolysis for other reasons (ovarian cyst, sterilization, etc.). The appearance of the myoma was noted. In eight cases, dense and fibrous adhesions were observed between the myoma and, most frequently, the small bowel and/or epiploon. After adhesiolysis, the myoma appeared white without any apparent vessels. In two cases, we decided to remove the myoma. Dissection of the myoma from the normal myometrium was surprisingly easy and the myomas were removed in order to evaluate histologically the efficacy of myolysis. There was necrosis in most myoma areas, characterized by edema and an absence of viable cells (Figure 8a, b and c). In other areas, giant cells and macrophages containing carbonized particles (Figure 9) very close to the necrotic sites suggested that necrosis was really induced by the laser coagulation.

MYOLYSIS WITH BIPOLAR NEEDLES

Use of the Nd : YAG laser for myoma coagulation has certain disadvantages: the laser creates a large amount of smoke, which can obscure visibility. Inexpensive bipolar needles were developed as an alternative to the Nd : YAG laser. First used in Hamburg in 1993 by Adolphe Gallinat[8], the bipolar needles were short (1.5 cm) and appropriate only for smaller myomas. Two years later, another bipolar needle instrument was designed by Goldfarb in the United States[9,10]. There are two forms of bipolar instrument: a 30-cm instrument with a 5-cm probe; and a 45-cm probe that can be passed through the operating laparoscope.

The 45-cm bipolar needle passed through the operating laparoscope enables the surgeon to coagulate a posterior myoma. Using the bipolar instrument, thorough coagulation of a 7-cm leiomyoma may be achieved in 20 min.

In 150 procedures performed laparoscopically, no serious complications were reported as a result of using this instrument; however, one patient developed a pelvic abscess and subsequently underwent hysterectomy. Another patient developed bacteremia and made an uneventful recovery after antibiotic therapy[6].

Coagulating the myoma with the bipolar needle devascularizes the leiomyoma, resulting in leiomyoma shrinkage of 30–50% beyond the effect attributable to gonadotropin releasing hormone (GnRH) therapy. Recent results in a series performed by Phillips[11,12] confirmed the efficacy of myoma coagulation. Prior to myoma coagulation, patients were pretreated with depot leuprolide. Leiomyomas were measured using a formula for the volume of an ellipsoid to achieve a volumetric evaluation of the leiomyoma before and after reduction. Within 6 months of surgery, satisfactory results were achieved in 97.4% of patients. Three to

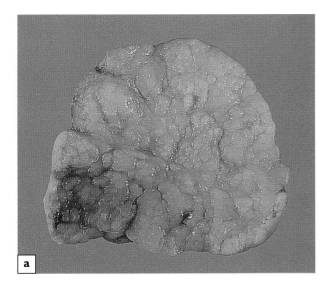

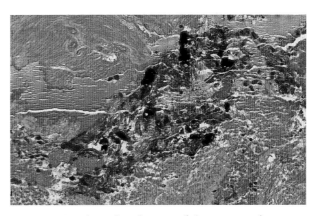

Figure 9 Histological evaluation of the myoma after myolysis: in some areas, giant cells and macrophages containing carbonized particles very close to the necrotic sites suggest that necrosis was really induced by the laser coagulation

MYOLYSIS WITH DIATHERMY

Chapman[13] reported on 18 patients with leiomyomas treated by myoma coagulation who were not ruled out if they wished to preserve fertility. Treatment involved exposing the myoma via laparotomy and then drilling holes with a CO_2 laser. To achieve coagulation, a diathermy electrode was inserted into each hole and the surrounding myoma was heated to achieve protein denaturation. Four of the 18 women subsequently became pregnant. Diathermy thus may be another promising method of treating myomas while minimizing adhesion formation.

CRYOMYOLYSIS

According to Zreik and colleagues[14], cryomyolysis maintains myomas at, or slightly reduces them to, post-GnRH agonist size, and all other uterine tissue returns to pretreatment size. The cryoprobe track begins as a small hole through the uterine serosa with a monopolar needle. The experience with cryomyolysis was limited to a prospective pilot study[14]. Fourteen patients were treated with a GnRH analog for 2 or more months to decrease myoma size, with initial magnetic resonance imaging (MRI) performed to determine shrinkage of the uterus. A second MRI was performed 4 months after surgery, with discontinuation of the GnRH analog therapy, when regrowth of the uterus to its original size would be expected.

Myoma volume decreased by 6% over 4 months postoperatively, with several patients having a decrease of over 50%. Thus, it appears that reduction in myoma size by GnRH agonists can be prolonged, or even enhanced, by cryomyolysis, despite the return to pretreatment size of normal uterine tissue. Four out of six women undergoing second-look office laparoscopy had adhesion formation at freezing sites. Most adhesions were filmy and easily lysed at laparoscopy, but they were severe in one patient.

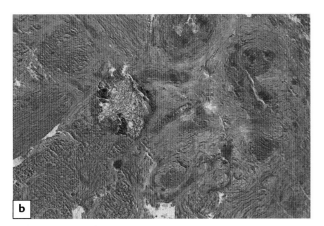

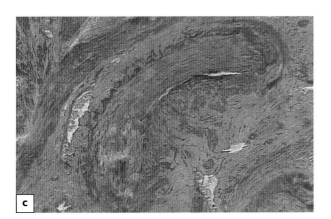

Figure 8 Specimen of myoma: (a) 6 months after myolysis; (b) and (c) there is necrosis characterized by edema and the absence of viable cells

six months postoperatively, there was an 83.1% decrease in mean total uterine volume, an 88.5% reduction in mean total leiomyoma volume, and a 60% reduction in the mean widest leiomyoma diameter (compared with premedication measurements).

Myoma interstitial thermo-therapy

Recently, Donnez and co-workers[15] presented, in Stockholm, the first cases of myomas treated by interstitial thermo-therapy using one specific laser fiber, as described in the endometrial laser intrauterine thermo-therapy (ELITT™) procedure[16] (Figure 10). After having made a hole in the myoma serosa with the help of a trocar (1.5 mm), the laser fiber was introduced into the myoma. The fiber consists of an optical light diffuser that is designed to transmit laser light in all directions to effect the destruction of the myoma by hyperthermia. Although this new method looks very promising to avoid adhesions, long-term results on myoma growth are necessary before proposing this method for myolysis. The procedure employs a laser light to destroy the myoma by thermal therapy, increasing the temperature of the myoma to induce coagulation. The laser light is diffused inside the myoma in all directions. The 830-nm wavelength laser light penetrates the myoma wall to a precise depth, and it is absorbed by the hemoglobin. The absorbed light is then transformed to heat; it warms the myoma and causes controlled coagulation (Figure 11). The inherent light scattering inside the myoma contributes positively to the uniformity of the light distribution and resultant coagulation. A compact tabletop 20-W, 830-nm diode laser is available for this kind of surgery.

REOPERATION

In the different studies published in the literature, the reoperation rate (hysterectomy) was found to vary from 3–5%[9,10] to 10% after 5 years[17].

PREGNANCY

Some authors have proposed this technique in order to reduce myoma size before pregnancy. In our group, we have always considered myolysis as a contraindication. Although Chapman[13] and Phillips[11] are in favor of attempting pregnancy after myolysis, recent papers reporting cases of uterine rupture during pregnancy[18,19] have strongly suggested that myolysis should be indicated only in women who do not desire further pregnancy.

DISCUSSION

Myomas are very common in women of reproductive age and may be responsible for menorrhagia, anemia, pelvic pain, compression, infertility or miscarriage. However, myomas are often asymptomatic and may not require treatment. In such asymptomatic patients, indications for myomectomy are debatable; therapy may be considered in some cases to prevent complications related to the growth

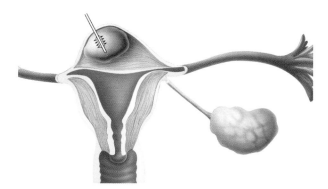

Figure 10 Interstitial thermo-therapy fibers can also be used to induce myoma shrinkage

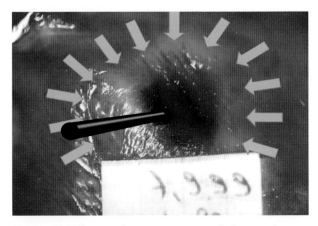

Figure 11 Efficacy of myoma interstitial thermo-therapy (MITT). The area of coagulation of the myoma by ITT is well visible (arrows)

of the myoma. Since the early 1990s, uterine fibroids can be treated endoscopically[1–4,20].

As previously described, in cases of submucosal uterine fibroids, hysteroscopic myomectomy[3,4] is carried out if the greater diameter of the leiomyoma is inside the uterine cavity. In cases of very large fibroids with the larger portion not inside the uterine cavity, the protruding portion is removed and the intramural portion is devascularized by introducing the laser fiber into the myoma, at a length depending on the depth of the remaining intramural portion[4,21]. This technique proved to be effective in provoking myoma shrinkage, with a dramatic decrease in size and a marked devascularization of the myoma. This concept of myolysis was thus first described in hysteroscopic techniques in the late 1980s and then applied to the laparoscopic approach in the treatment of intramural myomas in women who do not desire further pregnancy[5].

In cases of subserosal and intramural fibroids, myomectomy can also be carried out laparoscopically by an incision through the uterine serosa with a needle tip or knife electrode unipolar cautery, a KTP/YAG laser in KTP mode, or hook scissors. The exposed fibroid is separated from the myometrium and removed by a combination of traction, twisting and cutting[2]. Serosal reapproximation can be accomplished with a bipolar coagulator in cases of small fibroids (< 3 cm), sutures or fibrin glue (Tissucol® fibrin sealant, Immuno AG, Vienna, Austria). The excised fibroids are removed from the abdominal cavity via a posterior colpotomy, through suprapubic anterior wall incisions, or through the operating channel of the laparoscope after fragmentation, depending on the size of the tumor.

Sometimes, in cases of large intramural fibroids or multiple myomas, laparoscopic myomectomy can be difficult or time-consuming[20]. Laparoscopic myolysis can be proposed as an alternative to myomectomy, performed by laparoscopy or laparotomy in cases of large or multiple intramural fibroids[5]. The fibroids are not removed but coagulated with the help of the YAG laser[5], bipolar coagulation[9,10,22], cryoprobe[14], monopolar coagulation[13] or, very recently, diode laser (MITT)[17]. The myoma coagulation is followed by necrosis and the size of the myoma decreases dramatically. The success of myolysis in treating myomas has been reported by many investigators[5–11,13,22,23]. In the first report by Nisolle and colleagues[5], the Nd : YAG laser was used and a decrease of 50% was noted without regrowth of the myomas after 12 months. Since the first report, all authors have reported large series which have confirmed a leiomyoma shrinkage of 30–50%.

Concerning cost-effectiveness, myolysis has the obvious economic benefits of outpatient surgery and rapid recovery and return to a normal life-style. Moreover, the subsequent reoperation rates for recurrence or persistence of symptoms are quite low.

The final question is to establish whether myolysis can be offered to women who wish to bear children. According to the literature, this issue is controversial. Indeed, data published in the literature have clearly demonstrated that viable pregnancies are possible after laparoscopic myolysis[11,13,23,24], but the possibility of coagulation and devascularization of the myometrium exists, as does, at least theoretically, the possibility of uterine rupture in cases of pregnancy[18,19].

Patients must thus be selected; only those aged over 40 years or those not desiring to bear any more children but wishing to avoid a future hysterectomy should undergo myolysis.

Long-term follow-up has shown that there is no regrowth of the myoma[5,7]. Histology proved complete devascularization of the myoma with subsequent necrosis. However, when performed, the second-look laparoscopy demonstrated, in about 10–50% of cases, the presence of very dense adhesions. In order to reduce the risk of adhesions, Interceed was placed on the coagulated area[5,11,13]. Randomized studies must be carried out in the future in order to prove the efficacy of Interceed in this indication.

In order to reduce adhesions, new laser fibers (ITT fibers) are now being evaluated. In this type of fiber, diffusion of the heat-inducing necrosis occurs along the termi-

nal part of the fiber. Only one hole is required and this reduces the lesion in the myoma serosa.

In conclusion, myolysis is effective in the reduction of myoma size and can be proposed as an alternative to myomectomy, but only in selected patients. Because of the risk of bowel adhesions and of coagulation of the myometrium, this type of surgery must be reserved for large, intramural, symptomatic myomas if endoscopic myomectomy is considered to be too difficult or time-consuming.

REFERENCES

1. Daniell JF, Gurley LD. Laparoscopic treatment of clinically significant symptomatic uterine fibroids. *J Gynecol Surg* 1991;7:37–9

2. Dubuisson JB, Lecuru F, Foulot H, *et al.* Myomectomy by laparoscopy: a preliminary report of 43 cases. *Fertil Steril* 1991;56:827–30

3. Donnez J, Schrurs B, Gillerot S, *et al.* Treatment of uterine fibroids with implants of gonadotropin releasing-hormone agonist: assessment by hysterography. *Fertil Steril* 1989;51:947–50

4. Donnez J, Gillerot S, Bourgonjon D, *et al.* Neodymium : YAG laser hysteroscopy in large submucous fibroids. *Fertil Steril* 1990;54:999–1003

5. Nisolle M, Smets M, Gillerot S, *et al.* Laparoscopic myolysis with the Nd : YAG laser. *J Gynecol Surg* 1993;9:95–9

6. Goldfarb HA. Nd : YAG laser laparoscopic coagulation of symptomatic myomas. *J Reprod Med* 1992;37:636

7. Nisolle M, Smets M, Gillerot S, *et al.* Laparoscopic myolysis with the Nd : YAG laser. In Donnez J, Nisolle M, eds. *An Atlas of Laser Operative Laparoscopy and Hysteroscopy.* Carnforth, UK: Parthenon Publishing, 1994:187–93

8. Gallinat A, Lueken RP. Current trends in the therapy of myomata. In Leuken RP, Gallinat A, eds. *Endoscopic Surgery in Gynecology.* Berlin: Demeter Verlag GmBH, 1993:68–71

9. Goldfarb HA. Laparoscopic coagulation of myoma (myolysis). *Obstet Gynecol Clin North Am* 1995;22:807–19

10. Goldfarb HA. Bipolar laparoscopic needles for myoma coagulation. *J Am Assoc Gynecol Laparosc* 1995;2:175–9

11. Phillips D. Laparoscopic leiomyoma coagulation – myolysis. *Gynecol Endosc* 1995;4:5–11

12. Phillips DR, Nathanson HG, Milim SJ, *et al.* Experience with laparoscopic leiomyoma coagulation and concomitant operative hysteroscopy. *J Am Assoc Gynecol Laparosc* 1997;4:425–33

13. Chapman R. Treatment of uterine myomas by interstitial hyperthermia. *Gynecol Endosc* 1993;2:227

14. Zreik T, Rutherford T, Palter S, *et al.* Cryomyolysis: a new procedure for the conservative treatment of uterine fibroids. *J Am Assoc Gynecol Laparosc* 1998;1:33–8

15. Donnez J, Nisolle M, Polet R, *et al.* Laparoscopic myolysis. *Hum Reprod* 2000;6:609–13

16. Donnez J, Polet R, Squiffet J, *et al.* Endometrial laser intrauterine thermo-therapy (ELITT™): a revolutionary new approach to the elimination of menorrhagia. *Curr Opin Obstet Gynecol* 1999;11:363–70

17. Donnez J, Polet R, Squifflet J, *et al.* Laparoscopic myolysis. Proceedings of the ESGE meeting, Stockholm. *Gynecol Endosc* 1999:Abst 102

18. Arcangeli S, Pasquarette M. Gravid uterine rupture after myolysis. *Obstet Gynecol* 1997;89:857

19. Vilos G, Daly L, Tse B. Pregnancy outcome after laparoscopic electromyolysis. *J Am Assoc Gynecol Laparosc* 1998;5:289–92

20. Nezhat C, Nezhat F, Silfen SL, *et al.* Laparoscopic myomectomy. *Int J Fertil* 1991;36:275–80

21. Donnez J. Nd:YAG laser hysteroscopic myomectomy. In Sutton C, Diamond M, eds. *Endoscopic Surgery for Gynecology*. London: WB Saunders Company Ltd, 1993:331–7

22. Goldfarb HA. Myoma coagulation (myolysis). *Obstet Gynecol Clin North Am* 2000;27:421–30

23. Wood C, Maher P, Hill D. Myoma reduction by electrocautery. *Gynecol Endosc* 1994;3:163–5

24. Dubuisson JB, Chapron C, Fauconnier A, *et al.* Laparoscopic myomectomy and myolysis. *Curr Opin Obstet Gynecol* 1997;9:233–8

LASH: laparoscopic subtotal hysterectomy

23

J. Donnez, M. Nisolle, M. Smets, R. Polet and J. Squifflet

INTRODUCTION

The development of new accessories and improved technology has enabled gynecologists to perform laparoscopic hysterectomy. Reich and colleagues[1] described the technique of laparoscopic hysterectomy for the first time in 1989. Laparoscopy-assisted vaginal hysterectomy and bilateral salpingo-oophorectomy have been routinely performed since 1990[2] in cases of endometrial cancer and benign gynecological disease in our department, as well as in others[3–5]. Several series[2,6–8] have documented shorter hospital stays and recovery times in women having undergone laparoscopic hysterectomy.

In 1990, we performed the first laparoscopic subtotal (supracervical) hysterectomy (LASH) in our department and the first series of 32 cases was published in 1993[7]. Subsequently, a series of 500 cases was described[9]. From July 1990 to December 2000, 900 laparoscopic supracervical hysterectomies were performed in our department. The incidence of LASH in our series of hysterectomies was 31%. It increased from an incidence of 2% (1990) to 22% (1993) to 46% (1995) to 44% (1996) and then remained stable until 1999 (44%). These last 5 years, the incidence has remained stable (Table 1). A recent publication in the *New England Journal of Medicine* has demonstrated that the laparoscopic approach is not expensive if non-disposable material is used[10] (Table 2).

SURGICAL PROCEDURE

All patients had a standard Papanicolaou smear, colposcopy and hysteroscopic cervical canal evaluation, and all received general anesthesia. Following induction of

Table 1 A series of 1438 hysterectomies for benign uterine diseases

Procedures	June 1994–June 1996 n	(%)	July 1996–November 1997 n	(%)	December 1997–October 1999 n	(%)
LASH	236	(46)	170	(41.5)	228	(44)
LAVH or LH	130	(26)	90	(22)	162	(31)
Vaginal hysterectomy	82	(16)	113	(27.5)	104	(20)
Abdominal hysterectomy	60	(12)	37	(9)	26	(5)

LASH, laparoscopic subtotal hysterectomy; LAVH, laparoscopy-assisted vaginal hysterectomy; LH, laparoscopic hysterectomy

Table 2 Characteristics of 508 hysterectomies, according to the surgical procedure used

Procedure	Number of procedures (%)	Mean uterine weight (range) (g)	Cost per operation* ($)	Mean hospital stay (range) (days)
LASH	236 (46)	188 (44–810)	2.573	2.9 (2–5)
LAVH	130 (26)	208 (40–625)	2.832	4.5 (4–8)
Vaginal hysterectomy**	82 (16)	148 (40–613)	3.608	5.9 (5–12)
Abdominal hysterectomy***	60 (12)	412 (60–5780)	4.533	7.1 (5–14)

* Costs include hospital costs, medical and surgical supplies, and physicians' costs. Belgian francs were converted into US dollars at the exchange rate of 38 Belgian francs to $1 US[10]; ** with or without colporrhaphy; LASH, laparoscopic subtotal hysterectomy; LAVH, laparoscopy-assisted vaginal hysterectomy

general intratracheal anesthesia, the patient was placed in the dorsal lithotomy position. The abdomen and the vagina were prepared with a diluted iodine solution. A Foley catheter was inserted. Two Pozzi forceps were placed on the cervix and a non-metallic intrauterine cannula was inserted into the uterine cavity in order to manipulate the uterus easily. A four-puncture technique was used for LASH. Three 5-mm second-puncture trocars were inserted: one 3 cm above the symphysis pubis and the others 4–5 cm laterally, in each lower quadrant within the safety triangles (between the midline and the epigastric artery area).

A 10-mm laparoscope connected to a video camera was placed intraumbilically. After careful inspection of the entire peritoneal cavity, the patient was moved into the Trendelenburg position. Only one surgical method was used to transect pelvic ligaments and achieve hemostasis: bipolar coagulation and transection. Because endoscopic staplers are very expensive, bipolar coagulation (bipolar grasping forceps, Storz 3 mm wide) and transection were systematically used. Bipolar coagulation was used to desiccate the utero-ovarian ligaments and vessels and the isthmic portion of both Fallopian tubes (Figures 1 and 2). Scissors were then used to transect the structures within the coagulated areas. Meticulous hemostasis was achieved by repeated bipolar coagulation of transected vessels. If a bilateral (or unilateral) salpingo-oophorectomy was required, the infundibulopelvic ligaments were similarly coagulated and transected. The round ligaments were treated in the same way.

The anterior leaf and the posterior leaf of the broad ligament were then opened with scissors. Hydrodissection made the procedure easier and allowed the surgeon to expose the uterine vessels.

The vesico-uterine peritoneum was then opened with scissors (Figure 3). The vesicocervical space was dissected

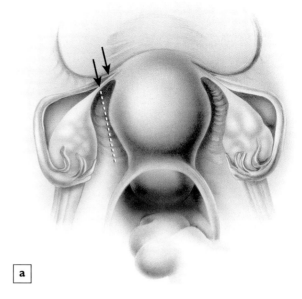

a

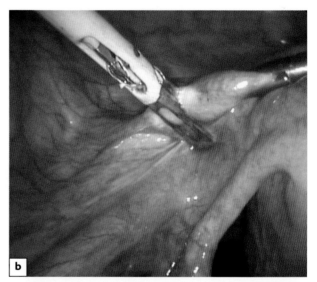

b

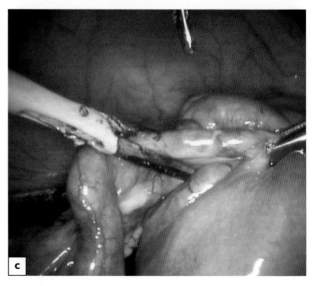

c

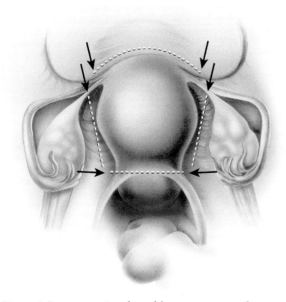

Figure 1 Laparoscopic subtotal hysterectomy technique

Figure 2 (a)–(c) Section of the round ligament, the Fallopian tube and the utero-ovarian ligament

234

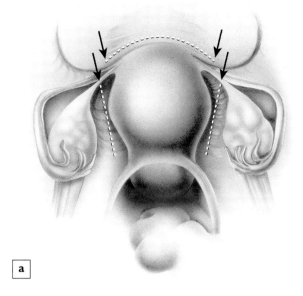

a

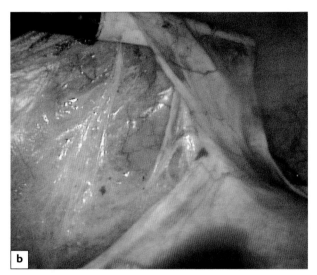

b

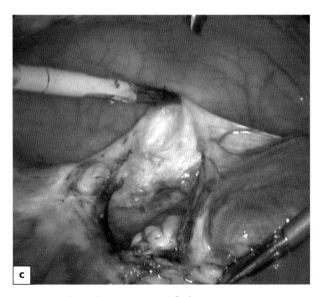

c

Figure 3 (a)–(c) Dissection of the vesico-uterine peritoneum

no more than 2 cm below the limit between the cervix and the corpus uteri.

After careful identification of the uterine vessels and ureters, the uterine vessels were electrocoagulated with the bipolar coagulation forceps and transected (Figure 4). The unipolar knife or unipolar scissors were then used to cut the cervix below the level of the internal os and separate the cervix from the corpus (Figure 5). Hemostasis was achieved by meticulous coagulation. Until November 1993, longitudinal (vertical or horizontal) posterior colpotomy was performed, either by laparoscopy or through the vagina. Since then, however, the uterus has been removed through a 12-mm trocar after morcellation using Steiner's morcellator[11] (Figure 6).

In the future, the new morcellator (20 mm in size) will enable the duration of morcellation to be reduced (Figure 7).

Irrigation fluid was instilled into the pelvis and the operative sites were inspected. A titanium clip was then applied to the uterine artery to insure complete hemostasis. The cervical stump was never reperitonealized. Saline solution with Rifocine® (300 ml) was left in the peritoneal cavity. The instruments were removed from the abdomen and the four incisions were reapproximated with 3-0 Nylon suture.

Prophylactic antibiotics (cephalosporin (Zinacef®) 2 g/dl were administered just before the procedure (5 min before the incision).

RESULTS

All of our LASH procedures were successful. The patients' ages ranged from 34 years to 57 years. The mean duration of surgery was 62 min (morcellation not included). In the majority of cases, in experienced hands, the average duration is about 60 min, although, in university teaching hospitals, the learning process of registrars leads to an increase in the surgery duration (Table 3).

The estimated blood loss was systematically less than 100 ml. There were no intraoperative complications such as bowel or ureteral injuries. No patients experienced fever. All patients were theoretically able to leave the hospital the first day following surgery. Many, nevertheless, preferred to stay 2 or 3 days, knowing that the Belgian insurance system offers reimbursement for up to 10 days' hospitalization (Table 2).

In our department, the length of hospital stay after surgery ranged from 4 to 5 days for vaginal hysterectomy, 3 to 4 days for laparoscopy-assisted vaginal hysterectomy (LAVH) and 5 to 8 days for abdominal hysterectomy (mostly dependent on the age of the patient). Patients who underwent LASH reported much less discomfort than patients who underwent other types of hysterectomy. No patients required major analgesic drugs. Only 8% of patients required analgesic drugs a few hours after surgery, but no patients required drugs the day after surgery.

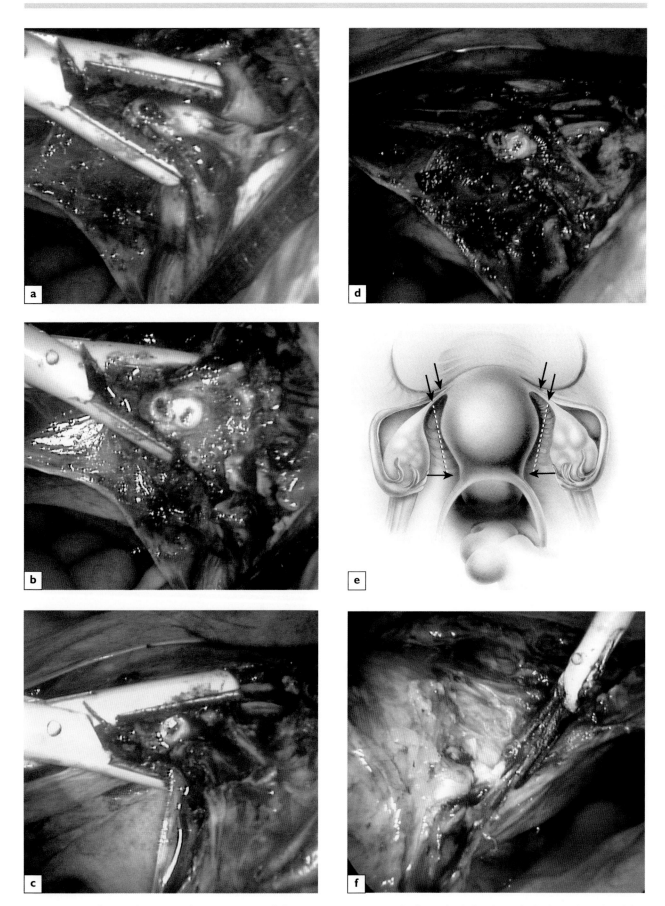

Figure 4 (a)–(f) Visualization and cauterization of the uterine artery, (a)–(d) show the left side and (f) the right side of the patient

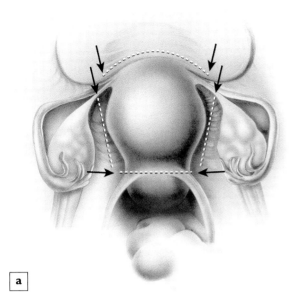

a

Patients were able to ambulate very soon after LASH (the same day), similar to patients who underwent laparoscopic adhesiolysis, ovarian cystectomy or salpingoneostomy. Sexual intercourse was permitted 2 weeks after surgery. There was only one case of cervical prolapse and no signs of enterocele were observed in patients reviewed in a 5-year follow-up ($n = 349$) (Table 4). There were no complaints of genuine urinary incontinence except in one case. This patient, however, had already complained of genuine urinary incontinence before LASH, and physiotherapy and biofeedback therapy were proposed at this time. As no improvement was seen after 1 year, surgery was required, and the patient underwent a laparoscopic Burch procedure in 1994. Six patients developed serous cysts ($n = 3$), a mucinous cyst ($n = 1$) or a dermoid cyst ($n = 2$). The laparoscopy allowed us to explore the pelvic cavity and to demonstrate the absence of severe adhesions on the

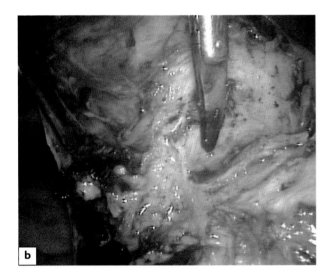

b

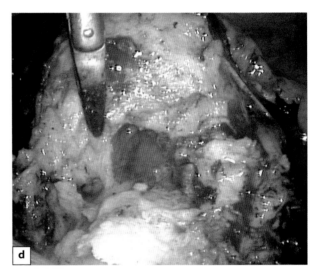

d

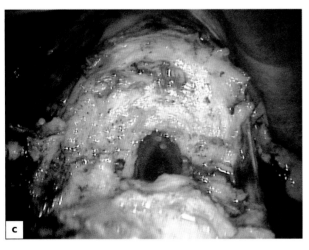

c

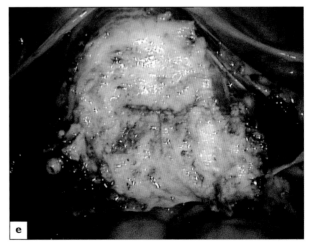

e

Figure 5 (a)–(d) Section of the cervix, taking care to cut the upper part of the cervix and to coagulate the upper endocervical canal. (e) Final view

Table 3 Preoperative and early postoperative complications in a series of 900 laparoscopic subtotal hysterectomies

Duration of surgical procedure (min)	62	(30–135)
including morcellation (min)	111	(40–168)
Uterine weight (g)	182	(60–810)
Complications		
Perioperative		
fever > 38°(after the second day)	0	
bladder incision (< 1 cm)	3*	(0.3%)
ureter	1**	
hemorrhage	0	
Postoperative		
urinary tract lesion**	2	(0.2%)
colon or rectal perforation	0	

* Sutured laparoscopically (in three patients with a previous history of two or three Cesarean sections); ** fistula caused by thermal damage treated by JJ stent (Figure 8)

Table 4 Late follow-up (> 5 years) (*n* = 349)

Fistula	0	
Cyclical bleeding	7	(2%)*
Cervical prolapse	1	
Pelvic pain or dyspareunia	0	
Abnormal smear	0	
Second-look laparoscopy		
Burch	1	
serous mucinous or dermoid ovarian cyst	6	(1.8%)
'forgotten' morcellated specimen	2	

* Since 1992, care has been taken to cut the cervix below the internal os so that no remaining endometrium persists. Laparoscopic coagulation of the upper part of the cervical canal is carried out

cervical stump. Patients were requested to undergo a Papanicolaou smear and a colposcopy every year. In two patients, the laparoscopy was performed because of a 'tumor' located in the pouch of Douglas, causing deep dyspareunia. Symptoms were due to a small piece (3 cm) of the morcellated uterus which had not been removed during the first laparoscopy (LASH). Laparoscopy allowed us to dissect the 'forgotten' specimen which was covered by peritoneum.

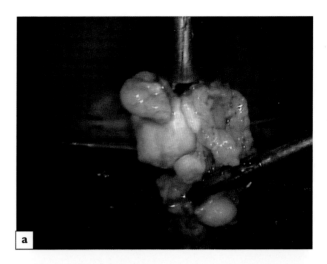

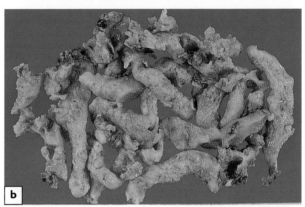

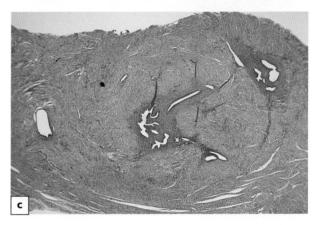

Figure 6 (a) Steiner morcellator: laparoscopic view; (b) uterus after morcellation; (c) histological analysis of a 'morcellated' specimen demonstrating adenomyosis

COMMENTS

The indications for laparoscopic surgery have expanded greatly over the past decades. Some expansion has also been seen in the field of hysteroscopic surgery. Endometrial ablation performed endoscopically has been proposed as an alternative to hormonal therapy or hysterectomy in dysfunctional bleeding without intrauterine lesions[12]. Hysteroscopic myomectomy has also been

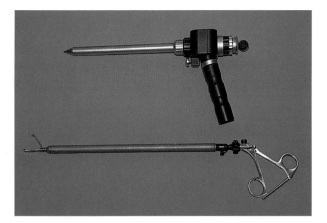

Figure 7 New Storz morcellator (2 cm in diameter): it allows a faster morcellation

proposed for large submucosal myomas. In a recent study, the long-term results of neodymium : yttrium–aluminum–garnet (Nd : YAG) laser hysteroscopic myomectomy were found to be excellent in cases of large submucosal fibroids less than three in number.

Indeed, in our series, recurrence of menorrhagia did not exceed 5% after a 2-year follow-up. However, in cases of multiple (more than four) submucosal fibroids, recurrence of bleeding due to recurrent myomas was found to be as high as 25%, even when endometrial ablation was performed concomitantly[12–15]. This is why hysteroscopic management of uterine bleeding cannot be systematically proposed and why an alternative surgical approach was suggested.

In 1990, the LASH technique was not frequently used in our department. Indeed, in a series of 204 hysterectomies carried out in the department in 1990, only four LASH (2%) were performed. At the time, the disadvantage of the technique, which is the remaining cervix, was considered as a potential risk factor for cervical cancer. It is obvious that the risk is low in some groups of the population. Moreover, this question is never asked when an endometrial ablation is performed. Subsequently, the incidence of LASH increased from just 2% to 44% of all hysterectomies (Table 1). Since the uterus can be removed laparoscopically with the help of Steiner's morcellator (Figures 6 and 7), LASH must be considered as a strictly laparoscopic approach to hysterectomy. No patients required major analgesics the day after surgery.

Numerous advantages were noted:

(1) Rapid recovery similar to that observed after laparoscopic surgery for infertility;

(2) Reduced postoperative discomfort and shorter hospital stay;

(3) Lower rate of complications when compared to laparoscopic hysterectomy (LH) and LAVH;

(4) Decreased risk of vaginal vault prolapse;

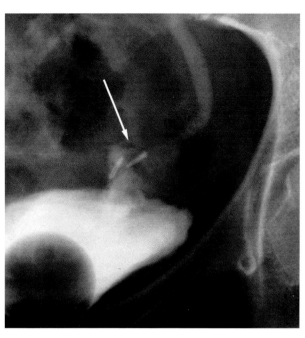

Figure 8 Ureteral fistula (arrow) provoked by thermal damage diagnosed 7 days after the procedure. A double JJ stent was placed for 2–3 months. Three months after removal of the JJ stent, intravenous pyelography revealed a normal ureter at the site of the fistula

(5) Decreased risk of post-hysterectomy urine incontinence;

(6) Absence of decreased libido.

Indeed, a serious complication rate of 3% was recently reported after LAVH and LH in a multicenter study in the UK (R. Garry, personal communication) as well as in Belgium[16]. Ureteral and/or bladder damage occurred at a rate of 2% after LH. In our series, as in the series carried out in Lyons[17], ureteral complications were rarely noted (only one case in our series). The LASH technique reduces the risk of ureteral injury, but does not eliminate it. Indeed, thermal damage due to the coagulation process can provoke ureteral fistula (Figure 8). Nevertheless, three cases of bladder injury (laparoscopically repaired) occurred in patients with a medical history of two or three Cesarean sections.

Sutton (personal communication) recently reported a high rate of complications after subtotal laparoscopic hysterectomy (SLH) in Paris; however, this high rate can only be explained either by an inappropriate surgical technique or by the 'learning' curve followed by some of the surgeons involved in the study. Indeed, the high rate of cyclical bleeding after SLH can only be accounted for by an inappropriate section of the upper part of the cervix, leaving in place the 'isthmic' portion of the uterus with the endometrium. Using our technique, we encountered this problem in the first series[7] of 32 cases and, therefore, frequently recommended cutting the cervix accordingly and coagulating the upper part of the cervical canal.

One other advantage of LASH is the preservation of the cardinal ligaments and the uterosacral ligaments which probably play a role in pelvic organ suspension and in bladder continence control[18].

According to Kilkku[19] and Virtanen[20] and their colleagues, the libido and orgasmic frequency are not affected by subtotal hysterectomy but are significantly reduced by total hysterectomy. Preliminary results of a prospective study carried out in our department confirm that sexual satisfaction is not affected by LASH.

Because of the feasibility of the technique, the very low morbidity rate and the fast recovery, LASH could be proposed as a 'strictly laparoscopic approach' in some indications and especially in cases where the uterus presents with multiple submucosal myomas. Indeed, we know that, in such cases, the recurrence rate of bleeding after hysteroscopic myoma resection and endometrial ablation is more than 25% after a 2-year follow-up[14] and therefore LASH could be proposed instead of hysteroscopic surgery to women with this type of pathology.

Failures of endometrial laser ablation and partial endometrial laser ablation for dysfunctional bleeding in a normal-sized uterus occur in about 3–5% of cases[12]. Failed endometrial ablation must also be considered as an indication for LASH. Because of the good results and the absence of complications, the LASH technique is proposed in our department in cases of:

(1) Enlarged uterus with multiple fibroids (up to a 13-week gestational volume) and normal cervix (even in nulligravida);

(2) Failures of endometrial ablation and/or myomectomy (failure demonstrated by the recurrence of menometrorrhagia);

(3) Myomatous uterus in women who have a medical history of Cesarean section;

(4) Multiple submucosal myomas even if the uterine volume is < 7 gestational weeks;

(5) As a step in laparoscopic sacrofixation in cases of uterine prolapse.

The risk induced by the preservation of the cervix has long been considered to be the development of a cervical stump carcinoma, though this risk is only 0.1–0.4%[19,21]. Historically, however, subtotal hysterectomy was condemned well before cervical smears became accepted.

Today, systematic cervical smears, colposcopy and biopsy, if required, are determining factors in the selection of the case and the postoperative follow-up of the patient. How many cases of invasive cervical carcinomas are observed in consultations every year? Because the incidence of this disease is very low in the group of women followed up every year by Papanicolaou smear, and because we now have accurate means to keep a close check on the cervix, the risk of encountering invasive cervical cancer is virtually nil.

We consider that patients suffering from uterosacral ligament endometriosis with dyspareunia and dysmenorrhea must be excluded. Indeed, total hysterectomy with resection of the uterosacral ligaments is more appropriate in these cases.

So far, more than 900 cases have been performed with an excellent follow-up to date because of the low rate of complications and good acceptance by the patient. This suggests that this strictly laparoscopic approach is the hysterectomy procedure of choice in selected cases.

REFERENCES

1. Reich H, De Caprio J, MacGlynn F. Laparoscopic hysterectomy. J Gynecol Coll Surg 1989;5:213
2. Nezhat C, Nezhat F, Silfen SL. Laparoscopic hysterectomy and bilateral salpingoooophorectomy using multifire GIA surgical stapler. J Gynecol Coll Surg 1990;6:287
3. Mage G, Canis M, Wattiez A, et al. Hystérectomie et coelioscopie. J Gynecol Obstet Biol Reprod 1990;19:573–6
4. Padial JG, Sotolongo J, Casey MJ, et al. Laparoscopy-assisted vaginal hysterectomy: report of seventy-five consecutive cases. J Gynecol Surg 1992;8:81
5. Liu CVY. Laparoscopic hysterectomy. Report of 215 cases. Gynecol Endosc 1992;1:73–7
6. Reich H, Mac Glynn F, Sekel L. Total laparoscopic hysterectomy. Gynecol Endosc 1990;2:59–63
7. Donnez J, Nisolle M. LASH: laparoscopic supracervical (subtotal) hysterectomy. J Gynecol Surg 1993;9:91–4
8. Phipps JH, John M, Hassanaien M, et al. Laparoscopic and laparoscopically assisted vaginal hysterectomy: a series of 114 cases. Gynecol Endosc 1993;2:7–12
9. Donnez J, Nisolle M, Smets M, et al. LASH: Laparoscopic supracervical (subtotal) hysterectomy. A first series of 500 cases. Gynecol Endosc 1997;6:73–6
10. Nisolle M, Donnez J. Alternative technique of hysterectomy. New Engl J Med 1997;336:291–2
11. Nisolle M, Grandjean P, Gillerot S, et al. Endometrial ablation with the Nd : YAG laser in dysfunctional bleeding. Min Invas Ther 1991;1:35
12. Steiner RA, Wight A, Tadir Y, et al. Electrical cutting device for laparoscopic removal of tissue from the abdominal cavity. Obstet Gynecol 1993;81:471–4
13. Donnez J, Gillerot S, Bourgonjon D, et al. Neodymium : YAG laser hysteroscopy in large submucous fibroids. Fertil Steril 1990;54:999
14. Donnez J, Nisolle M. Hysteroscopic surgery. Curr Opin Obstet Gynecol 1992;4:439
15. Donnez J. Nd : YAG laser hysteroscopic myomectomy. In Sutton C, Diamond M, eds. Endoscopic

Surgery for Gynecologists. London: WB Saunders Company Ltd, 1993:331–7

16. Cusumano PG, Deprest J, Hardy A, *et al*. Multicentric registration on laparoscopic hysterectomy: a one year experience. *Proceedings of the First European Congress of Gynecologic Endoscopy*. Clermont-Ferrand, France, September, 1992:46

17. Lyons TL. Laparoscopic supracervical hysterectomy using the contact Nd : YAG laser. *Gynecol Endosc* 1993;2:79–81

18. Parys BT, Haylen BT, Hutton JL, *et al*. The effects of simple hysterectomy on vesicourethral function. *Brit J Urol* 1989;64:594–9

19. Kilkku P, Gronroos M, Rauramon L. Supravaginal uterine amputation with peroperative electrocoagulation of endocervical mucosa. Description of the method. *Acta Obstet Gynecol Scand* 1985;64:175–7

20. Virtanen H, Makinen J, Tenho T, *et al*. Effects of abdominal hysterectomy on urinary and sexual symptoms. *Br J Urol* 1993;72:868–72

21. Storm HH, Clemmenson IH, Manders T, *et al*. Supravaginal uterine amputation in Denmark 1978–1988 and risk of cancer. *Gynecol Oncol* 1992;45:198–201

The Lap Loop – utilization for laparoscopic total and subtotal hysterectomy

24

J. Dequesne and N. Schmidt

INTRODUCTION

The first procedure described for laparoscopic removal of the uterus was total laparoscopic hysterectomy (TLH)[1–3]. However, supracervical, or subtotal, hysterectomy is a procedure that is now of renewed interest and is currently being evaluated in patients presenting with benign uterine disease but a healthy cervix.

Various techniques of partial laparoscopic hysterectomy have been described in the early 1990s[4,5]. The first classic supracervical laparoscopic hysterectomy (LASH) was described by Donnez and Nisolle[6]. Some of the potential advantages of this procedure include a shorter operating time, fewer complications and an earlier return to normal activity, including sexual function[6,7].

A difficult and time-consuming part of the laparoscopic procedure is the sectioning of the uterine cervix. Conditions are often far from optimal, due to the angle of approach of the cutting electrode or scissors and due to the proximity of neighboring structures, which are sometimes difficult to keep at a distance (Figure 1).

The authors have refined the technique by introducing an electrosurgical loop to cut the cervix during LASH[8]. This electrode loop consists of an 18-cm long stainless steel wire (disposable) which has been screwed on one side and is finished by a ball to facilitate its handling (Figure 2). In order to provide additional security, the device is also electrically isolated, except at the extremities of the introducer and in the middle portion which is used for cutting. After proper placement of the loop around the cervix at the correct level of the isthmus (over the ligation of uterine

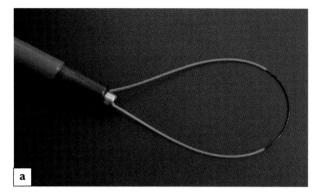
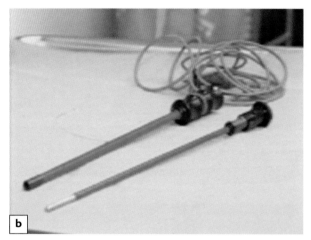
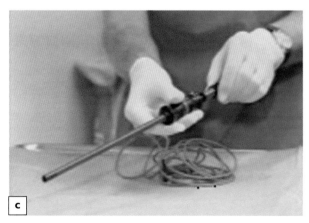

Figure 2 (a) The idea of a monopolar electrode designed like a lasso was developed in 1995. An 18-cm stainless steel wire covered by a teflon sheath (gray), interrupted for contact in the middle (black, 4 cm). At the end, a ball electrode permits easy reintroduction into the introducer; (b) view of the instument with the monopolar cable before use; (c) the introducer is placed into the sheath *(continued on next page)*

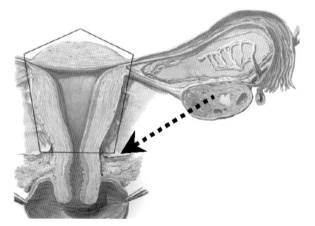

Figure 1 The separation of the uterus and the cervix was tedious, not precise and sometimes dangerous using ancillary instruments

vessels), monopolar current is applied, resulting in facilitated separation of the cervix from the corpus uteri, with less danger to neighboring structures.

SURGICAL TECHNIQUE

For subtotal laparoscopic hysterectomy, the preparation includes placement of a uterine manipulator and catheterization of the bladder. The surgical approach is through the usual laparoscopic ports: a primary port for the optic and two or three secondary ports (5 and 12 mm) for ancillary instruments. Treatment of the round ligaments and adnexae follows standard hysterectomy technique. The broad ligament and vesico-uterine fold are dissected to the superior cervix.

The various techniques for managing the uterine arteries have been described and are used as the basis of a classification system for supracervical hysterectomy[9,10]. Prior to applying the electrosurgical loop, the authors dissect and section the uterine vessels after occluding them with bipolar coagulation or placement of sutures. Treatment of the uterine arteries in this fashion corresponds to a type III

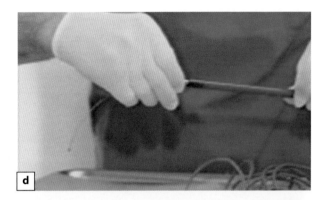

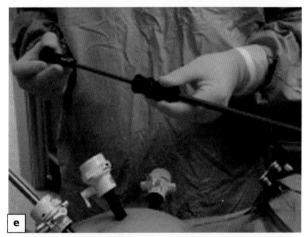

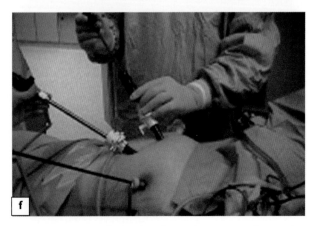

Figure 2 *Continued* (d) The electrode is screwed onto the introducer; (e) the introducer is then pulled back to protect the loop within the sheath before insertion into the abdomen; (f) the whole device is inserted through a 12-mm port

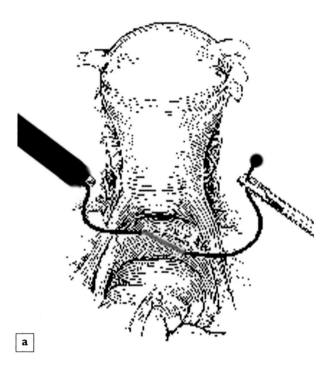

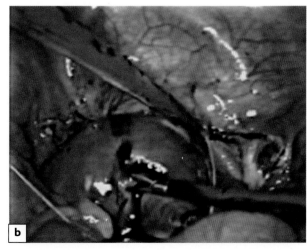

Figure 3 (a) and (b) After dissection of the broad ligament and ligation of the uterine arteries, the Lap Loop is fixed around the cervix (*continued on next page*)

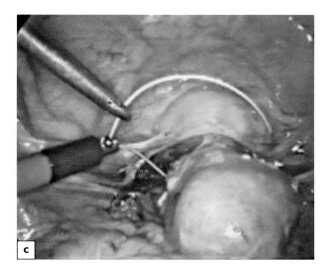

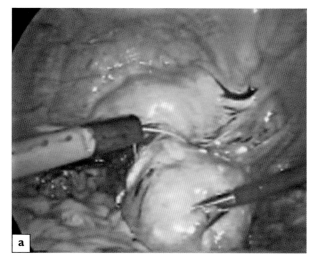

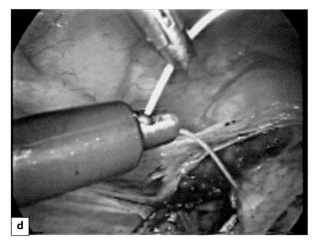

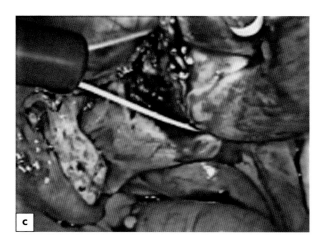

Figure 3 *Continued* (c) With a smooth forceps, the surgeon pushes the spheric tip into the sheath. When fixed, the loop is automatically aspirated into the sheath; (d) ball tip and easy plugging into the insertor

procedure, according to the Munro–Parker classification system.

Once the uterine arteries are cut, it is important to remove any manipulating device that has been placed in the uterus. The wire electrode loop is then introduced into the abdominal cavity and placed around the cervix (Figure 3a–d). The extremities are firmly held with the introducer to form a lasso around the cervix at the level of the isthmus. The uterus is retracted laterally by pulling on the stump of the round ligament in order to allow a clear view of adjacent structures: bladder, rectum, intestine, etc. (Figure 4a–c). Sectioning of the cervix is accomplished by applying high-frequency monopolar current to the electro-surgical loop while it is displaced horizontally (Figure 5a–d). It is often necessary to pause during cutting to remove smoke and, thus, maintain good vision during amputation. After the cervix has been cut, any residual bleeding may be treated with bipolar coagulation if necessary (Figure 6a and b). The minimal power setting of the

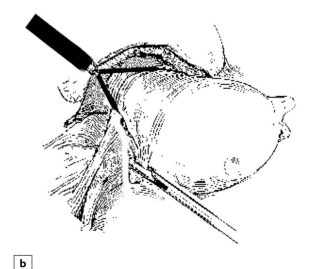

Figure 4 (a) The level of cutting is chosen after careful evaluation of the ligation of the uterine vessels; (b) the cable is fixed on the device and a pure cutting current is activated; (c) a bipolar forceps is ready in case of recurrent bleedings

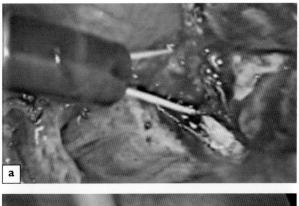

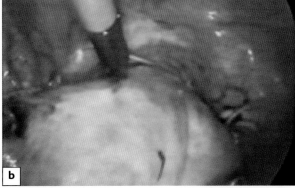

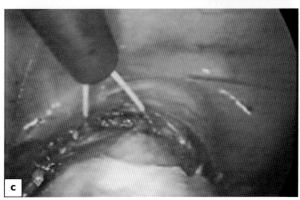

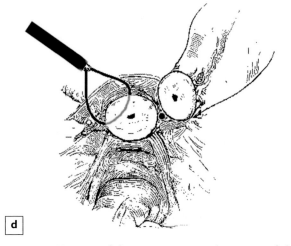

Figure 5 (a) View of the minute cutting, by means of the electrode (min. 100 W); (b) another approach for introduction, through the medial port; (c) during the cutting (notice the isolated part of the electrode); (d) view of the precision and the sharpness of the section

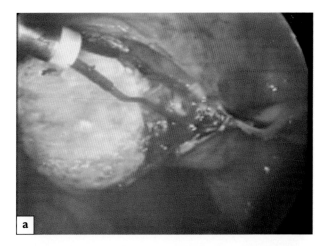

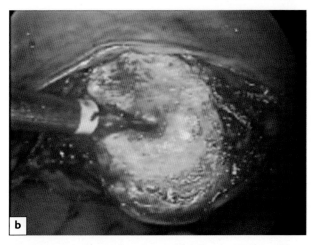

Figure 6 (a) In case of recurrent bleeding, a quick and easy correction is possible with a bipolar forceps; (b) coagulation of the endocervix

generator is 100 W in pure cutting mode (often 120 W). At the end of the procedure, the uterine corpus is removed from the abdominal cavity by morcellation.

For total laparoscopic hysterectomy, the technique is the same up to the uterine artery ligation; after that, the cervical dissection is performed with the help of the Clermont cannulator or, more easily, with the Australian tube (McCartney). A vaginal window is then made on the opposite side to anchor the loop (Figure 7a and b), strangle the vagina (Figure 7c) and permit precise cutting around the cervix when the monopolar current is activated (Figure 7d–f). At the end of the procedure the uterine corpus is removed from the abdominal cavity by either morcellation or vaginal extraction (Figure 7g–i).

This device is also very effective for pedunculated fibroids as described in Figure 8a–g. At the time of writing, it has been used only for pedicles less than 2 cm in size. The mode of utilization is, however, slightly different because we start by a coagulation (60 W) to ensure hemostasis and then apply the usual pure cutting power setting (100 W).

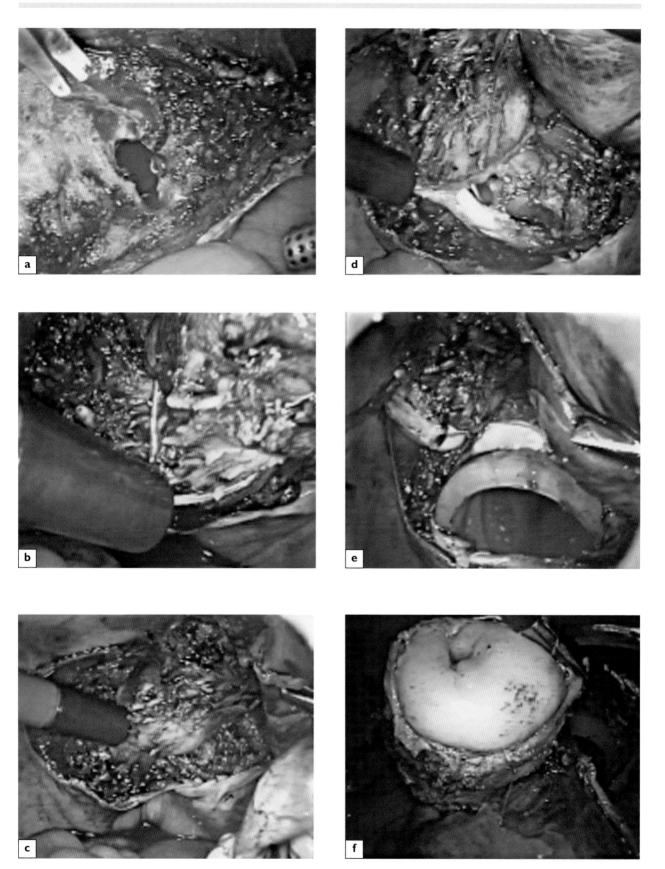

Figure 7 (a) For total hysterectomy, the dissection is performed further with the help of the Australian tube; (b) a window is made to fix the Lap Loop and the level of section; (c) the surgeon must strangle the dissected vagina before activating the current; (d) view during the section; (e) view after section, with the uterus above and the tube below; (f) sharp cut of the cervix *(continued on next page)*

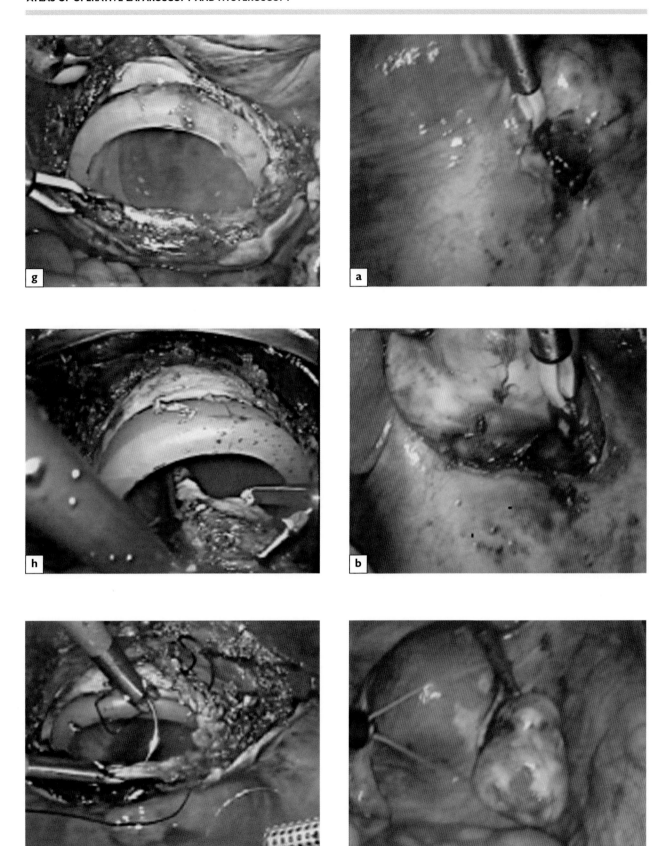

Figure 7 *Continued* (g) Pushing back the tube permits excellent control of hemostasis; (h) removal of the uterus through the tube; (i) suturing

Figure 8 (a) Dissection of the myoma into the broad ligament, with scissors and bipolar forceps; (b) further dissection of the myoma from the broad ligament; (c) the Lap Loop placed around the fibroid (*continued on next page*)

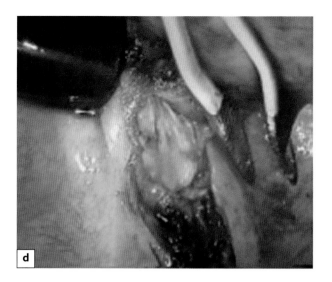

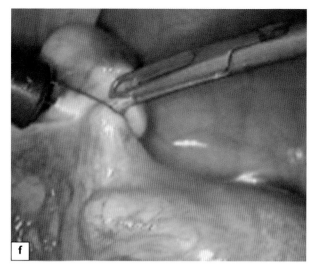

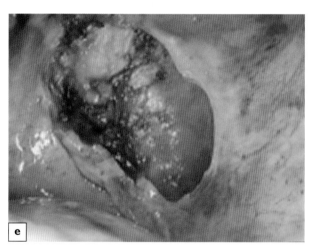

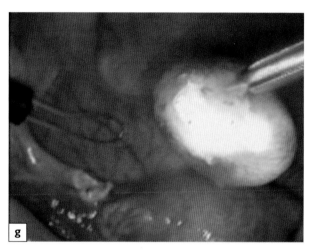

Figure 8 *Continued* (d) After careful control of the abdominal anatomy, i.e. uterine vessels, ureters, the current is activated (the traction device is a bipolar forceps); (e) status after section; (f) a pedunculate myoma fixed on the round ligament; (g) procedure on a pedunculate myoma, as in (f)

DISCUSSION

The authors have now successfully employed the Lap Loop technique in 132 patients for LASH, 18 cases of TLH and 15 cases of fibroids. No complications have been observed in any of these cases. The main advantages of the loop are safety, reduced operating time and precision of the section.

Safety has always been an important concern when indicating a supracervical procedure. By avoiding the risk of cervical dissection with possible ureteral lesions, the complication rate may be reduced with a supracervical technique[6]. However, when cutting the cervix with any monopolar instrument, there is an associated risk of damaging adjacent structures. This risk seems to be reduced considerably with the use of the electrosurgical loop because it is very precise and a large portion of the loop is electrically isolated (Figure 2a). The use of this monopolar device remains, however, an advanced laparoscopic technique and should be limited to only experienced laparoscopic surgeons.

Another advantage of laparoscopic supracervical hysterectomy is the reduced operating time[11–13]. A further decrease in operating time has been achieved with the loop technique for cervical amputation. Prior to the development of the electrosurgical loop, the time required to section the cervix was inconveniently long (around 16 min). With the introduction of this new device, the time we need has been greatly reduced, to about 4 min, with actual cutting time being less than 1 min. Section is also rapid in cases where the uterus is large or irregular.

No major complications have occurred, despite the need for a 100-W setting on the monopolar generator. Only five cases of recurrent bleeding of the uterine arteries occurred during the procedure. These were quickly corrected by bipolar coagulation. Smoke evacuation problems could also occur, which obliged the surgeon to stop the section briefly.

Some broken electrodes and deficient connections were found in the very beginning, with the prototype and before the commercialization of the actual device by the Medsys company (Gembloux, Belgium) in 1998.

CONCLUSION

An electrosurgical loop has been designed and successfully employed to decrease the time required for, and to facilitate, the section of the uterine cervix during LASH for benign uterine conditions. It has, more recently, been used successfully for total laparoscopic hysterectomy and for pedunculate myomas.

It facilitates and increases the safety of these procedures. It must, however, be emphasized that safe use of the electrosurgical loop requires an experienced staff and a surgeon aware of the proper management of electrical energy in laparoscopy.

REFERENCES

1. Reich H. New techniques in advanced laparoscopic surgery. *Clin Obstet Gynecol* 1989;3:655–81
2. Mage G, Wattiez A, Chapron C, *et al*. Hysterectomie per-coelioscopique: résultats d'une série de 44 cas. *J Gynecol Obstet Biol Reprod* 1992;21:436–44
3. Dequesne J, Waddle G. Presentation of the first total laparoscopic hysterectomies in Switzerland. Presented at *the Annual Congress of the SSGO*, Interlaken, 1991
4. Semm K. Hysterectomy via laparotomy or pelviscopy. A new CASH method without colpotomy. *Geburtshilfe Frauenheilkd* 1992;51:996–1003
5. Pelosi MA, Pelosi MA III. Laparoscopic supracervical hysterectomy using a single-umbilical puncture (mini-laparoscopy). *J Reprod Med* 1992;37:777–84
6. Donnez J, Nisolle M. LASH, laparoscopic supracervical hysterectomy. *J Gynecol Surg* 1993;9:91–4
7. Dequesne J. Avantages de l'hysterectomie subtotale par laparoscopie. Presented at *the 5th Laparoscopic Winter Course*, Champéry, Switzerland, January 1995
8. Dequesne J, Schmidt N, Frydman R. A new electrosurgical loop technique for laparoscopic supracervical hysterectomy. *Gynecol Endosc* 1998;7:29–32
9. Munro MG, Parker WH. A classification system for laparoscopic hysterectomy. *Obstet Gynecol* 1993;82:624–9
10. Munro MG. Supracervical hysterectomy: a time for reappraisal. *Obstet Gynecol* 1997;89:133–9
11. Lyons TL. Laparoscopic supracervical hysterectomy: a comparison of morbidity and mortality results with laparoscopically assisted vaginal hysterectomy. *J Reprod Med* 1993;38:763–7
12. Lalonde CJ, Daniell JF. Early outcomes of laparoscopic-assisted vaginal hysterectomy versus laparoscopic supracervical hysterectomy. *J Am Assoc Gynecol Laparosc* 1996;3:251–6
13. Richards SR, Simpkins S. Laparoscopic supracervical hysterectomy versus laparoscopic-assisted vaginal hysterectomy. *J Am Assoc Gynecol Laparosc* 1995;2:431–5

Laparoscopy-assisted vaginal hysterectomy and laparoscopic hysterectomy in benign diseases

25

J. Donnez, M. Nisolle, J. Squifflet and M. Smets

INTRODUCTION

In the United States, hysterectomy is one of the most commonly performed surgical procedures (656 000 hysterectomies in 1987 alone[1]). Approximately 70% are performed using the abdominal approach and 30% are performed vaginally[2]. Contraindications to vaginal hysterectomy depend essentially on the skill of the surgeon[2-5]. The most frequent contraindications are:

(1) Endometriosis (moderate or severe);

(2) Previous Cesarean section;

(3) Significant uterine enlargement or limited uterine mobility in a nulligravida;

(4) Previous pelvic surgery;

(5) Previous uterine suspension.

In many cases, however, careful examination of the pelvis by diagnostic laparoscopy reveals the absence of contraindications to vaginal hysterectomy. In addition, a large proportion of patients are candidates for vaginal hysterectomy after adhesiolysis.

Most of the endoscopic procedures can be applied to treat adhesions, extensive pelvic endometriosis, adnexal disease and myomas, and hysterectomies that require an abdominal approach may be performed with laparoscopic dissection (partial or total) followed by vaginal removal. A major benefit of both laparoscopic and vaginal hysterec-

tomy is the avoidance of an abdominal incision, which typically requires a longer hospitalization (5 days) and recuperation time (4–6 weeks) than does the combination of laparoscopy and vaginal removal.

Laparoscopic hysterectomy[6] is a substitute for abdominal hysterectomy and not for vaginal hysterectomy.

DEFINITIONS

Laparoscopic hysterectomy was first performed by Reich in January 1988[6]. According to Reich[6] and Mage and colleagues[7], there are at least four types:

(1) Type 1: laparoscopy performed for diagnostic purposes, where indications for a vaginal approach are equivocal, in order to determine whether vaginal hysterectomy is possible;

(2) Type 2: laparoscopy-assisted vaginal hysterectomy (LAVH), an initial laparoscopic surgical procedure after which vaginal hysterectomy is carried out;

(3) Type 3: laparoscopic hysterectomy, denoting the laparoscopic ligation of the uterine arteries[6];

(4) Type 4: complete laparoscopic hysterectomy; laparoscopic dissection continues until the uterus is free of all attachments in the peritoneal cavity.

Laparoscopic supracervical hysterectomy has recently regained advocates after Kilkku and co-workers[8] reported a reduction in orgasms after hysterectomy as compared with supravaginal amputation. Laparoscopic subtotal hysterectomy (LASH) was recently described by Donnez and Nisolle[9].

A staging system was devised in order to standardize the terminology (Table 1)[5].

INDICATIONS

The indications for laparoscopic hysterectomy include benign pathologies such as endometriosis, fibroids, adnexal masses, adhesions from a previous Cesarean section, inflammatory disease or previous surgery, which usually require an abdominal approach to hysterectomy. Laparoscopic hysterectomy may also be considered for stage I endometrial, ovarian and cervical cancer[7,10–12].

Table 1 Laparoscopy-assisted vaginal hysterectomy staging (according to Johns, 1993[5])

Stage	
0	diagnostic laparoscopy without laparoscopic procedure prior to vaginal hysterectomy
1	procedure including laparoscopic adhesiolysis and/or excision of endometriosis
2	one or both adnexa freed laparoscopically
3	bladder dissected from the uterus
4	uterine artery transected laparoscopically
5	anterior and/or posterior colpotomy or entire uterus freed

TECHNIQUES

All surgical procedures after uterine vessel ligation, including anterior and posterior vaginal incision, cardinal and intersacral ligament division, intact uterine removal and vaginal closure, can be performed vaginally or laparoscopically.

A Foley catheter is inserted during surgery to empty the bladder. Four laparoscopic puncture sites, including the umbilicus, are used: 10 mm umbilical, 5 mm right, 5 mm medial and 5 mm left lower quadrant. These are placed just above the pubic hairline; lateral incisions are made next to the deep epigastric vessels. A cannula is placed in the cervix for appropriate uterine mobilization. Abdominal and adnexal adhesions, if present, are lysed to mobilize the uterus, and the ureters are identified.

The adnexa are removed first. The infundibulopelvic ligament is identified and exposed by applying traction to the adnexa with an opposite forceps. The bipolar forceps is used to compress and desiccate the vessels (Figure 1), which are then cut with scissors (Figure 2). Bipolar coagu-

lation is used to coagulate the pedicle, or staples or sutures may be applied. Scissor division is carried out close to the line of desiccation to ensure that the pedicle remains compressed.

The peritoneum between the infundibulopelvic ligament and the round ligament is then cut (Figure 3). The round ligaments are desiccated (Figure 4) and cut with scissors (Figure 5). The leaves of the broad ligament are separated and cut (Figure 6).

The peritoneum of the vesico-uterine space is then grasped and elevated with a forceps while scissors are used to dissect the vesico-uterine space (Figure 7). Aquadissection may be used to separate the leaves of the broad ligament, distending the vesico-uterine space and defining the tendinous attachments of the bladder in this area; these are coagulated and cut. Sharp dissection can also be used to divide the peritoneum down to the uterosacral ligaments.

The uterine vessels are identified and skeletonized using aquadissection. When these are well identified, and after confirming the position of the ureters, the uterine

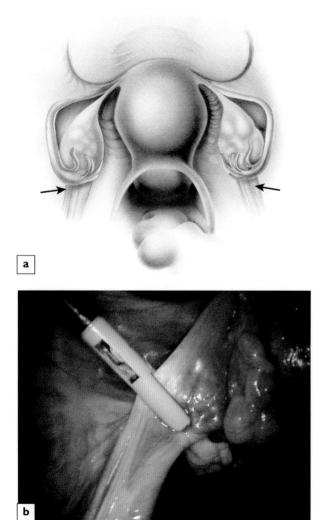

Figure 1 (a) and (b) Coagulation of the infundibulopelvic ligament

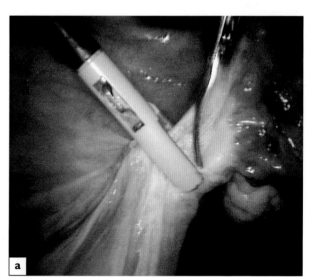

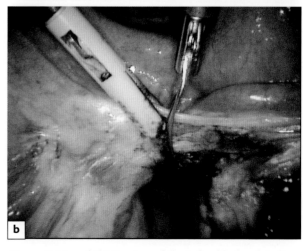

Figure 2 (a) and (b) Section of the infundibulopelvic ligament using the CO_2 laser. Scissors can also be used

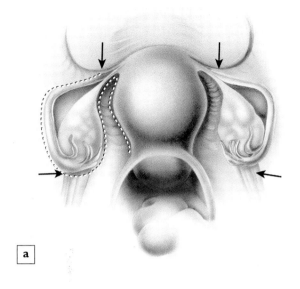

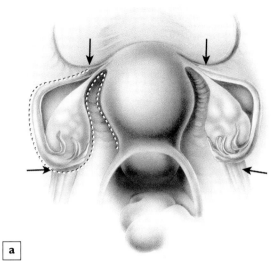

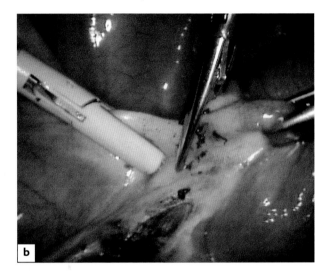

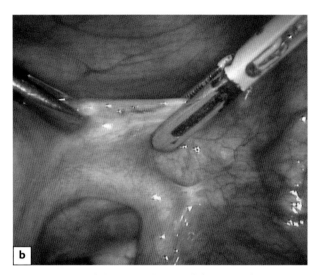

Figure 4 (a) and (b) Coagulation of the round ligament

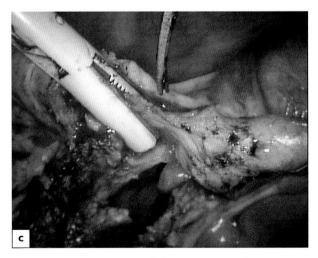

Figure 3 (a)–(c) Section of the peritoneum between the infundibulopelvic ligament and the round ligament

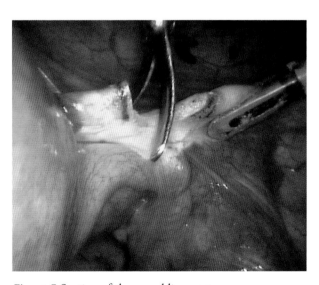

Figure 5 Section of the round ligament

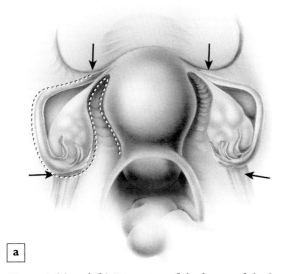

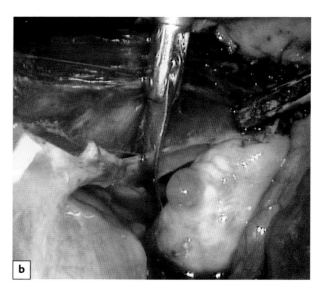

Figure 6 (a) and (b) Dissection of the leaves of the broad ligament

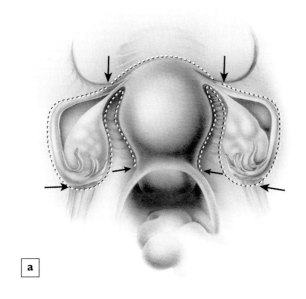

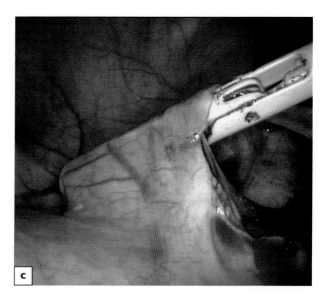

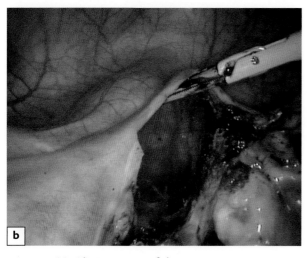

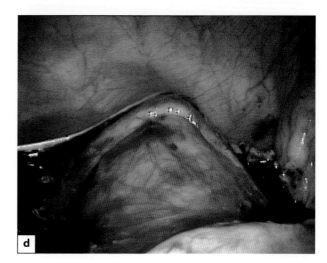

Figure 7 (a)–(d) Dissection of the vesico-uterine space

vessels are desiccated with bipolar coagulation (Figure 8) and cut (Figure 9). In some departments, staples are used, but this is very expensive. Some authors[13] prefer suture ligation of the vascular bundle. Ligation of the uterine vessels can also be performed by the vaginal approach.

The total procedure (type 4 according to Reich; stage 5 according to Johns) may be performed laparoscopically. Vaginal incision is achieved over a sponge placed between the vaginal anterior wall and the cervix (Figure 10).

The vagina is entered over a sponge using a unipolar cutting current or a CO_2 laser. The same procedure is performed posteriorly over a sponge, exposing the area in the cul-de-sac where an incision can be made. The vaginal incision is completed and the uterosacral and cardinal ligaments are clamped and divided.

The completely freed uterus is then pulled into the vagina. The vagina may be sutured from below (Figure 11) or laparoscopically with three sutures. The first joins the uterosacral ligament across the midline. The second brings the cardinal ligament and underlying vagina across the

midline. The third suture closes the anterior vagina and its fascia[5,6].

During laparoscopy, hemostasis is achieved by bipolar coagulation. Blood clots are removed. The pelvis is rinsed with an antiseptic solution which is left in the abdominal cavity for 2–3 h. The drain catheter is then opened without suction. Antibiotics (Zinacef® 2 g/day, Fasygin® 2 g/day) are given peroperatively.

SPECIFIC EQUIPMENT AND COMMENTS

Bipolar coagulation

Reich[13] suggests monitoring electrical current flow with a flow meter to ensure total coagulation of the tissue between the tips of the bipolar forceps. Current flow between the tips of the bipolar electrodes ceases only when complete desiccation (dehydration) has occurred. Kleppinger bipolar forceps are excellent for large-vessel

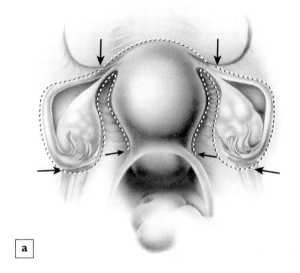

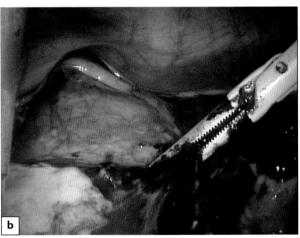

Figure 8 (a) and (b) Identification of the uterine vessels and coagulation with bipolar forceps

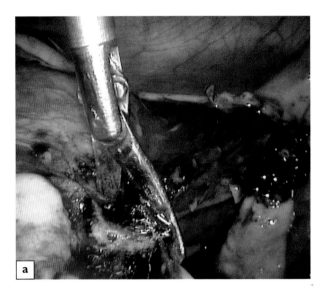

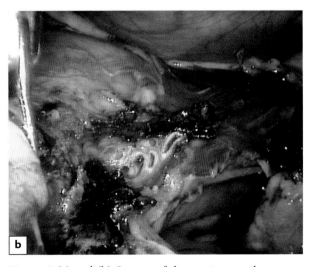

Figure 9 (a) and (b) Section of the uterine vessels

255

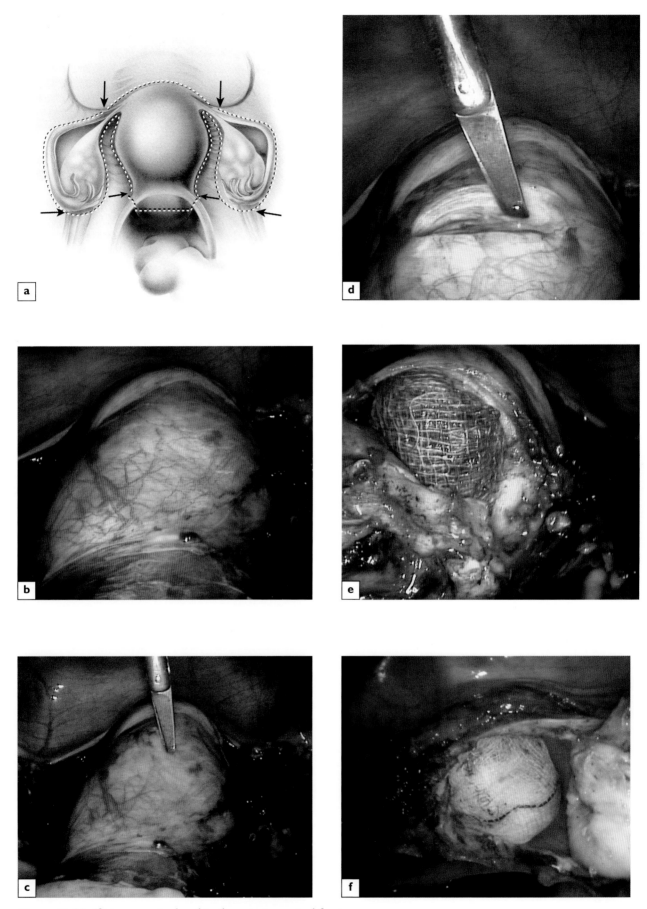

Figure 10 (a)–(f) A sponge is placed in the anterior vaginal fornix

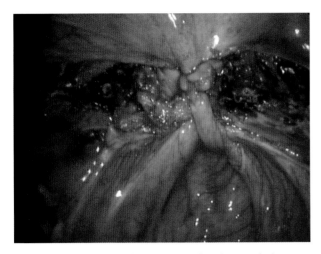

Figure 11 Final view after peritoneal and vaginal closure

hemostasis. Specially insulated bipolar forceps allow the current to pass only through their tips, so that precise hemostasis can be obtained. For Reich[13], the Kleppinger bipolar forceps with a matched power source is an indispensable tool for all operative laparoscopies. The visual current flow meter ensures that desiccation of the tissue held by the forceps is complete.

Uterine mobilizer

The uterine mobilizer is inserted to antevert the uterus and delineate the posterior vagina. Reich[13] uses the Valtchev uterine mobilizer. We prefer to use an intra-uterine cannula similar to that used for methylene blue injection and a sponge held in a forceps to delineate the 'anterior' and 'posterior' vaginal cul-de-sac. We have recently developed a new manipulator (Figure 12) which allows the mobilization of the uterus and the incision of the uterus and the incision of the vaginal cul-de-sac. The MacCartney tube (Figure 13) has been developed in Australia in order to facilitate the surgery.

Ureter dissection

Reich[6,13] begins surgery with identification of the ureters, usually at the pelvic brim, and their mobilization. Their dissection requires medial reflection of the rectosigmoid, to expose the ovarian vessels and the ureters as they cross over the iliac artery to enter the true pelvis.

The positions of the previously dissected ureters in the broad ligament are again checked before desiccation, stapling, or suturing of the uterine vessels. When the ureter is far from the uterine vessels, bipolar desiccation or stapling is carried out. Inspection of the ureter after positioning the stapler has been known to reveal entrapment of the ureter. Suture ligation of the vascular bundle is preferred by Reich[13]: this technique avoids such injury, as the ureter is visualized directly throughout the ligation process. Mage and colleagues[7,14] and Donnez and

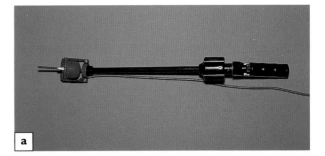

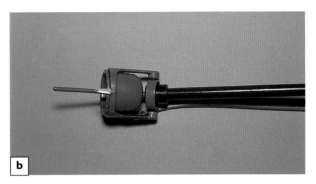

Figure 12 (a) and (b) The 'UCL' manipulator

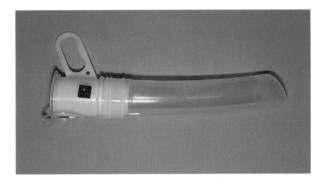

Figure 13 The MacCartney tube

colleagues[12] prefer bipolar coagulation. In our department, the ureter is identified but only dissected in cases of endometriosis.

Vaginal closure

Reich[13] proposes laparoscopic vaginal closure in which the ligaments and vaginal epithelium are brought together. In our department, the closure is performed through the vagina: the peritoneum and uterosacral ligaments are brought together, then the vaginal mucosa is closed. Laparoscopy is then used to inspect the operative sites.

Drainage

One of the intraoperative advantages of a laparoscopic approach to hysterectomy is the ability to achieve complete hemostasis and evacuate all blood clots at the end of the procedure. This removal of all remaining clots

257

Table 2 Methods of hysterectomy used in our department

Procedure	Number of procedures (%)		
	June 1994– June 1996	July 1996– November 1997	December 1997– October 1999
LASH	236 (46%)	170 (41.5%)	228 (44%)
LAVH or LH	130 (26%)	90 (22%)	162 (31%)
Vaginal hysterectomy	82 (16%)	113 (27.5%)	104 (20%)
Abdominal hysterectomy	60 (12%)	37 (9%)	26 (5%)

LASH, laparoscopic subtotal hysterectomy; LAVH, laparoscopy-assisted vaginal hysterectomy; LH, laparoscopic hysterectomy

and pelvic lavage may reduce postoperative infection associated with vaginal hysterectomy. At the end of surgery, we prefer to leave 300 ml iodine or Rifocine® solution in the abdominal cavity for 2–3 h. The drain is left in the Douglas pouch, closed for 2–3 h and then opened. In our series, no cases of infection were reported.

Is preoperative administration of a gonadotropin releasing hormone agonist useful?

Gonadotropin releasing hormone (GnRH) analogs may reduce the total uterine volume in patients with uterine leiomyomata by between 35% and 50%[15,16]. When hysterectomy is planned for the treatment of large myomas, women should be pretreated with a GnRH analog for at least 3 months, since shrinkage of the myoma should facilitate laparoscopic or vaginal hysterectomy. This preoperative therapy may also be used in women with an enlarged uterus of more than 13 weeks, but less than 17 weeks, in order to decrease the volume of the uterus.

CONCLUSION

Opponents of the concept of laparoscopic hysterectomy argue that vaginal hysterectomy is faster, less expensive, and results in a similar short hospital stay and convalescence. We have clearly demonstrated in a paper in the *New England Journal of Medicine* that laparoscopic hysterectomy was less expensive than the other approach if non-disposable instruments were used[17]. In the United States and in Europe, however, 75% of hysterectomies are performed by an abdominal approach. If laparoscopic hysterectomy is added to our surgical armamentarium, almost all hysterectomies (95%) will be carried out without an abdominal incision. In our department (Table 2), the rate of abdominal hysterectomy is less than 5%. The remaining indications for abdominal hysterectomy are myomas > 14–15 weeks (unless a GnRH agonist

can be administered in order to reduce the volume), malignant (or suspected to be malignant) ovarian masses and cervical cancer stage Ib (Wertheim–Meigs)[18], and frozen pelvis, when a hysterectomy is mandatory.

REFERENCES

1. Findlay S. The health-insurance factor. *US News World Rep* 1990;30:57
2. Kovak SR, Cruikshank SH, Retto HF. Laparoscopic assisted vaginal hysterectomy. *J Gynecol Surg* 1990;6:185–90
3. Isaacs JH. *Gynecology and Obstetrics. Clinical Gynecology*. Philadelphia: JB Lippincott, 1990;1: 1–11
4. Smith HO, Thompson JD. Indications and technique for sapinol hysterectomy. *Contemp Obstet Gynecol* 1986;125
5. Johns A. Laparoscopic assisted vaginal hysterectomy (LAVH). In Sutton C, Diamond D, eds. *Gynecologic Endoscopy for Gynecologists*. London, UK: Saunders, 1993:179–86
6. Reich H. New techniques in advanced laparoscopic surgery. *Clin Obstet Gynecol* 1989;3:655–81
7. Mage G, Wattiez A, Chapron C, *et al*. Hystérectomie per-coelioscopique: resultats d'une serie de 44 cas. *J Gynecol Obstet Biol Reprod* 1992;21:436–44
8. Kilkku P. Supravaginal uterine amputation vs hysterectomy: effects on libido and orgasm. *Acta Obstet Gynecol Scand* 1983;62:141–5
9. Donnez, J, Nisolle M. LASH: laparoscopic supracervical hysterectomy. *J Gynecol Surg* 1993;9:91–4
10. Querleu D, Leblanc E, Castelain G. Laparoscopic pelvic lymphadenectomy in the staging of early carcinoma of the cervix. *Am J Obstet Gynecol* 1991;164:579–81
11. Reich H, McGlynn F, Wickie W. Laparoscopic management of stage 1 ovarian cancer: a case report. *J Reprod Med* 1990;35:601

12. Donnez J, Nisolle M, Anaf V. Place de l'endoscopie dans le cancer de l'endomètre. In Dubuisson JB, Chapron CH, Bouquet de Jolinière J, eds. *Coelioscopie et Cancerologie en Gynecologie*. Paris: Arnette, 1993:77–82

13. Reich H. New laparoscopic techniques. In Sutton C, Diamond M, eds. *Endoscopic Surgery for Gynaecologists*. London, UK: W.B. Saunders, 1993:28–39

14. Canis M, Mage G, Wattiez A, *et al*. Vaginally assisted laparoscopic radical hysterectomy. *J Gynecol Surg* 1992;8:103–5

15. Donnez J, Sehrurs B, Gillerot S, *et al*. Treatment of uterine fibroids with implants of gonadotropin-releasing hormone agonist: assessment by hysterography. *Fertil Steril* 1989;51:947–50

16. Donnez J, Gillerot S, Bourgonjon D, *et al*. Neodymium : YAG laser hysteroscopy in large submucous fibroids. *Fertil Steril* 1990;54:999–1003

17. Nisolle M, Donnez J. Alternative techniques of hysterectomy. Letter to the Editor. *N Engl J Med* 1997;336:291–2

18. Canis M, Mage G, Wattiez A, *et al*. La chirurgie endoscopique a-t-elle une place dans la chirurgie radicale du cancer du col utérin? *J Gynecol Obstet Biol Reprod* 1990;19:921

Indications and techniques of laparoscopic hysterectomy 26

H. Reich

INTRODUCTION

Laparoscopic hysterectomy and laser surgery have become popular procedures due to media attention and consumer interest. Most hysterectomies (75%) are performed using an abdominal incision[1].

Laparoscopic hysterectomy, defined as the ligation of the uterine vessels, is a substitute for abdominal hysterectomy, with more attention to ureteral identification[2-4]. It was first performed in January 1988[5]. Laparoscopic hysterectomy stimulated a laparoscopic approach to hysterectomy, exemplified by laparoscopic-assisted vaginal hysterectomy (LAVH) as gynecologists not trained in vaginal or laparoscopic techniques struggled to maintain a market share of the large and lucrative hysterectomy market. LAVH has become an expensive procedure, performed for indications for which skilled vaginal surgeons rarely find laparoscopy necessary. Laparoscopic hysterectomy remains a substitute for abdominal hysterectomy.

Most hysterectomies currently requiring an abdominal approach may be performed by laparoscopic dissection of part or all of the abdominal portion followed by vaginal removal. There are many surgical advantages, particularly magnification of anatomy and pathology, easy access to the vagina and rectum, and the ability to achieve complete hemostasis and clot evacuation during underwater examination. Patient advantages are multiple and are related to the avoidance of a painful abdominal incision. They include reduced duration of hospitalization and recuperation and an extremely low rate of cuff infection and ileus.

The goal to be realized with vaginal hysterectomy, LAVH or laparoscopic hysterectomy is the safe avoidance of an abdominal wall incision. Vaginal hysterectomy should be performed if it is possible after ligation of the utero-ovarian ligaments. Laparoscopic inspection at the end of the procedure will still allow the surgeon to control any bleeding and evacuate any clots. Unnecessary operations should not be performed because of the surgeon's preoccupation with the development of new surgical skills. Laparoscopic hysterectomy is not indicated when vaginal hysterectomy is possible.

DEFINITIONS

There is a variety of operations in which the laparoscope is used as an aid to hysterectomy (Table 1).

Table 1 Laparoscopic hysterectomy classification

---

(1) Diagnostic laparoscopy with vaginal hysterectomy

(2) Laparoscopic-assisted vaginal hysterectomy (LAVH)

(3) Laparoscopic hysterectomy (LH)

(4) Total laparoscopic hysterectomy (TLH)

(5) Laparoscopic supracervical hysterectomy (LSH) including CISH (classical intrafascial Semm hysterectomy)

(6) Vaginal hysterectomy with laparoscopic vault suspension or reconstruction

(7) Laparoscopic hysterectomy with lymphadenectomy

(8) Laparoscopic hysterectomy with lymphadenectomy and omentectomy

(9) Laparoscopic radical hysterectomy with lymphadenectomy

It is important that these different procedures are clearly delineated:

(1) Diagnostic laparoscopy with vaginal hysterectomy indicates that the laparoscope is used for diagnostic purposes, when indications for a vaginal approach are equivocal, to determine whether *vaginal hysterectomy* is possible[6]. It also assures that vaginal cuff and pedicle hemostasis are complete and allows clot evacuation.

(2) Laparoscopic-assisted vaginal hysterectomy (LAVH) is a vaginal hysterectomy performed after laparoscopic adhesiolysis, endometriosis excision or oophorectomy[7-9]. Unfortunately, this term is also used when the upper uterine blood supply of a relatively normal uterus is staple-ligated. It must be emphasized that the easy part of both abdominal and vaginal hysterectomy is usually upper pedicle ligation.

(3) Laparoscopic hysterectomy (LH) denotes laparoscopic ligation of the uterine arteries, using electrosurgery desiccation, suture ligature or staples. All maneuvers after uterine vessel ligation can be performed vaginally or laparoscopically, including

anterior and posterior vaginal entry, cardinal and uterosacral ligament division, uterine removal (intact or by morcellation), and vaginal closure (vertically or transversely). Laparoscopic ligation of the uterine vessels is the *sine qua non* for laparoscopic hysterectomy. Ureteral isolation has always been advised.

(4)   Total laparoscopic hysterectomy (TLH) is a laparoscopic-assisted abdominal hysterectomy. Laparoscopic dissection continues until the uterus lies free of all attachments in the peritoneal cavity. The uterus is removed through the vagina, with morcellation if necessary. The vagina is closed with laparoscopically placed sutures.

(5)   Laparoscopic supracervical hysterectomy (LSH) has recently regained advocates after suggestions that total hysterectomy results in a decrease in libido[10]. The uterus is removed by morcellation from above or below.

Semm's version of supracervical hysterectomy is called the CISH procedure (classical intrafascial Semm hysterectomy). It leaves the cardinal ligaments intact while eliminating the columnar cells of the endocervical canal. After perforating the uterine fundus with a long sound-dilator, a calibrated uterine resection tool (COURT) that fits around this instrument is used to core out the endocervical canal. Thereafter, at laparoscopy, suture techniques are used to ligate the utero-ovarian ligaments. An Endoloop is placed around the uterine fundus to the level of the internal os of the cervix and tied. The uterus is divided at its junction with the cervix and removed by laparoscopic morcellation.

LASER DISSECTION

Most laparoscopic hysterectomy procedures can be performed with the CO_2 laser, whose main effect on tissue is vaporization. This can be used for direct vaporization of lesions, but is more often used for division or separation of adhesions and for excision of tissue in a manner similar to using scissors. As with electrosurgery, blood vessels less than 1 mm in diameter are often coagulated in the process, but application of the beam to an actively bleeding vessel usually results in burnt, black blood.

The major advantages of the CO_2 laser are its 0.1-mm depth of penetration and poor conduction through water, allowing a greater margin of safety when working around the bowel, ureter and major vessels, and its ability to work at a distance from tissue without contact while other instruments are used for traction. Backstops are rarely necessary because of this superficial penetration and the wet surgical field, especially, however, when the operator develops the skill of using the tissue to be treated as the backstop. It must be emphasized that laser surgery is still associated with a zone of thermal necrosis surrounding treated tissue and, in susceptible patients, adhesions will

form. Laser surgery does not result in a reduced rate of adhesion formation when compared to other thermal energy sources.

Use of the CO_2 laser through the operating channel of a laser laparoscope converts the umbilical incision into a portal for performing surgery, reducing the need for an additional incision. This delivery system allows the surgeon a panoramic field of vision to cut or ablate tissue in otherwise inaccessible locations in the deep pelvis perpendicular to and in the middle of this field. The invisible CO_2 laser beam, composed of photons of electromagnetic radiation of 10.6-µm wavelength, is delivered to the laparoscope through mirrors fixed in an articulating arm. This beam then travels down the 5–8-mm diameter operating channel of an operating laparoscope. The focal point is approximately 2 cm from the end of the laparoscope, and the beam remains in focus for several centimeters beyond this point. This beam is adjusted into a 1-mm helium–neon (HeNe) spot with a standard coupler or one with a micromanipulator joystick; the depth of tissue affected will be slightly greater than 1 mm. A useful technique is to align the beam and its surrounding symmetrical halo emanating from the laparoscope into the center of the operating channel, by using transparent tape or the cuff of the surgeon's glove over the scope tip to identify where the beam exits.

Major problems encountered when using CO_2 lasers through the operating channel of an operating laparoscope are jumping, blooming and loss of the beam. Tension on the laser laparoscope, as it traverses the trocar sleeve, will modify the beam spot, as will the extent of hydration of tissue being vaporized, irrigant on the scope tip, and smoke in the peritoneal cavity. The alignment of the articulating arm mirrors may require frequent adjustment to ensure a reproducible tissue effect. An ice pack between the laser-scope coupler and the surgeon's hand may be necessary to prevent skin burns when using lasers with large raw beams and beam–coupler mismatches.

Failure of the laser laparoscope coupler to connect with the laparoscope at precisely 90° causes asymmetric beam passage through the operating channel. The beam energy heats the CO_2 purge gas unevenly, causing it to act as an asymmetric lens and refracting the CO_2 laser energy to a spot other than where the HeNe aiming beam was located. Most new laser couplers correct this problem.

An effect similar to a blended current is accomplished with the CO_2 laser through the operating channel of an operating laparoscope when used at power settings > 50 W, as a large spot size with diameter from 2 to 4 mm is obtained. This is extremely coagulative and provides very good hemostatic cutting[11]. A similar tissue effect is obtained with a defocusing coupler. Heraeus LaserSonics (Milpitas, CA) and Sharplan Laser (Tel Aviv, Israel) have recently introduced defocusing couplers for laparoscopy. With the Sharplan CVD (continuously variable defocus) system, spot size can be controlled to obtain a 1-mm spot size for cutting and a much larger defocused spot for coagulation 0.6–4.0 mm).

The passage of CO_2 gas through the laparoscope lumen, presently a necessity to purge this channel of debris, decreases both the power delivered to tissue and the power density at tissue, because the 10.6-μm wavelength of the laser beam is absorbed and thus heats the CO_2 purge gas, which has the same wavelength. Power delivered to the tissue is reduced by 30–50% with a 7.2-mm laparoscopic operating channel (12-mm scope) and by 60% with a 5-mm operating channel (10-mm scope)[11]. While it is desirable to operate at high power density for a short time to minimize damage to surrounding tissue, heating of CO_2 gas in the laparoscope lumen increases spot size and thus reduces power density (the concentration of laser energy on the tissue) at higher power settings.

Considering these limitations, using a Sharplan 1100 laser through a 10-mm laparoscope with a 5-mm operating channel, a setting of 20–35 W in the superpulse mode is used for most procedures (<1000 W/cm^2 at the tissue). Between 80 and 100 W in the continuous mode is used to obtain a diffuse hemostatic effect for myomectomy and culdotomy.

Heraeus LaserSonics maintains a small spot size by performing rapid exchanges of gas through the operating channel of the laparoscope. The gas is exchanged faster than it can be heated up, a technique which also minimizes smoke in the peritoneal cavity during use of the laser.

Some new terms need defining. Superpulse mode implies very high power (500 W) released for brief surges (< 50 mJ), theoretically allowing tissue to cool between spikes to reduce surrounding thermal effects. Much higher energy pulses (> 200 mJ) are generated with Ultrapulse (Coherent, Palo Alto, CA) or Pulsar (Sharplan), allowing longer cooling intervals between pulses and resulting in char-free vaporization.

Coherent has recently advanced CO_2 laser technology by introducing the ^{13}C isotope of CO_2 to modify the 10.6-μm wavelength to 11.1 μm. This circumvents absorption of laser energy by the CO_2 purge gas in the operating channel of the laparoscope; the result is little interference in power transmission from the purge gas (Ultrapulse 5000L). A 6-mm raw beam enters the coupler from the end of the laser arm and emerges as a 1.5-mm spot 350–400 mm away. The 1.5-mm spot size is maintained at all settings. At high power settings, the power density at impact is 10 times more than at similar settings with a 10.6-μm wavelength beam that results in a 4-mm spot from heating of the CO_2 purge gas. With the isotope laser, cutting with minimal coagulation is obtained at 200 mJ/pulse. If more coagulation with cutting is required, < 100 mJ should be used. Power settings of 10–20 W ultrapulse are used for precise cutting and 50–80 W are used for extirpative procedures.

Using 200 mJ/pulse at 50 W with a conventional or ultrapulsed CO_2 laser, a beam spot size of 2–3 mm is obtained, resulting in excellent coagulation with cutting.

With the Coherent 5000L, a 1.5-mm beam spot size is maintained at all settings, and 200 mJ at 50 W results in cutting with little coagulation.

When a laser is used in the continuous wave mode of operation (non-pulsed), the most important predictor of thermal damage is power density at the tissue. It is generally accepted that, for continuous wave CO_2 lasers, the nature of the tissue interaction undergoes a gradual change as the power density crosses through a threshold at about 5000 W/cm^2. At or above this 'ablation threshold', cutting and ablation are achieved with minimal thermal damage. Below this threshold, more thermal damage is produced. With conventional CO_2 lasers and CO_2 purge gas, it is not possible to produce power densities > 1500 W/cm^2. Using isotopic $^{13}CO_2$, a power density of 3000 W/cm^2 can be reached.

For pulsed laser operation, the single pulse ablation threshold that also produces minimal thermal damage is 2.8 J/cm^2. Ultrapulse lasers produce higher energy pulses than superpulse lasers. At a pulse energy > 125 mJ, an energy density above the single pulse ablation threshold is reached. At 200 mJ/pulse, very little thermal effect occurs.

The 12-mm operating laparoscope with a 7.5-mm operating channel gives a smaller spot size and higher power transmission than a 10-mm operating laparoscope with 5-mm channel. This difference is due to the diffraction limit, a result of physical optics that describes the limiting focus spot diameter that can be achieved at the end of an opaque tube of given length and diameter, and which has little dependence on the laser itself.

Fiber lasers (KTP, argon, and YAG) are not used as they lack the versatility of electrosurgical electrodes for cutting, coagulation or fulguration. The energy from these lasers is converted in tissue to heat due to absorption by the tissue protein matrix. A much larger volume of tissue is involved in the laser thermal effect, with coagulation initially and vaporization only after protein is heated to > 100°C. In contrast, energy from the CO_2 laser is totally absorbed by water and converted rapidly to thermal energy, with a much smaller volume of tissue involved in the laser thermal effect as cutting proceeds.

INDICATIONS FOR LAPAROSCOPIC HYSTERECTOMY

Indications for laparoscopic hysterectomy presently include benign pathology such as endometriosis, fibroids, adhesions and adnexal masses, lesions which usually require an abdominal approach to hysterectomy. It is also appropriate when vaginal hysterectomy is contraindicated because of a narrow pubic arch, a narrow vagina with no prolapse, or severe arthritis that prohibits placement of the patient in a lithotomy position sufficient for vaginal exposure. Laparoscopic procedures in obese women allow the surgeon to make an incision above the panniculus and operate below it. Laparoscopic hysterectomy may also be considered for Stage I endometrial, ovarian and cervical cancer[12–14].

The most common indication for laparoscopic hysterectomy is a symptomatic fibroid uterus. Morcellation is often necessary. Fibroids fixed in the pelvis or abdomen without descent are easier to mobilize laparoscopically. Rectocele repair may be accomplished from above, but cystocele repair usually requires a perineal approach.

Uterine size and weight are important indicators of the appropriateness of laparoscopic hysterectomies: most small uteri can be removed vaginally. The normal uterus weighs 70–125 g. At the 12th week of pregnancy, the uterus weighs 280–320 g, and at 24 weeks the weight is 580–620 g.

Hysterectomy should not be undertaken for Stage IV endometriosis with extensive cul-de-sac involvement unless the surgeon has the capability and time to resect all deep fibrotic endometriosis from the posterior vagina, uterosacral ligaments and anterior rectum. Excision of the uterus using an intrafascial technique leaves the deep fibrotic endometriosis behind to cause future problems. It is much more difficult to remove deep fibrotic endometriosis when there is no uterus between the anterior rectum and the bladder; after hysterectomy, the endometriosis left in the anterior rectum and vaginal cuff frequently becomes densely adherent or invades the bladder and one or both ureters. In most cases, Stage IV endometriosis with extensive cul-de-sac obliteration is a reason to preserve the uterus to prevent future vaginal cuff, bladder and ureteral problems[15]. Obviously, this approach will not be effective when uterine adenomyosis is present. In these cases, after excision of cul-de-sac endometriosis, persistent pain will lead ultimately to hysterectomy. Oophorectomy is not necessary at hysterectomy; if the endometriosis is removed, it should not recur. Bilateral oophorectomy is rarely indicated in women under the age of 40 years undergoing hysterectomy for endometriosis.

Hysterectomy is performed in women of reproductive age for abnormal uterine bleeding, defined as excessive uterine bleeding or irregular uterine bleeding for > 8 days during more than a single cycle or as profuse bleeding requiring additional protection (large clots, gushes, or limitations on activity). There should be no history of a bleeding diathesis or use of medication that may cause bleeding. A negative effect on quality of life should be documented. The results of physical examination, laboratory data, ultrasound, and, if necessary, hysteroscopy and/or dilatation and curettage are frequently normal. Prior to hysterectomy, hormone treatment should be attempted and its failure, contraindication, or refusal documented. Any anemia should be corrected. If hysterectomy is chosen, a vaginal approach may be appropriate. Laparoscopic hysterectomy is performed when vaginal hysterectomy is not possible due to history of previous

surgery, lack of prolapse (nulliparous or multiparous), or inexperience of the operator with the vaginal approach.

EQUIPMENT

High-flow CO_2 insufflation up to 10–15 l/min is necessary to compensate for the rapid loss of CO_2 during suctioning. The ability to maintain a relatively constant intra-abdominal pressure between 10 and 15 mmHg during laparoscopic hysterectomy is essential.

Operating-room tables capable of achieving a 30° Trendelenburg position are extremely valuable for laparoscopic hysterectomy. Unfortunately, these tables are rare, and great difficulty can be encountered with the limited degree of body tilt produced by ordinary tables. The steep Trendelenburg position (20–40°), with shoulder braces and the arms at the patient's sides, has been used without adverse effects.

A Valtchev uterine mobilizer (Conkin Surgical Instruments, Toronto, Ontario) is the best available single instrument to antevert the uterus and delineate the posterior vagina. The uterus can be anteverted to about 120° and moved in an arc about 45° to the left or right by turning the mobilizer around its longitudinal axis. The 100-mm long, 10-mm thick or the 80-mm long, 8-mm thick obturator is used for uterine manipulation during hysterectomy. When this device is in the anteverted position, the cervix sits on a wide pedestal, making the cervicovaginal junction readily visible between the uterosacral ligaments when the cul-de-sac is inspected laparoscopically[16].

If a Valtchev uterine mobilizer is not available, a sponge on a ring forceps is inserted into the posterior vaginal fornix and a No. 81 French rectal probe (Reznik Instruments, Skokie, IL) is placed in the rectum to define the rectum and posterior vagina for excision of endometriosis, or to open the posterior vagina (culdotomy). In addition, a No. 3 or 4 Sims curette or Hulka uterine elevator is placed in the endometrial cavity to antevert the uterus markedly and stretch out the cul-de-sac. The rectal probe and intraoperative rectovaginal examinations remain important techniques even when the Valtchev mobilizer is available. Whenever rectal location is in doubt, it is identified by placing a probe.

Trocar sleeves are available in many sizes and shapes. For most cases, 5.5-mm cannulae are adequate. Newer electrosurgical electrodes which eliminate capacitance and insulation failures (Electroshield from Electroscope, Boulder, CO), require 7- or 8-mm sleeves. Laparoscopic stapling is performed through 12- or 13-mm Surgiports (US Surgical Corporation, Norwalk, CT).

A short trapless 5-mm trocar sleeve with a retention screw grid around its external surface (Richard Wolf Medical Instruments, Vernon Hills, IL; Apple Medical, Bolton, MA) is used on the left to facilitate efficient instrument exchanges and evacuation of tissue while allowing unlimited freedom during extracorporeal suture tying[17]. An experienced laparoscopic surgical team exchanges instruments so fast that little pneumoperitoneum is lost.

Bipolar forceps use a high-frequency low-voltage cutting current (20–50 W) to coagulate vessels as large as the ovarian and uterine arteries. The Kleppinger bipolar forceps (Richard Wolf) are excellent for large vessel hemostasis. Specially insulated bipolar forceps (Apple Medical) are available that allow current to pass only through their tips; so that precise hemostasis can be obtained. Microbipolar forceps contain a channel for irrigation and a fixed distance between the electrodes. They are used to irrigate bleeding sites, to identify vessels before coagulation and to prevent sticking of the electrode to the eschar. Irrigation is used during underwater examination to remove blood products and clots from the bleeding vessel, making its identification before coagulation more precise.

Disposable stapling instruments (US Surgical) are rarely used during laparoscopic hysterectomy because of their expense. A laparoscopic stapler (Multi-fire Endo GIA 30) places six rows of titanium staples, 3 cm in length, and simultaneously divides the clamped tissue. The standard staple compresses on firing to 1.5 mm, while the vascular cartridge compresses to 1 mm. The disposable handle is designed to fire up to six staple cartridges through a 12-mm cannula before being discarded.

PREOPERATIVE PREPARATION

The preoperative administration of gonadotropin releasing hormone (GnRH) analogs for at least 2 months before hysterectomy for large myomas is encouraged as it may reduce both the total uterine volume and the volume of the leiomyoma itself; making laparoscopic or vaginal hysterectomy easier[18,19]. During treatment with depot leuprolide (Lupron Depot) at a dose of 3.75 mg intramuscularly monthly for 3–6 months, anemia secondary to hypermenorrhea resolves, and autologous blood donation can be considered prior to laparoscopic hysterectomy. Packed red blood cells have a shelf life of 35 days if stored at 1–6°C. In addition, Lupron Depot is often administered after ovulation in the cycle preceding surgery to avoid operating on ovaries containing a corpus luteum.

Patients are encouraged to hydrate and eat lightly for 24 h before admission on the day of surgery. When extensive cul-de-sac involvement with endometriosis is suspected, a mechanical bowel preparation is ordered (polyethylene glycol-based isosmotic solution: Golytely or Colyte)[15]. Lower abdominal, pubic and perineal hair is not shaved. A Foley catheter is inserted during surgery and is removed the next morning. Antibiotics (usually cefoxitin) are administered in all cases.

POSITIONING OF PATIENT

All laparoscopic surgical procedures are performed under general anesthesia with endotracheal intubation. The routine use of an orogastric tube is recommended to diminish the possibility of a trocar injury to the stomach and to reduce small bowel distension. The patient is flat (0°) until after the umbilical trocar sleeve has been inserted and is then placed in steep Trendelenburg position (20–30°). Lithotomy position with the hip extended (thigh parallel to abdomen) is obtained with Allan stirrups (Edgewater Medical Systems, Mayfield Heights, OH) or knee braces, which are adjusted to each individual patient before she is anesthetized. A pelvic examination after the patient is anesthetized is always performed prior to preparing the patient.

Laparoscopy was never thought to be a sterile procedure before the incorporation of video, as the surgeon operated with his head in the surgical field, attached to the laparoscopic optic. Since 1983, this author has maintained a policy of not sterilizing or draping the camera or laser arm. Infection has been rare: fewer than 1/200 cases. The umbilical incision is closed with a single 4-0 Vicryl suture opposing deep fascia and skin dermis, the knot being buried beneath the fascia to prevent the suture from acting as a wick and transmitting bacteria into the soft tissue or peritoneal cavity.

HYSTERECTOMY TECHNIQUE

The technique described is for total laparoscopic hysterectomy (Figures 1–17).

Incisions

Three laparoscopic puncture sites, including the umbilicus, are used: 10- or 12-mm umbilical, 5-mm right, and 5-mm left lower quadrant. The left lower quadrant puncture is the major portal for operative manipulation. The right trocar sleeve is used for retraction with atraumatic grasping forceps. When a clip is applied or a stapler is used, it is inserted through the umbilical incision and the procedure is viewed through a 5-mm laparoscope in one of the 5-mm lower quadrant sites.

Placement of the lower quadrant trocar sleeves just above the pubic hairline and lateral to the deep epigastric vessels (and thus the rectus abdominis muscle) is preferred. These vessels, an artery flanked by two veins (venae comitantes), are located lateral to the umbilical ligaments (obliterated umbilical artery) by direct laparoscopic inspection of the anterior abdominal wall. The deep epigastric vessels arise near the junction of the external iliac vessels with the femoral vessels and make up the medial border of the internal inguinal ring. The round ligament curls around these vessels to enter the inguinal canal. When the anterior abdominal wall parietal peritoneum is thickened from previous surgery or obesity, the position of these vessels is judged by palpating and depressing the anterior abdominal wall with the back of the scalpel; the wall will appear thicker where rectus muscle is enclosed, and the incision site should be chosen lateral to this area near the anterior superior iliac spine.

Vaginal preparation

Hysteroscopy with CO_2 is performed during insufflation of pneumoperitoneum. This is especially useful for myoma hysterectomies to identify the location of the fibroids (Figure 1). Following hysteroscopy, the endocervical canal is dilated to Pratt number 25, and the Valtchev uterine mobilizer is inserted into the uterus.

Exploration

The upper abdomen is inspected, and the appendix is identified. If appendiceal pathology, such as dilatation, adhesions or endometriosis, is present, appendectomy is performed after ureteral isolation by mobilizing the appendix, desiccating its blood supply, and placing three Endo-loops at the appendiceal–cecal junction after desiccating the appendix just above this juncture. The appendix is left attached to the cecum and its stump is divided later in the procedure, after opening the cul-de-sac, so that removal from the peritoneal cavity is accomplished immediately after separation.

Ureteral dissection

Immediately after exploration of the upper abdomen and pelvis, each ureter is isolated deep in the pelvis, if possible. This is undertaken early in the operation before the pelvic side-wall peritoneum becomes edematous and/or opaque due to irritation by the CO_2 pneumoperitoneum or aquadissection and before ureteral peristalsis is inhibited by surgical stress, pressure, or the Trendelenburg position. The ureter and its overlying peritoneum are grasped deep

in the pelvis on the left to avoid division of the lateral rectosigmoid attachments required for high identification (Figure 2). An atraumatic grasping forceps is used from a right-sided cannula to grab the ureter (Figure 3) and its overlying peritoneum on the left pelvic side-wall below and caudal to the left ovary, lateral to the left uterosacral ligament. Scissors or a CO_2 laser at 10–30 W superpulse or ultrapulse are used to divide the peritoneum overlying the ureter and are then inserted into the defect created and spread (Figure 4). Thereafter one blade of the scissors is placed on top of the ureter, the buried scissors blade is visualized through the peritoneum, and the peritoneum is divided. This is continued into the deep pelvis where the uterine vessels cross the ureter, lateral to the cardinal ligament insertion into the cervix (Figure 5). Connective tissue between the ureter and the vessels is separated with scissors (Figure 6). Bleeding is controlled with micro-bipolar forceps.

Bladder mobilization

The left round ligament is divided at its mid-portion with minimal bleeding using a spoon electrode (Electroscope) at 150-W cutting current (Figure 7). Persistent bleeding is

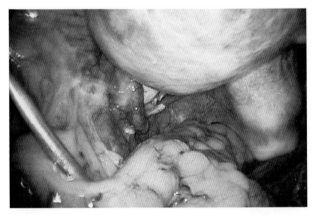

Figure 2 Left ureter is grasped from the right side. Valtchev retractor delineates junction of cervix with vagina

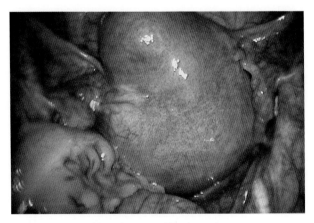

Figure 1 Large fibroid uterus fills the pelvis

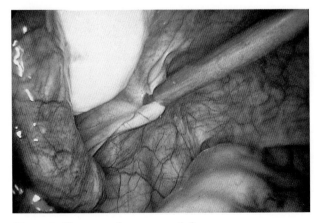

Figure 3 Close-up of grasper on left ureter

controlled with monopolar fulguration at 80-W coagulation current or bipolar desiccation at 30-W cutting current. Thereafter, scissors or a CO_2 laser are used to divide the vesicouterine peritoneal fold starting at the left side, continuing across the midline to the right round ligament. The right round ligament is divided, as was the left;

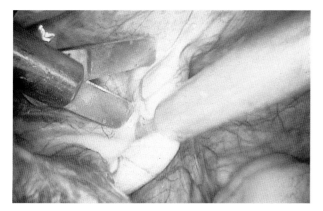

Figure 4 Scissors or CO_2 laser are used to divide peritoneum just above and lateral to ureter which has been placed on tension

with unipolar electrosurgery. The bladder is mobilized from the uterus and upper vagina using scissors.

Upper uterine blood supply

When ovarian preservation is desired, the utero-ovarian ligament and Fallopian tube pedicle are suture-ligated adjacent to the uterus with Vicryl-0 (Figure 8). When ovarian preservation is not desired, the infundibulopelvic ligaments and broad ligaments are coagulated until desiccated with bipolar forceps at 25–35-W cutting current and then divided.

Uterine vessel ligation

The broad ligament on each side is skeletonized down to the uterine vessels. Each uterine vessel pedicle is suture-ligated, with Vicryl-0 on a CT-l needle (70 cm). The needles are introduced into the peritoneal cavity by pulling them through a 5-mm incision. The curved needle is inserted on top of the unroofed ureter where it turns medially towards the previously mobilized bladder. A short

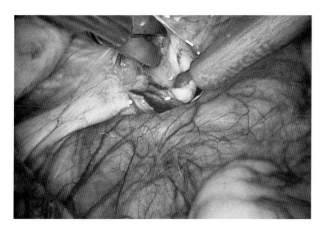

Figure 5 Dissection of left ureter continues to left uterine artery pedicle

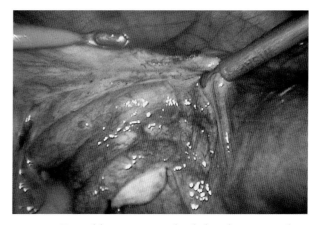

Figure 7 Round ligaments are divided with a spoon electrode at 150-W cutting current

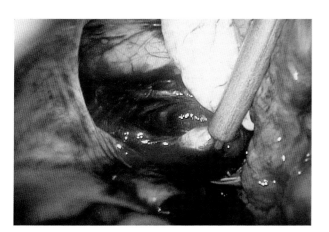

Figure 6 Uterine artery is isolated above the ureter

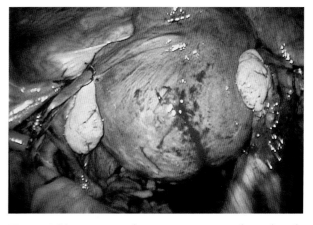

Figure 8 Utero-ovarian ligaments are suture ligated with Vicryl-0

267

---

rotary movement of the Cook oblique curved needle holder brings the needle around the uterine vessel pedicle. Sutures are tied extracorporeally using a Clarke knot pusher[20]. A single suture placed in this manner on each side serves as a 'sentinel stitch', identifying the ureter for the rest of the operation (Figures 9–11).

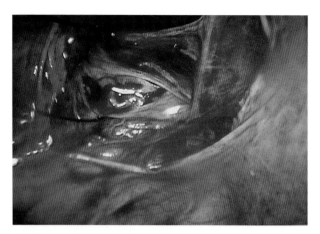

Figure 9 Suture ligature is placed around left uterine vessels with left ureter beneath

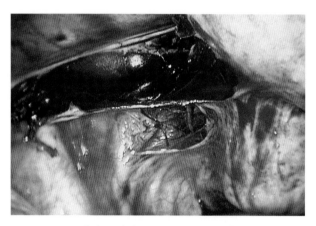

Figure 10 Left broad ligament is open to the bladder. Ligature is around left uterine artery

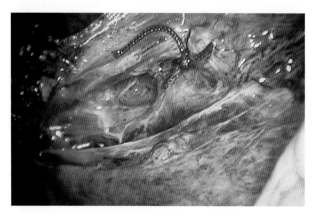

Figure 11 Close-up of ligature around left uterine artery with ureter beneath

Circumferential culdotomy (division of cervicovaginal attachments)

The cardinal ligaments on each side are divided with the CO_2 laser at high power. Control of bleeding is often necessary, using bipolar forceps. The vagina is entered posteriorly over the Valtchev retractor, which identifies the junction of cervix with vagina. A ring forceps inserted into the anterior vagina above the tenaculum on the anterior cervical lip identifies the anterior cervicovaginal junction, which is entered using the laser. Following the ring forceps or the aquapurator tip, and using them as backstops, the operator divides the lateral vaginal fornices. The uterus is morcellated if necessary and pulled out of the vagina (Figures 12–14). Alternatively, a 4-cm diameter operative colonoscope (Richard Wolf) is used to outline circumferentially the cervicovaginal junction; it also serves as a backstop for laser work.

Laparoscopic vaginal vault closure and suspension with McCall culdoplasty

Vaginal repair is accomplished after packing the vagina. The left uterosacral ligament and posterolateral vagina are

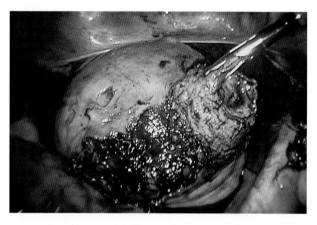

Figure 12 The uterus is free in the peritoneal cavity

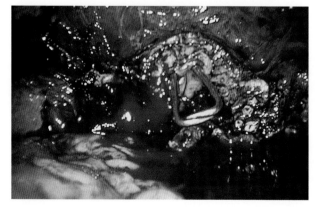

Figure 13 A single toothed tenaculum is used to pull the cervix into the vagina

first elevated. A suture is placed through this uterosacral ligament into the vagina, exits the vagina including posterior vaginal tissue near the midline on the left, and re-enters just adjacent to this spot on the right. Finally, an opposite-sided oblique Cook needle holder is used to fixate the right posterolateral vagina to the right uterosacral ligament. This suture is tied extracorporeally and gives excellent support to the vaginal cuff apex, elevating it superiorly and posteriorly toward the hollow of the sacrum (Figures 15–17). The rest of the vagina and overlying pubocervical fascia is closed vertically with a figure-of-eight suture.

Underwater examination

At the close of each operation, an underwater examination is used to detect bleeding from vessels and viscera tamponaded during the procedure by the increased intraperitoneal pressure of the CO_2 pneumoperitoneum. The CO_2 pneumoperitoneum is displaced with 2.5 l of Ringer's lactate solution, and the peritoneal cavity is vigorously irrigated and suctioned until the effluent is clear of blood products. Any further bleeding is controlled underwater using microbipolar forceps to coagulate through the

electrolyte solution, and at least 2 l of lactated Ringer's solution are left in the peritoneal cavity.

COMPLICATIONS

Complications of laparoscopic hysterectomy are the same as for hysterectomy in general: anesthetic accidents, post-operative pulmonary emboli, hemorrhage, injury to ureters, bladder and rectum, and infections, especially of the vaginal cuff[21]. Since the introduction of prophylactic antibiotics, vaginal cuff abscess, pelvic thrombophlebitis, septicemia, pelvic cellulitis and adnexal abscesses have become rare. Abdominal wound infection is rare, but the incidence of incisional hernias after operative laparoscopy is greatly increased if trocars of > 10 mm are placed at extra-umbilical sites.

Febrile morbidity following a vaginal hysterectomy is about half as common as after abdominal hysterectomy. Laparoscopic treatment with evacuation of all blood clots and the sealing of all blood vessels after removal of the uterus should reduce the infection rate further. Morcellation during laparoscopic or vaginal hysterectomy carries a slightly increased risk of fever, especially if prophylactic antibiotics are not used.

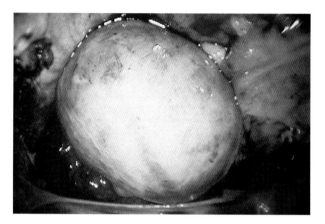

Figure 14 As the uterus is large, vaginal morcellation is required for removal

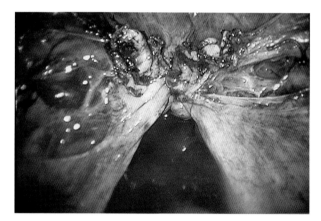

Figure 16 In the deep cul-de-sac, the uterosacral ligaments are together with the ureters lateral

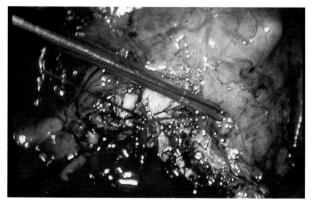

Figure 15 The uterosacral ligaments and posterior vagina are sutured together for vaginal apical support

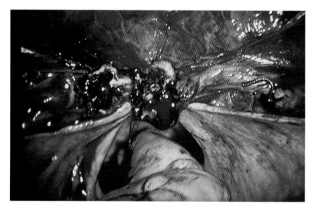

Figure 17 Excellent support of the vaginal cuff is noted with all anatomy visible

REFERENCES

1. Bachmann GA. Hysterectomy: a critical review. *J Reprod Med* 1990;35:839–62
2. Reich H. Laparoscopic hysterectomy. *Surg Laparosc Endosc* 1992;2:85–8
3. Liu CY. Laparoscopic hysterectomy: a review of 72 cases. *J Reprod Med* 1992;37:351–4
4. Liu CY. Laparoscopic hysterectomy. Report of 215 cases. *Gynaecol Endosc* 1992;1:73–7
5. Reich H, DeCaprio J, McGlynn F. Laparoscopic hysterectomy. *J Gynecol Surg* 1989;5:213–16
6. Kovac SR, Cruikshank SH, Retto HF. Laparoscopy-assisted vaginal hysterectomy. *J Gynecol Surg* 1990;6:185–9
7. Summit RL, Stovall TG, Lipscomb GH, *et al.* Randomized comparison of laparoscopy-assisted vaginal hysterectomy with standard vaginal hysterectomy in an outpatient setting. *Obstet Gynecol* 1992;80:895–901
8. Minelli L, Angiolillo M, Caione C, *et al.* Laparoscopically-assisted vaginal hysterectomy. *Endoscopy* 1991;23:64–6
9. Maher PJ, Wood EC, Hill DJ, *et al.* Laparoscopically assisted hysterectomy. *Med J Aust* 1992;156:316–18
10. Lyons TL. Laparoscopic supracervical hysterectomy. In Hunt RB, Martin DC, eds. *Endoscopy in Gynecology, Proceedings of the World Congress of Gynecologic Endoscopy*, AAGL 20th Annual Meeting, Las Vegas Nevada. Baltimore: Port City Press, 1993:129–31
11. Reich H, MacGregor TS, Vancaillie TG. CO_2 laser used through the operating channel of laser laparoscopes: *in vitro* study of power and power density losses. *Obstet Gynecol* 1991;77:40–7
12. Reich H. Laparoscopic extrafascial hysterectomy with bilateral salpingo-oophorectomy using stapling techniques for endometrial adenocarcinoma. Presented at the *AAGL 19th Annual Meeting*, Orlando, Florida, November 14–18, 1990
13. Reich H, McGlynn F, Wilkie W. Laparoscopic management of Stage I ovarian cancer. *J Reprod Med* 1990;35:601–5
14. Canis M, Mage G, Wattiez A, *et al.* Does endoscopic surgery have a role in radical surgery of cancer of the cervix uteri? *J Gynecol Obstet Biol Reprod* 1990;19:921
15. Reich H, McGlynn F, Salvat J. Laparoscopic treatment of cul-de-sac obliteration secondary to retrocervical deep fibrotic endometriosis. *J Reprod Med* 1991;36:516–22
16. Valtchev KL, Papsin FR. A new uterine mobilizer for laparoscopy: its use in 518 patients. *Am J Obstet Gynecol* 1977;127:738–40
17. Reich H, McGlynn F. Short self-retaining trocar sleeves. *Am J Obstet Gynecol* 1990;162:453–4
18. Schlaff WD, Zerhouni EA, Huth JA, *et al.* A placebo-controlled trial of a depot gonadotropin-releasing hormone analogue (leuprolide) in the treatment of uterine leiomyomata. *Obstet Gynecol* 1989;74:856–62
19. Freidman AJ, Hoffman DI, Comite F, *et al.* (Leuprolide Study Group). Treatment of leiomyomata uteri with leuprolide acetate depot: a double-blind, placebo-controlled, multicenter study. *Obstet Gynecol* 1991;77:720–5
20. Reich H, Clarke HC, Sekel L. A simple method for ligating in operative laparoscopy with straight and curved needles. *Obstet Gynecol* 1992;79:143–7
21. Woodland MB. Ureter injury during laparoscopy-assisted vaginal hysterectomy with the endoscopic linear stapler. *Am J Obstet Gynecol* 1992;167:756–7

27

Laparoscopic approach for prolapse

A. Wattiez

INTRODUCTION

From its beginnings in our department back in 1991, the laparoscopic approach for prolapse has changed considerably over the decade. Initially limited to strict reproduction of the techniques carried out by laparotomy, the addition of a number of complementary procedures has since enriched it so that, today, it provides an answer to all the situations encountered in the context of female prolapse repair.

The usual advantages of laparoscopy – less postoperative discomfort, shorter hospital stay, etc. – were rapidly eclipsed by the innovating aspect of this technique. By combining the precision of endoscopic vision and the positive pressure of the pneumoperitoneum, access has been gained to anatomical spaces that were difficult to exploit before, and the repair procedures can be adjusted under strict visual control. The results have been encouraging from the outset and are now excellent, with perfect anatomical correction and remarkable functional results. The time has now come to simplify the techniques and to render them reproducible by others, with acceptable operating times.

PREOPERATIVE WORK-UP

The preoperative work-up must be very meticulous. Thorough evaluation of the lesions is the only way to ensure a comprehensive repair under one anesthesia, thus preventing functional sequelae and recurrence.

Evaluating the prolapse

Clinical diagnosis of the lesions is the crucial phase of this evaluation. It is essential to stage the lesions for each sector. Standard clinical examination must seek to establish the degree to which the uterus, bladder and rectum are prolapsed. Lateral cystocele with vaginal folds still present must be distinguished from central cystocele with elimination of the vaginal folds. The former is due to detachment of the vagina from the arcus tendineus fasciae pelvis while the latter is due to a lesion in the vesicovaginal fascia. A systematic check must be made to detect any elytrocele.

The tone of the levator ani muscles should be assessed for both quality and quantity. A high rectocele corresponds to a fascia pathology, and must be distinguished from a low rectocele due to deficient levator muscle support.

The functional symptoms must be evaluated. Particular attention needs to be paid to urinary continence and three groups of patients need to be distinguished: patients in whom pure urinary stress incontinence is associated with the prolapse, patients presenting with masked urinary incontinence, and patients without any urinary problems.

Similarly, rectal problems must be surveyed, for example, constipation and/or incontinence of fecal matter or gas. The anal sphincter needs to be checked, using ultrasound investigation if necessary.

Modern imaging techniques associated with clinical examination enable these problems to be visualized. Thanks to the recent progress made with dynamic magnetic resonance imaging and when conditions are optimum, lesions in all three areas can be visualized simultaneously. Most importantly, any elytrocele can be detected.

Evaluation of urinary function

Urinary function needs to be assessed not only by questioning the patient but also by urodynamic investigation, which should be systematic. The main point to be determined is whether there is any deficit in the urethral sphincter which would require a change in the surgical strategy.

Evaluation of the feasibility of laparoscopy

Although the degree of feasibility of endoscopy has changed fundamentally over the past few years, it is still necessary to select the patients. Laparoscopic treatment of prolapse means that the patients have to undergo anesthesia that is generally protracted, a pneumoperitoneum and a protracted Trendelenburg position. The counter indications are most often connected with the anesthesia. However, the indications must also be established correctly for older patients and obese patients for whom the vaginal route should still be preferred.

PATIENT PREPARATION

The preparation of the patient is a crucial factor to obtain the best results from surgery. It must include preparation of the tissues to encourage healing and bowel preparation to optimize the endoscopic space.

Bowel preparation

The reason for this preparation is to empty the bowel and make it easier to push the loops of bowel out of the way and flatten them so as to enlarge the operating space. Preparing the bowel in case of accidental injury is not the prime purpose. Preparation starts with a standard low-residue diet which the patient is required to follow for the 5 days prior to the operation. Two days before the operation, the bowel is emptied by administering a laxative solution such as Xprep®. Finally, the day before the operation, the lower bowel should be cleaned with an enema. It is important to follow this chronological order in order to avoid any loss from the anus onto the table, which would give rise to a high risk of infection.

Vaginal estrogens

These should be prescribed for at least 1 month prior to surgery. The purpose is to improve the vaginal trophic condition. Improved tone will enable better healing.

Vaginal and parietal disinfection

Vaginal disinfection is essential. It should take place the day before surgery, by vaginal irrigation with an antiseptic solution and the installation of a pessary of Bétadine®. The abdominal wall must also be disinfected. After showering the day before the operation, the patient is shaved and then the abdominal wall is cleaned using an antiseptic solution, paying particular attention to the inner surfaces of the umbilicus. A dilute solution of Bétadine® is applied and the skin covered with a closed sterile dressing fixed in place.

INSTALLATION OF THE PATIENT

Endoscopic surgery is long and difficult. The procedure needs to be optimized and the operating time kept as short as possible by ergonomic organization of the operation, for which correct installation of the patient is of prime importance.

Anesthesia

Anesthesia is generally administered with endotracheal intubation. Curare is not systematically used but only when parietal distension is not obtained at 12 mmHg pneumoperitoneum pressure. This general anesthesia may be associated with locoregional anesthesia of the epidural or spinal block type to ensure the most comfortable post-operative conditions possible.

Installation

The patient is placed on her back with legs apart and half-bent. This position creates three operating spaces: one on the left occupied by the surgeon, another on the right occupied by the first assistant and the third between the legs for the second assistant. The patient's arms are placed along her body to avoid any brachial injury. It is best to have two shoulder rests level with the acromion, but without any pressure on the neck muscles. The patient's hands must be carefully arranged to avoid any compression of the fingers. A system to warm the patient can be used to avoid any chilling.

The patient must be placed right at the edge of the table to optimize the movements of the uterine manipulator. The greater the range of movement the manipulator has, the better the tissues will be exposed.

The patient's abdominal wall and vagina must be generously disinfected and the drapes installed before the Foley catheter and uterine manipulator. It is essential that the perineal area is in a sterile environment and accessible to the surgeon who will need to position the manipulator or carry out vaginal or rectal examination.

Bladder catheter

A permanent number 18 Foley catheter is installed; the balloon is filled with 15 ml normal saline and the catheter pulled back as far as possible in order to reveal the bladder neck as clearly as possible. The catheter is connected to a pouch placed where it can be seen easily, in order to keep a check on the urine (quantity, color, presence of any air in the pouch).

PREOPERATIVE ASSESSMENT

Clinical examination

It is essential to reassess the prolapse on the operating table once the patient has been anesthetized. This examination under general anesthesia may provide new information that might modify the operating strategy. It is carried out using vaginal valves and, most importantly, enables the appearance of the vaginal structure to be properly assessed together with the difference in collapse between the upper and lower areas. Similarly, any retroversion of the vagina can be better evaluated. If hysterectomy is to take place, the size and mobility of the uterus need to be assessed, and this element will guide the positioning of the trocars.

Appearance of the abdomen

The patient's general morphology and the appearance of the abdomen are decisive factors when deciding how to organize the operating field and position the trocars. The ergonomics of movements during the operation are highly dependent on this.

A number of elements need to be taken into account:

(1) The patient's morphology: the most important point to note is the distance between the pubis and the umbilicus. This governs the distance between the umbilical trocar and the suprapubic trocar. This suprapubic trocar needs to be located sufficiently high up to make it easy to approach the promontory, open the space of Retzius and perform the suturing. If the distance is short, the optics trocar will need to be placed above the umbilicus and the suprapubic trocar moved to the umbilical position.

(2) The distance between the iliac spines: suturing is easier when the trocars are spaced well apart. For a patient in whom this distance is short, the trocars should be moved up in order to gain more space.

(3) The quantity of fat present in the abdominal wall needs to be checked, so that the trocars can be positioned where the wall is thinnest. This will reduce the degree of rebound and the difficulty of reinsertion.

(4) The laxity of the abdominal wall will give an idea of how much operating space there will be, and will also affect the positioning of the trocars.

POSITIONING THE TROCARS

As a general rule, four trocars are needed: three suprapubic trocars and one umbilical trocar. The first trocar to be inserted is always the umbilical trocar. This is 10 mm in diameter. The final position of this trocar is decided after carrying out a visual internal inspection and comparison with known data (size of the uterus, patient's morphology). If the uterus is normal or below normal in size and there is sufficient distance between the pubis and umbilicus, this will be the optics trocar. If, on the other hand, there is a large uterus or a short pubo-umbilical distance, then it will be the central operating trocar.

In the great majority of cases, there are thus three suprapubic trocars and one umbilical trocar.

(1) For the suprapubic trocars, we prefer to use disposable trocars 5 mm in diameter. We have selected trocars made by mtp® (reference 020105 or 020106, Tuttlingen, Germany). They present the advantage of being light, transparent, with external tapping making them stable in the abdominal wall, and have a star-shaped valve which provides a leak-proof seal, even when making the sutures. Finally, they are reasonable in cost. The lateral trocars are positioned level with the anterior superior iliac spines, about two fingers inside the spines and outside the external edge of the rectus abdominis muscles. This means that they are located in the vicinity of the oblique and transversus abdominis muscles. The abdominal wall in this area is generally thin, making movements easier. The central trocar is located more or less halfway along the pubo-umbilical line. There should be about 6 cm at least between the umbilical optics trocar and the central trocar. In any case, the central trocar must be located no lower than the line running between the two external trocars.

(2) If the umbilical trocar is intended to hold the optics unit, a simple reusable steel trocar is used. We prefer the Karl Storz model (Tuttlingen, Germany), the reason being that it has a valve that the surgeon can lower when introducing the optics. This helps to keep the lens clean during insertion and consequently saves considerable time. If the umbilical trocar is to be the central operating trocar, we prefer to use a disposable trocar with a removable reducer device located at the top of the trocar. For reasons outlined above, we prefer the model by mtp® (reference 020174 or 020107, Tuttlingen, Germany).

Under standard conditions (three suprapubic trocars and one umbilical trocar), we prefer to start the operation with three 5-mm trocars for dissection procedures, replacing the central trocar later when suturing takes place (once hysterectomy has been completed).

ORGANIZATION OF THE OPERATING FIELD

Positioning the manipulator (Figure 1)

The uterine manipulator is an essential piece of equipment for presenting the uterus. It allows manipulation in all directions: pushing, anteversion, retroversion, lateralization and flexing of the uterus forwards and laterally. In addition, it enables the vaginal fornices to be presented and provides

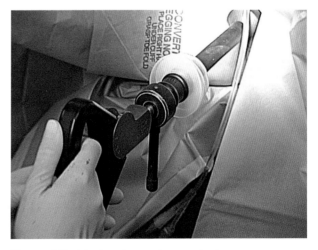

Figure 1 Positioning the uterine manipulator

a leak-proof seal for the pneumoperitoneum and a seal for the vagina after extraction of the uterus.

The device presents several concentric shafts. The central shaft has a screwed tip which is inserted in the uterus. Several sizes of screw are available but the size is chosen according to the size of the uterus. The end of the manipulator with the screw can be bent by tipping the distal handle. Around this shaft there is a valve, covered with ceramic material. This unique valve can rotate through 360°, and is used to expose the fornices. Finally, around the valve, there is a system of seals made up of three flexible disks. These are not introduced into the vagina until near the end of the operation when the vagina is opened.

Insertion

The Clermont-Ferrand manipulator (Karl Storz, Tuttlingen, Germany) must not be inserted until after the patient has been swabbed and draped. It needs to be manipulated by the surgeon under sterile conditions. After exposing the cervix, a hysterometer is used to measure the size of the uterine cavity. The screw is chosen according to the size found. The cervix is then dilated up to bougie no. 8; the device is locked in the zero position and presented at the opening of the cervix. It is important to screw the device home until the screw is completely inside the uterine cavity. Once this has been achieved, the handle-locking control lies on the right.

Exposure: the various possibilities for manipulation

In most cases, each manipulation is preceded by a movement thrusting the uterus towards the patient's head. Anteversion is achieved by combining two movements: pushing on the uterus and anteversion by lowering the handle of the device. This movement places the two uterosacral ligaments under tension and exposes the pouch of Douglas. Similarly, the adnexa are exposed by pushing and moving the handle laterally underneath the patient's legs, which are in a lithotomy position, being spread and half-bent. The valve can be manipulated at any time and enables the vaginal fornices to be exposed correctly.

Fixation of the intestine (Figure 2)

The operating field needs to be carefully organized right at the beginning of the operation. This helps to obtain stable exposure without the assistant needing to intervene. With this in mind, the pouch of Douglas is cleared by fixing the sigmoid to the abdominal wall. We use two different techniques to achieve this. The first technique uses a straight needle swaged to a length of nylon suture material. The needle is introduced through the abdominal wall about 5 cm above the left lateral trocar. The needle is then taken through the fatty tissues of the parasigmoid each side of the sigmoid itself, then back out through the abdominal

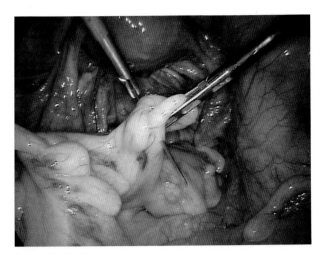

Figure 2 Fixation of the intestine so that the operating field is organized at the beginning of the operation

wall at the same place as before. The sigmoid is lifted with a forceps and the suture tightened over a pad, thus holding the sigmoid in position. The same effect can be achieved with a curved needle introduced into the abdominal cavity. The parasigmoid fatty tissue is taken up and the needle taken back out via the trocar. The needle is then cut, and a Reverdin's needle introduced through the abdominal wall above the left trocar, to grasp the ends of the suture inside the abdomen and bring them back out. They are then fixed using a forceps. After the hysterectomy, the vagina or stump of the cervix is suspended against the anterior abdominal wall in a similar fashion, using a Reverdin's needle.

Identification of the origin of the uterosacral ligaments

The origin of the uterosacral ligaments can be identified at the beginning of the operation. This is where culdoplasty will start. The means of identification may be a mark left by bipolar coagulation or, even better, by leaving a length of suture as a marker.

OPERATING STRATEGY

Strategic chronology of the phases

The strategic chronology of the operating procedures is important. A clear distinction must be drawn between the dissection and the fixing phases.

Dissection phases

The dissection phases take place in the following chronological order: dissection of the promontory, dissection of the right lateral peritoneum, dissection of the rectovaginal space and then the hysterectomy during which bladder dissection is taken very low. There is a good reason for this specific order. The promontory must be dissected first because it often needs the Trendelenburg position to be more marked. In many cases, this is possible only at the beginning of the operation. Once this part of the dissection has been completed, the patient can be laid flat if the anesthetist decides this is better. Dissection of the spaces where the prostheses are to be installed is made easier by the use of the uterine manipulator which improves the access to the various areas. Thus, this part of the dissection should be carried out prior to the hysterectomy.

Fixing phases

The posterior prosthesis is positioned first, then the culdoplasty takes place before the prosthesis is fixed at the front. Next comes peritonealization of the lower areas which continues until half of the right peritoneal opening has been closed. This is the point at which the timing of a Burch procedure needs to be discussed.

If it is desired to follow the traditional procedure and fix the bladder neck before fixing to the promontory, the prostheses are left waiting and the Burch procedure and any required paravaginal repair are carried out immediately. More often, the prosthesis is fixed to the promontory now, peritonealization is completed and cervicosuspension is carried out later.

The place of hysterectomy

In the classic procedure, the uterus was left in place to avoid opening the vagina with the consequent risks of infection for the prosthesis. This technique is possible with the laparoscopic approach, with dissection of the spaces taking place without sectioning the round ligaments and by taking the prostheses through the broad ligaments.

Today, the trend is to carry out hysterectomy. It may be subtotal or total. In our experience, subtotal hysterectomy is preferable because it offers the advantage of leaving the vagina closed. When the hysterectomy is total, vaginal closure should take place along two planes.

As we have said, the essential difference compared to a simple hysterectomy lies in the chronology of the operating phases. When treating a prolapse, dissection of the rectovaginal and vesicovaginal spaces goes further forward and the uterus is removed only after all these spaces have been dissected. We describe dissection of these spaces in more detail below.

Peroperative antibiotic therapy

We use peroperative antibiotic therapy. This consists of injections of the latest generation of cephalosporins as a 1-g flash which is repeated if the operation lasts more than 4 h.

OPERATING TECHNIQUE

Dissection of the promontory

The promontory is best approached for surgery by increasing the Trendelenburg position, after carefully pushing the loops of small intestine back and fixing the sigmoid. The desired position is opposite disc L5–S1, or the upper part of S1. The anterior common vertebral ligament is separated off. To the inside, the median sacral artery and vein are reclined or coagulated if necessary. Particular care must be taken concerning the left iliac vein in obese patients and those with a low bifurcation of the aorta (Figures 3 and 4).

The promontory is identified by palpation with the instruments. After the right ureter and the lower edge of the left primitive iliac vein have been identified, the posterior prevertebral parietal peritoneum is pulled upwards by the assistant and then incised vertically from the promontory, leaving the ureter to the outside. When the peritoneum is opened, the pneumoperitoneum gas rushes into the retroperitoneal space and initiates dissection. Those

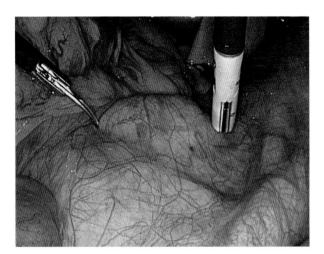

Figure 3 Laparoscopic view of the promontory

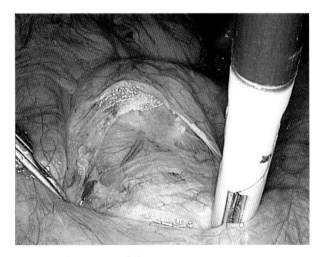

Figure 4 Dissection of the promontory

organs that adhere to the posterior plane remain fixed in place whereas all the elements that are free to do so move away from the promontory (Figure 5).

Incision of the right lateral peritoneum

Dissection continues vertically to reach the pouch of Douglas. During this dissection, the surgeon needs to pay particular attention to the internal iliac vein which must be crossed, and the uterosacral ligament area which does not detach easily. The purpose of this incision is to enable the prosthesis to be peritonealized, and it must leave the ureter free. Consequently, it is not enough simply to make an incision, but instead sufficient peritoneum must be freed to enable the prosthesis to be covered without imposing any constraints on the ureter.

Dissection of the rectovaginal space (Figure 6)

The point at which the two uterosacral ligaments join at the level of the torus uterinus is identified. The rectum is grasped by the assistant, using a bowel forceps, prior to applying strong traction downwards. The peritoneum

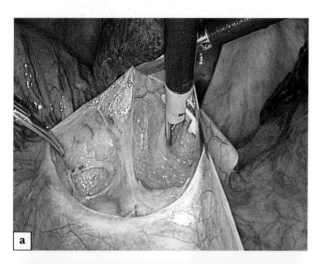
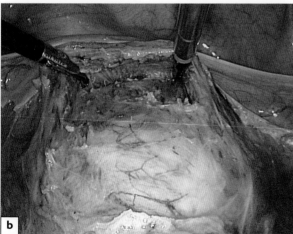

Figure 5 (a) and (b) Dissection of the promontory

opposite the torus uterinus tightens to form a fold, after which it is coagulated and sectioned 2 cm below its uterine insertion. Dissection then continues towards, and until it meets, the posterior wall of the vagina. The rectovaginal septum is now easier to tackle. Dissection is taken downwards, remaining in contact with the vagina to the front. It continues until the anal area is reached. At this point, dissection is directed outwards to the lateral wall of the pelvis, which is reached in the subobturator area. In this lateral area, the median rectal vessels will be found and can be left intact or coagulated according to the space available. Now the surgeon moves up towards the rectum in order to be sure of identifying the rectopubic bundles of the levator ani muscles.

When dissection has been completed, the levator ani muscles become visible. It is important for them to be seen clearly. The space dissected is now bordered by the following structures: the levator ani muscles and the pelvic wall to the outside, the anal area downwards, the vagina to the front, and the rectum to the rear.

Hysterectomy

The standard technique is used to carry out the hysterectomy:

(1) Installation of a uterine manipulator;

(2) The various dissection phases are part of the preparation for installing the prosthesis: vesicovaginal and rectovaginal spaces;

(3) Coagulation and preliminary section of the round ligaments and dissection of the lateral vesical spaces. Fenestration of the posterior layer of the broad ligament;

(4) The adnexa may be kept or not, depending on the patient's age. The utero-ovarian ligament, tube and adnexal vessels are coagulated and sectioned if the adnexa are to be spared, whereas the lumbo-ovarian

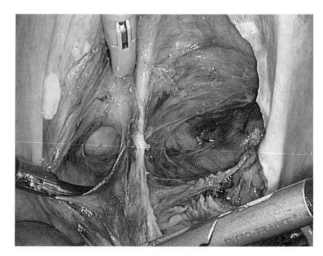

Figure 6 Dissection of the rectovaginal space

ligament is coagulated and sectioned if the adnexa are to be removed;

(5) Bladder dissection is taken lower to enable the prosthesis to be installed;

(6) The posterior layers of the broad ligament are dissected down to the origin of the uterosacral ligaments;

(7) The uterine pedicles are identified and then coagulated using the bipolar forceps, or taken up with a suture using Vicryl-0;

(8) Intrafascial dissection proceeds gradually with coagulation of the cervicovaginal vessels. For total hysterectomy, Halban's fascia needs to be separated off so that closure can be made along two planes;

(9) The vagina is opened through 360°, protected by the uterine manipulator;

(10) The uterus is extracted via the vagina;

(11) The vagina is closed along two planes. The first plane takes up solely the vaginal mucosa and the second plane covers the first using the pericervical fascias. These two planes are sutured using Vicryl-0. It is essential to suture in two planes in order to protect the prosthesis properly from any contamination via the vagina.

For subtotal hysterectomy, the cervix is sectioned at the isthmus after controlling the uterine arteries. Section can take place by various means. We prefer to use the cold knife in an endoscopic blade holder.

Fixation of the posterior prosthesis (Figure 7)

The strip is fixed at the back first. Once the hysterectomy has been completed, it is convenient to fix the vagina to the anterior abdominal wall in order to free the assistant's instrument so that it is more readily available for suturing.

Each of the levator muscles is taken up generously using a length of Ethibond 0 on a 30-mm needle. The prosthesis is fixed to the right and left. This is the point when myorrhaphy should take place. It is never total, but provides closure of the interlevator hiatus. This closure should be more or less complete depending on individual circumstances. It also forms the lower point of support against which the vagina will rest.

Once the prosthesis has been stretched between the two levator ani muscles, the hiatus between the prosthesis and the vagina is closed by suturing the prosthesis to the vagina, level with the anal area.

The prosthesis is then arranged over the posterior surface of the vagina and anchored to the cardinal ligaments using non-resorbable sutures (Ethibond 0). We avoid making any stitches in the posterior wall of the vagina to prevent any risk of transfixion. Once the prosthesis has been positioned at the back, a MacCall type culdoplasty is carried out.

Culdoplasty (Figure 8)

The aim of this procedure is to reposition the rectum higher up and restore tension for the vagina towards the back. The posterior part of the Douglas pouch needs to be closed. This can be achieved with or without Douglasectomy and can use one or two points. The suture material needs to be non-resorbable, and we recommend Ethibond 0.

The first step is to take up the fleshy part of the uterosacral ligament, fairly well to the rear. The cardinal ligament is taken up generously, after checking where the ureter is. Finally, the posterior prosthesis and the vagina are taken up and then the knot is tightened. This procedure is repeated on the other side.

Once this plasty has been completed, the vagina will have returned to its normal anatomical location. Consequently, no traction upwards will be needed any more.

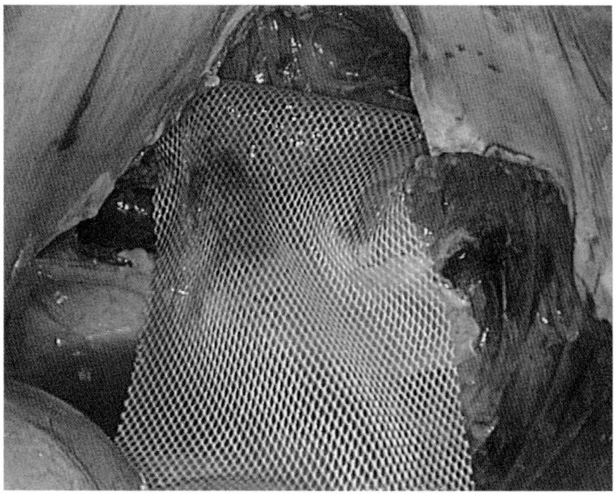

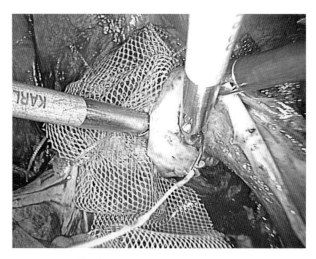

Figure 7 Fixation of the posterior prosthesis

Figure 8 Culdoplasty

Fixation of the anterior prosthesis (Figure 9)

The prosthesis is spread out in position in the anterior vesicovaginal space. If the uterus is to be kept, the two branches of the strip are taken down through windows created in the posterior layer of the broad ligament. Then they are knotted behind the isthmus, using a flat knot in the area deperitonealized when the rectovaginal space was opened up.

The prosthesis is fixed to the anterior vaginal wall by non-transfixing stitches of non-resorbable suture material (Ethibond gauge 2/0) with an 18-mm curved needle. These sutures are knotted using extracorporeal knots of the half-hitch type. Between four and six sutures are needed to ensure that the prosthesis is anchored firmly enough.

Peritonealization of the lower area (Figure 10)

At the vaginal level, the purpose of peritonealization is to exclude the prosthesis from the abdominal cavity and bring the bladder up onto the prosthesis. To do this, the surgeon starts on the left and, using Vicryl-0 suture swaged onto a 30-mm curved needle, takes up the supravesical peritoneal layer, the pillar of the bladder, the lateral vaginal peritoneum, and then the internal layer of the lateral incision, each in turn. Using the same suture, this procedure is repeated on the right. A series of half-hitches closes the purse formed, simultaneously closing the peritoneum and lifting the bladder.

Promontofixation (Figures 11 and 12)

Promontofixation is completed by fixing the anterior and posterior prostheses level with the promontory to the common anterior vertebral ligament, using two stitches of Ethibond 1 and a 30-mm curved needle, or staples or Tackers®.

The needle must remain visible by 'transparency' in order to avoid any risk of spondylodiscitis, only taking up the fibrous layer of the aponeurosis, which also means that there is no risk of perforating the substance of the disc itself. Once the stitches have been taken through, firm traction is applied to check that the anchorage is suffi-

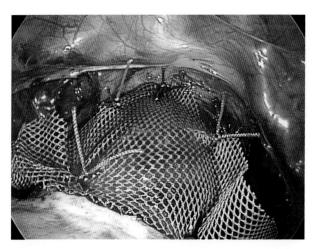

Figure 9 Fixation of the anterior prosthesis

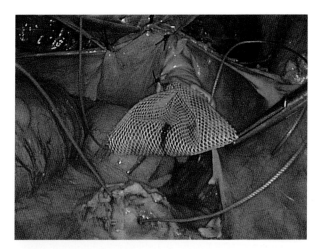

Figure 11 Promontofixation

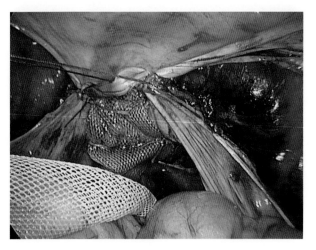

Figure 10 Peritonealization of the lower area

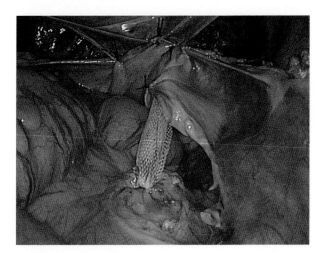

Figure 12 Lower peritonealization

ciently sturdy. The prosthesis needs to be fixed in position. This means that, once all the anatomical corrections have been made, the prosthesis is laid on the promontory and fixed *in situ*. The surgeon's experience is crucial at this point.

Upper peritonealization (Figure 13)

The prosthesis must be totally excluded in a retroperitoneal position. A running suture back and forth is therefore needed, taking up the internal and external layers of the lateral peritoneal incision. We use a length of Monocryl no. 0 suture swaged to a 30-mm curved needle. The slipping qualities of this material make this running suture in each direction easy to achieve, after which it is locked by half-hitches. However, several half-hitches are needed to ensure the knot remains stable.

These procedures complete the anterior stages. The later phases concern the space of Retzius only.

Opening the space of Retzius

With a transperitoneal incision, the operation starts by identification of the anatomical landmarks, the pubis, Cooper ligaments, and the upper edge of the bladder, identified by the beginning of the urachus.

The peritoneum is incised above the fundus of the bladder. The incision must run horizontally from one umbilical artery to the other. The assistant applies downwards traction on the peritoneum using a forceps, while the surgeon uses the instrument in his right hand to pull the plane vertically and incise it using the scissors in his left hand which are connected to the monopolar power source.

The urachus is coagulated then sectioned; the surgeon needs to progress vertically towards the abdominal wall, crossing the prevesical–umbilical aponeurosis to enter the space of Retzius. The space of Retzius is an avascular plane that is dissected by simple divergent traction. Pneumodissection helps to open the space. Remaining in contact with the aponeurosis, the surgeon will reach

several tissular planes in succession, which need to be broken down until the fatty tissues located in front of the Cooper ligament indicate that the upper limit of the space of Retzius has been reached. Now, the right and left Cooper ligaments need to be separated off. At this point, the space of Retzius is opened by simply breaking the tissues down until the arcus tendineus fasciae pelvis is found. Dissection continues backwards until just below the obturator fossa.

The vaginal walls are prepared with the help of a finger placed in the fornix. The edge of the bladder is often revealed by the presence of a vein running along it. This must then be carefully separated from the vagina which shows up pearly white.

Paravaginal repair (Figures 14 and 15)

At this point, the positive pressure from the pneumoperitoneum helps to reveal lateral defects which are nearly always present in complex prolapse cases. They show up as hernias running from the arcus tendineus fasciae pelvis to the vagina itself. If there is indeed a paravaginal hernia, it must be repaired. It is closed using separate stitches or a

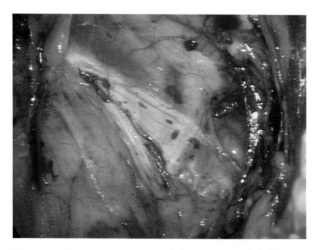

Figure 14 Laparoscopic view of the paravaginal defect

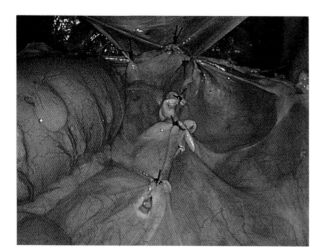

Figure 13 Upper peritonealization

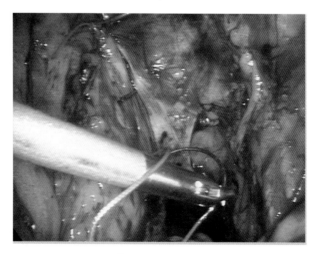

Figure 15 Paravaginal repair

running suture of Ethibond 0 with a size 18 needle. This suture should run from the pubo-urethral ligaments at the front to the sciatic spine at the back. It may be uni- or bilateral.

Burch bladder neck suspension (Figure 16)

Once the previous repair has been completed, bladder neck suspension is carried out. The material used is Ethibond gauge 3.5 (0) with a 26-mm needle.

The suture is taken through the Cooper ligament first, from top to bottom, then through the vagina from inside outwards, trying not to transfix. The passage through the vagina must be sufficiently broad to ensure that the construction will be sturdy. If there is any bleeding during the first passage through, an X-shaped stitch is made. In cases with promontofixation, a single suture is taken through each side. The tension applied must be moderate only. If there has also been paravaginal repair, this will prevent any hypercorrection by the cervicosuspension.

Peritonealization

This is systematic and complete. The purpose is to avoid any bowel becoming trapped in the space of Retzius. We use a length of Vicryl-0 swaged to a 36-mm curved needle. Closure is effected with three runs from right to left. The upper and lower edges of the peritoneum are taken up in turn, and then the suture is fixed using half-hitches.

Final procedures

Uterine morcellation

This is needed for subtotal hysterectomy. We use the Steiner morcellation device (Karl Storz, Tuttlingen, Germany). The uterus, which is usually small, is cut into a 10-mm diameter strip which is extracted through the device. It is then sent for examination by the pathologist.

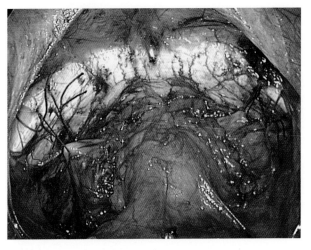

Figure 16 Burch bladder neck suspension

Releasing the attachments

The sutures holding the bowel out of the way are released under visual control and any bleeding areas are coagulated.

Peritoneal lavage

Ringer's lactate is the best substance to use for this cleaning phase, which must be thorough. All the blood clots are aspirated and any hemostasis still needed carried out. At the end of the operation, the rinsing liquid must return completely clear.

Cystoscopy

The ureters must be checked several times during the operation: after the hysterectomy, after peritonealization and after the Burch procedure. By checking after each phase to see whether there is an injury, it will be possible to identify what the cause was, thus helping to achieve the best repair possible. It is also important to keep a check on the color of the urine and any increase in volume of the pouch which could indicate a bladder or ureter injury.

The need for cystoscopy is the subject of debate. Some authors use it systematically whereas others use it only in case of doubt. The indications should be broad. It will confirm that the urine is correctly ejaculated from the utereral meatus and is the only way of certifying that the ureter is intact.

POSTOPERATIVE CARE

Antibiotic therapy

We do not use postoperative antibiotic therapy systematically. We treat only infections that are proven after sampling and an antibiogram.

Prevention of postoperative phlebitis

Our patients are given systematic treatment for the prevention of phlebitis. Low-dose heparin therapy is started on admission to the hospital the day before the operation, and is continued for 15 days.

Foley catheter

The Foley catheter is left in place for at least 24 h, and possibly for longer according to the patient's age and mobility. On removal, a systematic cytobacteriological examination is carried out. Antibiotic therapy is initiated in the event of urinary infection.

Hospital stay

This lasts between 3 and 5 days.

Postoperative regimen

The patient is asked to avoid undue exertion after the operation. No strain or carrying of heavy loads is allowed for 3 months. The recommended diet is normal with plenty of liquids in order to combat the constipation that is almost always experienced during the first 3 weeks postoperatively. Sexual relations can be resumed after 6 weeks.

CONCLUSIONS

Laparoscopy enables the advantages of prolapse treatment by laparotomy to be combined with the low morbidity of the vaginal route. The operating times, which initially were very long, have now been reduced to about 2 h in the hands of experienced surgeons. Naturally enough, studies are required on long-term efficiency and reliability in order to evaluate the technique fully.

BIBLIOGRAPHY

Addison WA, Livengood CH, Sutton GP, *et al.* Abdominal sacral colpopexy with Mercilene mesh in the retroperitoneal position in the management of posthysterectomy vaginal vault prolapse and enterocele. *Am J Obstet Gynecol* 1985;15:140–6

Addison WA, Timmons C, Wall LL, *et al.* Failed abdominal sacral colpopexy: observations and recommendations. *Gynecol Obstet* 1989;74:480–3

Ameline A, Huguier J. La suspension postérieure du disque lombo-sacré: techniques de remplacement des ligaments utéro-sacrés par voie abdominale. *Gynecol Obstet* 1957;56:94–8

Baker KR, Beresford JM, Campbell C. Colpo-sacropexy with Prolene mesh. *Gynecol Obstet* 1990;171:51–4

Caubel P, Lefranc JP, Foulkes H, *et al.* Traitement par voie vaginale des prolapsus génitaux récidivés. *J Chir* 1989;126:446–70

Hoff S, Manelfe A, Portet R, *et al.* Promonto-fixation ou suspension par bandelettes transversales? Etude comparée de ces deux techniques dans le traitement des prolapsus génitaux. *Ann Chir* 1984;38:363–7

Nichols D, Milley P. Significance of restoration of vaginal depth and axis. *Obstet Gynecol* 1970;36:251–5

Querleu D, Parmentier D, Delodinance P. Premiers essais de la coelio-chirurgie dans le traitement du prolapsus génital et de l'incontinence urinaire d'effort. In Blanc M, Boubli L, Baudrant E, D'Ercale C, eds. *Les Troubles de la Statiques Pelviennes*. Paris: Arnette 1995:155–8

Randall C. Surgical treatment of vaginal inversion. *Obstet Gynecol* 1971;38:327–32

Robert HG. Nouveau traité de techniques chirurgicales gynécologiques. *Masson et Cie* 1969:128–30

Sutton JP, Addison WA, Livengood CH, *et al.* Life threatening hemorrhage complicating sacral colpopexy. *Am J Obstet Gynecol* 1981;140:836–7

Wattiez A, Aimi G, Finkeltin F, *et al.* Cure chirurgicale des prolapsus vesico-uterins par voie cœlioscopie exclusive. *Gunaïkeia* 1997;2:50–5

Wattiez A, Boughizane S, Alexandre F, *et al.* Laparoscopic procedures for stress incontinence and prolapse. *Curr Opin Obstet Gynecol* 1995;7:317–21

Wattiez A, Canis M, Mage G, *et al.* Promontofixation dans le traitement des prolapsus: intérêt et technique de la voie cœlioscopie. *J Coeliochirugie* 1999;31:7–11

Wattiez A, Cucinella G, Giambelli F, *et al.* Laparoscopic burch procedure for retropubic colposuspension. *Ital J Gynaecol Obstet* 1997;9:114–17

28

Laparoscopic sacrofixation

J. Donnez, J. Squifflet, M. Smets and M. Nisolle

The surgical treatment of vaginal vault prolapse and cervical or uterine prolapse is a major challenge to the surgeon, especially when preservation of sexual function is sought. In patients with surgical contraindications, the placement of a vaginal pessary may offer great relief from symptoms without any surgical risk. But when surgery is possible, it is the preferable therapy.

Genital prolapse can be treated by various techniques, with or without synthetic material (prosthesis), by laparotomy, laparoscopy or vaginal surgery (Table 1). In vaginal surgery, hysterectomy is usually associated with the technique, except for the transposition of uterosacral ligaments in front of the cervix (Shirodkar technique). Some authors have described sacrospinal ligament vaginal fixation by the vaginal route[1]. Laparotomy techniques may be associated with total hysterectomy, subtotal hysterectomy, or uterus conservation. A synthetic material is then often used to attach the cervix, the uterus or the vagina to the sacrum or the prevertebral ligament. Alloplastic graft materials, such as polytetrafluoroethylene (Teflon®)[2,3], propylene (Marlex®)[2,4–6], polyester fiber (Mersilene®)[2,7–11], Gore Tex®[2,7] or polypropylene[12] have been used by many authors. Homologous materials, such as fascia[13–15] or dura mater[16], have also been used and are well tolerated, although unresorbable sutures covered with peritoneum have been reported too[17]. Since 1993, laparoscopic procedures have also been proposed in the management of vaginal, cervical or uterine prolapse[18–21]. All these recent techniques use a synthetic material which is attached to the vagina or the cervix towards the promontosacral space[18,20] or the anterosuperior iliac spine[19], according to the technique described by Kapandji[22]. The uterine promontosacropexy is, at present, the most frequently used technique in young women.

A series of 98 women (Table 2) underwent a simple combined vaginal and laparoscopic technique with or without uterus conservation, consisting of the sacral fixation of a tightened polypropylene prosthesis (mesh) attached to the posterior part of the cervix or the vaginal vault. This mesh was fixed to the body of either the first sacral vertebra or the fifth lumbar vertebra with the help of a novel tacking device (Origin Tacker™ Fixation Device, Origin Medsystems, Inc., Menlo Park, CA). All the women had a preoperative front and profile lumbosacral junction X-ray to check the promontory.

Table 1 Sacrofixations carried out in the department since 1985

Laparotomy	$n = 22$	1985–1994
Laparoscopy	$n = 107$	
Mackar®	$n = 9$	1994–1995
Tacker®	$n = 98$	1995–2000
(Origin, Autosuture)		

Table 2 Number of laparoscopic sacrofixations (SF) carried out in 5 years using the 'Tacker' procedure

Vaginal vault prolapse	$n = 31$
Uterine prolapse	$n = 67$
uterus	$n = 6$
cervix	$n = 4$
LASH + SF	$n = 57$

LASH, laparoscopic subtotal hysterectomy

OPERATIVE TECHNIQUE

Cervical or uterine sacrofixation

The patient is placed in the Trendelenburg position. The surgeon is on the left of the patient and holds the laparoscope in his right hand. The assistant is between the legs of the patient. Single-tooth vulsellum forceps are placed on the anterior lip of the cervix and a cannula is inserted into the cervix for uterine mobilization if the cervix is present. A Foley catheter is inserted into the bladder. Three 5-mm suprapubic trocars are introduced: one in the midline and two lateral to the epigastric vessels.

First step: exploration

The abdominal cavity is explored first. The peritoneum, the uterus and the adnexa are inspected; the ureters are traced along the pelvic side-wall and the major iliac vessels are carefully located. Adhesiolysis is performed if necessary. A laparoscopic subtotal hysterectomy (LASH) may be performed if indicated[23,24]. The uterine corpus should then be removed during the second step (colpotomy) (Figure 1).

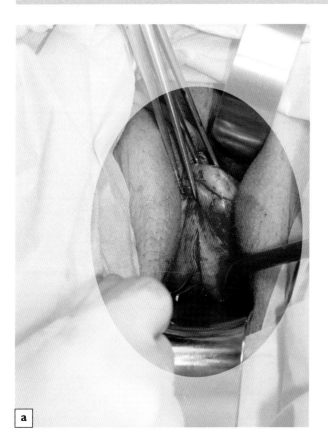

a

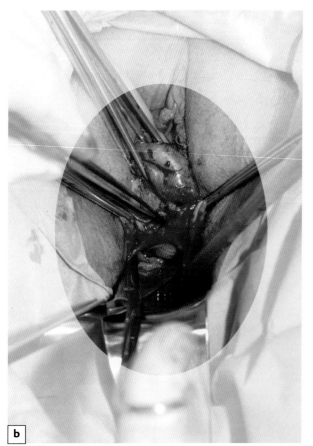

b

Figure 1 (a) and (b) Posterior colpotomy and dissection of the enterocele

Second step: cervical fixation of the mesh by posterior colpotomy (Figure 2)

After careful disinfection of the pouch of Douglas and the vagina with an iodine solution, a posterior colpotomy is performed along a sagittal vaginal incision over a length of 4–5 cm (Figure 1a and b). After the dissection and opening of the posterior peritoneal cul-de-sac, a right-angled retractor is placed on the posterior lip of the vagina. Another vulsellum holds the posterior lip of the cervix to provide exposure. If LASH was performed during the first step, the uterus will already have been removed (Figure 2). A polypropylene mesh is then tightly stitched to the posterior part of the cervix with two non-absorbable stitches (Figure 3) (Nylon O, Ethicon, Somerville, USA). The mesh is placed in the abdominal cavity. Two round circumferential sutures are then placed high on the peritoneum in order to carry out a culdoplasty to treat associated enterocele (Figure 4). The highest suture brings both uterosacral ligaments to the medial line to prevent any future occurrence. The culdotomy is then closed. Separate points or a running suture are applied to both vaginal lips.

Third step: laparoscopic dissection of the presacral tissue (Figure 5)

The patient, still in the Trendelenburg position, is placed slightly in left lateral decubitus. After careful coagulation of the peritoneum, an opening is made with scissors from the lumbosacral joint towards the cervix. The prevertebral space is opened. The presacral peritoneum is grasped with two atraumatic forceps on the right lateral side of the rectum. The right ureter is situated 1–2 cm from the presacral peritoneal incision and is systematically checked over the length of this incision. The sigmoid is pushed laterally and careful dissection and hemostasis of the presacral tissue provide exposure of the anterior common vertebral ligament. Coagulation and section of the medial sacral artery and vein are sometimes necessary. The most prominent point of the space is the lumbosacral joint (the mesh must be fixed either to the anterior wall of the corpus of the first sacral vertebra or to that of the fifth lumbar vertebra).

Fourth step: sacral fixation of the polypropylene mesh (Figure 6)

Two grasping forceps hold the edges of the parietal posterior peritoneum to give access to the anterior wall of the first sacral vertebra. The Origin Tacker is introduced through the medial suprapubic trocar. This tacking device utilizes a helical coil of 3.9-mm diameter to achieve secure fixation to the vertebra (Figure 7). Forceps grasp the prosthesis, which is then tightened until the cervix or the uterus recovers its anatomical position. The tip of the Tacker is placed on the mesh, in front of the anterior wall of the first sacral vertebra, and several tacks are inserted

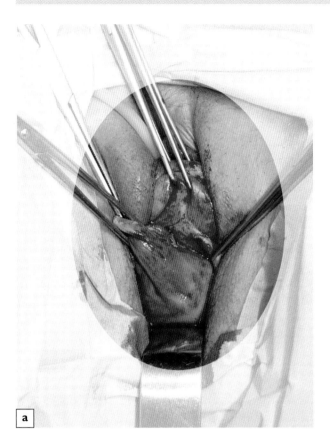

a

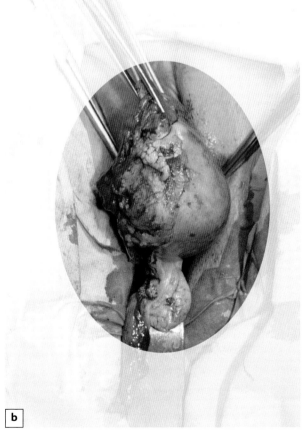

b

Figure 2 (a) The uterus is grasped; (b) the uterus is removed through the posterior colpotomy

through the mesh into the periosteum of the vertebra and the common vertebral ligament. Excess mesh is cut away and removed.

Fifth step: reperitonealization (Figure 8)

Both folds of the peritoneum are sutured with a resorbable material or stapled with endoscopic staples. Careful washing of the peritoneal cavity is then performed and an antiseptic solution of Rifocine (Rifamycin, Merrel Dow, Kansas City, USA) is instilled into the pelvis. Finally, a Douglas catheter is placed through one of the suprapubic trocars. It will be clamped for 2–4 h and removed the day after surgery.

Vaginal vault sacrofixation

Fixation of the mesh to the vagina can be performed either vaginally or laparoscopically using the tacking technique, but the vaginal route is preferred because it allows quick repair of the enterocele.

Using the vaginal route, the vagina is opened along its posterior wall with a 4–5-cm incision, perpendicular to the vaginal vault. Dissection is performed to enter the abdominal cavity. The enterocele is then dissected and the excess peritoneum is cut away.

The polypropylene mesh is fixed to the vaginal vault through the vaginal incision by two or three nonabsorbable stitches. The mesh is introduced into the peritoneal cavity. The peritoneum is then closed with two high, continuous, round circumferential sutures to close the pouch of Douglas (Douglasorrhaphy). The vagina is finally closed.

It is important to note that none of the patients underwent a concomitant Burch procedure. After surgery, a pessary is placed. It will be removed 1 month later at the postoperative check-up. On postoperative day 3, radiography of the sacrum (Figure 9) confirms the correct position of the coils.

COMPLICATIONS

We did not observe any intraoperative complications. No bleeding occurred during the procedure among the 98 patients in this study. There was one immediate postoperative complication (Table 3). One patient complained of difficulty moving her left foot straight after leaving the operating room. It was associated with severe pain in the left buttock and in the upper part of the left thigh. An electromyography concluded that the fifth left lumbar neural root or one of the first left sacroneural roots was affected. A radiography of the sacrum showed that one coil was too laterally placed on the left, near the neural root (Figure 10a). After magnetic resonance imaging (MRI) (Figure 10b) had confirmed that one spring had been placed in the foramen intervertebrale of the second sacral

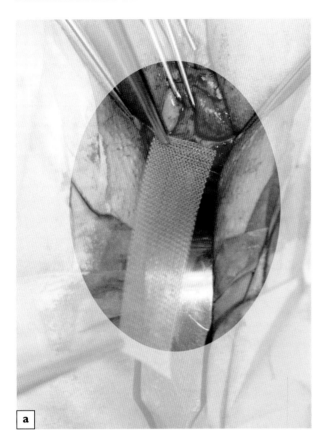

a

root, we decided to perform a laparotomy and the spring was carefully removed. The patient made a rapid recovery and now has (6 months after surgery) only a slight mobility defect of her left foot.

Postoperative discomfort was similar to that observed after any straightforward laparoscopy. Bowel function resumed within 24 h and the patients were able to leave hospital on average on day 4 postoperatively. Sexual intercourse was allowed 3 weeks after surgery. Patients were reviewed every 6 months. The average follow-up is now 1–6 years. No patients have complained of dyspareunia or urinary stress incontinence.

Table 3 Complications and recurrence after laparoscopic sacrofixation ($n = 98$)

Complications $n = 2$ (2%)
    compression of sciatic nerve (wrong insertion)
    spondylodiscitis (9 months postoperatively)

Recurrence $n = 2$ (2%)
    defective application on the cervix
    enterocele after vaginal vault prolapse without enterocele repair

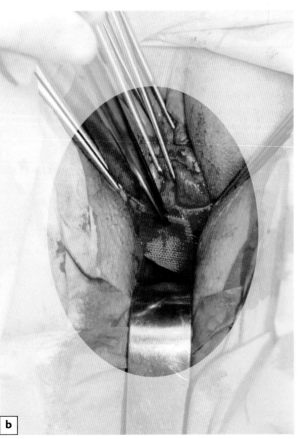

b

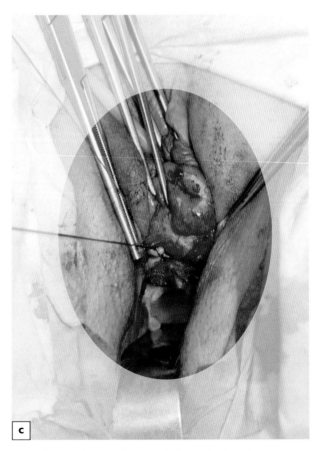

c

Figure 3 (a)–(c) Cervical fixation of the mesh by posterior colpotomy. The polypropylene mesh is stitched to the posterior part of the cervix with two non-absorbable stitches (Nylon 0)

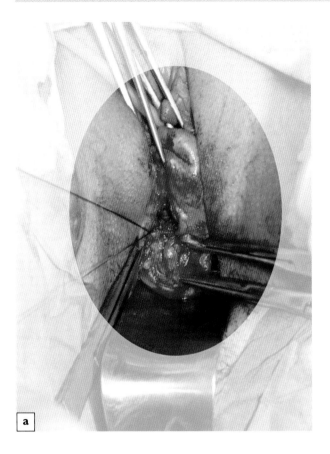

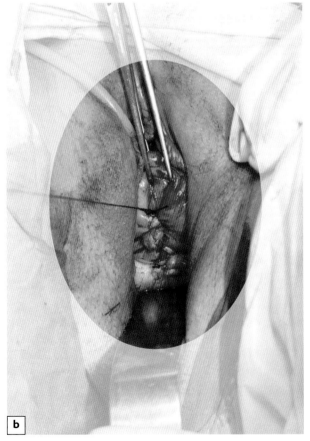

Figure 4 (a) Two round circumferential sutures are then placed high on the peritoneum; (b) final view

One patient experienced spondylites 9 months post-operatively. She underwent laparotomy with disc resection and bone transplantation.

We have observed two cases of recurrence. The first case was observed 8 months after surgery in one patient from Group II. The patient underwent another laparoscopy which showed that the mesh was well fixed to the sacrum but was detached from the cervix. The mesh was separated from the covering peritoneum and then fixed to the cervix with the help of two non-absorbable sutures. The second case of recurrence was due to incomplete surgery. Indeed, this patient, who had undergone fixation of the vaginal vault, developed a severe enterocele several months later. She underwent surgery a second time and laparoscopy showed that the vaginal vault was well fixed to the mesh but an enterocele had developed below the point of fixation of the mesh to the vagina. Vaginal surgery of the enterocele was easily carried out. There has been no recurrence in more than 2 years of follow-up.

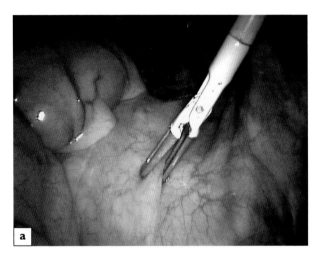

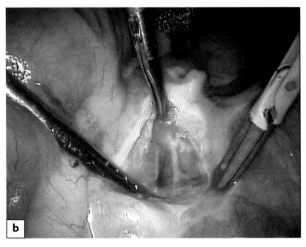

Figure 5 (a) and (b) Laparoscopic dissection of the presacral tissue. The presacral peritoneum is grasped with two atraumatic forceps on the right lateral side of the rectum. Careful hemostasis of the presacral tissue provides exposure of the anterior common vertebral ligament

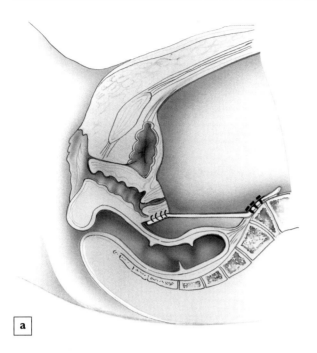

a

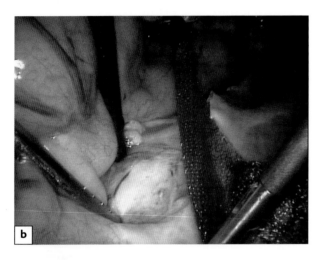

b

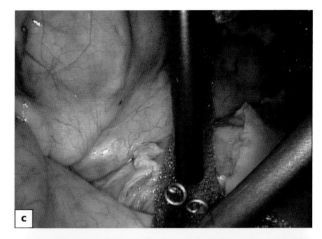

c

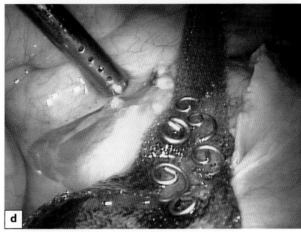

d

Figure 6 (a) Sacral fixation of the polypropylene mesh; (b) and (c) a polypropylene mesh is fixed vaginally to the cervix or the vaginal vault. The tip of the Tacker System (Origin, Autosuture) is placed on the mesh, in front of the anterior wall of the first sacral vertebra and several tacks are inserted through the mesh into the periosteum of the vertebra; (d) the anatomical position of the vagina is restored

COMMENTS

The goal of pelvic reconstruction is to restore normal anatomy, maintain or restore normal bladder and bowel function, and provide a vagina of normal length to ensure pain-free coitus[25]. A well-supported vagina lies on the rectum and levator plate with its axis directed towards the hollow of the sacrum and its apex at or above the ischial spines. It is suspended from the sacrum by the paracolpium. Vaginography[26] and contemporary MRI demonstrate this anatomical fact. Vaginal eversion and uterine prolapse are a result of disruption of the upper paracolpium, which includes the fibromuscular tissue of the cardinal and uterosacral ligaments[20]. Many different corrective procedures use this anatomical principle and anchor the vaginal apex or the cervix to the available supporting tissue at this level, including the sacrospinal

ligaments, cliococcygeus or coccygeus fascia, uterosacral ligaments, or sacrum.

Many authors have advocated vaginal surgery as the only method for this type of pathology. The main problem is that, in cases of severe attenuation of both uterosacral ligaments, which is frequent in vaginal vault prolapse, vaginal repair of cystocele and rectocele often fails[27]. The technique, first proposed by Amreich[28] and later modified by Richter and Albrich[1], consists of the fixation of the vaginal vault to the sacrospinal ligament. One of the disadvantages of sacrospinal ligament fixation is that the marked vaginal retroversion subsequent to this type of fixation may predispose patients to recurrent support defects in the anterior vagina, resulting in cystocele, urethral hypermobility, or both[29,30]. Holley and co-workers[30] reported a 92% incidence of cystoceles (76% first-degree and 24% second-degree) in 36 women who underwent sacrospinous ligament fixation or repair of associated pelvic support defects

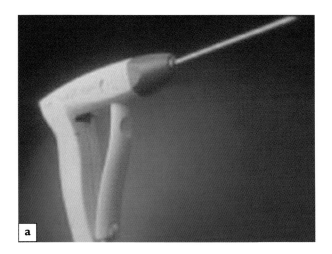

a

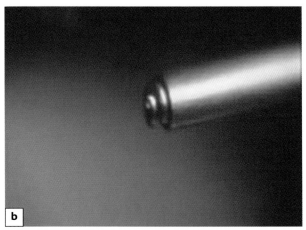

b

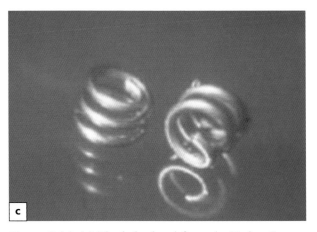

c

Figure 7 (a)–(c) The helical coil from the Tacker System (Origin, Autosuture)

with a mean follow-up of 42 months. The majority of cases were asymptomatic, however, and only a small number required a subsequent surgical procedure (5.5%). A second disadvantage of sacrospinous ligament fixation is the possible neuropathy produced by vaginal dissection[31]. Such neuropathy may have an effect on subsequent muscle strength and integrity of muscular tissue support. It can also be related to dysfunction of the lower urinary tract and explain the higher incidence of incontinence after

sacrospinous ligament fixation than after sacrofixation[32]. In a prospective study comparing the vaginal versus the abdominal approach, Benson and colleagues[32] demonstrated that the abdominal approach is more effective in treating uterovaginal prolapse, with the probability for an optimal surgical outcome being twice as great with an abdominal operation and the probability for an unsatisfactory surgical outcome twice as great with a vaginal operation.

Among the transabdominal approaches described so far, the most frequently published is the fixation of the vaginal vault to the midsacrum or sacral promontory using an artificial material.

Sacral colpopexy has a high success rate (85–99%) in repairing vault prolapse and does not shorten the vagina[5,6,8,17,33,34]. Recently, laparoscopic approaches to sacrofixation[12,20,35] have been described. The advantage of sacrofixation is that it ensures vaginal length with a larger-caliber, normal horizontal vaginal axis and a more anatomical repair[32]. Sacral colpopexy is performed to correct severe vaginal vault eversion by replacing the upper paracolpium with synthetic mesh, which results in a stronger fixation than a simple culdoplasty[20]. According to Ameline and Huguier[36], the only physiological suspension involves placement of suture material into the ligamentous and periosteal fibrous connective tissue in the midline of the anterior sacrum. Although sacral segments 3 and 4 are anatomically ideal, control of the tip of the needle deep in the hollow of the sacrum is difficult and laceration of presacral veins is an ever-present risk, leading to life-threatening hemorrhages which are extremely difficult to control[37]. Fixation to the first vertebra (beyond the sacrolumbar joint) or the lower part of the fifth lumbar vertebra gives back the genital tube its triple angulation: a postero-ascending vaginal obliquity, an anteflexion of the cervix over the uterine corpus and an anteversion, and thus correctly restores the anatomy. In our series of cases where sacrofixation was performed by laparotomy or by laparoscopy[12] using the Macker™ staple, more severe cystoceles were not observed (except in two cases) even after long-term follow-up. This is probably due to the more anatomical reconstruction. Like Hoff and colleagues[38], we believe that, in the great majority of cases, anterior colporrhaphy with sacrofixation is not needed to treat an associated cystocele. Nevertheless, we believe that posterior colporrhaphy can be helpful treating even a huge rectocele completely. We performed posterior colporrhaphy only in cases where the rectocele was so large that simple fixation of the cervix or vagina did not allow a sufficient reduction.

Like Smith[6], we believe that osseous anchorage of the prosthesis is stronger than sacrospinous ligament stitching (Tables 4 and 5). In one of our previous series of 20 patients who underwent osseous anchorage of a prosthesis using Mackar staples by laparotomy or laparoscopy between 1985 and 1995, the long-term results were excellent and no recurrence was noted[12]. The tacking technique described here allows fixation of the mesh to the vertebra

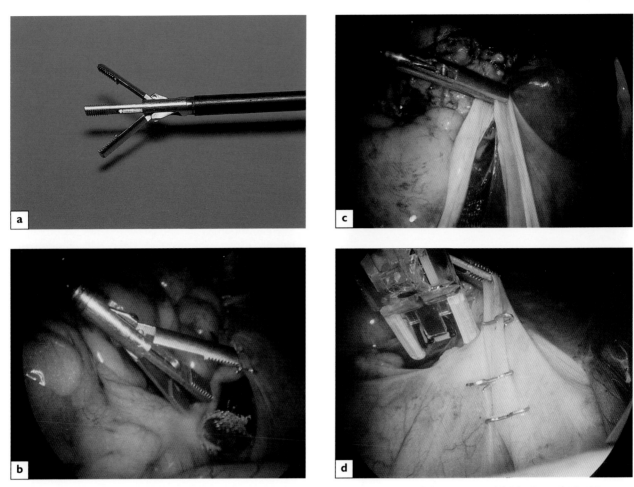

Figure 8 (a) A 'double' grasping forceps (5 mm in size) allows an approximation of the peritoneal folds (b) and (c); (d) using five or six titanium clips (Endohernia®)

Table 4 Advantages of osseous anchorage (Tacker) versus stitching

Osseous anchorage of the prosthesis is stronger than sacrospinal stitching

Less risk of bleeding than with presacral stitching

Table 5 Advantages of laparoscopic subtotal hysterectomy-associated sacrofixation compared to laparoscopic hysterectomy-associated sacrofixation

Vaginal vault	*Cervix*
No strong tissue	Stronger tissue for prosthesis
Mesh erosion risk	fixation
Difficult visualization of	By traction, better
uterosacral ligaments	visualization of uterosacral
	ligaments
	Better repair during
	peritonealization

with the same reliability. It is less invasive (no penetration of the bones but only the periosteum) and thus reduces the risk of bone infection. It enables us to avoid difficulties related to a prevertebral suture. The most common complications of sacropexy are intraoperative bleeding and a postoperative temperature. Spondylodiscitis and bleeding due to presacral vessel lesions are rarely observed[37,39,40]. The mesh should be reperitonealized to prevent bowel adhesions[41,42]. Undue tension must be avoided to prevent pain[5].

We have observed two prolapse recurrences among the 98 patients who underwent sacrofixation (2.4%). The first occurred in a patient in whom the mesh had been fixed to the cervix using a coil. It was the cervical fixation of the mesh that had given way, while the sacral fixation remained intact. The consistency of the cervix does not favor a solid fixation of the mesh using tacking springs and strongly suggests fixing the mesh with the help of non-absorbable sutures by posterior colpotomy. This allows the surgeon to perform a Douglasorrhaphy, shorten the uterosacral ligaments and treat the enterocele, if present. The second case of recurrence that we encountered, with secondary development of an enterocele, was explained by

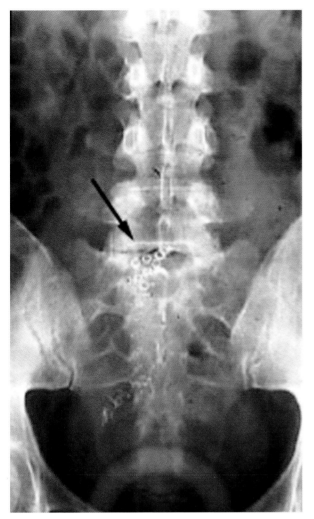

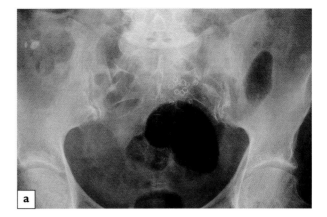

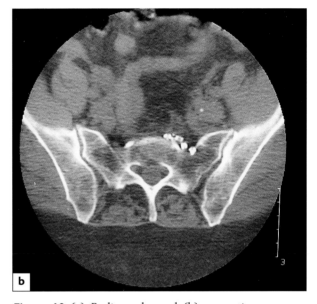

Figure 9 Radiogram of the pelvis on postoperative day 3 checks the correct position of the coil (arrow) at the level of the first sacral vertebra (profile and face)

Figure 10 (a) Radiography and (b) magnetic resonance imaging confirm the presence of a coil in the foramen intervertebrale of the second sacral root

the fact that simple fixation of the mesh to the vagina is not sufficient because it could favor, as in this case, the development of a more severe enterocele by 'sliding' under the site of fixation. For this reason, Douglasorrhaphy and enterocele repair must be systematically carried out in cases of vaginal vault repair.

In contrast to sacrospinous fixation, because of its more anatomical repair, sacrofixation does not favor the development of secondary cystoceles, does not cause vaginal shortening and, providing that particular care is taken to insert the springs into the central part of the body of the vertebra, is without risk for nerves if the prevertebral area dissection is easy and well performed. In overweight women, in whom there is a wide area (with fatty tissue) between the prevertebral peritoneum and the vertebral bone itself, we believe that intraoperative X-rays are indicated in order to determine the exact site of coil insertion.

Like Vancaillie[43], we would like to conclude this Chapter bearing in mind that sacrocolpopexy remains a potentially high-morbidity procedure with invasion of the

presacral space, and that laparoscopy does not reduce this kind of morbidity.

CONCLUSION

A combined (vaginal and laparoscopic) approach can be proposed in cases of uterine or vaginal vault prolapse. Fixation of the mesh by posterior colpotomy has several advantages. First, it allows easy use of non-absorbable sutures. Second, associated surgical procedures can be performed to resolve or prevent enterocele. Third, this technique provides the quickest surgical resolution when compared to a purely laparoscopic approach.

Laparoscopic fixation of the mesh to the sacrum with the help of springs (Origin Tacker System) also has several advantages. It avoids the risk of presacral vein laceration by the use of a needle. It provides an easy and quick fixation of the mesh to the fifth lumbar vertebra or the first sacral vertebra. Finally, it gives an extremely good-quality fixation. For these reasons, we believe that this type of approach can provide a good alternative for the treatment of genital prolapse.

REFERENCES

1. Richter K, Albrich W. Long-term results following fixation of the vagina on the sacrospinal ligament by the vaginal route (vaginal fixation sacrospinalis vaginalis). *Am J Obstet Gynecol* 1981;141:811–16

2. Virtanen H, Hirvonen T, Mäkinen J, *et al.* Outcome of thirty patients who underwent repair of posthysterectomy prolapse of the vaginal vault with abdominal sacral colpopexy. *J Am Coll Surg* 1994;178:283–7

3. Birnboum SJ. Rational therapy for the prolapsed vagina. *Am J Obstet Gynecol* 1973;115:411–15

4. Grundsell H, Lorsson G. Operative management of vaginal vault prolapse following hysterectomy. *Br J Obstet Gynaecol* 1984;91:808–11

5. Drutz HP, Cha LS. Massive genital and vaginal vault prolapse treated by abdominal vaginal sacropexy with the use of Marlex Mesh. Review of the literature. *Am J Obstet Gynecol* 1987;156:387–92

6. Smith MR. Colposacropexy: an alternative technique. *Am J Obstet Gynecol* 1997;176:1374–5

7. Snyder TE, Krantz KE, Litt D. Abdominal retroperitoneal sacral colpopexy for the correction of vaginal prolapse. *Obstet Gynecol* 1991;77:944–9

8. Addison WA, Timmons MC, Wall LL, *et al.* Failed abdominal sacral colpopexy: observations and recommendations. *Obstet Gynecol* 1989;74:480–2

9. Rust JA, Botte JM, Howlett RJ. Prolapse of the vaginal vault. Improved techniques for the management of the abdominal approach or vaginal approach. *Am J Obstet Gynecol* 1976;125:768–73

10. Creighton SM, Stanton SL. The surgical management of vaginal vault prolapse. *Br J Obstet Gynaecol* 1991;98:1150–4

11. Timmons MC, Addison WA, Addison SB, *et al.* Abdominal sacral colpopexy in 163 women with posthysterectomy vaginal vault prolapse and enterocele. *J Reprod Med* 1992;37:323–7

12. Smets M, Donnez J. Mackar staple fixation for uterus prolapse. *Gynecol Endosc* 1995;4:18–19

13. Maloney JC, Dunton CJ, Smith K. Repair of vaginal vault prolapse with abdominal sacropexy. *J Reprod Med* 1990;35:6–10

14. Hendee AE, Berry CM. Abdominal sacropexy for vaginal vault prolapse. *Clin Obstet Gynecol* 1981;24:1217–26

15. Kauppila O, Punnonen R, Teisala K. Operative technique for the repair of posthysterectomy vaginal prolapse. *Ann Chir Gynecol* 1986;75:242–4

16. Lansman HH. Posthysterectomy vault prolapse: sacral colpopexy with dura mater graft. *Obstet Gynecol* 1984; 63: 577–82

17. Grünberger W, Grünberger V, Wierani F. Pelvic promontory fixation of the vaginal vault in sixty-two patients with prolapse after hysterectomy. *J Am Coll Surg* 1994;178:69–72

18. Querleu D, Parmentier D, Debodinance P. Premiers essais de coeliochirurgie dans le traitement du prolapsus génital et de l'incontinence urinaire d'effort. In Blanc B, Boubli L, Baudrant E, d'Ercale C, eds. *Les Troubles de la Statique Pelvienne.* Paris: Arnette Editions, 1993:155

19. Cornier E, Madelenat P. Hystéropexie selon M. Kapandji: technique percoelioscopique et résultats préliminaires. *J Gynecol Obstet Biol Reprod* 1994;23:378–85

20. Ross JW. Techniques of laparoscopic repair of total vault eversion after hysterectomy. *J Am Assoc Gynecol Laparosc* 1997;4:173–83

21. Godin PA, Nisolle M, Smets M, *et al.* Combined vaginal and laparoscopic sacrofixation for genital prolapse using a tacking technique: a series of 45 cases. *Gynecol Endosc* 1999;8:277–85

22. Kapandji M. Cure des prolapsus uro-génitaux par colpo-isthmo-cystopexie par bandelettes transversales et la Douglassoraphie ligamento-péritonéale étagée et croisée. *Ann Chir* 1967;21:32

23. Donnez J, Nisolle M. LASH: laparoscopic supracervical (subtotal) hysterectomy. *J Gynecol Surg* 1993;9:91–4

24. Donnez J, Nisolle M, Smets M, *et al.* Laparoscopic supracervical (subtotal) hysterectomy. A first series of 500 cases. *Gynecol Endosc* 1997;6:73–6

25. Shull BL, Capen CV, Riggs MW, *et al.* Preoperative and postoperative analysis of site-specific pelvic support defects in 81 women treated with sacrospinous ligament suspension and pelvic reconstruction. *Am J Obstet Gynecol* 1992;166:1764–71

26. Nichols DH, Milloy AS, Randall CL. Significance of restoration of normal vaginal depth and axis. *Obstet Gynecol* 1970;36:251–5

27. Symmonds RE, Williams TJ, Lee RA, *et al.* Posthysterectomy enterocele and vaginal vault prolapse. *Am J Obstet Gynecol* 1981;140:852–9

28. Amreich J. Actrologie und Operation des Schidenstrumpf-Prolapses. *Wien Klin Wodenschr* 1951;63:74

29. Cruikshank S, Cox D. Sacrospinous ligament fixation at the time of transvaginal hysterectomy. *Am J Obstet Gynecol* 1990;162:1611–19

30. Holley RL, Varner RE, Gleason BP, *et al.* Recurrent pelvic support defects after sacrospinous ligament fixation for vaginal vault prolapse. *J Am Coll Surg* 1995;180:444–80

31. Benson JT, McClellan E. The effect of vaginal dissection on the pubertal nerve. *Obstet Gynecol* 1993;82:387–9

32. Benson JT, Lucente V, McClellan E. Vaginal versus abdominal reconstructive surgery for the treatment of pelvic support defects: a prospective randomized study with long-term outcome evaluation. *Am J Obstet Gynecol* 1996;175:1418–22

33. Arthure HG, Savage D. Uterine prolapse and prolapse of the vagina treated by sacropexy. *J Obstet Gynaecol Br Commonw* 1957;64:355–60

34. Creighton S, Stanton S. The surgical management of vaginal prolapse. *Br J Obstet Gynaecol* 1991;98:1150–4

35. Nezhat CH, Nezhat F, Nezhat C. Laparoscopic sacral colpopexy for vaginal vault prolapse. *Obstet Gynecol* 1994;84:885–8

36. Ameline A, Huguier J. La suspension postérieure aux disques lombo-sacrés: technique de remplacement des ligaments utéro-sacrés par voie abdominale. *J Gynecol Obstet Biol Reprod* 1957;56:94

37. Sutton JP, Addison WA, Livengood CH, *et al.* Life-threatening hemorrhage complicating sacral colpopexy. *Am J Obstet Gynecol* 1981;140:836

38. Hoff S, Manelfe A, Portet R, *et al.* Promontofixation ou suspension par bandelettes transversables? Etude comparée de ces deux techniques dans le traitement des prolapsus génitaux. *Ann Chir* 1984;38:363

39. Baker KR, Beresford JM, Campbell C. Colposacropexy with Prolene mesh. *Obstet Gynecol* 1990;171:51–4

40. Addison WA, Livengood CH, Sutton GP, *et al.* Abdominal sacral colpopexy with Mercilene mesh in the retroperitoneal position in the management of posthysterectomy vaginal vault prolapse and enterocele. *Am J Obstet Gynecol* 1985;15:140–6

41. Soichet S. Surgical correction of total genital prolapse with retention of sexual function. *Obstet Gynecol* 1970;36:69–75

42. Todd JW. Mesh suspension for vaginal prolapse. *Int Surg* 1978;63:91–3

43. Vancaillie Th. The role of laparoscopy in the management of pelvic floor relaxation. *J Am Assoc Gynecol Laparosc* 1997;4:147–8

Part 4
Oncology

Borderline tumors of the ovary or epithelial ovarian tumors of borderline malignancy

29

A. Münschke, M. Nisolle and J. Donnez

INTRODUCTION

In 1929, Taylor[1] first described borderline tumors of the ovary (BOT), also known as 'epithelial ovarian tumors of low malignant potential'. These neoplasms occupy a position somewhere between benign and clearly malignant ovarian epithelial tumors. As a consequence of this histological peculiarity, they were recognized as a special, clinical entity by the International Federation of Gynaecologists and Obstetricians (FIGO) and included in its classification in 1971, with the World Health Organization (WHO) following 2 years later.

When compared to the 'classic' malignant ovarian tumor, they are characterized by the following features[2]:

(1) Younger age at time of diagnosis (approximately 10 years earlier);

(2) Earlier stage when first diagnosed (almost 70% of all borderlines are being discovered when still at stage I[3]);

(3) Infrequent and late recurrence (recurrence possibly up to 20 years after surgery);

(4) Excellent long-term survival.

EPIDEMIOLOGY, PROGNOSIS AND RISK FACTORS

Borderline tumors account for approximately 10–15% of all epithelial ovarian cancers in Caucasian populations. Mean age at the time of diagnosis ranges (according to different studies) from 38 to 56 years, which is approximately 10 years younger than in malignant tumors of the ovary[4].

Link and colleagues[3] found, in their review, the following distribution at the time of diagnosis: 69.6% at stage I, 10.3% at stage II, 19.2% at stage III, and 0.6% at stage IV.

The most important pejorative factors are[3,5]:

(1) High FIGO stage;

(2) Greater size;

(3) Pseudomyxoma peritonei;

(4) Patient's age at time of diagnosis;

(5) Presence of a residual mass after surgery;

(6) Ploidy of the tumor: aneuploidy;

(7) High mitotic index;

(8) Cell atypia;

(9) Presence of invasive peritoneal implants.

It appears that women with invasive implants have worse survival rates, and that such tumors behave more typically like malignant ones (with recurrence rates of up to 45% in serous BOTs, if invasive implants are present, and only 4.8% in cases of non-invasive implants[6]). The presence of such implants might be considered as an indication for adjuvant chemotherapy, because of the poor outcome.

Survival

The survival rate depends more on the FIGO stage than on the histological type of the lesion. A review of more than 1000 cases by Massad and colleagues[7] showed the following 5-year survival rates: stage I, 98.1%; stage II, 94.1%; stage III/IV, 79.0%; with an overall survival rate of 94.6%.

Because of the risk of late recurrence inherent in this disease, overall survival at 20 years drops to approximately 80%[3]. It worsens when considering patients with pseudomyxoma peritonei; their 10-year survival rates are estimated to be as low as 40%. The chances of recurrence or persistent disease depend on the FIGO stage and on the nature of the peritoneal implants[3,7,8]. In the same study, Massad and colleagues[7] encountered the following rates: stage I, 2.1 % of recurrence or persistent disease; stage II, 7.1 %; stage III/IV, 14.4 %. Lin and co-workers[8] found 11% recurrence if peritoneal implants were non-invasive (III) and 45% if they were invasive.

Risk factors

The same prognostic factors as for malignant tumors have been evaluated, but they do not all seem to be equally relevant[9]. No relationship has been found with the following parameters:

(1) Family history;

(2) Hormone replacement therapy (HRT);

(3) Menstrual history;

(4) Body mass index (BMI);

(5) Use of intrauterine devices (IUD).

The same protective effects as for invasive cancers have been confirmed[9]:

(1) Pregnancy and birth (relative risk: 0.7);

(2) Breastfeeding (relative risk: 0.5);

(3)   Use of oral contraceptives (relative risk: 0.4).

Infertility and infertility treatment as a risk factor for border-line tumors of the ovary

Borderline tumors are encountered more often in patients who suffer from infertility. As a consequence of this observation, some authors[10–13] initially blamed the infertility treatments. They suggested that the recurrent micro-traumas associated with multiple induced ovulations might be responsible for the higher risk of malignancies. Nevertheless, recent evidence[14,15] shows an equal increase in the incidence of BOT in groups of patients suffering from infertility without any treatment, as in those being treated; furthermore, many BOTs are discovered during infertility work-ups. Therefore, it is possible that an underlying problem of the ovary itself, and not the attempts to bypass this problem, might be the cause of BOT. However, further studies are necessary to prove that ovulation-inducing treatments are not implicated in the genesis of BOT.

HISTOLOGY

Histological criteria used to make the diagnosis of border-line tumors of the ovary include[9]:

(1)   Epithelial budding;

(2)   Multilayered epithelium;

(3)   Mitotic activity;

(4)   Nuclear atypia;

(5)   Absence of any signs of stromal invasion.

To make sure that this last and most important criterion is fulfilled, there must be a close investigation of a large number of slides by an experienced anatomopathologist. Otherwise, the risk of mistaking a BOT for an invasive epithelial cancer, or worse, for a benign cystadenoma, is high.

Different subspecies of BOT: (Hart–Norris–Scully classification)

The most frequent types of tumors of low malignant potential are the serous and mucinous forms. Together, they account for more than 95% of all BOTs and are, therefore, the most widely studied and understood.

Serous BOT

Fifty-five per cent of all BOTs are of the serous subtype (15% of all serous tumors of the ovary being borderline variants). They are often bilateral (38%[8]), cystic, and have a mean diameter between 6 and 12 cm, (which is generally smaller than mucinous BOTs). At the time of diagnosis,

the serous BOT is confined to the ovaries in 75% of all cases. Ascites is uncommonly encountered, at least in the early stages of this disease. The most common lesion is a unilocular cyst, often filled with clear liquid (Figure 1), with microscopic papillary structures bordering the inner walls (Figure 2). These structures are generally covered with low-grade proliferative epithelium (Figure 3).

Exterior vegetations are found more often than in the mucinous BOT, but they do not seem to constitute an unfavorable element. Psammomas may be present, even extensively in some cases.

Recently, some authors[8,16–19] have proposed a subdivision of the serous BOT into two groups: atypical proliferative epithelial cystadenoma, with a benign character, and non-invasive intraepithelial carcinoma, or micropapillary serous carcinoma. This latter form behaves more like a malignant tumor and might benefit from a more aggressive treatment.

Mucinous BOT

The mucinous form accounts for approximately 40% of all borderline tumors. Its spread tends to be limited to one ovary at the time of diagnosis (80–90% of stage I lesions,

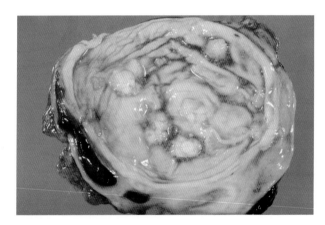

Figure I Several papillomatous foci can be seen inside a borderline cystic serous tumor of the ovary

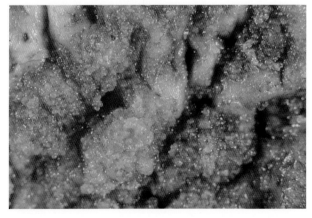

Figure 2 A close-up shows the micropapillary pattern of borderline foci in another cystic serous tumor

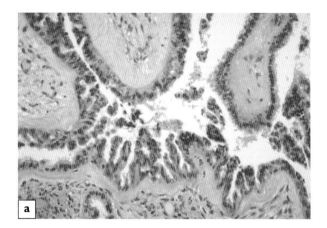

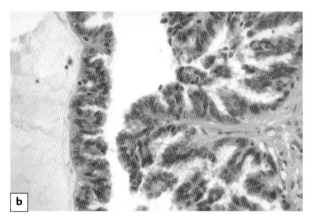

Figure 3 (a) and (b) Papillae covered with low-grade proliferative epithelium showing micropapillary tufting. Note the well-differentiated ciliated cells

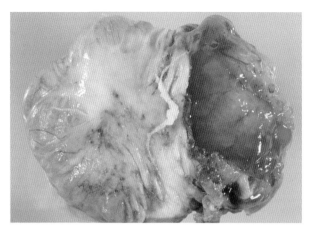

Figure 4 A large borderline tumor of the ovary with its mucinous content extruding through the right opening

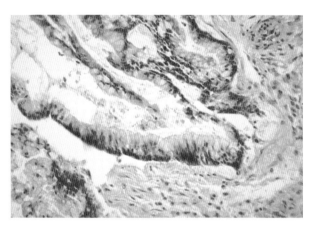

Figure 5 Pseudostratified epithelial lining of the cyst showing hyperchromatic nuclei and several goblet cells

only 5% of bilateral lesions), but these tumors seem to have a greater malignant potential than the serous forms.

Mucinous borderline neoplasms are typically large multilocular cysts (Figure 4), with a mean diameter over 15 cm. Areas of necrosis and hemorrhage can be seen, as well as small papillations or nodules. The presence of surface vegetations is not uncommon, but ascites is rarely present. Histologically, the pseudostratified epithelium shows nuclear atypia (Figure 5).

The presence of stromal invasion (by atypical cells) excludes them by definition from the borderline subgroup, but in some cases mucin can be found dissecting the stroma (pseudomyxoma ovarii).

Mucinous tumors of low malignant potential can be divided into two different subgroups with different histological characteristics: the Müllerian, endocervical type, and the intestinal type.

A particular form is the pseudomyxoma peritoneii. It may occur as a complication in all mucinous neoplasms and is characterized by a more or less chronic form of mucinous ascites with peritoneal implants, producing a gelatinous substance. It is generally associated with a defect in the primary cyst wall, leading to spontaneous spillage.

This condition may lead to abdominal pain or discomfort, and even to bowel obstruction.

A concomitant appendix lesion is often found, especially when pseudomyxoma peritoneii is present. Careful surgical exploration of the appendix is thus necessary, and routine appendectomy should be performed if necessary.

Endometrioid tumors

These tumors are often associated with peritoneal or ovarian endometriosis (in 30–50% of cases). But peritoneal implants can be distinguished from endometriosis by the lack of hemorrhage and endometriotic stroma. Two different subtypes are known. The first develops on an adenofibrous background. The second consists of back-to-back glands and shows no adenofibrous matrix. Both types tend to be cystic and recurrence seems to be infrequent.

Brenner tumors

This very rare variant seems to generally behave as a benign tumor, and stromal invasion is exceptionally infrequent. This BOT is usually cystic and bordered by epithelium formed of several cell layers, resembling a non-invasive papillary urothelial cell carcinoma.

Clear cell tumors

Clear cell tumors are another rare subspecies of borderline tumors, consisting of mostly fibrous tissue with glandular and tubal elements in a one-cell layer epithelium.

Peritoneal implants

If focal invasion is present in the primary ovarian lesion, it should be classified and treated as malignant cancer. On the other hand, the presence of microinvasive implants on the peritoneal surface is often encountered in higher stage disease[18]. The impact on long-term survival is still uncertain with this type of implant, but they seem to constitute one of the most unfavorable elements in disseminated disease[3,6].

Some authors consider these peritoneal lesions not as local metastases but as independent primary lesions. This theory of multifocal disease[20] is supported by the polyclonal origin of these lesions.

DIAGNOSIS

Symptoms

BOTs are responsible for the same clinical symptoms as invasive epithelial cancers[3,15,16]:

(1) Abdominal discomfort or pain;

(2) Abdominal enlargement;

(3) Sensation of an abdominal mass;

(4) Menometrorrhagia.

Many patients have no complaints, and the ovarian mass is detected during a routine check-up, or investigation for an infertility problem. Any newly discovered ovarian mass (mostly cysts) should be carefully evaluated.

Ultrasound scans

The first examination should be a transvaginal ultrasound scan[21]. The proximity of the probe to the ovary allows relatively precise resolution. This examination has high sensitivity (87–95%) if performed by an experienced operator using the latest technology.

Criteria used to evaluate the benign nature of a cyst by ultrasound scan are the following[16]:

(1) The cyst diameter: size below 5 cm suggests a benign nature. A diameter above 10 cm, on the other hand, suggests either a malignant cyst or a benign mucinous cyst.

(2) The homogeneity of the cyst content: a homogeneous content of low echogenicity in a unilocular cyst is in favor of a non-malignant lesion. On the contrary, the presence of hyperechogenic areas and septa is suspect (Figure 6).

(3) The absence of intracystic vegetations: the presence of such vegetations is certainly not proof of malignancy but is at least suspect (Figure 7).

(4) The thickness and regularity of the cyst wall: a cyst with a wall thick enough to be easily visible on ultrasound or computerized tomography (CT) scan is a sign of malignancy (Figure 8). Figure 9 shows the CT scan image of the same patient.

(5) The presence of ascites: the presence of a small amount of ascites in the posterior cul-de-sac can be encountered in physiological circumstances, but a larger volume is suspicious.

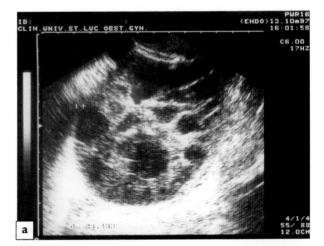

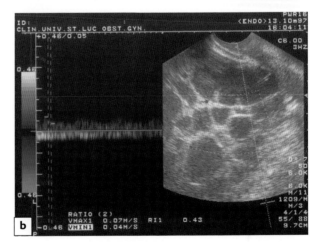

Figure 6 (a) and (b) These echographic images show the presence of a cyst of 83 mm in diameter. No normal ovarian cortex can be seen. Hypo- and hyperechogenic areas are visible, with the presence of septa. The visible vascularization is of venous type, RI 0.43. Histological results proved that this cyst was a mucinous borderline tumor of the ovary

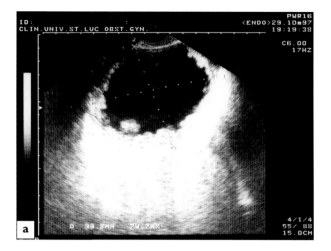

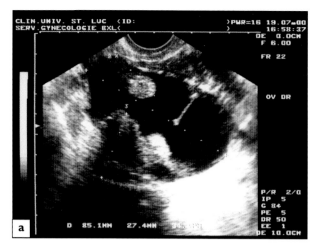

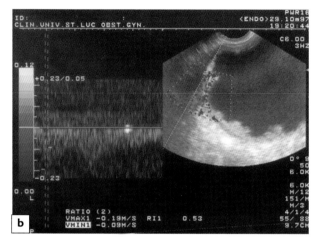

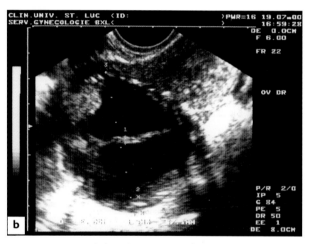

Figure 7 (a) and (b) Right ovary with a serous borderline tumor of the ovary: a cyst with an irregular wall is visible with the presence of multiple vegetations. RI = 0.43/0.53

Figure 8 (a) and (b) These images show a serous borderline tumor of the ovary of 88.5 × 55 mm. The cyst wall is 6.5 mm thick and a heterogeneous area of 34 mm in diameter can be seen. A 2.5 mm-thick septum is also visible

The use of Doppler ultrasound[21] (Figures 6 and 7) allows investigation of intracystic blood flow, a sign of proliferative pathology inside this cyst. Pulsed Doppler analysis can be used to measure flow velocity and resistance index (RI). RI values lower than 0.4 (or 0.5) are considered as abnormal.

CT scans

Further evaluation of the lesion is possible using CT scanning (Figures 10 and 11) with injection of contrast medium. This allows a closer evaluation of the limits of the ovarian mass. Invasion of the surrounding tissue often results in unrecognizable limits. Detection of significant invasion of the omentum and lymph nodes is possible within the bounds of resolution of this technology. The CT scan is, however, an excellent way to evaluate the presence of ascites and metastatic lesions. Therefore, CT evaluation is required for an adequate staging process.

CA-125

CA-125[21], a tumor marker used to investigate and follow invasive carcinoma of the ovary, is only of limited use for early-stage borderline tumors.

High serum levels of CA-125 in stage I serous borderline tumors are relatively uncommon. In some cases (35%), an intermediate value is found (35–100 U/ml). In stage III lesions, elevated levels are encountered more often (89%)[21].

In mucinous borderline tumors of stage I, CA-125 levels are even more frequently below the 35 U/ml limit. Disseminated lesions tend to have higher levels, but not as often as serous tumors.

In all cases, the CA-125 dropped to normal levels after surgical resection of most of the tumor tissue.

The low sensitivity of this test makes it of little use as a diagnostic tool for BOTs on its own. However, it can still be useful in association with other tests and can help to distinguish BOTs from invasive epithelial cancers.

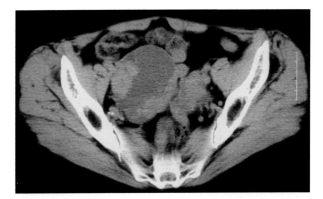

Figure 9 The computerized tomography scan confirmed the echographic findings and showed irregularity of the cyst wall. No calcifications or ascites or lymph node invasions were visible

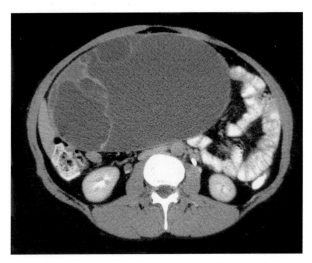

Figure 10 The computerized tomography scan shows a large, hypodense cystic tumor of ovarian origin. Multiple septa can be seen. The cyst wall is, in some areas, thick enough to be easily visible. The suspected mucinous nature of this borderline tumor of the ovary was confirmed later by histological evaluation

Magnetic resonance imaging

Malignant and most borderline tumors are formed of cells containing a higher than normal amount of triglyceride in their membrane. They show a characteristic spectrum in magnetic resonance imaging (MRI). Therefore, MRI is useful for evaluating the potential malignant character of suspect ovarian masses or peritoneal implants of a certain size[9].

Today, there is still no non-invasive technique available that can predict the malignant nature of the lesion with 100% accuracy. The best results are achieved with an association of transvaginal ultrasound scanning, CA-125 levels and intracystic blood flow measurement (sensitivity of over 93%[16,21]). Of course, only microscopic analysis can provide a definitive diagnosis.

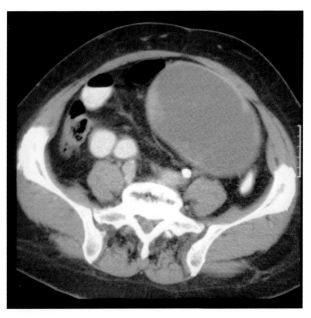

Figure 11 The computerized tomography scan shows a large, cystic ovarian mass. The cyst is bordered by an irregular wall with some vegetations visible. No ascites or lymph nodes can be seen. The mass later proved to be a serous borderline tumor of the ovary

Laparoscopic staging

A laparoscopic procedure allows visual exploration of the abdominal cavity and sample taking, necessary to perform adequate staging[8,9]. Because of the more benign-like behavior of borderline tumors and the absence of effective adjuvant therapy, staging procedures do not need to be as extensive as for malignant ovarian cancers.

Even if lymph node invasion is not uncommon (14–23%), it has no significant impact on survival or recurrence rates[8,22,23], so lymph node sampling does not seem to be an absolute necessity. On the other hand, the search for peritoneal implants, their biopsy and cytological analysis of ascites, if present, are required. Awareness of dissemination of the disease can determine the therapeutic approach of the surgeon and histological analysis of the implants is useful to evaluate whether they are of invasive nature, which is an important negative prognostic factor.

TREATMENT

Surgery

Treatment of invasive epithelial cancer of the ovary includes total hysterectomy, bilateral adnexectomy, removal of the omentum and lymphadenectomy, completed usually by chemotherapy. Because of the excellent prognosis of borderline tumors such extensive treatment is not necessary and a less aggressive approach is generally sufficient[9,16,22,24,25].

The choice of adequate surgical treatment depends on the following factors:

(1) The stage of the disease;

(2) The age of the patient;

(3) A potential desire for pregnancy;

(4) The nature of the peritoneal implants, if present (invasive or non-invasive).

The borderline nature must, of course, be proven, otherwise one cannot decide upon conservative surgery. The only way to ensure a precise diagnosis is histological analysis of the whole tumor by an experienced anatomopathologist.

Stage I lesions

Women of childbearing age

BOTs occur more often in younger women than invasive tumors. Many of these patients have a desire to preserve their fertility. In carefully staged cases with a borderline lesion confined to one ovary, a more conservative treatment is possible.

Unilateral adnexectomy. This operation preserves fertility, leaving one functional ovary and the uterus. Several groups have reported pregnancies after such treatment[9,16,26]. This operation can be performed by laparoscopy. The greatest risks of this procedure are intra-abdominal spillage and contamination of the abdominal wall. The use of a lap-sac and abundant peritoneal lavage might reduce this risk to an acceptable level, if performed by an experienced surgeon. Of course, there is a relatively small risk of recurrence in the contralateral ovary (15%)[24,25].

We, therefore, propose the following security measures:

(1) Close follow-up: frequent transvaginal ultrasound check-ups and controls of CA-125 levels should be performed on a regular basis (every 6–12 months) and over a long period of time because of the late recurrence of this slowly progressive pathology. (Morice and colleagues[26] encountered no recurrence in their study that escaped diagnosis during routine follow-up.)

(2) Removal of the remaining ovary, once childbearing is completed, to reduce the risk of a recurrent contralateral lesion. (Of the nine recurrences after conservative surgery, observed by Morice and colleagues[26], all occurred in the remaining contralateral ovary.)

(3) 'Second-look' laparoscopy should be carried out some time (3–6 months) after the first conservative operation to ensure the absence of residual or recurring disease requiring a complementary procedure.

Re-operation after diagnosis of recurrence is still possible and even another conservative procedure might be possible in some cases. Morice and colleagues[26] reported five cases of second, fertility-sparing operations, without relapse during follow-up. In their study, they found no changes in overall survival rate, even if they encountered higher recurrence rates after conservative management (20.5% versus 5.7% after radical treatment).

Cystectomy. A simple cystectomy might be a tempting solution. It preserves women's fertility better than unilateral adnexectomy because of the removal of less ovarian tissue. The great danger of this option is the risk of leaving behind some malignant cells without noticing.

Therefore, this procedure should only be performed in the following circumstances:

(1) Young patients;

(2) Normal CA-125 levels;

(3) Loosely attached cysts;

(4) No suspicious ultrasound findings;

(5) No other unfavorable factors;

(6) Patient compliance; this important factor should not be overlooked if conservative treatment is considered.

Many borderline tumors are incidental, histological discoveries after cystectomy for a supposed benign cyst with no presurgical suspicion of malignancy. No further, more radical, surgical procedure is generally needed and a very close follow-up should be sufficient if the following criteria are met:

(1) Complete macroscopic exploration of the abdominopelvic cavity has been carried out;

(2) The complete complementary work-up is negative;

(3) The borderline lesion is on the inner side of a cyst;

(4) There are no vegetations on the outer side;

(5) There is enough healthy tissue between the lesion and the surgical section.

The recurrence rates after this type of surgery vary in the literature. Barnhill and colleagues[27] and Gotlieb and colleagues[15] did not find higher recurrence rates, when considering cystectomy versus adnexectomy in carefully selected patients. Morice and colleagues[26], on the other hand, encountered 36.3% of relapse (versus 15.1% after unilateral adnexectomy).

Bilateral adnexectomy or cystectomy. In borderline tumors involving both ovaries, bilateral adnexectomy should be performed, otherwise there is an unacceptably high risk of recurrence. However, in certain cases, incomplete resection of one ovary might be possible (cystectomy or partial adnexectomy). The same precautions as for simple cystectomy apply here. Even in these cases, there might still be a chance for future pregnancy, if the uterus can be spared, using embryo cryopreservation, oocyte cryopreservation or oocyte donation.

Embryo cryopreservation. In some cases, an *in vitro* fertilization (IVF) procedure might be performed[28], before the surgical removal of both ovaries. This is, of course, only possible in borderline pathology; for women suffering from malignant cancer, this approach is too dangerous. Indeed a delay in treatment for at least 2 months of IVF cycles with high hormone levels can lead to further, life-threatening growth of a malignant tumor. BOTs generally develop slowly enough to justify a certain delay before surgery.

Embryos obtained in this way can be frozen for later implantation after treatment or, in some carefully selected cases, pregnancy can even be continued until delivery, under strict surveillance[28]. This procedure is, of course, not possible for women without a male partner and cases requiring urgent treatment must be recognized and treated properly.

Ovarian cryopreservation. Another way of preserving a patient's fertility might be ovarian cortex cryopreservation, even if the thawing process remains problematic with today's technology. There are two possible uses for banking ovarian tissue[28–30]. A first possibility is autotransplantation of the ovarian cortex, after complete and lasting recovery. A potential risk of this procedure is, of course, the possible grafting of malignant cells and the resulting relapse. This risk is considered to be very low in BOTs, if the area where the biopsy was taken has been chosen carefully and if histological analysis has been performed. An advantage of this procedure would be the presence of functional ovarian tissue, with its hormone secretion. Exogenous hormone therapy might, therefore, not be necessary. Another option is the isolation of oocytes, contained in the frozen cortex. Theoretical *in vitro* maturation and IVF procedures may then later be proposed. This procedure rules out the risk of grafting cancer cells back into the patient[29,30].

In case of adnexectomy for a unilateral BOT, it might be interesting to remove, during first-look surgery, part of the contralateral ovarian cortex for cryopreservation. The chances of recurrence are real and, as shown by the case reports, might affect the whole remaining ovary, compromising the survival of enough oocytes to perform effective cryopreservation[28]. Gynecologists should, therefore, propose this procedure early in borderline pathologies, even if conservative surgery seems possible. This might help to preserve fertility, even if further treatment is necessary due to recurrence of the initial tumor.

Oocyte donation. This is the last option offering patients a chance of childbearing after bilateral adnexectomy. This procedure should, of course, only be applied if, for any reason, no other option was possible. Chances of success are even lower, but pregnancy still remains possible.

Postmenopausal period

In elderly women, bilateral adnexectomy should be sufficient for lesions confined to the ovary. A total hysterectomy for low-stage disease, as proposed by some authors, seems to be more aggressive than necessary; this type of operation causes higher morbidity and there is still no evidence of any improvement in survival rates when compared to adnexectomy.

Lesions of stage II or higher

One of the most unfavorable factors is the presence of residual malignant tissue after surgery. Therefore, lesions with intra-abdominal extension should be treated more aggressively than localized stages. Total hysterectomy with bilateral adnexectomy is generally proposed with resection of the omentum and generous peritoneal lavage. This procedure should be performed by laparotomy to reduce the risk of contamination and assure complete removal of all malignant tissue. Sometimes, in carefully selected cases of young women, the uterus can be spared (after bilateral salpingo-oophorectomy and omentectomy). The treatment might be completed by adjuvant chemotherapy.

Pseudomyxoma peritoneii

This particular form of disseminated mucinous BOT requires frequently repeated surgical removal of as much tumor tissue and mucous ascites as possible. The prognosis of this form is relatively poor, when compared to simple mucinous BOT, even after optimal surgical management.

Because of the frequent association between appendix lesions and pseudomyxoma peritoneii, removal of the appendix should be performed.

ADJUVANT TREATMENT

There is still no consensus on the need to perform adjuvant treatment (mostly cyclophosphamide and carboplatin) in cases of high-stage lesions[3,20,22,27]. There is no evidence of longer disease-free survival or better long-term survival. Yet, there might be a subgroup of patients who could benefit from such treatment because of the presence of negative prognostic factors such as invasive peritoneal implants or aneuploidy[6,17]. Clinical research may confirm this in future studies.

HORMONE REPLACEMENT THERAPY AFTER SURGERY

There is no clinical evidence of any adverse effect of hormone replacement therapy. Therefore, such treatment should be administered to prevent the known negative side-effects (higher cardiovascular risks, osteoporosis) of the lack of endogenous estrogen[9].

FERTILITY

Because of the young age of many patients with borderline tumors, fertility-sparing treatment has been proposed by some surgeons for low-stage disease. This type of procedure (mostly unilateral salpingo-oophorectomy) allows childbearing in younger patients even if the loss of half the oocyte reserve might reduce their fertility. Several authors have reported normal pregnancies after surgery without any complications (22 pregnancies in 15 patients out of 39[15]). Some cases of successful IVF have recently been reported after conservative surgery in young women, who subsequently gave birth to normal babies[26,31]. The safety of ovarian stimulation after conservative surgery is still a matter of debate. Several authors reported no recurrence after stimulation in their series[26], but, because of the theoretical risk of relapse, this sort of treatment should be reserved for low-stage disease, and the number of IVF cycles should be limited.

This shows that conservative treatment in carefully chosen cases might be worth the risk. Because of the small numbers of patients treated this way in the different studies, it is difficult to conduct a statistical analysis of the remaining fertility of these women, especially because of the higher rate of infertility in borderline groups (13% of infertility[15] before diagnosis). Whether this is a consequence or cause of the borderline tumor is still controversial. The implication of ovulation-inducing drugs in the genesis of this pathology is still unproven and some authors blame the underlying infertility more than its treatment.

CASE REPORTS

A 19-year-old single woman underwent unilateral, laparoscopic adnexectomy (with use of a lap-sac) for a cystic lesion with a diameter of 12 cm. Histological analysis confirmed the diagnosis of a serous borderline tumor. Second-look laparoscopy was performed 6 months later to assess the absence of residual or recurrent disease. No suspect lesions were encountered and even the biopsy, taken from the remaining ovary, showed only normal ovarian tissue. Surprisingly, 4 months later, during a transvaginal ultrasound check-up, an ovarian cyst of 9 cm in diameter was discovered. During a third laparoscopic procedure, the remaining ovary was removed in a lap-sac. Histological analysis revealed the presence of another borderline tumor. The well-informed patient accepted ovarian tissue cryopreservation as a chance of maintaining her fertility. Unfortunately, the remaining ovarian cortex was already very thin due to distortion by the large cyst.

Histological examination of the cortex failed to show the presence of oocytes, but the tissue has been stored for further use nevertheless.

A 28-year-old married, nulliparous woman underwent unilateral salpingo-oophorectomy for a serous BOT (suggested by frozen slide analysis during surgery and confirmed later by complete histological analysis). Peritoneal biopsies were taken, along with a biopsy of the contralateral ovary. No other lesions were found. Three months later, a 1.2-cm cyst was discovered on the remaining ovary by transvaginal ultrasound scan. Because of the possibility of a contralateral relapse of the BOT, requiring another surgical procedure, it was decided to perform an IVF attempt as fast as possible under close surveillance. In order to confirm the diagnosis of an intraovarian tumor and prepare for the IVF, gonadotropin releasing hormone agonist was administered for 3 months. The cyst persisted at the same size and it was decided to start the IVF cycles. Pregnancy was obtained after two stimulation cycles. During the first 3 months of pregnancy, no modification of the cyst was visible. Later, evaluation by ultrasound scanning became impossible. Delivery was performed by Cesarean section for obstetric reasons. Surgical exploration during the same procedure only revealed a macroscopically normal-looking ovary, but ultrasound scan showed a persisting cyst of 1.2 cm. The patient insisted on preserving at least part of her ovary, so partial ovariectomy was carried out (with complete removal of the tumor, of course). During this procedure, a biopsy of the remaining ovarian cortex was taken for cryopreservation, because of the risk of recurrence and further surgery. One year later, a second, spontaneous pregnancy led to the birth of another healthy baby. The patient did not desire any further pregnancy, so we performed a resection of the remaining ovary 2 months later. No relapse has been noted so far (follow-up: 3 years).

A 15-year-old girl suffered from acute pelvic pain caused by ovarian torsion. Vaginal echography during work-up also revealed a cystic lesion of the right ovary, measuring 8 cm in diameter, showing intracystic vegetations. A laparoscopic procedure was performed to reverse the torsion and a cystectomy was carried out. Histological analysis revealed a serous borderline tumor within the cyst. The patient underwent another laparoscopic procedure to check for residual or contralateral disease. A right salpingo-oophorectomy was performed and contralateral biopsies of the left ovary were taken. Histological results came up negative. After obtaining informed consent from the patient and her parents, cryopreservation of one of the biopsies was performed, in order to assure fertility in case of later recurrence.

A nulliparous woman, aged 19 years, underwent diagnostic laparoscopy after the ultrasonic discovery of two bilateral ovarian cysts, with diameters of 6 cm and 5.3 cm. Intracystic vegetations were noted during echography. During the surgical procedure, multiple peritoneal implants were discovered on the omentum and in the posterior cul-de-sac. Biopsies were taken and histological analysis revealed a multifocal serous borderline tumor (FIGO stage II). The patient was then referred to our institution for further treatment. We performed bilateral adnexectomy and omentectomy by laparotomy (Figure 12). Further analysis revealed a genetic aberration of the *p53* gene in this tumor. CA-125 levels dropped from 2434 U/ml before surgery to 19.3 and stayed below 20 during follow-up. After interdisciplinary discussion, the decision was made to complete the surgical treatment with chemotherapy, because of the advanced stage and the young age of the patient. Six cycles of Carboplatin® (Faulding Pharmaceuticals, Belgium) and Taxol® (Bristol-Myers Squibb, Belgium) were administered. During follow-up, another diagnostic laparoscopy was performed 8 months later. No relapse of the initial pathology was noted, only the presence of three white peritoneal lesions, which proved to be of non-malignant nature. Because of the disease-free status, hormone replacement therapy was administered using Livial® (Organon, Belgium). Due to the aggressive nature of this BOT, the patient is still under close surveillance. CA-125 measurements and ultrasound check-ups are performed every 2 months and another laparoscopy is scheduled in 6–9 months. Future fertility-restoring treatment by oocyte donation has already been discussed with the patient.

During an infertility work-up, an ovarian cyst was discovered in a 35-year-old nulliparous patient. The cyst measured 7 cm in diameter when removed by laparoscopic adnexectomy. The definitive histological diagnosis was a serous borderline tumor. A second laparoscopic procedure was carried out 4 weeks later, in our institution, to perform multiple biopsies of the peritoneum and the remaining ovary. Resection of an additional endometriotic nodule of the rectovaginal septum was also carried out. During the operation, a small ovarian cyst of 1.5 cm was discovered. It contained mucinous fluid and papillary vegetations. Analysis of frozen slides suggested a contralateral relapse of the initial borderline pathology, which was confirmed

later. Because of the antecedent of unilateral salpingo-oophorectomy, the decision was made to perform a cystectomy. Additional biopsies of the ovarian section were taken and ovarian cortex was removed for cryopreservation. No further progression of this borderline disease has been noted so far.

RESULTS

We performed a retrospective analysis of patients treated in our hospital for borderline tumors over the past 15 years.

Patients

Fifty-one patients underwent surgical procedures for borderline pathology of the ovary. The mean age in our population was 52.2 years (± 19.3 years) with a range from 19 to 90 years. Fifteen (29.4%) of these patients were under 40 years of age.

In the subgroup of patients who underwent conservative surgery, the mean age was, of course, lower, ranging from 20 to 37 years, with a mean age of 27.2 years (± 5.6 years).

Patient distribution according to FIGO stage can be seen in Table 1.

Histology

Mucinous borderline tumors accounted for 47.1% of all tumors (24 cases). All but one (95.8%) were stage I lesions (70.8% stage Ia, 8.3% Ib, 8.3% Ic, and 8.3% not clearly specified stage I). One lesion was stage III (4.2%) and one case of pseudomyxoma peritoneii was found.

Serous borderline tumors were encountered in 25 cases (49.0%). Of these BOTs, 21 (84.0%) were stage I (Ia

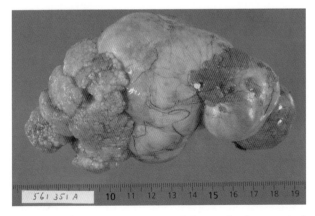

Figure 12 A cystic ovary, removed during the first surgical procedure. Papillary vegetations and neovascularization can be seen on the outer surface of the ovary

Table 1 Patient classification according to FIGO stage. Prevalence of conservative and radical treatment in a series of 51 women

FIGO stage	Total	Conservative treatment	Radical treatment
Stage I total	46 (90.2%)	9 (90%)	37 (90.2%)
a	31 (60.8%)	7 (70%)	24 (58.5%)
b	7 (13.7%)	1 (10%)	6 (14.6%)
c	4 (7.8%)	1 (10%)	3 (7.3%)
unknown	4 (7.8%)	0 (0%)	4 (9.8%)
Stage II	2 (3.9%)	1 (10%)	1 (2.4%)
Stage III	3 (5.9%)	0 (0%)	3 (7.3%)
Total	51	10	41

52.0%, Ib 20.0%, Ic 4.0%, Ix 8.0%). Two patients suffered from stage II disease (8.0%) and two cases of stage III disease (8.0%) were encountered.

One patient had a stage Ia mixed (serous–mucinous) tumor (1.9%) and one stage Ic endometrioid BOT was discovered (1.9%).

Treatment

Surgery

Forty-one (80.4%) women underwent a radical treatment, defined as bilateral adnexectomy and hysterectomy. Omentectomy was generally associated. Of course, none of these procedures was carried out by laparoscopy.

In ten patients (19.6%), conservative, fertility-sparing treatment was performed. This group accounted for 66.6% of all women aged under 40 years in our population. As conservative treatment, the following procedures were considered:

(1) Unilateral cystectomy (one patient, 10%);

(2) Unilateral adnexectomy (seven patients, 70%);

(3) Unilateral adnexectomy and contralateral cystectomy (two patients, 20%);

(4) Bilateral cystectomy (no patients in our series, 0%).

Omentectomy was performed in three of ten cases (30%). Four out of ten procedures were performed by laparoscopy (40%).

Chemotherapy

Chemotherapy was added systematically in 13 out of 51 cases (25.5%). These included one case of conservative management and one case of pseudomyxoma peritoneii. One relapse in a patient who underwent conservative surgery was treated with adjuvant chemotherapy.

Recurrence

After radical treatment, there were no recurrences in our series. One patient, who died from recurrent, progressive disease, was ruled out of our study because of the presence of focal invasive carcinoma, shown after complete examination of the removed ovary.

In the conservatively treated cohort, two patients (20%) suffered relapse, one of them twice (Table 2). In the first patient, recurrence occurred 1 year after the initial surgical procedure, a unilateral adnexectomy, associated with a contralateral cystectomy. Six cycles of chemotherapy were administered (Carboplatin®, Faulding Pharmaceuticals, Belgium and Endoxan®, Asta Medica, Belgium). This patient remained disease-free for another 6 years. Then a second relapse was diagnosed and an extended hysterectomy with omentectomy was performed, completed by another six cycles of adjuvant therapy

Table 2 Recurrence rates among patients after either conservative or radical treatment

Treatment	n	Patients with recurrent disease (%)	Disease-related death (%)
Conservative	10	2 (20%)	0 (0%)
Radical	41	0 (0%)	0 (0%)

(Cisplatine Efeka®, AHP Pharma, Belgium and Taxol®, Bristol-Myers Squibb, Belgium). No further recurrence has been noted during follow-up.

The second patient with recurrent disease (see second case report) was initially treated by unilateral adnexectomy. A small cystic lesion was noted 1 year later, during infertility work-up. A partial adnexectomy was performed several months later, following pregnancy achieved 2 months after diagnosis. After a second spontaneous pregnancy, the remaining ovarian tissue was removed to reduce the risk of further relapse as the patient did not desire further pregnancy. No recurrence has been noted so far (3 years of follow-up).

Survival

No disease-related deaths occurred in our series, either in the conservatively treated group, or after radical procedures. The only deaths we can report occurred in borderline diseases, excluded from our study because of the presence of focal invasive carcinoma in the ovaries.

Fertility

In the group treated by conservative surgery, six pregnancies occurred in four patients (one after a second conservative surgical procedure for recurrent disease). No disease recurrence was noted after pregnancy (Table 3).

One patient presented with a fertility problem after treatment. Ovarian stimulation was carried out using Clomide® (Hoechst Marion Roussel, Belgium) without success.

It is difficult to estimate the real rate of infertility in this group of patients. The pregnancies obtained in four patients probably underestimate the remaining fertility potential in this group. This is because of the short follow-up of three patients treated recently (end of 1999 and mid-2000). Nothing is known about the desire for pregnancy in four of the women.

Nevertheless, these results show that childbearing is possible in a considerable number of cases, after conservative treatment, without affecting survival rates (40% of all women treated conservatively or 66% of women with a known desire for pregnancy).

Table 3 Fertility outcome in conservatively treated women ($n = 10$, mean age 27.2 years)

	Number of patients	%
Conservative treatment	10	100
Infertility work-up before diagnosis	1	10
Known desire for pregnancy	6	60
Pregnant patients	4/6	66.6
total pregnancies	6	
total deliveries	6	
Recurrent disease	2	20
before pregnancy	2	20
after pregnancy	0	0

Comparison with other studies

Morice and colleagues[26] came to similar conclusions in their recent study. They studied 174 cases, treated in their institution over the last 32 years. The mean age of their patients was 42.3 years (± 15.8 years). The subgroup treated conservatively was, on average, older than the patients we selected for conservative surgery (mean age: 32 years versus 27 years in our series).

In their series, conservative treatment was performed in 49 patients (28%) and consisted of unilateral adnexectomy (38 cases, 77.6%), unilateral adnexectomy and contralateral cystectomy (five cases, 10.2%), unilateral cystectomy (five cases, 10.2%), bilateral cystectomy (one case, 2.0%). Additional treatment was given in several cases: namely, omentectomy (20 cases, 40.8%), pelvic or para-aortic lymphadenectomy (four cases, 8.2%), chemotherapy (four cases, 8.2%).

The recurrence rates encountered after radical treatment (5.7%) were significantly lower than after fertility-sparing treatment (20.5%). Even if we did not perform lymphadenectomy in any of our patients, we observed approximately the same recurrence rates after conservative management in our study (20%).

The highest recurrence rates were observed after cystectomy (36.3% versus 15.1% after unilateral adnexectomy), suggesting that this procedure should only be performed in carefully selected cases and only if close surveillance can be assured.

Despite the more frequent relapse after conservative treatment, they found no tumor-related deaths in this group. Therefore, no negative effect on the survival rates of these women could be demonstrated.

Seventeen pregnancies were observed in 14 (28%) women out of 49 who underwent fertility-sparing surgery.

Table 4 Management of borderline tumor of the ovary (BOT) in young women

Stage I tumors
Vaginal echography
    presence of intracystic vegetations
Laparoscopy
    papillary vegetation biopsy
        $\Rightarrow$ frozen slide analysis
        $\Rightarrow$ suspicion of BOT
Unilateral salpingo-oophorectomy*
    + contralateral biopsies
        $\Rightarrow$ histology
        $\Rightarrow$ cryopreservation
    + peritoneal biopsies
Histological confirmation of the borderline nature
    $\Rightarrow$ if stage I confirmed $\rightarrow$ surveillance

Stage II or higher tumors
Bilateral adnexectomy + omentectomy $\pm$ hysterectomy
In some cases, adjuvant chemotherapy should be administered
        $\Rightarrow$ second-look laparoscopy and re-evaluation
        $\Rightarrow$ CA-125 and ultrasound surveillance

* Cystectomy should only be performed in carefully chosen cases

All but two were spontaneous pregnancies; the other two were obtained after ovarian stimulation. Infertility problems after surgery were observed in another four (8.2%) cases. Nothing is known about the desire for pregnancy of the other 31 patients.

The birth rates observed in our series were higher (40% versus 28.6%). A possible explanation for this might be the younger age of our patients or stricter criteria applied in selecting women for conservative surgery.

However, one must bear in mind that fertility estimation remains difficult because nothing is known about the desire for pregnancy in a significant number of patients in both studies (40% in our series and 62.3% in Morice's study).

In conclusion, suggested management for BOT in young women is given in Table 4.

ACKNOWLEDGEMENT

We especially thank Dr Marbaix and his colleagues in the Department of Anatomopathology of the Catholic University of Louvain, Cliniques Universitaires St. Luc, for providing the illustrations and for useful advice.

REFERENCES

1. Taylor HC. Malignant and semimalignant tumors of the ovary. *Surg Gynecol Obstet* 1929;48:204

2. Morrow CP, Curtin JP, Townsend DE. *Synopsis of Gynecologic Oncology*, 4th edn. New York: Churchill Livingstone, 1993

3. Link CJ, Reed E, Sarosy G, *et al*. Borderline ovarian tumors. *Am J Med* 1996;101:217–25

4. Auranen A, Grénman S, Mäkinen J, *et al*. Borderline ovarian tumors in Finland: epidemiology and familial occurrence. *Am J Epidemiol* 1996;144:548–53

5. Trope CG, Kristensen G, Makar A. Surgery for borderline tumors of the ovary. *Semin Surg Oncol* 2000;19:69–75

6. Gershenson DM, Silvia EG, Levy L, *et al*. Ovarian serous borderline tumors with invasive peritoneal implants. *Cancer* 1998;15:1096–103

7. Massad LSJ, Hunter VJ, Szpak CA, *et al*. Epithelial ovarian cancers of low malignant potential. *Obstet Gynecol* 1991;78:1027–32

8. Lin PS, Gershenson DM, Bevers MW, *et al*. The current status of surgical staging of ovarian serous tumors. *Cancer* 1999;85:905–11

9. Markmann M, Hoskins WJ. *Cancer of the Ovary*. New York: Raven Press, 1993

10. Goldberg GL, Runowicz CD. Ovarian carcinoma of low malignant potential, infertility and induction of ovulation: is there a link? *Am J Obstet Gynecol* 1992;166:853–4

11. Atlas M, Meriger J. Massive hyperstimulation and borderline malignancy carcinoma of the ovary: a possible association. *Acta Obstet Gynecol Scand* 1982;61:261–3

12. Parazzini F, Negri E, La Vecchia C. Treatment for fertility and risk of ovarian tumors of borderline malignancy. *Gynecol Oncol* 1998;68:226–8

13. Grimbizi G, Tarlatzis BC, Bontis J, *et al*. Two cases of ovarian tumors in women who had undergone multiple ovarian stimulation attempts. *Hum Reprod* 1995;10:520–3

14. Mosyard BJ, Lindegaard O, Kjaer S. Ovarian stimulation and borderline tumors: a case control study. *Fertil Steril* 1998;70:1049–55

15. Gotlieb WH, Flikker S, Davidson B, *et al*. Borderline tumors of the ovary: fertility treatment, conservative management, and pregnancy outcome. *Cancer* 1998;82:141–6

16. Nicoloso E, d'Ercole C, Boubli L, *et al*. Tumeurs borderline et cancer de l'ovaire: evaluation coelichirurgicale. *Presse Méd* 1995;24:1421–4

17. Seidman JD, Kurman RJ. Subclassification of serous borderline tumors of the ovary into benign and malignant types. *Am J Surg Pathol* 1996;20:1331–45

18. Prat J. Ovarian tumors of borderline malignancy (tumors of low malignant potential): a critical appraisal. *Adv Anat Pathol* 1999;6:247–274

19. Lawrence WD. The borderland between benign and malignant surface epithelial ovarian tumors: current controversy over the nature and nomenclature of 'borderline' ovarian tumors. *Cancer* 1995;76:2138–42

20. Kehoe S, Powell J. Long-term follow up of women with borderline ovarian tumors. *Int J Gynecol Obstet* 1996;53:139–43

21. Gotlieb WH, Soriano D, Achiron R, *et al*. CA-125 measurement and ultrasonography in borderline tumors of the ovary. *Am J Obstet Gynecol* 2000;183:541–6

22. Kennedy AW, Hart WR. Ovarian papillary serous tumors of low malignant potential (serous borderline tumors). *Cancer* 1996;78:278–86

23. Laeke JF, Currie JL, Rosenshein NB, *et al*. Long-term follow-up of serous ovarian tumors: a case control study. *Gynecol Oncol* 1992;47:150–8

24. Gershenson DM. Contemporary treatment of borderline ovarian tumors. *Cancer Invest* 1999;17:206–10

25. Trope C, Kaern J. Management of borderline tumors of the ovary: state of the art. *Semin Oncol* 1998;25:372–80

26. Morice P, Camatte S, El Hassan J, *et al*. Clinical outcomes and fertility after conservative treatment of ovarian borderline tumors. *Fertil Steril* 2001;75:92–6

27. Barnhill DR, Kurman RJ, Brady MF, *et al*. Preliminary analysis of the behavior of stage I ovarian serous tumors of low malignant potential: a Gynecologic Oncology Group Study. *J Clin Oncol* 1995;13:2752–6

28. Donnez J, Bassil S. Indications for cryopreservation of ovarian tissue. *Hum Reprod Update* 1998;4:248–59

29. Aubard Y, Newton H, Oktay K, *et al*. Follicle freezing and autografting. A new method of medically assisted procreation? *Presse Méd* 1996;25:921–3

30. Oktay K, Newton H, Aubard Y, *et al*. Cryopreservation of immature human oocytes and ovarian tissue: an emerging technology? *Fertil Steril* 1998;69:1-7

31. Hoffman JS, Laird L, Benadiva C, *et al*. *In vitro* fertilization following conservative management of stage 3 borderline tumor of the ovary. *Gynecol Oncol* 1999;74:515–18

Gonadal cryopreservation in the young patient with gynecological malignancy

30

J. Donnez, J.P. Qu, O. De Hertogh and M. Nisolle

INTRODUCTION

Advances in the diagnosis and treatment of childhood, adolescent and adult cancer have greatly enhanced the life expectancy of premenopausal women with cancer. As a result, there is a growing population of adolescent and adult long-term survivors of childhood malignancies[1]. For the majority of women, ovarian damage caused by radiotherapy and/or chemotherapy will result in premature menopause.

Sperm or oocyte cryopreservation, therefore, has important applications in the field of oncological medicine. Because it halts the cell's biological rhythm, cryopreservation has already been extensively applied to fertilized oocytes at pronucleate or embryo stages. This process, widely used in *in vitro* fertilization (IVF) programs, is also applied for sperm cryopreservation. Although the first pregnancy consequent upon the fertilization of a frozen–thawed oocyte was reported in 1986[2], and the first live birth in 1987[3], there have only been a few further pregnancies resulting from the fertilization of cryopreserved oocytes[4–7]. The reason for the poor results of oocyte cryopreservation has been linked to spindle damage and, hence, to chromosomal abnormalities[8], the pathogenesis of oocytes[9], zona hardening and low oocyte survival rates after thawing[8]. Oocyte cryopreservation is still at the experimental stage; it cannot be considered yet as a routine option for female patients before chemo- and radiotherapy. Embryo cryopreservation, however, is a routine procedure in all IVF units. Before cancer treatment, patients can undergo IVF and embryos can then be cryopreserved. However, this is not an ideal solution because superovulation is needed, it is time-consuming and not without unpleasant side-effects. Moreover, some patients may be without a male partner.

Recently, following the success of animal experiments[10,11], reports have been published about ovarian tissue cryopreservation for such patients[12–14]. Storage of ovarian tissue may provide a means of restoring long-term fertility to patients undergoing treatment that may irreversibly damage the oocyte population. Also, tissue obtained before any systemic or local treatment may provide more security with regard to genetic abnormalities for future offspring[15–18]. There are a number of possible motives for banking ovarian tissue. First, it could be performed with a view to autotransplantation at a later date. Second, it could be a means of storing oocytes prior to their isolation and maturation *in vitro*. However, there are still considerable technical and biological hurdles to overcome, principally in the field of follicular maturation.

INDICATIONS FOR CRYOPRESERVATION IN THE CASE OF GYNECOLOGICAL MALIGNANCY

In this field, there has been no major modification since our review published in 1998[19] (Table 1).

In the case of gynecological malignancies, a conservative fertility approach is only valuable if the uterus can be spared during surgery. This includes cases of early cervical carcinoma[20], early vaginal carcinoma[21], ovarian tumors of low malignancy[22] and some selected cases of unilateral

Table 1 Indications for cryopreservation of ovarian tissue in cases of malignant disease

---

Extrapelvic diseases

Bone cancer (osteosarcoma – Ewing sarcoma)

Thyroid, kidney cancers

Breast cancer

Melanoma

Neuroblastoma

Bowel malignancy

Pelvic diseases

Non-gynecological malignancy

    pelvic sarcoma

    sarcoblastoma

    rhabdomyosarcoma

    sacral tumors

    rectosigmoid tumors

Gynecological malignancy

    early cervical carcinoma

    early vaginal carcinoma

    early vulvar carcinoma

    selected cases of ovarian carcinoma (stage IA1)

    ovarian borderline tumors

Systemic disease

    Hodgkin's disease

    non-Hodgkin's lymphoma

    leukemia

    melanoblastoma

---

ovarian carcinoma (stage IA1)[19,23]. The choice of a possible conservative surgical approach in these patients, and the issue of implementing such treatment alone, remain controversial, and all the results were obtained on the basis of retrospective studies and/or case reports. The fertility outcome is conditioned by the adjuvant therapy, i.e. local radiotherapy and/or chemotherapy. For chemotherapy, the risk appears to be dose- and age-dependent[24-27]. Complete amenorrhea was reported after a dose of 5 g of cyclophosphamide in women over 40 years of age, and after doses of 9 g and 20 g, respectively, in women of 30–40 and 20–30 years of age[28].

A combination of many chemotherapeutic agents increases the gonadal toxicity.

For radiotherapy, it has already been stated that a dose of 5–20 Gy administered to the ovary is sufficient to completely impair gonadal function[29,30], whatever the age of the patient. Even if ovarian transposition has been performed, this cannot be considered completely safe because patients receive infradiaphragmatic irradiation[31] and, in many cases, there is an association between radio- and chemotherapy[31,32].

Ovarian tissue cryobanking offers two advantages: the possibility of removing both ovaries for more accurate management and the possibility of administering pelvic radiation in selected cases for the completion of treatment. There are other possible indications but the practitioner should be aware of the effect of radiotherapy on the uterus, and also that such patients may not be good candidates for ovarian tissue grafting. Future experiments should enable us to answer questions about the relevance of replacing residual malignant cells with grafted tissue in such cases.

OVARIAN TISSUE CRYOPRESERVATION, THAWING AND FOLLICULAR MATURATION

In order to achieve a pregnancy after cryopreservation, it is essential to obtain acceptable rates of oocyte survival after the freeze–thawing process.

Oocyte survival after cryopreservation

The primordial follicle is the earliest form of ovarian follicle, consisting of an oocyte surrounded by a single layer of pregranulosa cells[33]. These follicles are located in the cortex of the ovary, and progressively enter the next phase of development under an unknown initiation signal. Only a few follicles develop to the Graafian follicle stage, when they are able to ovulate. The mechanism involved in the recruitment of primordial follicles to pre-antral follicles is unclear. It may require the presence of a factor secreted by the ovary or an extragonadal source, which selectively causes some primordial follicles to enter the growth phase while keeping the others quiescent.

Primordial follicles are more abundant in the ovary and are thus a more appropriate source for cryopreservation. Lass and colleagues[34] demonstrated that primary-stage and secondary-stage follicles represent only 8% and 4%, respectively, of the total number of follicles in the ovarian cortex. Only a little is known about the effect of freezing on the primordial follicle and its further maturation and development after cryopreservation.

A cryoprotectant is essential to minimize ice formation, to ensure the survival of ovarian tissue after freezing and thawing. Newton and colleagues[11] demonstrated that cryopreservation with ethylene glycol or dimethyl sulfoxide produced survival rates of 84% and 74% of the follicles, respectively, compared to only 44% with propylene glycol and 10% with glycerol in frozen–thawed ovarian tissue grafted into the renal capsule of severe combined immunodeficient (SCID) mice. The extent of follicular survival was presumed to be partly related to the speed of cryoprotectant permeation in ovarian tissue specimens[35].

Recently, Gook and co-workers[9] demonstrated that the incidence of oocyte abnormalities encountered on histological analysis was significantly higher at high cooling rates than low.

Thus, primordial follicles constitute the most realistic source for cryopreservation and later use because these follicles are the most abundant and survive the cryopreservation process at a rate of 70–80%.

Effect of cryopreservation on thawing of primordial follicles

Only a little is known about the effect of freezing on the primordial follicle and its further maturation and development after cryopreservation. Even if Porcu and colleagues[6], describing the first birth of a healthy female using a combination of mature oocyte cryopreservation and intracytoplasmic sperm injection (ICSI), demonstrated that cryopreservation of mature oocytes could be an alternative to ovarian tissue cryopreservation, and, even if there are advantages of storing isolated follicles at low temperatures, the use of slices of ovarian cortex may be another practicable method for storing human follicles[36,37]. The storage of primordial-stage follicles seems to be better because these germ cells are more abundant. Oocytes in primordial follicles are far smaller than at metaphase II, less differentiated, possessing fewer organelles and lacking a zona pellucida and cortical granules. All these characteristics render them less susceptible to adverse effects of low temperature storage. In all these studies, however, no attention has been paid to analyzing the stromal tissue. In a recent study, Nisolle and colleagues[38] tried to evaluate the follicular density, the fibrosis and the angiogenesis in the graft, comparing transplantation with human fresh cortical slices and human frozen–thawed slices.

Evaluation after cryopreservation

According to a recent paper[39], each square millimeter of ovarian surface in women aged approximately 30 years contains 35 primordial follicles. By comparing the follicular density (number of primordial and primary follicles/mm^2 of ovarian tissue) in fresh and frozen–thawed cortical slices, Nisolle and colleagues[38] did not observe any significant decrease after cryopreservation. They also investigated the distribution of follicles in fragments of human ovarian tissue before and after cryopreservation. A great variation in follicular distribution in ovarian tissue was observed between individual patients and also between different fragments obtained from the same patient. They also found that primordial follicles were distributed predominantly in the ovary (78–82%), that primary follicles were sparsely scattered and that secondary follicles could only be found occasionally.

Using electronmicroscopy, Oktay and colleagues[40,41] demonstrated that the majority of cells lacked ultrastructural signs of damage after isolation and cryopreservation. In contrast, in another study[38], frozen–thawed human ovarian tissue in some cases revealed follicles which appeared to be degenerating, being largely vacuolated and, in other cases, revealed follicles showing well-preserved structures. It must be emphasized that secondary follicles showed signs of degeneration, such as lysis of the nuclear matrix and fragmentation of the cytoplasm, more frequently than did primordial follicles.

Evaluation after transplantation

Ovarian xenografts in immunodeficient mice are useful models for testing follicular viability and development. Candy and colleagues[35] demonstrated that freezing and thawing do not substantially damage marmoset ovarian tissue and that the cryopreserved tissue retains its ability to support the development of large antral follicles after transfer beneath the kidney capsules of immunodeficient mice. In the study of Nisolle and co-workers[38], the follicular density was found to be significantly lower in transplanted ovarian tissue than in fresh ovarian tissue. Their results confirm that cryopreservation itself is not responsible for the decreased follicular density; it is a result of the tissue being grafted. Indeed, fresh and frozen–thawed ovarian tissue grafts demonstrated the same decrease in follicular density. Probably, the interval before revascularization of the graft takes place should be considered as the key factor. Nevertheless, even if their number was reduced, the residual follicles appeared normal by light microscopy.

This study also demonstrated that primordial follicles xenografted into nude mice could survive if they were transplanted without vascular anastomosis, subcutaneously or intraperitoneally, fresh or frozen–thawed. By light microscopy, the follicles that we observed in xenografts after freezing and thawing seemed to be normal even when

they were surrounded by fibrotic tissue but, on the other hand, transmission electron micrographs (TEM) revealed signs of degeneration in some cases. Recently, Oktay and colleagues[40,41] demonstrated the development of primordial follicles to antral stages in human ovarian tissue xenografted into immunodeficient (SCID) and hypogonadic (hpg) mice, stimulated with follicle stimulating hormone (FSH). They also demonstrated that, grafted into humans after cryopreservation, the ovarian tissue retained steroid secretion activity. But even if normal follicles with the capacity for growth can be observed, there is still a need to determine whether or not the oocyte itself is altered by cryopreservation. Further studies are thus needed in order to evaluate the influence of fibrosis on follicular development and fertilization potential.

By studying the rate of fibrosis in fresh and frozen–thawed cortical slices xenografted into immunodeficient nude mice, an average of 40% of the graft was found to be fibrotic after 24 days. A significantly higher fibrosis-related surface area (68%) was observed in frozen–thawed xenografted tissue, regardless of the site of transplantation (either subcutaneous or intraperitoneal).

Neovascularization of the graft remains one of the key factors for its survival. Ovarian tissue is a rich source of angiogenic factors which encourage rapid migration of endothelial cells into the grafts and early restoration of blood circulation.

The transplanted ovary is able to produce substances that promote direct angiogenesis and it has been demonstrated in animal models that the autotransplantation of ovaries can result in a prompt ovarian revascularization[42]. According to Dissen and colleagues[43], gonadotropin secretion after ovarian transplantation contributes to revascularization of the grafts in the rat by up-regulating the gene expression of two major angiogenic factors, vascular endothelial growth factor (VEGF) and transforming growth factor β_1 (TGF-β_1). By morphometric study, Nisolle and colleagues[38] demonstrated a vascular network located at the periphery of the graft, but macroscopic and microscopic differences were observed according to the site of transplantation. Indeed, when ovarian grafts were implanted subcutaneously, they observed macroscopic differences between fresh and frozen–thawed grafts. Indeed, fresh ovarian grafts were systematically well revascularized and small vessels were visible on the graft surface after 3 weeks, confirming that small pieces of fresh ovarian tissue (2 mm) rapidly become revascularized.

Maturation of primordial follicles

There are two ways to achieve maturation of primordial follicles. The first is to perform transplantation of ovarian cortical slices (homologous or heterologous transplantation, orthotopic or heterotopic grafting). The second is through *in vitro* follicular maturation.

Growth factors and cyopreserved tissue

Qu and colleagues[36,37] intend to set up a bank of cryo-preserved ovarian tissue for IVF programs. Their observation of the expression of transforming growth factor-α (TGF-α), epidermal growth factor (EGF) and EGF receptors in human follicles leads to the assumption that it may be useful to add TGF-α or EGF to the culture of cryopreserved ovarian tissue to promote the maturation of follicles *in vitro*. Investigating the possible influence of freezing and thawing on the immunoreactivities of TGF-α, EGF and EGF receptor in frozen ovarian tissue, they observed that there was no significant difference in immunostaining for TGF-α, EGF and EGF receptor between fresh and frozen ovarian tissues, indicating that human ovarian tissue could be frozen without substantially altering the immunoreactivities of TGF-α, EGF and EGF receptors in the follicles.

TGF-α and EGF receptor were simultaneously expressed in early follicles of human ovarian tissue. TGF-α might play a role in the regulation of folliculogenesis through binding to EGF receptor by an autocrine or paracrine mechanism. EGF was expressed in a different pattern from TGF-α and EGF receptor in follicles. These growth factors may be useful to promote the *in vitro* maturation of follicles from cryopreserved ovarian tissue, for potential uses in the treatment of infertile patients and in IVF programs in the future[36,37].

Like insulin-like growth factors (IGF), TGF-βs are important intra-ovarian regulators of folliculogenesis. TGF-β was localized immunocytochemically in ovarian granulosa and theca-interstitial cells[44–46]. The dominant form present in granulosa cells is TGF-β_1[44,45,47]. Both theca-interstitial and granulosa cells secreted TGF-β in cultures[44]. An increase in TGF-β levels was recently observed in ovarian follicular fluid in women following ovarian hyperstimulation for IVF[48]. TGF-β differentially regulated DNA synthesis and the proliferation of granulosa cells[49] and induced apoptosis in rat theca-interstitial cells[50]. TGF-β enhanced basal and gonadotropin-stimulated steroidogenesis in granulosa and thecal cells[51–53], although both inhibin and TGF-β suppressed luteinizing hormone (LH)-induced oocyte maturation in preovulatory follicles[54].

In another study, Qu and colleagues[37] observed that the expression of TGF-β type II receptor was distinct from that of the type I receptor with respect to cellular distribution in ovarian tissue. TGF-β type II receptor stained only in oocytes of primordial and primary follicles, and faintly in thecal cells; but no significant staining was observed in oocytes and granulosa cells in preantral and antral follicles. These results are not consistent with the report by Roy and Kole[55] on the expression of TGF-β type II receptor in granulosa, thecal and interstitial cells in the ovary. The reason for the discrepancy is unknown. The significance of the concomitant presence of TGF-β receptors and IGF type I receptor in early follicles is yet to be illuminated, but it has been suggested that both IGF-I and TGF-β may be involved in a sophisticated paracrine–autocrine network in the regulation of oocyte maturation and follicular growth in the ovary, and it could be worthwhile further investigating the possibility of using IGFs and TGF-βs to regulate the *in vitro* or *in vivo* growth of oocytes in early follicles from cryopreserved ovarian tissue.

Results from Qu and co-workers[36,37] showed that there was no significant difference in immunostaining for either IGF type I receptor or TGF-β types I and II receptors in follicles of frozen ovarian tissues, compared to fresh tissues from pair-controlled samples. It seems that freezing does not significantly alter the immunoreactivity of IGF type I receptor and TGF-β type I and II receptors in follicles after ovarian tissue cryopreservation.

In vivo maturation of follicles after transplantation of ovarian cortical slices

As already discussed in this Chapter, growth and maturation of cryopreserved human primordial and primary follicles have been achieved by homologous transplantation of frozen–thawed ovarian tissue[29]. However, the best site for ovarian tissue transplantation, enabling revascularization and providing easy access to mature follicles, has not yet been determined[38]. The kidney capsule of immunodeficient mice serves as a site for transplantation of ovarian slices from various species and as a model for the development of follicles, since the transplants are not rejected and receive a rich blood supply[56–61].

Sheep and cat ovarian cortical slices were transplanted to this site and developed to late antral stages[10]. Candy and associated[35] demonstrated that freezing and thawing do not substantially damage marmoset ovarian tissue and that the cryopreserved tissue retains its ability to support the development of follicles at all stages of folliculogenesis, including large antral follicles, 21–32 weeks after transplantation. Recently, Oktay and colleagues[41] reported that human primordial follicles could develop to antral–secretory stages in ovarian tissue xenografts in SCID/hpg mice.

Xenografts, nevertheless, pose major ethical problems because of the possibility of alterations in the human genome or transmission of hitherto unknown infectious agents.

The transmission of lymphoma was reported, via grafts of both fresh and frozen–thawed ovarian tissue, from diseased donor mice to healthy recipients. This study highlighted the risks of the clinical transplantation of ovarian biopsy samples to women recovering from cancer, especially a blood-borne cancer[62,63]. However, there are certain circumstances where the risk of cancerous involvement of the ovary is absent or minimal[64] and where autografting would thus pose no or little danger[65,66].

In vitro follicular maturation

The risks of ovarian tissue transplantation could be eliminated by obtaining unilaminar follicles from frozen–thawed tissue and growing the follicles *in vitro*, followed by routine IVF[65].

Secondary follicles

Secondary mammalian follicles have been matured *in vitro* and live pups have been born from fertilized oocytes[67–70]. Recently, fresh and frozen–thawed ovine ovarian tissue has been cultured[71]. It was possible to maintain a three-dimensional structure for oocyte–cumulus complexes greater than 190 μm in size throughout 30 days of culture. Twenty-five per cent of the cumulus units formed antral-like cavities.

Secondary human follicles isolated enzymatically were cultured for 4 days to antral stages[72] and mechanically isolated and human secondary and early-antral follicles were cultured for a few weeks[73]. However, the oocyte recovery rate from these cultures remained poor. Only 20% of the follicles contained an oocyte on histological analysis.

Primordial follicles

The number of secondary follicles in the human ovarian cortex is small[74,75] and there is a substantial natural atretic loss of early-antral human follicles[73]. Therefore, maturing the more abundant unilaminar follicles presents a more favorable option. Unfortunately, the signal that initiates their growth into secondary preantral follicles is unknown. It is possible that this information comes from the surrounding stroma. Some serum factors present in culture medium could have an inhibitory effect[76,77].

Once the primordial follicles commence their growth *in vitro*, it takes 85 days for them to reach the Graafian stage[78].

There are two possible approaches to the culture of primary and primordial follicles: *in situ* follicle culture and isolated follicle culture.

The first (organ culture) consists of culturing whole slices of ovarian tissue so that the structural integrity of the ovarian tissue is maintained and, thus, the interaction between the surrounding stromal cells and follicles is retained. Different authors have described primary mouse follicle culture to the preantral or preovulatory stage in the mouse[79,80]. A live newborn was reported after continuous culture of mouse follicles from the primordial stage[80], indicating that it will one day be possible to produce mature oocytes for IVF by growing primordial follicles *in vitro*. Slices of fresh and frozen–thawed adult human ovarian tissue were placed in organ cultures, and unilaminar follicles survived for up to 3 weeks[81]. Picton and colleagues[82] recently demonstrated that *in vitro* growth of human primordial follicles can be initiated in this *in situ* condition, but intact follicle survival is limited (only 20%).

The cumulus set-up for primordial human follicles will probably require a very dynamic system, providing several growth factors and physical stimuli for each of the different stages of follicular maturation. So far, none of the research on human primordial follicles has led to the demonstration of an increase in oocyte diameter in culture[83]. Most groups demonstrate the autonomous proliferation of granulosa cells, but the oocyte diameters stagnate and show signs of atresia after a few days of culture[76,79,81,82]. Until now, complete *in vitro* development from a primordial follicle has only been possible in mice.

The second approach involves the culture of isolated unilaminar follicles. Enzymatically isolated mouse and pig[84–86] and mechanically isolated bovine[87] unilaminar follicles have been cultured to multilaminar stages. Oktay and colleagues[40,41] described morphologically normal human follicles that were isolated by a combined enzymatic and mechanical method and studied by electron microscopy and fluorescent viability markers. Primordial human follicles from fresh and frozen–thawed ovarian tissue survived in culture for up to 5 days.

Since follicles cultured as isolated units can at present only develop to early antral stages when their starting diameter is > 190 μm, it is not yet possible to obtain antral follicles from primordial or primary follicles.

CONCLUSION

Cryopreservation of ovarian tissue should be seriously considered for any patient undergoing treatment likely to impair future fertility, the indications being pelvic, extra-pelvic and/or systemic diseases. The age of the patient should also be taken into consideration, because the contents of the ovary are not the same in prepubertal and postpubertal women. Because a decline in fertility is now well documented after the age of 38 years, the procedure should probably be restricted to patients below this limit, although, whatever the disease in question, when surgery can preserve the genital tract, irradiation and/or chemotherapy appears to be less harmful to the gonads of prepubertal than those of postpubertal women[88,89].

There may be many potential indications for ovarian tissue cryopreservation. Indeed, careful evaluation of all the parameters, such as the type of disease, the survival prognosis, the age, the dose and type of treatment, should be carried out before candidate selection for such procedures. On the other hand, respecting the code of good practice, all patients who may become infertile have the right to receive proper consideration of their interests for future possibilities in the field of ovarian function preservation. The selection of cases should be carried out on the basis of a multidisciplinary staff discussion including oncologists, gynecologists, biologists, psychologists and pediatricians. Counselling should be given and informed consent obtained from the patient.

We believe that it is preferable to remove only one ovary if possible, to avoid the psychological stress of surgical castration in a young patient, because cases of spontaneous pregnancy have been described after total body irradiation[90,91] and because, in many cases, the remaining ovary will be able to resume all endocrine functions after some years. Moreover, the thousands of primary follicles that are contained in a single ovary of a young patient are more than sufficient to ensure fertility after cryopreservation.

After unilateral ovariectomy and cryopreservation of multiple cortical slices, different options would be available:

(1) Isolation of immature oocytes or preantral follicles and in vitro maturation to metaphase II oocytes;

(2) Autotransplantation. One can wait for restoration of natural fertility after orthotopic transplantation, or practice ovarian stimulation and IVF after heterotopic transplantation;

(3) Heterotransplantation to women for restoration of natural fertility or for IVF (e.g. patients suffering from premature ovarian failure, patients after chemotherapy or radiotherapy for malignant disorders, etc).

It has been demonstrated that cryopreserved primordial follicles can survive after thawing and that growth and maturation are possible under certain conditions. Research must now focus on the best way to use thawed tissue. It is probable that the answer lies in the use of culture environments adapted to each stage of follicular development. The encouraging results presented here raise hopes in the area of clinical application of banked ovarian tissue[66,83,92,93]. Great effort in the research programs is still required in order to restore fertility with a view to obtaining healthy babies from cryopreserved ovarian tissue[19,83,84,94].

If autografting is the aim of the cryopreservation of ovarian tissue, testing for malignant cells in the tissue must be carried out using adequate techniques. This is especially the case for malignant lymphoma, since these disorders are not limited to single organs, but can arise in all body tissue. The idea of 'oocyte banking' is attractive but it requires continued efforts to achieve better results with ovarian tissue cryopreservation techniques and in vitro oocyte maturation procedures. Although animal studies have proved that ovarian tissue cryopreservation may restore fertility, there is no evidence that cryopreservation of ovarian tissue could restore fertility in humans, at least by means of transplantation. More information is needed to determine whether human oocytes are competent enough after cryopreservation and transplantation to achieve full maturation, fertilization and embryo development and to determine if active angiogenesis can be induced to accelerate the process of neovascularization of the graft.

REFERENCES

1. Byrne J, Kessler LG, Devesa SS. The prevalence of cancer among adults in the United States. Cancer 1987;69:2154–9

2. Chen C. Pregnancy after human oocyte cryopreservation. Lancet 1986;1:884–6

3. Van Hem JFHM, Siebrehnrube ER, Schub B, et al. Birth after the cryopreservation of unfertilised oocyte. Lancet 1987;1:752–3

4. Al-Hassani S, Ludwig M, Gagsteiger F, et al. Comparison of cryopreservation of supernumerary pronuclear human oocytes obtained after intracytoplasmic sperm injection (ICSI) and after conventional in-vitro fertilization. Hum Reprod 1996;11:604–7

5. Hwang JL, Liu YH, Tsori YL. Pregnancy after immature oocyte donation and intracytoplasmic sperm injection. Fertil Steril 1997;68:1139–40

6. Porcu E, Fabri R, Seracchiali R, et al. Birth of healthy female after intracytoplasmic sperm injection of cryopreserved human oocytes. Fertil Steril 1997;68:724–6

7. Tucker MJ, Wright G, Morton PC, et al. Birth after cryopreservation of immature oocytes with subsequent in vitro maturation. Fertil Steril 1998;70:578–9

8. Fuller BA. Cryopreservation of human oocytes. A review of current problems and perspectives. Hum Reprod Update 1996;2:193–207

9. Gook DA, Osborn SM, Johnson WIH. Pathogenic activity of human oocytes following cryopreservation using 1,2-propandiol. Hum Reprod 1995;10:654–8

10. Gosden RG, Boulton M, Grant R, et al. Follicular development from ovarian xenografts in SCID mice. J Reprod Fertil 1994;11:619–23

11. Newton H, Aubard J, Rutherford A, et al. Low temperature storage and grafting of human ovarian tissue. Hum Reprod 1996;11:1487–91

12. Bahadur G, Steele SJ. Ovarian tissue cryopreservation for patients. Hum Reprod 1996;11:2215–16

13. Gosden RG. Freezing ovary tissue may help cancer patients to preserve fertility. J Natl Cancer Inst 1996;88:1181–5

14. Law C. Freezing ovary tissue may help cancer patients preserve fertility. J Natl Cancer Inst 1996;88:1184–5

15. Byrne J, Mulvihill JJ, Meyers MH, et al. Effects of treatment on infertility in long term survivors of childhood or adolescent cancer. N Engl J Med 1987;317:1315–21

16. Green DM, Hall B, Zevon MA. Pregnancy outcome after treatment for acute lymphoblastic leukemia during childhood or adolescence. Cancer 1989;64:2235

17. Mulvlhill JJ. Sentinel and other mutational effects in offspring of cancer survivors. Prog Clin Biol Res 1990;340C:179

18. Aisner J, Wiernik PH, Pearl P. Pregnancy outcome in patients treated for Hodgkin's disease. J Clin Oncol 1993;11:507

19. Donnez J, Bassil S. Indications for cryopreservation of ovarian tissue. Hum Reprod Update 1998;4:248–59

20. Schneider A, Krause N, Kuhne-Heid R, *et al.* Preserving fertility in early cervix carcinoma trachelectomy with laparoscopic lymphadenectomy. *Zentralbl Gynakol* 1996;118:6–8

21. Kicks M, Pizer M. Conservative surgery plus adjuvant therapy for vulvovaginal rhabdomyosarcoma diethylstilbestrol clear cell adenocarcinoma of the vagina and unilateral germ cell tumors of the ovary. *Obstet Gynecol Clin North Am* 1992;19:219–33

22. Link C, Reed E, Sarosy G, *et al.* Borderline ovarian tumors. *Am J Med* 1996;101:217–25

23. Kleine W. Results of fertility preserving operations in malignant ovarian tumors. *Zentralbl Gynakol* 1996;18:317–21

24. Chapman R, Sutcliffe S, Malpas J. Cytoxic-induced ovarian failure in women with Hodgkin's disease. I. Hormone function. *J Am Med Assoc* 1979;242:1877–81

25. Horning S, Hoppe R, Kaplan H, *et al.* Female reproductive potential after treatment for Hodgkin's disease. *N Engl J Med* 1981;304:1377–82

26. Whitehead E, Shalet S, Blackledge G, *et al.* The effect of combination chemotherapy on ovarian function in women treated for Hodgkin's disease. *Cancer* 1983;52:988–93

27. Nicholson S, Blasck A, Markle B, *et al.* Uterine anomalies in Wilm's tumor survivors. *Cancer* 1996;78:887–91

28. Shalet S. Effects of cancer chemotherapy on gonadal function of patients. *Cancer Treat Rev* 1980;7:41

29. Lushbaugh C, Casaren G. The effect of gonadal irradiation in clinal radiation therapy: a review. *Cancer* 1976;37:1111–20

30. Muvihill J, McKeen E, Rosner F, *et al.* Pregnancy outcome in cancer patients. Experience in a large cooperative group. *Cancer* 1987;60:1143–50

31 Baker T. Radiosensitivity of mammalian oocyte with particular reference to the human female. *Am J Obstet Gynecol* 1971;110:746–61

32. Hodel K, Rich W, Austin P, *et al.* The role of ovarian transposition in conservation of ovarian function in radical hysterectomy followed by pelvic radiation. *Gynecol Oncol* 1982;13:195–202

33. Adashi EY. The ovarian follicular apparatus. In Adashi EY, Rock JA, Rosenwacks Z, eds. *Reproductive Endocrinology, Surgery and Technology*. Philadelphia: Lippincott-Raven Publishers, 1996:17–40

34. Lass A, Silye R, Abrams DC, *et al.* Follicular density in ovarian biopsy of infertile women: a novel method to assess the ovarian reserve. *Hum Reprod* 1997;12:1028–31

35. Candy CJ, Wood MJ, Whittingham DG. Effect of cryoprotectants on the survival of follicles in frozen mouse ovaries. *J Reprod Fertil* 1997;110:11–19

36. Qu J, Godin PA, Nisolle M, *et al.* Distribution and epidermal growth factor receptor expression of primordial follicles in human ovarian tissue before and after cryopreservation. *Hum Reprod* 2000;15:302–10

37. Qu J, Godin PA, Nisolle M, *et al.* Expression of receptors for insulin-like growth factor-I and transforming growth factor-β in human follicles. *Mol Hum Reprod* 2001;6:137–45

38. Nisolle M, Godin PA, Casanas-Roux F, *et al.* Histological and ultrastructural evaluation of fresh and frozen–thawed human ovarian xenografts in nude mice. *Fertil Steril* 2001;in press

39. Meirow D, Fasouliotis S, Nugent D, *et al.* A laparoscopic technique for obtaining ovarian cortical biopsy specimens for fertility conservation in patients with cancer. *Fertil Steril* 1999;71:948–51

40. Oktay K, Nugent D, Newton H, *et al.* Isolation and characterization of primordial follicles from fresh and cryopreserved human ovarian tissue. *Fertil Steril* 1997;67:481–6

41. Oktay K, Newton H, Mullan J, *et al.* Development of human primordial follicles to antral stages in SCID/hpg mice stimulated with follicle stimulating hormone. *Hum Reprod* 1998;13:1133–8

42. Gosden RG. Restitution of fertility in sterilized mice by transferring primordial ovarian follicles. *Hum Reprod* 1990;5:499–504

43. Dissen GA, Lara HE, Fahrenbach WH, *et al.* Immature rat ovaries become revascularized rapidly after autotransplantation and show a gonadotropin-dependent increase in angiogenic factor gene-expression. *Endocrinology* 1994;134:1146–54

44. Mulheron G, Bossert N, Lapp J, *et al.* Human granulosa–luteal and cumulus cells express transforming growth factors-beta type 1 and type 2 mRNA. *J Clin Endocrinol Metab* 1992;74:458–60

45. Gangrade B, Goteher E, Davis J, *et al.* The secretion of transforming growth factor-beta by bovine luteal cells *in vitro*. *Mol Cell Endocrinol* 1993;93:117–23

46. May J, Stephenson L, Turzcynski C, *et al.* Transforming growth factor-beta expression in the porcine ovary: evidence that theca cells are the major secretory source during antral follicle development. *Biol Reprod* 1996;54:486–96

47. Teerds K, Dorrington J. Immunohistochemical localization of transforming growth factor-beta 1 and -beta 2 during follicular development in the adult rat ovary. *Mol Cell Endocrinol* 1992;84:R7–17

48. Fried G, Wramsby H, Tally M. Transforming growth factor-β1, insulin-like growth factor, and insulin-like growth factor binding proteins in ovarian follicular fluid are differentially regulated by the type of ovarian hyperstimulation use for *in vitro* fertilization. *Fertil Steril* 1998;70:129–34

49. May J, Gotcher E, Gangrade B, *et al.* Secretion of transforming growth factor-beta (TGF-β) by porcine theca and granulosa cells *in vitro* and differential effects upon cell proliferation. *Endocrinology* 1994;2:1045–54

50. Foghi A, Teerds K, Van der Donck H, *et al.* Induction of apoptosis in rat thecal/interstitial cells by transforming growth factor-α plus transforming growth factor-β *in vitro. J Endocrinol* 1997;153:169–78

51. Dodson W, Schomberg D. The effect of transforming growth factor-β on follicle-stimulating hormone-induced differentiation of cultured rat granulosa cells. *Endocrinology* 1987;120:512–16

52. Magoffin D, Gancedo B, Erickson G. Transforming growth factor-β promotes differentiation of ovarian thecal/interstitial cells but inhibits androgen production. *Endocrinology* 1989;12:1951–8

53. Fournet N, Weitsman S, Zachow R, *et al.* Transforming growth factor-beta inhibits ovarian 17 alpha-hydroxylase activity by a direct noncompetitive mechanism. *Endocrinology* 1966;137:166–74

54. Tsafriri A, Vale W, Hsueh A. Effect of transforming growth factors and inhibin-related proteins on rat preovulatory graafian follicles *in vitro. Endocrinology* 1989;125:1857–62

55. Roy S, Kole A. Ovarian transforming growth factor-β (TGF-β) receptors: *in vitro* effects of follicles stimulating hormone, epidermal growth factor and TGF-β on receptor expression in human preantral follicles. *Mol Hum Reprod* 1988;4:207–14

56. Gosden KG, Baird DT, Wade JC, *et al.* Restoration of fertility to oophorectomized sheep by ovarian autografts stored at −196°C. *Hum Reprod* 1994;9:597–603

57. Harp R, Leibach J, Balck J, *et al.* Cryopreservation of marine ovarian tissue. *Cryobiology* 1994;31:336–43

58. Cox SL, Shaw S, Jenkin G. Transplantation of cryopreserved fetal ovarian tissue to adult recipients in mice. *J Reprod Fertil* 1996;107:315–22

59. Aubard Y, Newton H, Scheffer G, *et al.* Conservation of the follicular population in irradiated rats by the cryopreservation and orthotopic autografting of ovarian tissue *Eur J Obstet Gynecol Reprod Biol* 1998;79:83–7

60. Salle B, Lornage J, Franck M, *et al.* Freezing, thawing and autograft of ovarian fragments in sheep: preliminary experiments and histologic assessment. *Fertil Steril* 1998;71:124–8

61. Nugent D, Meirow D, Brook PF, *et al.* Transplantation in reproductive medicine: previous experience, present knowledge and future prospects. *Hum Reprod Update* 1997;3:267–80

62. Shaw SM, Bowles S, Koopman P, *et al.* Fresh and cryopreserved ovarian tissue samples from donors with lymphoma transmit the cancer to graft recipients. *Hum Reprod* 1996;11:1668–73

63. Shaw J, Trounson A. Oncological implications in the replacement of ovarian tissue. *Hum Reprod* 1997;12:403–5

64. Meirow D, ben Yehuda D, Prus D, *et al.* Ovarian tissue banking in patients with Hodgkin's disease: is it sure? *Fertil Steril* 1998;69:996–8

65. Gosden RG, Rutherford AJ, Norfolk DR. Ovarian banking for cancer patients: transmission of malignant cells in ovarian grafts. *Hum Reprod* 1997;12:403–5

66. Moomjy M, Rosenwaks Z. Ovarian tissue cryopreservation: the time is now. Transplantation or *in vitro* maturation: the time awaits. *Fertil Steril* 1998;69:999–1000

67. Gosden RG, Boland NI, Spears N, *et al.* The biology of follicular oocyte development *in vitro. Reprod Med Rev* 1993;2:129–52

68. Hartshorne GM. *In vitro* culture of ovarian follicles. *Rev Reprod* 1997;2:94–104

69. Eppig DG, Schroeder AC. Capacity of mouse oocytes from preantral follicles to undergo embryogenesis and development to live young after growth, maturation and fertilization *in vitro. Biol Reprod* 1989;41:268–76

70. Spears N, Boland NI, Murray AA, *et al.* Mouse oocytes derived from *in vitro* grown primary ovarian follicles are fertile. *Hum Reprod* 1994;9:527–32

71. Newton H, Picton H, Gosden RG. *In-vitro* growth of oocyte–granulosa cell complexes isolated from cryopreserved ovine tissue. *J Reprod Fertil* 1999;115:141–50

72. Roy SK, Treacy BJ. Isolation and long term culture of human preantral follicles. *Fertil Steril* 1993;59:783–90

73. Abir R, Franks S, Mobberley MA, *et al.* Mechanical isolation and *in vitro* growth of preantral and small antral human follicles. *Fertil Steril* 1997;68:682–8

74. Hovatta O, Silye R, Kraustz T, *et al.* Cryopreservation of human ovarian tissue by using dimethylsulphoxide and proandiol-sucrose as cryoprotectants. *Hum Reprod* 1996;11:1268–72

75. Hughesdon PE. Morphology and morphogenesis of the Stein-Leventhal ovary and so-called 'hyperthecosis'. *Obstet Gynecol* 1982;37:59–77

76. Wandji SA, Srsen V, Voss AK, *et al.* Initiation *in vitro* of growth of bovine primordial follicles. *Biol Reprod* 1996;55:942–8

77. Wandji SA, Srsen V, Nathanielsz PW, *et al.* Initiation of growth of baboon primordial follicles *in vitro. Hum Reprod* 1997;12:1993–2001

78. Gougeon A. Dynamics of follicular growth in the human: a model from preliminary results. *Hum Reprod* 1986;1:81–7

79. Qvist R, Blackwell LF, Bourne H, *et al.* Development of mouse follicles from primary to preovulatory stages *in vitro. J Reprod Fertil* 1990;89:169–80

80. Eppig JJ, O'Brien M. Development *in vitro* of mouse oocytes from primordial follicles. *Biol Reprod* 1996;54:197–207

81. Hovatta O, Silye R, Abir R, *et al.* Extracellular matrix improves the survival of human primordial and primary fresh and frozen-thawed ovarian follicles in long-term culture. *Hum Reprod* 1997;12:1032–6

82. Picton HM, Mkandla A, Salha O, *et al.* Initiation of human primordial follicle growth *in vitro* in ultrathin slices of ovarian cortex. 15th annual Meeting of ESHRE, Tours, France. *Hum Reprod* 1999;14 (Abstract Book 1):0-020p11

83. Smitz J, Cortvrindt R. Oocyte *in-vitro* maturation and follicle culture: current clinical achievement and future directions. *Hum Reprod* 1999;14:145–61

84. Torrance C, Telfer E, Gosden RG. Quantitative study of the development of isolated mouse pre-antral follicles in collagen gel culture. *J Reprod Fertil* 1989;87:367–74

85. Greenwald GS, Moor RM. Isolation and preliminary characterization of pig primordial follicles. *J Reprod Fertil* 1989;87:561–71

86. Morbeck DE, Flowers WL, Britt JH. Response of granulosa cells isolated from primary and secondary follicles to FSH,8-bromo-cAMP and epidermal growth factor *in vitro*. *J Reprod Fertil* 1993;99:577–84

87. Hulshof SCJ, Figueiredo JR, Beckers JF, *et al.* Effects of fetal bovine serum, FSH and 17β-estradiol on the culture of bovine preantral follicles. *Theriogenology* 1995;44:216–26

88. Haie-Meder C, Mlika-Cabanne N, Michel G, *et al.* Radiotherapy after ovarian transposition ovarian function and fertility preservation. *Int J Radiat Oncol Biol Phys* 1993;25:419–24

89. Sanders J, Hawley J, Levy W, *et al.* Pregnancies following high-dose Cyclophosphamide with or without high-dose Busulfan or total body irradiation and bone marrow transplantation. *Blood* 1996;87:3045–52

90. Spinelly S, Chiodi S, Bacigalupo A, *et al.* Ovarian recovery after total body irradiation and allogenic transplantation: long term follow-up of 79 females. *Bone Marrow Transplant* 1994;14:373–80

91. Atkinson HG, Apperley JF, Dawson K, *et al.* Successful pregnancy after allogenic bone marrow transplantation for chronic meyloid leukemia. *Lancet* 1994;344:199

92. Newton H, Fisher J, Arnold JRP, *et al.* Permeation of human ovarian tissue with cryoprotective agents in preparation for cryopreservation. *Hum Reprod* 1998;13:378–80

93. Weissrnan A, Gotlieb L, Colgan T, *et al.* Preliminary experience with subcutaneous human ovarian cortex transplantation in the NOD-SCID mouse. *Biol Reprod* 1999;60:1462–7

94. Ludwig M, Al-Hasani S, Felberbaum R, *et al.* New aspects of cryopreservation of oocytes and embryos in assisted reproduction and future perspectives. *Hum Reprod* 1999;14:162–85

Ovarian tissue cryopreservation: technical aspects and existing alternatives

31

O. De Hertogh, J.P. Qu, M. Nisolle and J. Donnez

A BRIEF HISTORY OF TIME . . . AND CRYOBIOLOGY

The idea that life could be brought back to a human body after freezing was first put forth over 200 years ago by John Hunter, Scottish surgeon and anatomist[1]. His experiments, using rabbits' ears in which he injected the arteries with a dye to assess the tissue damage related to freezing, testify to his interest in tissue viability, which nowadays remains the prime concern of cryobiology. However, preserving a whole body of which Hunter dreamt (or even a whole organ, as most surgeons involved in transplantation dream) remains a seemingly unattainable goal.

Living cell cryopreservation only became possible with the (accidental) discovery of cryoprotectants in the mid-twentieth century, and was first performed by Audrey Smith and her colleagues who froze spermatozoa at −80°C, using glycerol to prevent cellular damage[2]. Nature best imitates itself, as it appears some insects withstand sub-zero temperatures by using sugar-based molecules[3].

Other cryoprotective agents, such as dimethylsulfoxide, ethylene glycol and propylene glycol, which possess a higher water solubility and an ability to penetrate cells more rapidly[4], were discovered and used after glycerol.

ADVANTAGES AND DISADVANTAGES OF OOCYTE, FOLLICLE, WHOLE OVARIAN TISSUE AND EMBRYO CRYOPRESERVATION

The will to ensure reproductive potential in those young patients whose gonadal function is threatened (either by premature menopause, or by treatments such as pelvic radiotherapy, gonadotoxic chemotherapy, or surgical castration) raises several issues about the germinal cells one would aim to store.

Do these cells have to be fertilized? Do the unfertilized cells have to be separated from their functional environment? Or do they even have to be isolated from the surrounding tissue?

Fertilized cells

Embryo cryopreservation has become a routine technique in any *in vitro* fertilization (IVF) center, and has proven its efficacy in terms of pregnancy and 'take-home-baby rate'; in our own experience, the latter reaches about one-third of all cycles (for detailed results see Table 1).

Although this method has already been used for young cancer patients[5], all questions regarding its applicability in this particular situation are far from being answered.

On the one hand, medical reasons might impede its application, either if the beginning of the treatment cannot be delayed, making it impossible to spend several weeks on the completion of a proper IVF cycle, or if the malignancy has proven hormonal sensitivity, implying a risk for high sex steroid blood levels (linked to the ovarian stimulation protocol) to increase malignant cell growth. Even if IVF can theoretically be undertaken on the basis of a spontaneous ovarian cycle[6], the small number of obtainable oocytes (and subsequently of viable embryos eligible for transfer) still does not make it possible to obtain any live births in these conditions.

On the other hand, what one could call 'human factors' can also make it impossible, or useless. If the patient is not involved in a stable relationship with a male partner, the only – but somewhat odd – solution would be to use donor sperm to ensure fertilization of her oocytes. Even if such a relationship does exist, the young couple might be bothered by the idea of the 'embryos joint ownership', meaning they belong to the couple but not to its separate members. If destroying the embryos in cases of divorce or death of a spouse is part of the 'contract' in standard IVF cycles, this practice raises legal, ethical and moral issues in the case of cancer patients. If the female partner died, destroying the embryos might be much more difficult for an already afflicted spouse. Also, it would leave no alternative but to transfer the embryos to a surrogate mother. If the male partner died, our surviving patient could not then use the embryos, which would in fact represent her only chance of becoming a mother.

Unfertilized cells

In contrast to the male situation, where obtaining an able spermatozoon only implies the growth and maturation of a single germinal cell, the long route leading from primordial follicle to fertilizable oocyte goes hand in hand with the development of a specific functional entity, which is the ovarian follicle. One might then raise the question about how extensive a 'woman's germinal entity' is: does it make sense to isolate oocytes from their surrounding follicles, or does it even make sense to isolate such follicles from the surrounding tissue (as long as autocrine and paracrine mechanisms seem to be implicated, within the ovary itself, in oocyte maturation)?

Table I Université Catholique de Louvain, Brussels (Belgium) *In Vitro* Fertilization Unit: global results for 1999 (whole year) and 2000 (first semester)

	1999	2000
Patients' age (mean ± SD) (years)	32.6 ± 5.4	32.0 ± 5.5
Number of attempted cycles per patient (mean ± SD)	2.1 ± 1.4	2.0 ± 1.4
Performed cycles (C)	671	345
Ovarian punctures (OPU)	642 (95.7% C)	335 (97.0% C)
Global fertilization rate	60.2%	65.0%
Embryo transfers (ET)	582 (90.6% OPU) (86.7% C)	312 (93.0% OPU) (90.4% C)
Number of transferred embryos per patient (mean ± SD)	2.1 ± 1.0	2.1 ± 0.8
Pregnancies (2 consecutive blood tests, with positive and increasing β-hCG)	228 (39.0% ET) (35.5% OPU) (34.0%C)	147 (47.0% ET) (43.8% OPU) (42.6% C)
Implantation rate	17.3%	26.2%
Ongoing clinical pregnancies or deliveries	162	113
Not including:		
biochemical pregnancies	28	16
miscarriages	33	15
extrauterine pregnancies	5	3
Take-home-baby rate	27.8% ET 24.1% C	36.2% ET 32.8% C

hCG, human chorionic gonadotropin

Isolated oocytes, in metaphase II

Mature oocyte freezing appeared to be the logical way to store female germ cells, when compared to the routinely performed sperm banking. Still, this procedure has mainly brought disappointment. At present, the oocyte survival rate after freezing and thawing only stands at about 30%, although fertilization and embryonic evolution rates do not seem to decrease dramatically once oocyte survival has been achieved. Moreover, case reports on patients benefiting from this procedure and obtaining pregnancies are still sporadic.

There are three main reasons for failure. First, the zona pellucida hardens during the freezing process, probably as a consequence of premature exocytosis of the cortical granules. It could then act as a fence, impairing spermato-zoan penetration (although micromanipulation techniques can, to a certain extent, bypass this problem)[7–10]. Second, the cellular cooling process induces a depolymerization of the meiotic spindle, which is a dynamic structure (microtubules being continually assembled at one of its ends, and separated at the other). Although chromosomes gather at the spindle equator during cellular warming, the cell is at risk of losing chromosomes and suffering aneuploidy during the first maturation cellular division. This is the main reason why mature oocyte cryopreservation has been put aside in clinical use[11,12], although studies do not agree on the extent of the problem; some even argue that spindle alterations do not systematically imply the presence of stray chromosomes[13], and that a higher rate of aneuploidy is encountered in any IVF process. Third, the damage caused to the cytoskeleton is able to modify the organites and molecular organization of the oocyte[14].

Isolated oocytes, in prophase I (at the diplotene stage, or 'germinal vesicle stage')

One could say that these oocytes, obtained from DeGraaf follicles, are 'competent but less fragile'. These cells have reached full size and complete meiotic competence, but have not yet resumed their maturation process and initiated their second metaphase. Although the risk of hardening of the zona pellucida or damage to the cytoskeleton cannot be avoided, the absence of spindles guarantees the absence of cytogenetic anomalies during forthcoming cellular divisions.

This technique might thus be considered feasible for clinical practice, but only in the somewhat distant future, available data still being insufficient to initiate oocyte banking. Indeed, even if the cells appear to tolerate freezing and thawing (with high survival and maturation resumption rates), the required *in vitro* maturation of the oocytes might explain the disappointing embryonic development rates[15–17] (for detailed results see Table 2 and Figure 1).

Furthermore, the question of cumulus cells remains open. On the one hand, isolating the oocyte makes the frozen structure smaller, and could thus increase cellular resistance to the freezing–thawing process[12].

On the other hand, although preserving the cumulus cells surrounding the oocyte might include a risk of neoplastic disease transmission through the 'graft', it should also enhance oocyte meiosis and maturation, oocyte fertilization and embryo quality. Numerous studies are currently being conducted on animals about the importance of the cumulus–oocyte complex (COC) in oocyte cultures, and the gap junctional channels (GJCs) mediating its actions[18].

Oocyte maturation. Granulosa cells and cumulus cells appear to play a regulatory role in oocyte meiosis, in a complex way (possibly both stimulating and inhibiting, see Table 3)[19–23].

Oocyte fertilization. Inhibition of the GJCs does not seem to interfere with the penetrability of the oocytes by the spermatozoa, but it appears to interfere with the oocytes' capacity to shed the nuclear envelope of spermatozoa. In 'GJC-deprived oocytes' (treated with heptanol), there is an increase in spermatozoa arrested at stage 1, and a decrease in spermatozoa proceeding to stages 4 and 5[18] (for detailed results, see Figure 2). Finally, it could also interfere with the ability of the oocyte to form male pronuclei, this being strongly related to the presence of cumulus cells during maturation and fertilization[24–30], and promoted in 'cumulus-free oocytes' by cysteamine (which also increases the oocyte glutathione content)[31].

Embryo development. It appears that *in vitro* maturation with cumulus cells improves the development of 'corona-enclosed oocytes' to the blastocyst stage, but has no effect on oocytes denuded from their somatic cells, and that this effect is dependent on the density of the cumulus cells in the culture medium[32].

Isolated primordial follicles

The idea behind this technique is to both preserve the 'functional germinal entity' (meaning the follicle) past the germ cell alone, and to enhance the resistance of the isolated structure to freezing and thawing by having:

(1) A smaller cellular volume (of both the oocyte and the follicle). Assuming that 'the smaller, the better', is true, this would improve the quality of the freezing process *per se*.

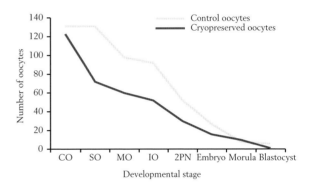

Figure 1 Evolution of prophase I oocytes collected during stimulated cycles. CO, collected oocytes; SO, surviving oocytes; MO, matured oocytes; IO, inseminated oocytes; 2PN, two pronuclei. From Toth[17]

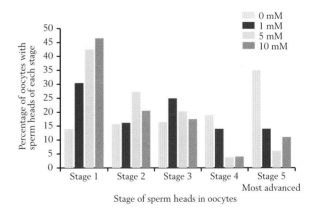

Figure 2 Most advanced stage of sperm heads in porcine oocytes, according to heptanol concentrations in the culture medium and the subsequent degree of gap junctional channel (GJC) inhibition. Reproduced with permission from Mori[18]

Table 2 Maturation, fertilization and early embryo development achieved after *in vitro* culture of prophase I oocytes

| | Toth et al.[16,17] | | | |
	Control[17]	Unstimulated cycles[17]	Stimulated cycles[16]	Mandelbaum et al.[15]
Treatment of isolated oocytes	no freezing	cryopreservation in 1.5 mm 1,2 propanediol	cryopreservation in 1.5 mm 1,2 propanediol	cryopreservation
Collected oocytes (CO)	131	123		
Surviving oocytes (SO) after freezing and thawing	no freezing	72/123 (58.5% of CO)	43%	37%
Matured oocytes (MO) to metaphase II stage	98/131 (74.8% of CO)	60/72 (48.8% of CO) (83.3% of SO)	27%[†]	20%
Inseminated oocytes (IO)	92/98	52/60		
Two pronuclei (2PN)	52/92 (56.5% of IO)	30/52 (57.7% of IO)		
Three pronuclei (3PN)	2/92 (2.2% of IO)	2/52 (3.8% of IO)		
Two- to eight-cell embryos	27/52 (52.0% of 2PN)	16/30 (53.3% of 2PN)		
Morula	8/52 (15.4% of 2PN)*	10/30 (33.3% of 2PN)*		
Blastocyst	6/52 (11.5% of 2PN)*	1/30 (3.3% of 2PN)*		

* The question has been raised whether prophase I oocytes collected after ovarian stimulation could possibly be of a lesser quality. Whatever the answer, there appears to be an influence of the ovarian stimulation protocol on the developmental potential of these immature oocytes. Actually, the larger the cohort of immature oocytes (collected from the patient), the greater their cleavage potential after IVF (44% of maturation to morula and blastocyst stage for prophase I oocytes coming from a predominantly immature cohort, versus 25% of maturation for prophase I oocytes coming from a predominantly mature cohort). This could possibly be due to an inadequate ovarian stimulation protocol, and insufficient exposure of the oocytes to gonadotropins to achieve full maturation[17].

† The low maturation rate of prophase I oocytes collected from non-stimulated follicles, when compared to same-stage oocytes collected from stimulated follicles, could be related to the harvesting of these oocytes outside the cohort normally recruited by the ovaries during the menstrual cycle; being at stages of growth or atresia, they are either more susceptible to cryodamage, or have a lesser *in vitro* maturation potential[16]

(2) A lower differentiation degree. This implies less fragile cellular structures (fewer organites, no zona pellucida, no cortical granules), and more time for the oocyte to repair (through a long forthcoming maturation process) all the sub-lethal damage it might have suffered.

(3) A cellular cycle stopped at the prophase stage. This implies a lesser risk of cytogenetic anomalies.

Nevertheless, several drawbacks exist. Isolating the oocyte with a single layer of surrounding pre-granulosa cells can only be achieved by mechanical dissection (which remains virtually impossible) or enzymatic digestion incubating the follicles into proteolytic enzymes such as collagenase (which diminishes the oocyte survival rate, and could impair its further development by altering the external cell layer)[33,34]. Moreover, none of these isolation methods are completely specific. Being unable to guarantee the absence of neoplastic cells in a dissected follicle culture could be sufficient reason to refuse to use these follicles in the case of former cancer patients, although detecting the residual neoplastic cells through increasingly sensitive polymerase chain reaction methods, or eliminating them through specific culture conditions, might help to bypass the problem[33,35–38].

Table 3 Suspected regulatory roles of cumulus–oocyte complexes (COCs) on oocyte meiotic abilities

Potential roles of the GJCs	Underlying physiological processes	Animal source of oocytes
Inhibition of oocyte meiosis	production of a meiosis-arresting substance by the mural granulosa cells, transported into the oocyte through granulosa–cumulus and cumulus–oocyte GJCs	bovine oocytes[19] cattle oocytes co-cultured with pig membrane granulosa cells[20]
	resumption of oocyte meiosis, following disruption of the cumulus–oocyte GJCs	pig oocytes[21] rat oocytes[22]
Stimulation of oocyte meiosis	mediation of the action of concanavalin A and FSH (that induce meiotic resumption in the mouse), through gap junctional coupling	mouse oocytes[23]

GJC, gap junctional channels; FSH, follicle stimulating hormone

Eventually, one has to prepare these immature oocytes for fertilization. *In vitro* maturation is still a distant prospect, as long as all endocrine, paracrine and autocrine mechanisms implicated in oocyte development are not fully explained. *In vivo* autograft raises concerns, as previously discussed, about the presence of residual neoplastic cells if performed in former cancer patients. Xenografts of human tissue into immunodeficient animals, such as hpg/SCID mice[39,40], used as living culture medium to bring oocytes to full maturity, again raise more questions than answers about the fertilization of the matured oocytes, the quality of the resulting embryos and the ethics of using an animal as an incubator.

Ovarian tissue biopsy

At first sight, this method appears to be a clinician's dream: feasible whenever, however and wherever one wants. One can harvest the ovarian tissue at any time, with no concern about the phase of the menstrual cycle, or the need for any hormonal treatment. The biopsy can be made by means of a simple laparoscopy (see Technical aspects). It can even provide very small amounts of ovarian cortex (a few square millimeters), this tissue containing hundreds of thousands of primordial follicles in young women. However, one must bear in mind that ovarian follicles are randomly distributed inside the cortex, and that the contents of any biopsy, in terms of follicles, does not reflect more than itself (so that no biopsy will ever reflect the global follicular population of a woman).

Moreover, whole ovarian tissue is far easier to 'isolate' than mature oocytes (obtainable only in small number, for a limited period of the menstrual cycle, and very fragile when facing freezing and thawing procedures), immature follicles (requiring a difficult isolation process) and embryos (implying a long hormonal stimulation protocol and the presence of a spouse, and raising ethical issues, as previously mentioned).

Still, even though full pregnancies have been achieved in mice and sheep after autografting of frozen–thawed ovarian tissue, even though primate ovarian tissue resumes maturation up to the production of antral follicles after xenografting in nude mice, even though the same experiment has been successfully achieved with human tissue, and even though ovulation has been observed in a frozen–thawed ovarian fragment after autografting in a patient, *nothing* proves, at present, that such grafts will enable the recovery of fertility, or even of a normal hormonal status in castrated women.

Moreover, the notion of grafting itself raises questions about the risk of transmission of infectious (such as HIV or hepatitis) and malignant diseases. Frozen–thawed bone marrow has been proven to be the source of residual leukemia in the human more than 10 years after allogeneic transplantation for chronic myelogenous leukemia, and both fresh or frozen–thawed ovarian tissue seem to transmit lymphoma from donors to recipients in mice. Ovarian tissue samples might thus be at risk for transmission of ovarian malignancies, hematological malignancies such as leukemia, and systemic malignancies such as lymphoma or metastatic cancers, although there is no proof that all cancers will present the same risks as lymphoma, which is known to be quite aggressive. Again, these notions bring us back to selecting the cells for use (primordial follicle culture) or not using the patient as a graft recipient (xenografting into immunodeficient animals).

Finally, assuming that the procedure is feasible and risk-free, the ovarian graft would have to be transplanted in a carefully chosen site, to allow sufficient angiogenesis in the graft, echographical visualization of the growing follicles and sampling of the mature oocytes. These criteria would seem to designate the abdomen, excluding any region that would have been previously irradiated or would depend on the enteric blood vessels.

TECHNICAL ASPECTS OF WHOLE OVARIAN TISSUE CRYOPRESERVATION

Obtaining the ovarian biopsy

Follicles are located inside the ovarian cortex, so that tissue samples collected for cryopreservation have to be from this particular compartment of the organ. The biopsy can be performed during any gynecological procedure, by laparoscopy or laparotomy, and can be composed of one or several cortical fragments, or even of a whole ovary, depending on the surgical indication. Nevertheless, if no widespread surgery (mainly occurring in the treatment of pelvic malignancies) is needed, biopsies should be obtained by simple laparoscopy performed under general anesthesia. Palmer forceps (see Figure 3) are inserted through one of the 5-mm trocars placed in the iliac fossa, and are used to grasp the ovary and cut a fragment of its surface (meaning a piece of cortex with a variable amount of the underlying medulla) (ovarian tissue biopsy, using Palmer forceps, see Figure 4).

As soon as the biopsy is performed, the tissue sample is collected in a sterile BlueMax 50-ml polypropylene conical tube (Falcon, Becton Dickinson and Company; Franklin Lakes, NJ, USA) containing 20 ml Leibovitz medium (L-15) supplemented with L-alanyl-L-glutamine (Gibco BRL, Life Technologies Ltd., Paisley, UK), and kept at 4°C in melting ice. To minimize any tissue damage due to ischemia, the sample is transferred within minutes to the laboratory for processing.

Processing the ovarian biopsy for freezing

The whole procedure is performed on a laminar air flux table, using sterile disposable material, to ensure optimal sterility to the tissue fragments.

Isolating fragments of ovarian cortex

The samples are transferred one by one to a Petri dish containing a sterilized glass slide and 1–2 ml of L-15 medium; tissue temperature is kept close to 4°C by putting the dish on top of a glass box containing crushed ice. The ovarian medulla is then separated from the cortex using forceps and a scalpel blade, and thrown away. The remaining cortex is cut on the glass slide, into strips of 1 mm^2 of section and 3–5 mm in length.

These strips are transferred into 2-ml Cryovials (Simport Plastics, Beloeil Quebec, Canada) containing 800 µl of L-15 medium and kept close to 0°C in a cooler box (Nalgene LapTop Cooler, Cat. No. 5116-0032, USA), each of these tubes containing four to eight strips. A few of these strips are randomly put aside and used for histological examination, two to four strips being put in a 37%

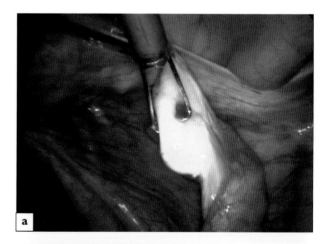

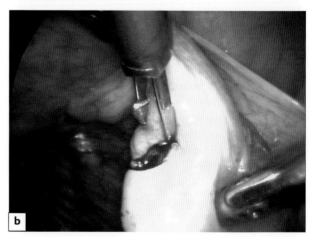

Figure 4 Laparoscopic view of Palmer forceps inserted through a 5-mm trocar, and used to grasp the ovary and cut a fragment of its surface

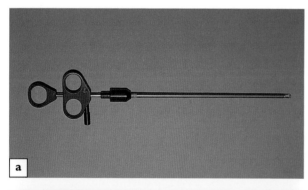

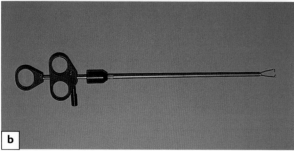

Figure 3 Palmer forceps are used to grasp the ovarian cortex, and to perform the biopsy. (a) Palmer forceps shown in closed position; (b) Palmer forceps shown in open position

paraformaldehyde solution, and one to two strips in a Bouin solution.

Preparing the fragments for freezing

Leibovitz medium is then twice replaced by freshly prepared SF-S solution, containing: 88% L-15 medium, 2% human albumin (Albumine humaine 20%, Département central de fractionnement de la Croix Rouge SCRL, Brussels, Belgium) and 10% dimethylsulfoxide (Sigma-Aldrich Co Ltd., Irvine, UK).

This aims to ensure optimal penetration of the tissue strips by the cryoprotective agent. Cryoprotective agents (CPAs) share the common goal of maximizing the cellular survival after freezing and thawing, although their action is based on different mechanisms of physics.

One class of cryoprotective agents permeate the tissue. They minimize the lethal effect of ice formation on the cells41 and reduce the induced build-up of extracellular salts42,43. These two phenomena are believed to be responsible for ovarian loss during the freezing process. One can easily understand that, when compared to single-cell freezing, whole tissue cryopreservation would need a longer exposure time to the CPA, thereby allowing it to reach an adequate concentration in the center of the tissue fragment but possibly increasing its toxicity on the 'over-exposed' near-surface cells44.

Several molecules are eligible as 'permeating CPA', such as ethylene glycol, dimethylsulfoxide, propylene glycol and glycerol. These four were studied in terms of CPA permeation rate and follicular population survival rate, taking the incubation time and the temperature into account44.

When considering the follicular population survival rate, it appears that the extent of follicular survival depends on the speed of CPA permeation, and on the final CPA tissue concentration achieved45; ethylene glycol and dimethylsulfoxide permeate the ovarian tissue more efficiently (dimethylsulfoxide being slightly better, but also much more toxic46), and subsequently allow better follicular survival than propylene glycol and glycerol (for detailed results, see Figure 5).

When considering the CPA permeation rate, it appears that CPA penetration is quicker when tissue is incubated at 37°C rather than 4°C. Maintaining physiological temperature during CPA exposure maximizes CPA entry into the cell by increasing the membrane fluidity48, and avoids inducing shock to the oocyte. However, this method has never been applied for clinical use, considering the fact that it does not affect the tissue concentration of CPA achieved after 30 min of incubation, and that it increases the CPA toxicity49.

A second class of CPAs does not permeate the cells. This class includes sugars (such as sucrose) and polymers (such as hydroxethyl starch)50. Their course of action is unclear, and their efficacy lower. They could act as osmotic buffers against the stress incurred by the cells on addition

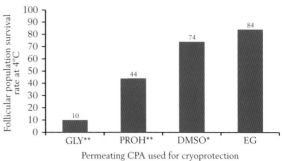

* No significant difference with EG value
** Significant difference with EG value

Figure 5 Follicular population survival rate at 4°C, according to the permeating cryoprotective agent (CPA) used for ovarian tissue cryoprotection. GLY, glycerol; PROH, propylene glycol; DMSO, dimethylsulfoxide; EG, ethylene glycol. From Newton *et al.*47

and removal of the 'permeating CPA', giving a plausible explanation for the better survival of single cells and embryos after freezing–thawing when a non-penetrating sugar, such as sucrose or mannitol, is added to the cryopreservation medium15,51,52.

Disappointingly, this method did not offer any improvement in the quality of ovarian tissue fragments after freezing and thawing; neither did it increase cell survival44, nor improve tissue structure at histology50.

Nevertheless, some authors consider sucrose to be a valuable addition to the freezing medium, as long as it induces a slight decrease in lactate dehydrogenase release; this could be the sign of lesser cell damage, which should be extensively studied to assess its actual importance in terms of further oocyte maturation and fertilization.

Freezing the tissue

The tissue samples are then transferred to a programmable freezer (Kryo 10, Planer Biomed, Sunbury on Thames, UK) and cooled down following the sequence:

(1) From 10°C to 0°C, at a rate of –2°C/min;

(2) Stable at 0°C for 15 min;

(3) From 0°C to –8°C, at a rate of –2°C/min;

(4) Stable at –8°C for 8 min for soaking;

(5) Manual induction of the formation of ice crystals, by grasping the cryovials (for 15–20 s each) with forceps pre-chilled in liquid nitrogen;

(6) Stable at –8°C for 8 min;

(7) From –8°C to –40°C, at a rate of –0.3°C/min;

(8) From –40°C to –150°C, at a rate of –30°C/min.

They are then transferred in liquid nitrogen (–196°C) for storage.

When thawing is needed, the patient's cryovials are taken out of the liquid nitrogen, and left at room temperature for 2 min. Thawing is subsequently completed by immersing the cryovials in a warm (37°C) water bath for 2 min. The tissue samples are grasped with small forceps and put in a Petri dish containing L-15 medium, thrice replaced to completely remove the cryoprotectant.

Ovarian tissue morphology and viability after freezing and thawing

One may wonder what influence a 240°C shift in temperature could have on ovarian tissue.

Although an increase in the relative surface area of fibrosis can be observed in frozen–thawed fragments of human ovarian tissue after grafting them into nude mice (when compared to fresh tissue grafted in the same conditions), it does not seem to impair either the viability or implantation capacity of the ovarian graft (angiogenesis), or its primordial and primary follicular population.

Indeed, no difference between fresh and frozen–thawed tissue is observed regarding follicular density, active angiogenesis (proved by both immunohistochemical staining for vascular endothelial growth factor and morphometric analysis of the vascular network) or ultrastructural characteristics. Moreover, neither the primordial follicle morphology, nor their proportion when compared to the entire follicular population, seem to differ (for detailed results, see Table 4). (For illustration of the identity of primordial and primary follicle morphology between fresh and frozen–thawed ovarian tissue, see Figures 6 and 7. When compared to Figure 6, Figure 7 identically shows the presence of morphologically intact primordial and primary follicles.)

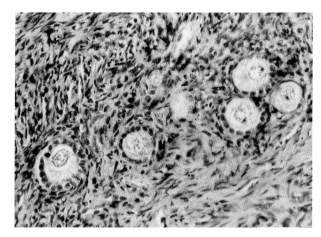

Figure 6 Primordial and primary follicle morphology in fresh ovarian tissue

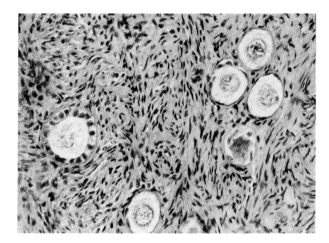

Figure 7 Primordial and primary follicle morphology in frozen–thawed ovarian tissue

Table 4 Follicular density in ovarian biopsies and fresh and frozen–thawed ovarian transplants. Fibrosis relative surface area and vascularization of the ovarian grafts. Reproduced with permission from Nisolle[53]

	Biopsy		Subcutaneous graft		Intraperitoneal graft	
	Fresh	Frozen–thawed	Fresh	Frozen–thawed	Fresh	Frozen–thawed
Fibrosis relative surface area (%)	NA	NA	40.7 ± 19.1	$68.35 \pm 28.7^*$	45.4 ± 6.5	$69.5 \pm 16.3^*$
Capillary relative surface area (%)	NA	NA	2.68 ± 1.62	271 ± 2.30	2.68 ± 1.08	4.85 ± 3.90
Mean area of capillaries (μm²)	NA	NA	234	518	112	305**
Number of capillaries per mm²	NA	NA	95	47	188	108†
Number of primordial follicles per mm²	2.66 ± 3.5	1.55 ± 1.7	$0.32 \pm 0.98^{\dagger\dagger}$	$0.31 \pm 0.5^{\dagger\dagger}$	0.45 ± 0.38	$0.43 \pm 0.45^{\dagger\dagger}$
Number of primary follicles per mm²	0.58 ± 0.75	0.25 ± 0.27	0.25 ± 0.5	0.47 ± 0.72	0.50 ± 1.4	0.65 ± 1.57

Values are mean ± SD or median. * The fibrosis relative surface area was significantly higher in frozen–thawed grafts than in fresh transplanted ovarian tissue ($p < 0.03$); ** the mean area of capillaries was significantly higher in frozen–thawed grafts than in fresh transplanted ovarian tissue ($p < 0.05$); † the number of capillaries per mm² was significantly lower in frozen–thawed grafts than in fresh transplanted ovarian tissue ($p < 0.05$); †† the follicular density was significantly lower than that observed in ovarian biopsies before grafting ($p < 0.05$)

These various elements suggest an acceptable tolerance of ovarian cortex and follicles regarding their morphology and function, although there is no proof concerning the maturation and fertilization potential of the immature oocytes contained in the frozen tissue.

REFERENCES

1. Oktay K, Newton H, Aubard Y, et al. Cryopreservation of immature human oocytes and ovarian tissue: an emerging technology? Fertil Steril 1998;69:1–7
2. Smith AU. Biological Effects of Freezing and Supercooling. London: Edward Arnold, 1961
3. Pegg DE. Cryobiology: life in the deep freeze. Biologist 1994;41:53–6
4. Gosden RG, Aubard Y. Transplantation of Ovarian and Testicular Tissues. Austin, TX: RG Landes Co, 1996
5. Winkel CA, Fossum GT. Current reproductive technology: considerations for the oncologist. Oncology Huntingt 1993;7:40–5 (discussion 46–8, 51)
6. Brown JR, Modell E, Obasaju M, et al. Natural cycle in-vitro fertilisation with embryo cryopreservation prior to chemotherapy for carcinoma of the breast. Hum Reprod 1996;11:197–9
7. Vincent C, Pickering SJ, Johnson MH. The hardening effect of dimethylsulfoxide on the mouse zona pellucida requires the presence of an oocyte and is associated with a reduction in the number of cortical granules present. J Reprod Fertil 1990;89:253–9
8. Trounson A, Kirby C. Problems in the cryopreservation of unfertilised eggs by slow cooling in dimethylsulfoxide. Fertil Steril 1989;52:778–86
9. Nagy ZP, Cecile J, Liu J, et al. Pregnancy and birth after intracytoplasmic sperm injection of in-vitro matured germinal vesicle stage oocytes: case report. Fertil Steril 1996;65:1047–50
10. Gook DA, Schiewe MC, Osborn SM, et al. Intracytoplasmic sperm injection and embryo development of human oocytes cryopreserved using 1,2-propanediol. Hum Reprod 1995;10:2637–41
11. Pickering SJ, Braude PR, Johnson MH, et al. Transient cooling to room temperature can cause irreversible disruption of the meiotic spindle in the human oocyte. Fertil Steril 1990;54:102–8
12. Gook DA, Osborn SM, Johnston WI. Cryopreservation of mouse and human oocytes using 1,2-propanediol and the configuration of the meiotic spindle. Hum Reprod 1993;8:1101–9
13. Gook DA, Osborn SM, Bourne H, et al. Fertilization of human oocytes following cryopreservation: normal karyotypes and absence of stray chromosomes. Hum Reprod 1994;9:684–91
14. Vincent C, Johnson MH. Cooling, cryoprotectants, and the cytoskeleton of the mammalian oocyte. Oxf Rev Reprod Biol 1992;14:73–100
15. Mandelbaum J, Junca AM, Plachot M, et al. Cryopreservation of human embryos and oocytes. Hum Reprod 1988;3:117–19
16. Toth TL, Lanzendorf SE, Sandow BA, et al. Cryopreservation of human prophase I oocytes collected from unstimulated follicles. Fertil Steril 1994;61:1077–82
17. Toth TL, Baka SG, Veeck LL, et al. Fertilisation and in-vitro development of cryopreserved human prophase I oocytes. Fertil Steril 1994;61:891–4
18. Mori T, Amano T, Shimizu H. Roles of gap junctional communication of cumulus cells in cytoplasmic maturation of porcine oocytes cultured in vitro. Biol Reprod 2000;62:913–19
19. De Loos FA, Zeinstra E, Bevers MM. Follicular wall maintains meiotic arrest in bovine oocytes cultured in vitro. Mol Reprod Dev 1994;39:162–5
20. Kalous J, Sutovsky P, Rimkevicova Z, et al. Pig membrana granulosa cells prevent resumption of meiosis in cattle oocytes. Mol Reprod Dev 1993;34:58–64
21. Isobe N, Maeda T, Terada T. Involvement of meiotic resumption in the disruption of gap junctions between cumulus cells attached to pig oocytes. J Reprod Fertil 1998;113:167–72
22. Dekel N, Beers WH. Development of rat oocytes in vitro: inhibition and induction of maturation in the presence or absence of cumulus-oophorus. Dev Biol 1980;75:247–54
23. Fagbohun CF, Downs SM. Metabolic coupling and ligand-stimulated meiotic maturation in the mouse oocyte-cumulus cell complex. Biol Reprod 1991;45:851–9
24. Mattioli M, Galeati G, Seren E. Effect of follicle somatic cells during pig oocyte maturation on egg penetrability and male pronuclear formation. Gamete Res 1988;20:177–83
25. Mattioli M, Galeati G, Bacci ML, Seren E. Follicular factors influence oocyte fertilizability by modulating the intercellular co-operation between cumulus cells and oocytes. Gamete Res 1988;21:223–32
26. Moor RM, Mattioli M, Ding J, et al. Maturation of pig oocytes in vivo and in vitro. J Reprod Fertil Suppl 1990;40:197–210
27. Fukui Y. Effect of follicular cells on the acrosome reaction, fertilization, and developmental competence of bovine oocytes matured in vitro. Mol Reprod Dev 1990;26:40–6
28. Vanderhyden BC, Armstrong DT. Role of cumulus cells and serum on the in vitro maturation, fertilization, and subsequent development of rat oocytes. Biol Reprod 1989;40:720–8

29. Kikuchi K. Effect of follicular cells on *in vitro* fertilization of pig follicular oocytes. *Theriogenology* 1993;39:593–9

30. Ka HH, Sawai K, Wang WH, *et al.* Amino acids in maturation medium and presence of cumulus cells at fertilization promote male pronuclear formation in porcine oocytes matured and penetrated *in vitro*. *Biol Reprod* 1997;57:1478–83

31. Yamauchi N, Nagai T. Male pronuclear formation in denuded porcine oocytes after *in vitro* maturation in the presence of cysteamine. *Biol Reprod* 1999;61:828–33

32. Hashimoto S, Saeki K, Nagao Y, *et al.* Effects of cumulus cells density during *in vitro* maturation on the developmental competence of bovine oocytes. *Theriogenology* 1998;49:1451–63

33. Eppig JJ. Further reflections on culture systems for the growth of oocytes *in vitro*. *Hum Reprod* 1994;9:974–6

34. Oktay K, Nugent D, Newton H, *et al.* Isolation and characterisation of primordial follicles from fresh and cryopreserved human ovarian tissue. *Fertil Steril* 1997;67:481–6

35. van Rhee F, Lin F, Cross NC, *et al.* Detection of residual leukaemia more than 10 years after alllogenic bone marow transplantation for chronic myelogenous leukaemia. *Bone Marrow Transplant* 1994;14:609–12

36. Roy SK, Treacy BJ. Isolation and long-term culture of human pre-antral follicles. *Fertil Steril* 1993;59:783–90

37. Lion T. Clinical implications of qualitative and quantitative polymerase chain reaction analysis in the monitoring of patients with chronic myelogenous leukaemia. *Bone Marrow Transplant* 1994;14:505–9

38. Roy DC, Perreault C, Belanger R, *et al.* Elimination of B-lineage leukaemia and lymphoma cells from bone marrow grafts using anti-B4-blocked-ricin immunotoxin. *J Clin Immunol* 1995;15:51–7

39. Gosden RG, Boulton MI, Grant K, *et al.* Follicular development from ovarian xenografts in SCID mice. *J Reprod Fertil* 1994;101:619–23

40. Oktay K, Gosden RG. Human primordial follicles can grow to early-antral stage in a novel xenograft model using the hpg/SCID mouse. *Fertil Steril* 1996;66:S6–7

41. Mazur P. Kinetics of water loss from cells at subzero temperatures and the likelihood of intracellular freezing. *J Gen Phys* 1963;47:347–69

42. Meryman HT. Modified model for the mechanism of freezing injury in erythrocytes. *Nature* 1968;218:333–6

43. Lovelock JE. The haemolysis of human red blood cells by freezing and thawing. *Biochem Biophys Acta* 1953;10:414–26

44. Newton H, Fisher J, Arnold JR, *et al.* Permeation of human ovarian tissue with cryoprotective agents in preparation for cryopreservation. *Hum Reprod* 1998;13:376–80

45. Candy CJ, Wood MJ, Whittingham DG. Effect of cryoprotectants on the survival of follicles in frozen mouse ovaries. *J Reprod Fertil* 1997;110:11–19

46. Vincent C, Pickering SJ, Johnson MH, *et al.* Dimethylsulfoxide affects the organisation of microfilaments in the mouse oocyte. *Mol Reprod Dev* 1990;26:227–35

47. Newton H, Aubard Y, Rutherford A, *et al.* Low temperature storage and grafting of human ovarian tissue. *Hum Reprod* 1996;11:1487–91

48. Isachenko V, Soler C, Isachenko E, *et al.* Vitrification of immature porcine oocytes: effects of lipid droplets, temperature, cytoskeleton, and addition and removal of cryoprotectant. *Cryobiology* 1998;36:250–3

49. Aigner S, Van der Elst J, Siebzehnrubl E, *et al.* The influence of slow and ultra-rapid freezing on the organisation of the meiotic spindle of the mouse oocyte. *Hum Reprod* 1992;7:857–64

50. Meryman HT. Cryoprotective agents. *Cryobiology* 1971;8:173–83

51. Hovatta O, Silye R, Krausz T, *et al.* Cryopreservation of human ovarian tissue using dimethylsulfoxide and propanediol-sucrose as cryoprotectants. *Hum Reprod* 1996;11:1269–72

52. Lassalle B, Testart J, Renard JP. Human embryo features that influence the success of cryopreservation with the use of 1,2-propanediol. *Fertil Steril* 1985;44:645–51

53. Nisolle M, Casanas-Roux F, Qu J, *et al.* Histologic and ultrastructural evaluation of fresh and frozen-thawed human ovarian xenografts in nude mice. *Fertil Steril* 2000;74:122–9

32

Laparoscopic ovarian transposition

M. Nisolle, J. Squifflet and J. Donnez

INTRODUCTION

Pelvic radiotherapy is frequently used to treat pelvic tumors in premenopausal women. It has already been stated that a dose of 5–20 Gy administered to the ovary is sufficient to completely impair gonadal function[1-3], whatever the age of the patient. Iatrogenic destruction of the follicular reserve by radiation therapy may be avoided by ovarian transposition into the paracolic gutter. Ovarian transposition performed by laparotomy was first described by McCall and colleagues in 1958 in patients treated for cervical carcinoma[4]. Nowadays, ovarian suspension is laparoscopically performed before irradiation[5-7]. However, it has also been demonstrated that, even if ovarian transposition is performed, it cannot be considered completely safe because patients receive infradiaphragmatic irradiation[8] and, in many cases, there is an association between radiation and chemotherapy[8,9]. For women who are to receive chemotherapy and/or radiotherapy, not only ovarian transposition but also cryopreservation of ovarian tissue should be proposed, even if *in vitro* maturation of oocytes has not yet been proved to be routinely efficacious after cryopreservation.

All patients need to be informed of the long-term consequences of cancer and its therapy even if not all treatments cause infertility.

SURGICAL TECHNIQUES

The procedure is performed under general endotracheal anesthesia. After induction of a pneumoperitoneum, a 12-mm trocar is inserted subumbilically. The laparoscope is connected to a video camera. Three 5-mm trocars are systematically inserted suprapubically: one in the mid-line approximately 3 cm above the symphysis pubis, and the other two, a few centimeters on either side, taking care to avoid the epigastric vessels. The surgical procedure of laparoscopic ovarian transposition is identical to that performed by laparotomy[10].

Usually, the right ovary is preferred for transposition because of easier access, as the bowel may be pushed out of the way. But if radiotherapy is localized on the right, the left ovary is transposed.

The right adnex is grasped and mobilized. The isthmic portion of the tube and the utero-ovarian ligament are coagulated using bipolar forceps and cut off at their uterine origin (Figure 1). The peritoneum is incised along the infundibulopelvic ligament to mobilize the adnex

completely. The course of the ureter is visualized and care is taken to avoid damage to the ureter. Dissection of the infundibulopelvic vessels using bipolar coagulation and scissors is continued until adnexal transposition to the paracolic gutter is achieved, without any traction or torsion of the ovarian vascular pedicle (Figure 2). Using Vicryl-1,

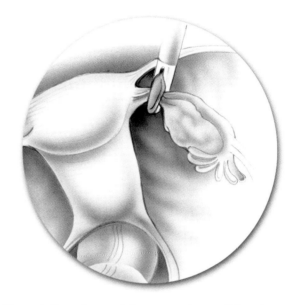

Figure 1 Coagulation of the proximal part of the adnex

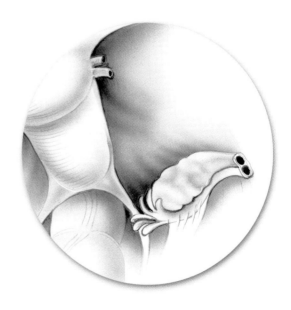

Figure 2 Adnexal transposition avoiding traction to the ovarian vascular pedicle

the right ovary is anchored to the peritoneum of the anterior abdominal wall very high in the right paracolic gutter. In order to facilitate the fixation of the ovary, a curved needle is inserted in the right lateral flank in front of the desired anchoring of the ovary.

Titanium clips are placed on the two opposite borders of the ovary to allow radiological identification prior to radiotherapy (Figure 3a and b). To avoid bowel incarceration between the transposed ovary and the abdominal wall, the vascular pedicle is attached to the anterolateral abdominal wall with three or four titanium clips.

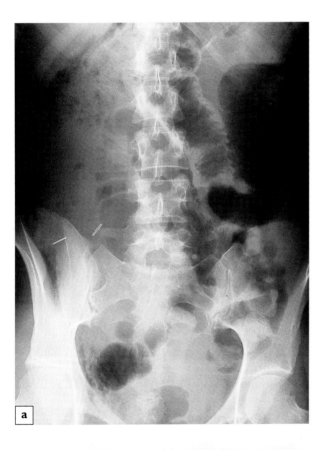

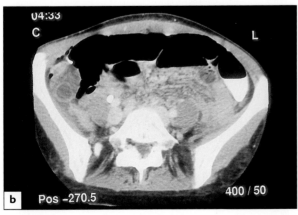

Figure 3 Postoperative identification of the transposed ovary before radiotherapy using (a) radiography and (b) computerized tomography

INDICATIONS

Laparoscopic ovarian transposition should be indicated in all women requiring radiotherapy for gynecological or non-gynecological malignancy.

All the indications for laparoscopic ovarian transposition should also be indications for ovarian tissue cryopreservation and ovarian tissue-banking facilities should be available. Indeed, even if chemotherapy is not initially proposed to the patient, it must always be considered as a possibility after surgery, which could impair gonadal function even in a transposed ovary.

In our department, ovarian cryopreservation has been available since April 1997 and it has been performed in 76 patients suffering from different types of cancer. In this series of 76 patients, five underwent ovarian transposition because of the indication for radiotherapy. The ovarian transposition was performed laparoscopically in three cases and by laparotomy in two cases.

The indications for radiotherapy were: two cases of recto-sigmoid tumors, one case of cervical carcinoma, one case of quadriceps liposarcoma, and one case of medulloblastoma. The classic indications for ovarian transposition in cases of malignant disease are summarized in Table 1.

The main indication for ovarian transposition in gynecological malignancy is the detection of early cervical carcinoma. Transposition is usually performed during the surgical treatment of the cervical carcinoma.

Concerning detection of rectosigmoid tumors in young patients, laparoscopic ovarian transposition is usually performed before radiotherapy indicated to decrease tumor size and before removal of the tumor.

DISCUSSION

Radiotherapy and ovarian function: risk factors

Irradiation, which is required as treatment for different types of cancer, exposes the patient to the risk of castration. Several procedures have been proposed[1,9,11,12] to preserve ovarian function when radiotherapy is needed in the pelvis. In 1993, Haie-Meder and colleagues[3] reported the outcome of ovarian preservation after lateral transposition in young women requiring radiotherapy with or without chemotherapy. In their study, the predictive factors of ovarian function preservation after radiotherapy were age, the irradiation fields and doses, and the association with chemotherapy.

Age and hormonal status at diagnosis

Age in itself is a predictive factor of ovarian function. The physiological decrease in the number of primordial

Table I Indications for ovarian transposition in cases of malignant disease

Gynecological malignancy
Early cervical carcinoma
Early vaginal carcinoma
Early vulvar carcinoma

Non-gynecological malignancy
Rectosigmoid tumors
Pelvic or extrapelvic sarcoma
Bone cancer (osteosarcoma, Ewing's sarcoma)
Lymphoma
Medulloblastoma

Table 2 Toxicity of radiotherapy according to irradiation fields

Site of radiotherapy	Risk of premature ovarian failure (%)
Supradiaphragmatic	10
Infradiaphragmatic	35
Total body irradiation	> 50

follicles during life makes the ovaries more sensitive to any aggressive treatment, such as chemotherapy and/or radiotherapy. In patients treated for Hodgkin's disease, Schilsky and colleagues[13] reported a significantly shorter time from diagnosis to amenorrhea in patients > 25 years of age. Gradishar and Schilsky[14] suggested that patients < 25 years of age would not experience any significant therapy-related dysfunction for 5–10 years following completion of chemotherapy.

From the literature published to date, it is impossible to determine whether the prepubertal ovary is less susceptible to the effects of irradiation than the adult ovary. An alternative explanation for an apparently increased resistance to damage of a girl's ovary may simply be a reflection of the earlier age and larger number of oocytes within the ovary, rather than any effect of puberty. Furthermore, in addition to direct gonadal damage, irradiation may also affect the uterus, thus decreasing the chance of successfully carrying a pregnancy to full term.

Irradiation fields and doses

Ovarian preservation according to the type of irradiation is determined by measurements on the phantom[3]. There is a significant difference in ovarian preservation according to the irradiation fields. Pelvic irradiation and inverted irradiation carry the highest probability for ovarian failure (Table 2).

In cases of supradiaphragmatic irradiation, the risk of impairment of gonadal function is ± 10% and in cases of infradiaphragmatic irradiation, this risk increases to 35%[3]. These percentages are dependent on the total dose and distribution of the dose administered. The risk of ovarian failure according to the dose of radiotherapy is summarized in Table 3.

Women who received a dose of ≤ 5 Gy of ovarian irradiation had a higher probability of ovarian function preservation than patients who received > 5 Gy[3]. In addition to dose, age also has an impact on ovarian function preserva-

tion. Lushbaugh and Casaren[1] suggested that the total dose inducing menopause was 6 Gy in women ≥ 40 years of age, while it could reach 20 Gy in girls. In the study by Haie-Meder and colleagues[3], all the impubescent girls became pubescent, while the same range of doses caused menopause in 32% of patients > 25 years of age. The dose to the ovaries, however, was the most important predictive factor of ovarian function preservation (≤ 5 versus > 5 Gy).

Association with chemotherapy

Association of radiotherapy and chemotherapy is indicated in many cancers, mostly arising during adolescence, including Hodgkin's disease, non-Hodgkin's lymphoma, leukemia, medulloblastoma and other systemic malignant conditions. In such cases, bone marrow transplantation may be indicated.

The most frequent chemotherapy combination is mechlorethamine, vincristine, procarbazine and prednisone (MOPP). When associated with radiotherapy, the incidence of ovarian function failure was found to be significantly higher than in patients who had other or no chemotherapy[3].

Radiotherapy after ovarian transposition: are ovarian function and fertility preserved?

Byrne and colleagues[15] showed very little diminution in women's fertility after treatment for cancer (relative fertility 0.93). Fertility was decreased by 25%, however, when infradiaphragmatic radiotherapy was performed. Haie-Meder and co-workers[3] found that the measured dose to the transposed ovaries was 10% of the delivered dose when the ovaries were located under shielding blocks and 4.4% when the ovaries were outside the irradiation field. Nevertheless, results in terms of pregnancy outcome must be evaluated with caution. In the series of Haie-Meder's group[3], the pregnancy outcome was 19%, although ovarian function was apparently preserved. This rate was significantly lower than the rate in the general population. Interpretation is difficult, however, because this low rate could also reflect a patient's personal choice, or an effect of radiotherapy on the uterus itself which could affect implantation.

333

Table 3 Risk of ovarian failure according to the dose of radiotherapy

Ovarian dose (rads)	Results
60	no deleterious effect
150	no deleterious effect in young women some risk for women > 40 years
250–500	in women aged 15–40 years, 60% permanent POF
	in women > 40 years, 100% permanent POF
500–800	in women aged 15–40 years, 60–70% permanent POF
> 800	100% permanent POF

POF, premature ovarian failure

Ovarian transposition appears to be a good technique to protect ovaries from the risk of castration.

A very large prospective series of ovarian transposition in patients with cervical carcinoma treated by a radiosurgical combination was recently published[16]. Ovarian transposition to the paracolic gutters with radical hysterectomy and lymphadenectomy was performed on 107 patients (bilaterally in 98% of cases). This procedure was recommended for patients < 40 years of age with a small invasive cervical carcinoma (≤ 3 cm) treated by initial surgery. The rates of ovarian preservation were 90% in patients treated by postoperative vaginal brachytherapy and 60% in patients treated by postoperative external radiation therapy and vaginal brachytherapy.

Thus, ovarian transposition could not prevent ovarian failure after vaginal brachytherapy and ovarian cryopreservation must be systematically proposed to patients when surgery spares the female genital tract[17,18].

In conclusion, there is a place for ovarian transposition in cases of radiotherapy exclusively directed at the lowest parts of the pelvis, but there is still a lack of knowledge concerning the effect of radiotherapy on uterine receptivity. There is also an indication for ovarian tissue cryopreservation in cases where radiotherapy is associated with chemotherapy.

REFERENCES

1. Lushbaugh CC, Casaren GW. The effect of gonadal irradiation in clinical radiation therapy: a review. Cancer 1976;37:1111–20

2. Mulvihill JJ, McKeen EA, Rosner F, et al. Pregnancy outcome in cancer patients. Experience in a large cooperative group. Cancer 1987;60:1143–50

3. Haie-Meder C, Mlika-Cabanne N, Michel G, et al. Radiotherapy after ovarian transposition: ovarian function and fertility preservation. Int J Radiat Oncol Biol Phys 1993;25:419–24

4. McCall ML, Keaty EC, Thompson JD. Conservation of ovarian tissue in the treatment of the carcinoma of the cervix with radical surgery. Am J Obstet Gynecol 1958;75:590–600

5. Tulandi T, Al-Took S. Laparoscopic ovarian suspension before irradiation. Fertil Steril 1998;70:381–3

6. Hart R, Sawyer E, Magos A. Case report of ovarian transposition and review of literature. Gynecol Endosc 1999;8:51–4

7. Yarali H, Demirol A, Bukulmez O, et al. Laparoscopic high lateral transposition of both ovaries before pelvic irradiation. J Am Assoc Gynecol Laparosc 2000;7:237–9

8. Baker TG. Radiosensitivity of mammalian oocytes with particular reference to the human female. Am J Obstet Gynecol 1971;110:746–61

9. Hodel K, Rich WM, Austin P, et al. The role of ovarian transposition in conservation of ovarian function in radical hysterectomy followed by pelvic radiation. Gynecol Oncol 1982;13:195–202

10. Morice P, Castaigne D, Haie-Meder C, et al. Laparoscopic ovarian transposition for pelvic malignancies: indications and functional outcomes. Fertil Steril 1998;70:959–60

11. Nahhas WA, Nisce LZ, D'Angio GJ, et al. Lateral ovarian transposition. Obstet Gynecol 1971;38:785–8

12. Leporrier M, Van Theobald P, Roffe JL, et al. A new technique to protect ovarian function before pelvic irradiation. Heterotopic ovarian transplantation. Cancer 1987;60:2001–4

13. Schilsky RL, Sherins RJ, Hubbard SM, et al. Long-term follow up of ovarian function in women treated with MOPP chemotherapy for Hodgkin's disease. Am J Med 1981;71:552–6

14. Gradishar WJ, Schilsky RL. Effects of cancer treatment on the reproductive system. CRC Crit Rev Oncol Hematol 1988;8:153–71

15. Byrne J, Mulvihill JJ, Meyers MH, et al. Effects of treatment on infertility in long term survivors of childhood or adolescent cancer. N Engl J Med 1987;317:1315–21

16. Morice P, Juncker L, Rey A, et al. Ovarian transposition for patients with cervical carcinoma treated by radiosurgical combination. Fertil Steril 2000;74:743–8

17. Donnez J, Qu J, Nisolle M. Gonadal cryopreservation in the young patient with gynecological malignancy. Curr Opin Obstet Gynecol 2000;12:1–9

18. Donnez J, Bassil S. Indications for cryopreservation of ovarian tissue. Hum Reprod Update 1998;4:248–59

33

The place of endoscopy in malignancy

J. Donnez, M. Berlière, J. Squifflet and M. Nisolle

Indications for gynecologic surgery have, in recent years, increased. In the case of gynecologic malignancies, the use of laparoscopy is still in its infancy.

More clinical data are required before laparoscopic techniques are accepted as new surgical standards. Ongoing prospective clinical studies will help answer many of the questions regarding the safety and efficacy of gynecologic laparoscopy. Until more data are available, operative laparoscopy will remain a promising but unproven tool in the management of patients with gynecologic malignancies.

INDICATIONS FOR LAPAROSCOPIC PROCEDURES IN ENDOMETRIAL CANCER

Evaluation of the anatomosurgical stage is crucial in the therapeutic strategy of endometrial cancer. Lymph node involvement plays a major role in this evaluation, as an indicator of both prognosis and the need for adjuvant therapy. Lymph node metastasis is related to tumor size and grade, tumor stage and invasion of the myometrium (Table 1). In our department, bilateral laparoscopic adnexectomy and laparoscopic hysterectomy are performed in atypical hyperplasia and in cases of stage 0–1, grade 1 endometrial cancer. Stage I, grade 2–3 endometrial cancer requires additional lymphadenectomy (Table 2). Laparoscopic lymphadenectomy is also performed 2 weeks after laparoscopic hysterectomy, when histology reveals either myometrial invasion of more than two-thirds of the depth of the myometrium, histological invasion of the cervix, or a histological grade more severe than that suspected from the preoperative biopsy.

Table 1 Prevalence of lymph node metastasis in relation to tumor size and tumor grade in endometrial cancer

Tumor grade	Tumor size		
	≤ 2 cm diameter	> 2 cm diameter	Entire surface
1	0/15 (0%)	0/14 (0%)	0/3 (0%)
2	0/10 (0%)	4/12 (33%)	1/3 (33%)
3	2/10 (20%)	6/20 (30%)	3/4 (75%)

Table 2 Indications for laparoscopic procedures in endometrial cancer

Diagnosis	Proposed therapy
Atypical hyperplasia Adenocarcinoma stage 0–I; grade 1	laparoscopic adnexectomy and hysterectomy
Adenocarcinoma stage I; grade 2–3	laparoscopic adnexectomy and hysterectomy + laparoscopic lymphadenectomy
Adenocarcinoma stage II	laparoscopic lymphadenectomy followed by radical vaginal hysterectomy (Schauta)
Adenocarcinoma stage III–IV	+ multiple biopsies?

Stage II endometrial cancer requires laparoscopic lymphadenectomy, followed by radical vaginal hysterectomy, as described by Schauta[1]. This technique should only be attempted by experienced surgeons who are experts in the vaginal approach. In many departments, stage II endometrial cancer is treated by a Wertheim–Meigs surgical procedure with lymphadenectomy.

In stage III and IV endometrial cancer, the role of laparoscopy is not yet clearly defined. It may be an indication for performing multiple biopsies in different sites of the peritoneal cavity.

In patients with endometrial cancer, initial laparoscopic lymphadenectomy, together with bilateral adnexectomy, allows the subsequent hysterectomy to be performed, either vaginally or laparoscopically[2,3]. The few studies which have been reported[2,4] suggest that more extensive investigation is needed to determine the possible future role of laparoscopic surgery in the treatment of endometrial cancer.

In our department, laparoscopic bilateral adnexectomy and laparoscopic hysterectomy are the procedures of choice in the treatment of stage I endometrial cancer. Laparoscopic lymphadenectomy is also performed in cases of non-differentiated endometrial cancer.

INDICATIONS FOR LYMPHADENECTOMY IN VAGINAL CANCER

Primary carcinoma of the vagina is a malignant lesion that appears in the vagina and does not involve the cervix or vulva. It is rare, representing 1–2% of all gynecologic malignancies. In an extensive review of the literature, Plentl and Friedman[5] found that 51.7% of primary vaginal cancers occurred in the upper third of the vagina and 57.6% were on the posterior wall. Tumors originating in the vagina may spread along the vaginal wall to involve the cervix or the vulva. However, if biopsies of the cervix or the vulva are positive at diagnosis, the tumor cannot be considered a primary vaginal lesion.

Lymphatic drainage of the vagina involves an extensive intercommunicating network. The lymphatics in the upper portion of the vagina drain primarily via the lymphatics of the cervix, whereas those in the lower portion of the vagina drain either to cervical lymphatics or follow drainage patterns of the vulva into femoral and inguinal nodes. The anterior vaginal wall usually drains into the deep pelvic nodes, including the interiliac and parametrial nodes.

The incidence of positive pelvic nodes at diagnosis varies with the stage and location of the primary tumor. Because the lymphatic system of the vagina is so complex, any of the nodal groups may be involved, regardless of the location of the lesion. Involvement of inguinal nodes is most common, however, when the lesion is located in the lower third of the vagina. The reported incidence of clinically positive nodes at diagnosis varies from 5.1%[7] to 20.8%[6]. Radiation therapy is the preferred treatment for most carcinomas of the vagina. Surgical procedures may be reserved for the treatment of irradiation failures and for non-epithelial tumors. For tumors of the upper third of the vagina (Figures 1 and 2), surgery can be an excellent alternative, especially if the tumor is near the cervix. In this case, laparoscopic lymphadenectomy (Figure 3) can be performed before radical hysterectomy (Figure 4).

CERVICAL CANCER

Laparoscopic surgery offers two possible options to avoid laparotomy in cervical cancer:

(1) Laparoscopic lymphadenectomy followed by the vaginal operative approach according to the Schauta technique[7–10];

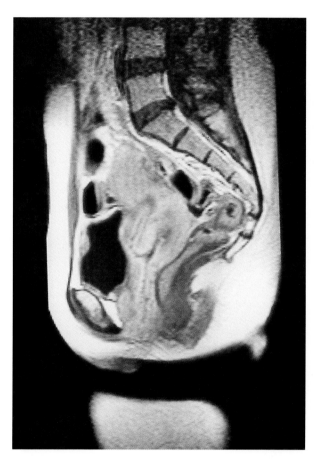

Figure 2 Magnetic resonance imaging (same patient as in Figure 1) provides an excellent view of vaginal involvement

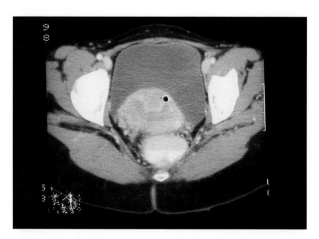

Figure 1 Computerized tomography (CT) scan: cancer of the vagina located in the upper third on the posterior wall

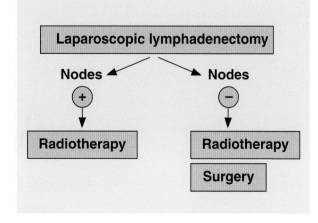

Figure 3 Proposed therapy for carcinoma of the upper third of the vagina

(2) Lymphadenectomy followed by an extended laparoscopic hysterectomy[10,11].

The presence of lymph node metastasis is the most significant prognostic factor in cervical cancer. Squamous carcinoma of the cervix spreads principally by direct local invasion to adjacent tissue and by lymphatics[12,13], and less commonly through blood vessels. Initially, the tumor grows by direct continuity along tissue spaces of least resistance, the perineural and perivascular tissues, into the paracervical and parametrial areas and into the cardinal and uterosacral ligaments. Ultimately, lateral spread may reach the bony pelvis and obstruct one or both ureters.

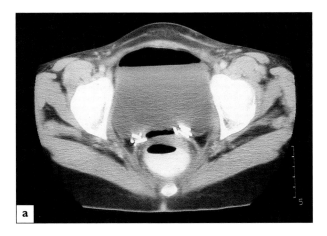

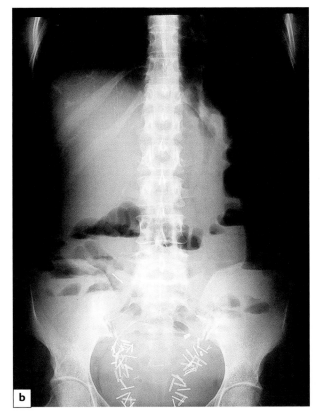

Figure 4 Computerized tomography (CT) scan (a) and radiography (b) after hysterectomy and colpectomy in cases of primary carcinoma (same patient as in Figure 1)

Direct extension may also involve the uterine cavity and vagina, with extension into the urinary bladder and rectum, resulting in vesicovaginal and rectovaginal fistulas.

The spread of cervical cancer via lymphatics occurs relatively early in the course of the disease and is found in 25–50% of patients with stage Ib and II carcinomas. The preferential course of dissemination is via the paracervical hypogastric, and external iliac lymph nodes followed by extension to lateral sacral, common iliac, para-aortic and inguinal nodes. Isolated invasion of the sacral, external iliac, and hypogastric nodes is occasionally observed. Metastases to distant lymph nodes above the diaphragm, including the supraclavicular lymph nodes, are uncommon and are a feature of widespread disease. In these cases, cancer cells are transported from the para-aortic nodes into the mediastinum and then into the thoracic duct. Diagnosis of lymph node metastasis can be made by lymphography, computerized tomography and/or nuclear magnetic resonance (Figure 5). The low sensitivity of lymphography (< 30%)[14], computerized tomography (Figure 6) (between 30 and 70%)[14–16], nuclear magnetic resonance and lymphoscintigraphy[8] in the detection of potentially malignant adenopathies has prompted some authors to perform retroperitoneal lymph node sampling[17,18]. Positron emission tomography (PET) (Figure 7) provides a view of lymph node involvement and is, at the present time, under evaluation.

The first laparoscopic lymphadenectomies were performed by Dargent[18], Reich[19], Querleu and colleagues[2,8,20], Canis and colleagues[12] and Nezhat and co-workers[11]. Results are very encouraging, with a 100% sensitivity rate in a series of 75 patients and a very low postoperative complication rate[2,8]. The first indication for laparoscopic lymphadenectomy in gynecological oncology is the staging of early, operable, carcinoma of the cervix[2]. The risk of 'skip' metastases to the para-aortic nodes without pelvic node involvement is very low (< 1%); this occurs almost exclusively in patients with large tumors (> 4 cm). Patients with stage Ib, IIa or IIb disease and nega-

Lymph node metastasis
=
prognostic factor of cervical carcinoma

| Diagnosis |

1. Lymphangiography
2. Computerized tomography (Figure 6)
3. Nuclear magnetic resonance imaging
4. PET tomography (Figure 7)
5. Laparoscopic lymphadenectomy

Figure 5 Diagnosis of lymph node metastasis. PET, positron emission tomography

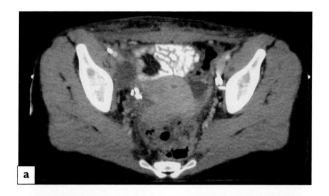

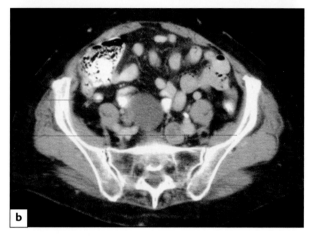

Figure 6 (a) and (b) Computerized tomography (CT) scan reveals a necrotic metastatic lymph node

tive pathological staging may be cured by radical or abdominal surgery.

However, radical hysterectomy does not seem justified when nodes are invaded by metastatic disease[15,19] (Figure 8).

In stage IV carcinoma extension (extension into the urinary bladder) (Figure 9), laparoscopic lymphadenectomy must be carried out before performing an anterior pelvectomy. A new technique[13] for the detection of the sentinel lymph node is being investigated in early stage cervical cancer and this procedure is described in another chapter by Dargent.

INDICATIONS FOR LAPAROSCOPIC PROCEDURES IN OVARIAN CANCER

In advanced ovarian cancer, laparoscopy might prove to be a valuable tool when evaluating patients prior to debulking surgery[21]. Retrospective analyses suggest that a subgroup of patients with stage III and IV ovarian carcinoma can – after staging by laparoscopy – be treated by neoadjuvant chemotherapy, followed by interval debulking surgery[21].

For patients with advanced ovarian cancer who can be treated, the feasibility and reliability of a laparoscopic second-look procedure and comparison with second-look laparotomy have been investigated in a French study[22].

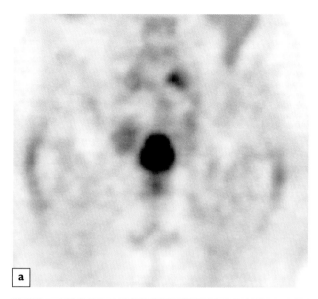

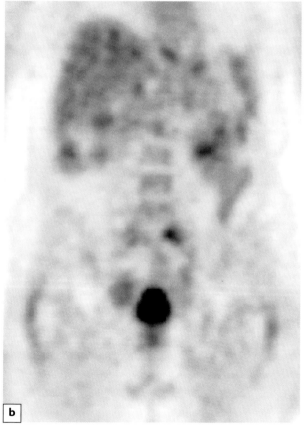

Figure 7 (a) and (b) Positron emission tomography (PET) provides a view of lymph node involvement

The conclusions are that, after treatment of ovarian cancer, second-look laparoscopy appears to be less reliable than second-look laparotomy. The presence of severe postoperative adhesions is the main obstacle to an exhaustive, reliable and safe laparoscopic second-look procedure.

Current guidelines for the surgical staging of ovarian cancer (stage I and II) include the removal of retroperitoneal lymph nodes (pelvic and aortic)[23–25]. In most

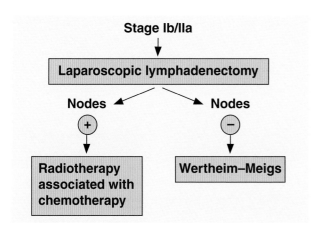

Figure 8 Proposed therapy for cervical carcinoma stage Ib, IIa and IIb

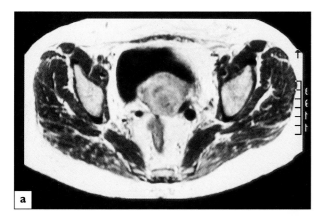

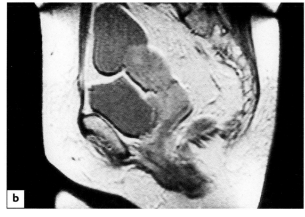

Figure 9 (a) and (b) Magnetic resonance imaging of stage IV cervical carcinoma. The involvement of the urinary bladder wall is clearly seen

centers, this is achieved by means of laparotomy but advanced laparoscopic techniques have been performed[24].

If laparoscopy is useful in the staging of established and advanced ovarian cancer, it may also play a role in early-stage epithelial ovarian carcinoma[25].

Especially for young women, the laparoscopic procedure allows fertility-sparing surgery and appears safe and promising. Finally, the laparoscopic procedure also seems to be the surgical procedure most adopted for prophylac-

tic oophorectomy in patients with an inherited risk of ovarian cancer[26] (carriers of BRCA1-BRCA2 mutations).

The laparoscopic procedure could be converted into laparotomy if ovarian cancer is discovered during the procedure.

The fields of laparoscopic surgery in malignant ovarian pathology offer encouraging results but need confirmation by prospective randomized trials and studies of long-term survival.

TECHNIQUE

Laparoscopic hysterectomy

Endometrial cancer typically occurs in obese, high-risk women. The use of the laparoscope precludes an abdominal incision wound infection in these patients. Atypical hyperplasia and stage 0–I, grade 1 endometrial cancer do not require lymphadenectomy. Treatment may be by laparoscopically assisted vaginal hysterectomy (LAVH) or a laparoscopic hysterectomy (LH) (see Chapter 25): all maneuvers following internal vessel ligation can be performed vaginally or laparoscopically, including anterior and posterior vaginal entry, cardinal and intersacral ligament division, intact uterine removal and vaginal closure.

The adnexa are removed first. The infundibulopelvic ligament is identified and exposed by applying traction to the adnexa with an opposite forceps. The bipolar forceps are used to compress and desiccate the vessels which are then cut with scissors. Alternatively, staples or sutures may be applied. The other steps are described in Chapter 19. Ligation of the uterine vessels can also be performed by the vaginal approach. Some authors prefer suture ligation of the vascular bundle. If LAVH is being performed, the rest of the operation is done vaginally, as is suturing of the vaginal vault.

Laparoscopic lymphadenectomy

The preparation of the patient for surgery follows standard procedures. In order to avoid any possible disturbance due to an overdistended large bowel, cleansing of the digestive system must be undertaken. A pneumoperitoneum is achieved through the subumbilical incision. Three suprapubic incisions are made. The operation begins with a peritoneal cytology and abdominopelvic exploration. The ureters are visualized. The peritoneum is incised between the round and the lumbo-ovarian ligament. The subperitoneal space is opened using scissors and the iliac vessels are identified (Figure 10).

During the whole operation, the round ligament is grasped and kept in an elevated and medial position. This allows identification of the umbilical artery, the internal limit of node sampling. The obturator nerve is then identified, located against the pelvic wall under the iliac vessels.

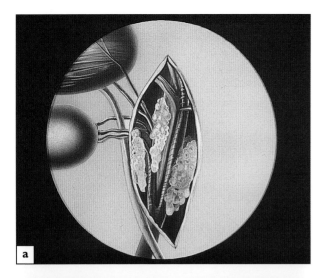

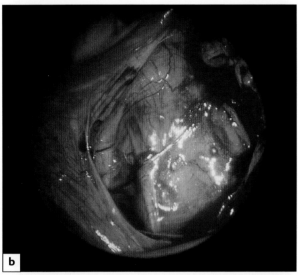

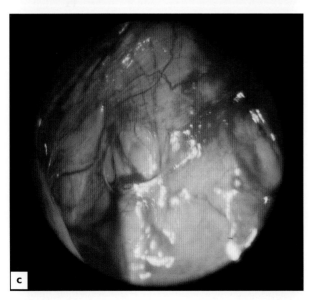

Figure 10 (a)–(c) Incision of the peritoneum between the round ligament and the lumbo-ovarian ligament. The iliac vessels are identified behind the lymph nodes and the retroperitoneal fatty tissue

Node sampling can begin with the subvenous group, which is the lowest one; this ensures that any bleeding does not make further dissection more difficult.

The operation can also begin by the sampling of the supra-arterial nodes. Dissection is performed towards the origin of the external iliac vein (Figure 11) with gentle traction on the nodes. Careful lymphostasis with clips is performed throughout the dissection when a large lymphatic canal is encountered.

Once the space between the pelvic wall and the inferior side of the internal iliac vein has been treated, dissection of the internal retrocrural nodal group is begun (Figure 12). The obturator nerve is clearly seen (Figure 13). During this procedure, an anastomosis between the external iliac vein and the obturator vein may be encountered; careful dissection is required to avoid venous injury.

A forceps (celioextractor)[9–19] can be used to remove nodes from the abdominal cavity without any risk of abdominal wall contamination. They can also be removed through the laparoscope trocar or through a 25-mm trocar (Figure 14) with a forceps (Figure 15). Analysis of suspect nodes may be indicated in order to avoid further dissection in cases of node positivity. Querleu and colleagues[7] reported false-negative analyses in 14 cases of cervical cancer. The duration of lymphadenectomy varies from 75 to 150 min, depending largely on the associated surgical procedures, such as hysterectomy. The number of nodes removed varies; the average number of lymph nodes has been reported as 13–22, 10, 19–34, while in our series of lymphadenectomies, the number of nodes ranged from 20 to 37.

COMPLICATIONS

Vascular injury is the major potential risk of laparoscopic pelvic lymphadenectomy, but is much less frequent than expected. Significant bleeding may occur due to injury to pelvic arteries or veins. Injury to the branches of the hypogastric artery (uterine artery, superior vesical artery or umbilical artery) is managed by direct application of vascular clips or bipolar hemostasis to the vessel. Injury to the external iliac vein or a main branch of the internal iliac veins is the most serious potential complication of pelvic lymphadenectomy because its management is more difficult than for arterial injury.

When fixed lymph nodes are encountered, any attempt at their dissection is hazardous and cytological examination (needle aspiration) must be carried out in order to prevent a vein injury[20]. If bleeding of the external iliac vein occurs, compression may be successful; a closed forceps may be firmly applied in order to compress the vessel against the pelvic side wall. If hemorrhage persists, the use of clips or coagulation may worsen the laceration; laparotomy must be performed in order to manage an external iliac vein laceration.

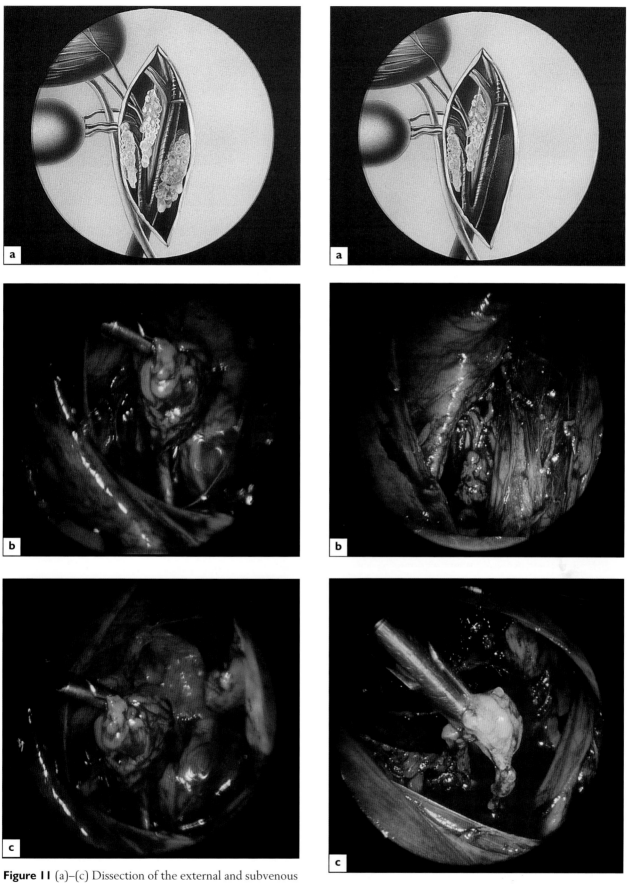

Figure 11 (a)–(c) Dissection of the external and subvenous groups. Using gentle traction on the nodes, the dissection is performed. The external iliac vein is then visible

Figure 12 (a)–(c) Dissection of the internal retrocrural and obturator group

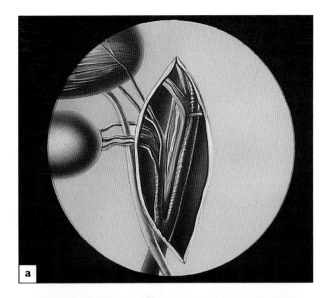

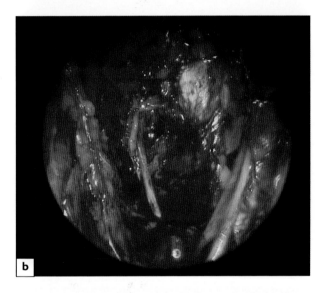

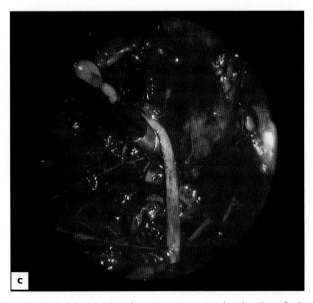

Figure 13 (a)–(c) The obturator nerve is clearly identified

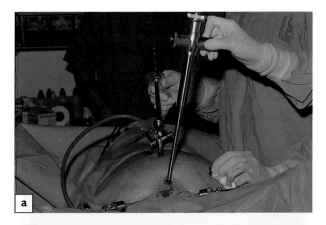

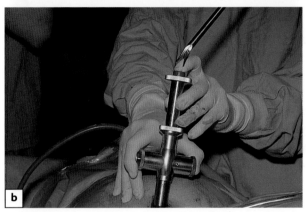

Figure 14 (a) A 25-mm trocar is inserted suprapubically; (b) a forceps is introduced via a trocar reducer

The risk of accidental section of the obturator nerve is very low.

Ureteral injury during lymphadenectomy is extremely infrequent; indeed, the ureter is not in the operative field. The ureter may, however, be identified under the peritoneum and dissected free.

Lymphocyst formation is a complication of lymph node sampling. This may be prevented by using surgical clips during lymph node dissection and by drainage of the retroperitoneum. Querleu and Leblanc[20] do not, however, place preventive clips for lymphastasis or any drain in the dissection area, and report no case of significant lymphocyst formation.

Scarring may follow peritoneal or retroperitoneal repair. The peritoneum usually heals with minimal scarring and no or minimal adhesions (Figure 16). The tissue in the retroperitoneal space heals with a dense fibrosis, making subsequent dissections difficult. If indicated, radical hysterectomy must be performed no more than 7 days after laparoscopic lymphadenectomy[9,20].

CONCLUSION AND DISCUSSION

The main advantage of the laparoscopic approach is that bilateral adnexectomy can be carried out laparoscopically,

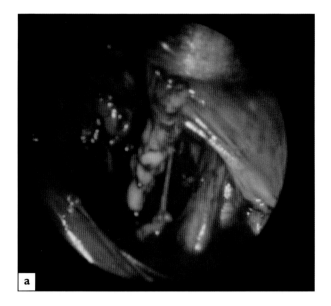

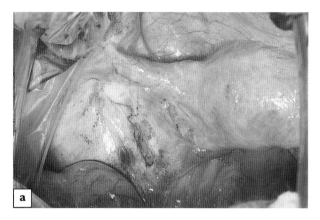

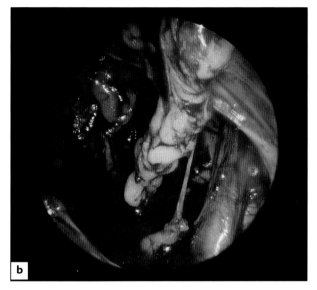

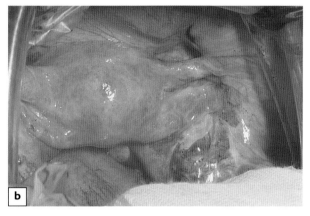

Figure 16 (a) and (b) Peritoneal healing after laparoscopic lymphadenectomy

Figure 15 (a) and (b) The lymph nodes are systematically removed after their dissection in order to avoid their loss in the peritoneal cavity and to determine their exact location (in cases of metastasis)

making a laparotomy unnecessary. Hysterectomy can then be performed either by the vaginal approach or by laparoscopy. The intraoperative advantages of this laparoscopic approach are numerous. It allows ureteral identification, complete hemostasis and evacuation of all the blood clots at the end of the procedure. Removal of blood clots and the instillation of intra-abdominal antiseptics or antibiotics may reduce the incidence of postoperative infection associated with vaginal hysterectomy, thus decreasing the postoperative hospitalization and recovery time.

The results of radical laparoscopic hysterectomy ('Wertheim' procedure) performed with lymphadenectomy are clearly less optimistic. In spite of the less painful

postoperative convalescence, a significantly faster recovery of bowel movement, a less pronounced drop in the hemoglobin rate and reduced hospitalization costs[27], the procedure has several disadvantages. The relatively long operating time (6–8 h) and the rather difficult technical approach of this procedure[12,27] lead us to conclude that this technique (of which only a few cases have been published) still requires further research and evaluation, especially in oncological surgery. Continued studies involving greater numbers of women should thus demonstrate the potential advantages of laparoscopic surgery compared to laparotomy, but also its harmful effects, such as tumor dissemination due to internal trauma during uterine mobilization or lymph node removal.

All surgical maneuvers are more or less feasible by laparoscopy; the important thing to consider with regard to this new approach to radical uterine surgery is not its feasibility, but rather whether it is justifiable and safe[27].

As already stated in this Chapter, lymphangiography is unable to visualize internal iliac and other medical node groups. Computerized tomography scanning and magnetic resonance imaging are not sensitive if the nodes are not macroscopically enlarged. PET seems to be an interesting tool and is being evaluated in different malignancies. It is probably a very sensitive method but not specific enough[28]. As a consequence, lymph node biopsy remains the only reliable method for appraising the status of pelvic nymph nodes..

Pelvic lymph node sampling by a retroperitoneal endoscopic approach has been described[18]. Progress in laparoscopic surgery allows a surgically satisfactory pelvic lymphadenectomy to be performed, removing the obturator, external iliac and hypogastric lymph nodes. Dargent and Salvat[18] have described a panoramic retroperitoneal approach. Querleu and Leblanc have described the technique of pelvic lymphadenectomy[7,20] and para-aortic lymphadenectomy by laparoscopy[20].

The indication for laparoscopic lymphadenectomy in gynecological oncology is the staging of carcinoma of the cervix[7]. The risk of involvement of para-aortic nodes is very low (< 1%) if the pelvic nodes are negative histologically. Stage Ib-IIa-IIb cancer with negative pathological staging may be cured by radical vaginal or abdominal surgery. However, radical hysterectomy does not seem justified when metastatic nodes are present.

Pretreatment laparoscopic staging of stage I endometrial carcinomas is not very useful since the prevalence of lymph node metastasis is very low in this condition. Laparoscopic lymphadenectomy may be included in the surgical step of treatment, in association with vaginal surgery[3].

REFERENCES

1. Schauta R. Techniques chirurgicales. In *Encyclopedie Medico Chirurgicale*. Paris: Elsevier Science, 1961:41–735
2. Mage G, Wattiez A, Chapron C, *et al.* Hystérectomie per-coelioscopique: résultats d'une série de 44 cas. *J Gynecol Obstet Biol Reprod* 1992;21:436–44
3. Donnez J, Nisolle M, Anaf V. Place de l'endoscopie dans le cancer de l'endomètre. In Dubuisson JB, Chapron C, Bouquet de Joliniere J, eds. *Coelioscopie et Cancerologie en Gynecologie*. Paris: Arnette, 1993:77–82
4. Photopulos GJ, Stovall TG, Summitt RL Jr. LAVH, bilateral salpingoophorectomy, and pelvic lymph node sampling for endometrial cancer. *J Gynecol Surg* 1992;8:91–4
5. Plentl AA, Friedman EA. *Lymphatic System of the Female Genitalia: The Morphologic Basis of Oncologic Diagnosis and Therapy*. Philadelphia: WB Saunders, 1971:57–74
6. Perez CA, Korba A, Sharma S. Dosimetric considerations in irradiation of carcinoma of the vagina. *Int J Radiol Oncol Biol Phys* 1977;2:639–45
7. Querleu D, Leblanc E, Castelain G. Laparoscopic pelvic lymphadenectomy in the staging of early carcinoma of the cervix. *Am J Obstet Gynecol* 1991;164:579–81
8. Querleu D, Leblanc E, Castelain B. Lymphadénectomie pelvienne sous contrôle coelioscopique. *J Gynecol Biol Reprod* 1990;19:576–8
9. Dargent D. A new future for Schauta's operation through presurgical retroperitoneal pelviscopy. *Eur J Gynecol Oncol* 1987;8:292–6
10. Svardi J, Vidaurreta J, Bermudez A, *et al.* Laparoscopically assisted Schauta operation: learning experience at the gynecologic oncology unit, Buenos Aires, University Hospital. *Gynecol Oncol* 1999;75:361–5
11. Nezhat GR, Burrel MO, Nezhat FR, *et al.* Laparoscopic radical hysterectomy with para-aortic and pelvic node dissection. *Am J Obstet Gynecol* 1992;166:864–5
12. Canis M, Mage G, Wattiez A, *et al.* La chirurgie endoscopique a-t-elle une place dans la chirurgie radicale du cancer du col utérin? *J Gynecol Obstet Biol Reprod* 1990;19:921–6
13. Dargent D, Martin X, Mathevel P. Laparoscopic assessment of the sentinel lymph node in early stage cervical cancer. *Gynecol Oncol* 2000;79:411–15
14. Vercamer R, Janssens J, De P Usewils RI, *et al.* Computerised tomography and lymphography in the presurgical staging of early carcinoma of the uterine cervix. *Cancer* 1987;60:1745–50
15. King LA, Talledo OE, Gallup DG, *et al.* Computed tomography in evaluation of gynecological malignancies: a prospective analysis? *Am J Obstet Gynecol* 1986;60:1055–61
16. Walsh JM, Goplerud DR. Prospective comparison between clinical and CT staging in primary cervical carcinoma. *Am J Roentgenol* 1981;137:997–1003
17. Wurtz A, Mazman E, Gosselin B, *et al.* Bilan anatomique des adénopathies rétropéritonéales par endoscopie chirurgicale. *Ann Chir* 1987;41:258–63
18. Dargent D, Salvat J. *L'envahissement Ganglionnaire Pelvien*. Paris: Midsi/MacGraw Hill, 1989
19. Reich H. New techniques in advanced laparoscopic surgery. *Clin Obstet Gynecol* 1989;3:655–81
20. Querleu D, Leblanc E. Laparoscopic pelvic lymphadenectomy. In Sutton C, Diamond M, eds. *Endoscopic Surgery for Gynecologists*. London: Saunders, 1993:172–8
21. Vergote I, De Wever I, Tjalma W, *et al.* Neoadjuvant chemotherapy or primary debulking surgery in advanced ovarian carcinoma: a retrospective analysis of 285 patients. *Gynecol Oncol* 1998;71:431–6
22. Clough KB, Ladonne JM, Nos C, *et al.* Second look for ovarian cancer: laparoscopy or laparotomy? A prospective comparative study. *Gynecol Oncol* 1999;72:411–17
23. Reich H, McGlynn F, Wickie W. Laparoscopic management of stage 1 ovarian cancer: a case report. *J Reprod Med* 1990;35:601

24. Dexus S, Cusido MT, Suris JC, *et al.* Lymphadenectomy in ovarian cancer. *Eur J Gynaecol Oncol* 2000;21:215–22

25. Leblanc E, Querleu D, Narducci F, *et al.* Surgical staging of early invasive epithelial ovarian tumors. *Semin Surg Oncol* 2000;19:36–41

26. Morice P, Pautier P, Mercier S, *et al.* Laparoscopic prophylactic oophorectomy in women with inher-

ited risk of ovarian cancer. *Eur J Gynaecol Oncol* 1999;20:202–4

27. Canis M, Mage G, Wattiez A, *et al.* Vaginally assisted laparoscopic radical hysterectomy. *J Gynecol Surg* 1992;8:103–5

28. Anderson H, Price P. What does positron emission tomography offer oncology? *Eur J Cancer* 2000;36:2028–35

Place of laparoscopic surgery in the management of cervical cancer

34

D. Dargent and P. George

INTRODUCTION: WARNING

It is in the field of cervical cancer management that laparoscopic surgery first entered the realm of oncology. It was in 1986 that we started using the laparoscope to assess the pelvic lymph nodes, before taking the decision in the management of early stage cervical cancer[1]. In the following years, the 'staging laparoscopy' became more and more popular, and spread to the management of other intraperitoneal or retroperitoneal malignancies. At the same time, laparoscopy also started being used to assist extirpative surgery, the role played by laparoscopic preparation becoming larger and larger.

As soon as laparoscopy was used in the dissection of malignant tumors, it appeared that the chances for abdominal recurrence and intraperitoneal tumor seeding were increased[2]. Adenocarcinomas are more likely to give rise to such complications, but these complications can also occur in the handling of epidermoid cancers. The use of the open technique (which includes the necessity of an abdominal closure) and the use of the gasless technique could lessen the risk. However, it is clear that laparoscopic surgery is dangerous in itself because tumor manipulation is more important. For these reasons, laparoscopy can only be accepted if the dissections are carried out at a distance from the tumor bulk[3].

Laparoscopic lymphadenectomy is an acceptable operation, providing the lymph nodes are not enlarged and not infiltrated and fixed. An accurate imaging is necessary before taking the decision. The endoscopic dissection has to be discussed in the case of suspicious findings, or similarly, if suspicious symptoms appear at the beginning of the endoscopic assessment. It is only in the cases where the nodes are of normal size that the dissection can be carried out using the laparoscope. One knows that metastasis can exist in normal-size nodes (that is the reason why systematic lymphadenectomy is scheduled), but the chances are low for an involvement and, even more, for rupture of the capsule.

Assistance by radical surgery is also an acceptable operation, the condition being that the surgical divisions are also made at a distance from the tumor itself. This rule, in fact, is not different from the rules of conventional radical surgery. As far as cervical cancer is concerned, it means that radical surgery must be limited to early-stage cases. If the laparoscopic technique is chosen, the use of a uterine manipulator must be prohibited as this increases the chances for peritoneal diffusion[4]. On the other hand, it is

better to use laparoscopic vaginal radical surgery than purely laparoscopic surgery, since, by starting the surgery while making a vaginal cuff and closing it with appropriate forceps, one completely isolates the tumor for the remainder of the operation.

LAPAROSCOPIC LYMPHADENECTOMY

Pelvic and aortic lymphadenectomies are part of the current standard management of cervical cancer. They can be carried out with the laparoscope. Before undertaking the laparoscopic dissection, one has to make sure, using magnetic resonance imaging (MRI) for the pelvic area and computerized tomography (CT) scan for the aortic area, that lymph nodes more than 2 cm in size are not present. If not, the laparoscope can be used on the condition that its use is stopped if unexpected obvious metastatic involvement is found.

Laparoscopic pelvic lymphadenectomy

The most popular technique used for performing laparoscopic pelvic lymphadenectomy is the transumbilical, transperitoneal one. The set-up is the same as for routine laparoscopy. The ancillary ports are opened rather high (just underneath the line joining the two iliac spines): one in the midline (10–12 mm) and the other two medial to the iliac spines, lateral to the inferior epigastric vessels (5 mm). A fourth port (5 mm) is required in the paraumbilical area, either on the right or the left side, if para-aortic lymphadenectomy has to be carried out.

The surgeon intending to perform the pelvic dissection stays on the patient's left side. The video monitor is put at the foot of the operating table. The peritoneum is divided alongside the pelvic brim (Figure 1) between the round ligament and the infundibulopelvic ligament, which is best left undivided until the dissection is finished. Prior to peritoneal opening, the umbilical ligament is located which lifts an oblique peritoneal fold on the posterior surface of the abdominal wall. By following this 'Ariadne's thread' from front to back, it is easy, once the broad ligament is opened, to identify the superior vesical artery of which the umbilical ligament is a ventral continuation (Figure 2). The superior vesical artery is the first surgical landmark in the pelvic dissection. Pushing it medially enables one to open the paravesical space and free up the pelvic side wall. This also reveals the external iliac vessels at the point at which they cross the Cooper's ligament. In obese patients, whose anatomical structures are covered with fatty tissue, it is recommended to first locate the Cooper's ligament (Figure 3). This can be identified by palpation with a blunt instrument driven on the posterior surface of the abdominal wall, lateral to the umbilical ligament – acting the same way as the blind man seeking the edge of the pavement with his white stick.

The dissection is started by grasping the tissues located caudally to the external vein and gently pulling on them, while at the same time a second instrument tears the connective fibers and lymphatic channels joining the node-bearing tissues to the surrounding structures. It is common to find an inferior obturator vein at this level which crosses the nodes that are required; blunt dissection is generally enough to circumvent this. Once the subvenous nodes are freed, revealing the obturator nerve, the external iliac vein is traced back to the point where it meets the internal iliac vein. The same is done for the tissues located between the external iliac artery and the external iliac vein. The ascend-

ing dissection leads to the bifurcation of the common iliac artery.

The next step concerns the node-bearing tissues located between the external iliac artery and the psoas muscle. One starts ventrally, at the level of the origin of the circumflex artery, and continues dorsally to the level of the common iliac artery. At this time, it is often necessary to make a lateral peritoneal incision in order to reflect upwards the ileocecal junction on the right side and the sigmoid colon on the left side. The ureter is identified at the level it crosses the vessels. If the infundibulopelvic ligament has not been divided and the posterior sheet of the broad ligament is intact, the ureter remains attached to its natural support. Both are pushed medially. The pararectal space is then opened (Figure 4). The node-bearing tissues alongside the inferior aspect of the common iliac artery and posterior aspect of the internal iliac artery are freed up.

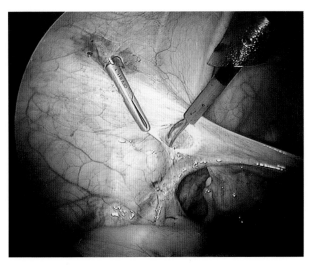

Figure 1 Incision of the peritoneum between the round ligament and the infundibulopelvic ligament (left side)

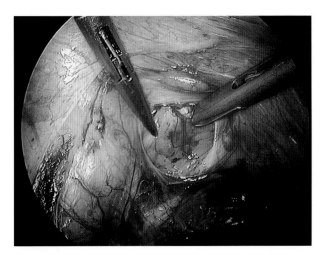

Figure 3 Identification of the Cooper's ligament which is crossed vertically by a collateral of the external iliac vein: the inferior obturatic vein

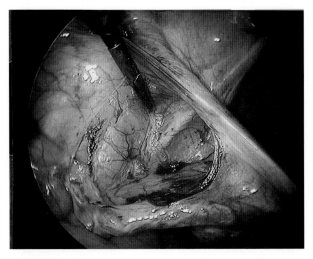

Figure 2 Identification of the superior vesical artery: traction medially onto the umbilical ligament

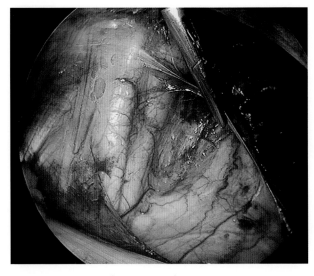

Figure 4 Opening the pararectal space

The order in which the landmarks are identified and the different steps and techniques of dissection are performed vary from surgeon to surgeon. As for the technique of dissection, the simplest is the best, i.e. grasping the nodes with 'grasping forceps' (crocodile forceps) and tearing the surrounding structures with 'dissecting forceps' (cobra forceps). Such a technique (Figure 5) requires skill, but once this skill is acquired it is certainly less bloody: only the resistant structures, the blood vessels, have to be controlled before being divided and they are few if the dissection is made in the appropriate way, not too far from and not too close to the nodes.

Two options are offered for removal of the nodes. The first is gathering them somewhere (in the uterovesical space, for example) and extracting them at the end of the procedure using an extracting bag. The second, and our preferred technique, is to use the Coelio-extractor® which enables us to deliver the nodes one by one without contaminating the abdominal wall.

Querleu and colleagues[5] were the first to give data concerning the feasibility and safety of transumbilical transperitoneal laparoscopic pelvic dissection. For the 39 procedures they performed on patients affected by cancer of the cervix, stage Ib/IIb, the mean duration of the procedure was 80 min. No conversion to laparotomy was needed. The mean yield of nodes was 8.7. Positive nodes were found in five patients who were submitted to exclusive radiotherapy, as the 34 other patients were operated on and submitted either to abdominal radical hysterectomy (32 patients) or to vaginal radical hysterectomy (two patients). All the patients were reassessed after 5 years. The 5-year life table survival rate was similar to the survival of a historical group matched for age, stage and therapy. Childers and co-workers[6] reported data collected from 18 procedures performed for cervical cancer, among whom five were immediately submitted to abdominal radical hysterectomy and 13 were assessed before radiotherapy.

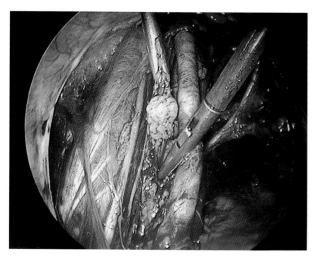

Figure 5 Dissection of the dorsal external iliac nodes: 'two forceps technique'

No complications were observed. The duration of the staging procedure was 75–175 min for the patients assessed before radiotherapy. The lymph node yield was medially 31.4 (17–37) for the patients submitted to abdominal radical hysterectomy. One year later, data about 53 patients affected by endometrial cancer were presented[7]. All the patients were assessed with the laparoscope and 29 of them were submitted to pelvic lymphadenectomy plus aortic sampling. Three intraoperative complications occurred (one pneumothorax, one transection of the ureter and one bladder lesion) and three postoperative complications (two bowel obstructions and one left-side pulmonary collapse). The issue was addressed again 5 years later[8] for 125 patients. The rate of complications did not vary. However, the rate of conversion to laparotomy dropped from 8% (2/25) to 0% (0/100). At the same time, the operative time decreased from 196 min to 128 min ($p < 0.02$) and the hospital stay from 3.2 days to 1.8 days ($p < 0.0001$).

Since 1993, most of the published series[9–18] include data concerning the low aortic lymph node sampling, which was added to the pelvic dissection. Summarizing the data (Table 1), one can assume that the mean number of nodes retrieved with the scope was about 25 (plus five to ten aortic nodes). This number is close to the number of nodes retrieved in open surgery. Comparative studies confirmed that the numbers were about the same. Fowler and colleagues[9] pointed out that 25% of the pelvic nodes were still present at laparotomy after the patient had undergone a laparoscopic lymphadenectomy. However, no patient with negative nodes at laparoscopy had positive nodes at laparotomy. Moreover, Spirtos and co-workers[13], in a comparative study, obtained medially 20 pelvic nodes (plus eight para-aortic) in 13 patients operated on with a laparoscope versus 22 (plus seven para-aortic) in 16 patients operated on by laparotomy.

Concerning the safety of laparoscopic lymphadenectomy, the data collected in the Gynecologist Oncologist Group (GOG) study[19] are the most informative. The mean number of retrieved nodes is 32.1 (16.6 on the left side and 15.5 on the right side). In spite of this record number, the results were judged incomplete in six of the 40 patients submitted to laparotomy after the laparoscopic lymphadenectomy. In fact, removing a high number of nodes is meaningless. The point is to remove the significant nodes. The extreme rarity of pelvic side-wall recurrences in laparoscopically pN_0 patients managed without laparotomic lymphadenectomy or radiotherapy indicates that laparoscopy enables us to remove the significant nodes, even if the total number of nodes is low (see later). If a criterion of safety had to be elected, photographic records taken at the end of the laparoscopic procedure would be the best. In the GOG study, the result was judged inadequate in three of the patients whose photographic records were reviewed by two independent observers. If the requirement of identifying clearly the dorsal part of the obturator nerve and lumbosacral nerve is fulfilled, the risk

Table I Lymph node yield after laparoscopic pelvic lymphadenectomy

Reference	Number of cases	Cancer	Associated OP	Number of nodes +/– aortic
Querleu[5]	39	cervix I II	ARH 32	8.7 LAVRH 2
Childers et al.[6]	18	cervix	ARH 5	31.4
Childers et al.[7]	29	endometrium	LAVRH 29	?
Fowler et al.[9]	12	cervix Ib	ARH 12	23.5 + 6.5
Nezhat et al.[10]	19	cervix Ia IIa	LAVRH 11 LRH 7	21.5 + 5.5
Spirtos et al.[11]	40	endometrium	LAVH 38	20.8 + 7.9
Hatch et al.[12]	37	cervix	LAVRH 37	35.5 + 11.3
Spirtos et al.[13]	10	cervix Ia2 Ib	LAVRH 10	18.3 + 6.5
Roy et al.[14]	25	cervix Ia2 IIa	LAVRH 27	27
Chu et al.[15]	34	cervix Ia2 Ib	LAVRH 6	26.7
Possover et al.[16]	150	cervix 96 endometrium 41 ovary 13	LAVRH 70 LAVH 24 LARH 2	26.8 ± 7.3
Yoon Soon Lee[17]	19	cervix 17 vagina I endometrium I	ARH 9 LAVRH 10	AR 23.9 LAVRH 23.2
Lee et al.[18]	24	cervix Ia IIa	LAVRH 24	13.2 (macroscopic)

ARH, abdominal radical hysterectomy; LAVRH, laparoscopically assisted vaginal radical hysterectomy; LRH, laparoscopic radical hysterectomy; LAVH, laparoscopically assisted vaginal hysterectomy; LARH, laparoscopically assisted radical hysterectomy

of missing a positive pelvic node is nil, at least in cervical cancer and endometrial cancer.

Besides the transumbilical transperitoneal technique, an extraperitoneal approach can be used for performing pelvic lymphadenectomy. New trocars, designed for entering the successive layers of the abdominal wall, and the visual control (Visiport Tyco®, Optiview Ethicon®) enable penetration of the extraperitoneal space, starting with a curved low umbilical incision. Once entered, the space is insufflated with CO_2. An ancillary port is opened on the midline in the suprapubic area. The peritoneum is separated from the abdominal wall using a forceps introduced through this trocar and two more ancillary ports are opened. Then the pelvic dissection can be performed, following a technique similar to the standard one. The extraperitoneal approach has the advantage of respecting the peritoneal serosa and lessening the chances for postoperative adhesions. However, the risk of postoperative collections (hematoma, seroma, lymphocyst) is increased.

On the other hand, the operating room time is more because of the 15–20 min one needs for the development of the extraperitoneal space.

Laparoscopic aortic lymphadenectomy

Laparoscopic aortic dissection is, from the technical view point, just the opposite of pelvic dissection. Transumbilical transperitoneal techniques can be used but the extraperitoneal route is surely the better one.

The transumbilical technique uses the same set-up used for pelvic lymphadenectomy. As far as the aortic lymphadenectomy is concerned, two techniques are available. In the first[6], the set-up is the same as that used for pelvic dissection. Two details, only, differ: the video monitor is put on the side of the patient opposite the side where the surgeon stays and the video camera is turned clockwise through 90° so that the axis of the aorta appears horizontal. The intestinal loops are pushed into the diaphragmatic domes. The dorsal peritoneum is opened longitudinally beside this axis. The upper peritoneal flap is developed upwards. The right ovarian vessels and the right ureter are identified and pushed upwards. The ventral aspect of the vena cava is cleared out, then the inter-aorticocaval space. Finally, the anterior aspect of the aorta is cleared out. The origin of the inferior mesenteric artery is identified, then the nodes lying on the left side of the aorta are mobilized and delivered.

In the second technique[20], the surgeon stands in between the patient's legs with the monitor at the head of the bed. The dorsal peritoneum is opened transversally alongside the axis of the right common iliac vessels. The upper peritoneal flap is pushed cranially at the same time as the last ileal loop. The right gonadal vessels are identified at the same time as the third part of the duodenum. After having mobilized it (and eventually divided the ovarian vessels), one finds the left renal vein and can start the dissection, which is performed alongside the anterior aspect of the vena cava, then continued in the inter-aorticocaval space, alongside the ventral aspect of the aorta and, finally, alongside the left aspect of the aorta. Obtaining access to the retro-aortic and retrocaval spaces necessitates mobilizing the vessels laterally and medially in order to clear out each of the spaces in two steps. The lumbar arteries and veins represent a great danger during this final part of the job.

The extraperitoneal approach to aortic dissection[21] is performed with the patient in the dorsal decubitus position, the surgeon standing to the left of the patient and the assistant to the left of the surgeon. The surgeon and assistant watch the monitor placed to the right of the patient. A 15-mm incision is performed at the left MacBurney point, i.e. 3 cm medial to the left anterior superior iliac spine. Skin, subcutaneous fat and fascia are opened sharply along the same oblique axis. Large muscles are opened bluntly while separating their horizontally orientated bundles lateral to their fascial insertion. The fascia parietalis must be opened, but the fascia peritonealis is preserved, as far as possible, to protect the peritoneum. The surgeon introduces his right forefinger into the incision to develop the extraperitoneal space under the control of transperitoneal laparoscopy. Digital dissection is performed caudally until the anterior surface of the psoas muscle is identified. Dissection is then continued cranially along the psoas muscle to the level of the iliac crest and then laterally. Once the preperitoneal space has been prepared, a 10-mm Blunt Tip trocar (Origin) is introduced and the laparoscope is transferred to this point. The preperitoneal space is insufflated through the trocar sheath and the peritoneal cavity is simultaneously exsufflated. The extraperitoneal insufflation pressure is identical to that used for transperitoneal laparoscopy (12 mmHg). Two additional trocars are then introduced in the mid-axillary line, in the preperitoneal space, under laparoscopic guidance. A 5-mm trocar is placed immediately above the iliac

crest for introduction of a cannula, to which the insufflation tube is connected. This cannula is used to extend the preperitoneal cavity cranially and a 10-mm trocar is then introduced just below the ribs. The left psoas muscle is released from the peritoneum by using these two ancillary trocars and by extending the peritoneum medially. The left ureter, identified on the anterior surface of the psoas muscle, is retracted with the peritoneum. Extending more medially, the left common iliac artery and aorta are identified and dissection is continued cranially as far as the inferior mesenteric artery and left renal vein. Lymph node dissection is commenced below the left renal vein. This dissection is performed bluntly using two forceps, one grasping forceps (Manhes 'Crocodile' forceps) and one dissection forceps (Manhes 'Cobra' forceps). Scissors and monopolar and bipolar diathermy are rarely used. A celio-extractor (Lépine) enables the retrieval of the dissected nodes. All nodes between the aorta and psoas muscle are removed. The left and ventral surfaces of the aorta and left common iliac artery are then dissected, while preserving collateral vessels (ovarian, inferior mesenteric and lumbar arteries). The next step of dissection involves the dorsal aspect of the aorta. The fourth and/or fifth lumbar arteries are clipped and cut to open the retrovascular space. As soon as the lumbar vessels are divided, the space between the aorta and the common vertebral ligament opens and it is often possible to go on and join the interaorticocaval space and, further, the dorsal and ventral aspects of the vena cava. If not, a third ancillary port must be opened as medially as possible, in order to introduce a third instrument to elevate the aorta.

Our 1992–1998 experience[22] enables the feasibility and safety of the elected technique to be assessed. During this period, we attempted to achieve access to the aortic nodes in 44 patients affected by advanced or recurrent cervical cancer. In the first part of the study, the transumbilical access was the favorite access; we met with two failures (conversion to laparotomy) in nine attempts. Then we moved to the extraperitoneal approach, which led, in a population of 35 patients, to a failure in two additional cases. Among the 35 operations performed using the extraperitoneal approach, the first 14 were carried out using two successive incisions and the 21 successive operations used only the left-side incision. In the cases where a systematic dissection was accomplished, the operating room time was less in the unilateral approach (12 cases) than in the bilateral approach (six cases; 119 ± 14 min versus 153 ± 22 min) while the number of retrieved nodes was about the same (15 ± 3 versus 16 ± 2). However, one has to mention that the right-side aortic nodes were fewer in number (2.4 ± 2 versus 7.7 ± 1.7). When assessing patients affected by cervical cancer, this under-representation of the right-side aortic nodes (and the subsequent 'over'-representation of the left-side aortic nodes) is not crucially important because the aortic metastases of cervical cancer in three out of four cases are located on the left side.

LAPAROSCOPICALLY ASSISTED HYSTERECTOMIES

The aim of laparoscopic assistance in the frame of cancer hysterectomy is to lessen the aggression of the procedure, whilst not violating the rules of radical surgery. Laparoscopically assisted simple hysterectomy will not be described here because the indications for simple hysterectomy are few in cervical cancer (stage Ia1 only) and the technique is not different from the routine technique. As far as laparoscopically assisted radical hysterectomy is concerned, we will not describe the purely laparoscopic radical hysterectomy because we disagree with the use of a uterine manipulator, which cannot be avoided when carrying out this operation. We will only describe here the different techniques of laparoscopically assisted vaginal radical hysterectomy.

Schauta operation after laparoscopic lymphadenectomy

In the combination 'laparoscopic pelvic lymphadenectomy–Schauta operation', the laparoscope is used in the same way as it is used in those patients one intends to submit to vaginal hysterectomy for benign disease, since they are in a situation which, theoretically, prevents the use of the vaginal approach: previous laparotomic pelvic surgery, for example. In fact, most of the alleged contraindications to the vaginal approach do not actually prevent its use and laparoscopy provides evidence of that. It is the same for early-stage cervical cancer, where the vast majority of the patients can be submitted to the vaginal radical hysterectomy since the cancer does not spread outside the uterus. That was the rationale we followed at the time we started using the laparoscope: performing, at first, the laparoscopy to be sure the regional lymph nodes were not involved and, if positive (85% of the cases), performing the vaginal radical hysterectomy.

During the years 1986–1992, we operated on 146 patients affected by primary infiltrative cancer using the combination 'laparoscopic pelvic lymphadenectomy–vaginal radical hysterectomy'. In 98 cases, the hysterectomy was carried out as usual. In the remaining 48 cases, it was done while leaving in place the uterine body, the tubes and the ovaries (radical trachelectomy, see later). In 68 patients, the radical hysterectomy was carried out following the Amreich technique, which includes a paravaginal incision and is similar in radicality to the Piver 3 abdominal operation. In the 78 other patients, a modified radical hysterectomy was performed following the Stoeckel technique, carried out without a paravaginal incision and removing a specimen like the one retrieved after a Piver 2 abdominal operation. For the patients operated on after

Amreich operation, the mean operating room time was 139 min and the rates of blood transfusion, visceral injuries (one cystotomy, four ureterotomies and one rectotomy), re-operation and bladder dysfunction (retention and/or incontinence) persisting more than 6 months after the surgery were 8.8%, 14.7%, 8.8% and 59%, respectively. For the patients operated on after a Stoeckel operation, the mean operating room time was 132 min and the rates of blood transfusion, visceral injuries, re-operation and persisting bladder dysfunction were 13.3%, 0%, 6%, 7% and 26.7%, respectively. No fistula occurred in either population.

Schauta–Amreich operation assisted by laparoscopy

Rather than being used only as a tool enabling us to select the indications to vaginal radical surgery, the laparoscope can also be used for preparing for radical surgery. This has been proposed by both us[23] and Kadar and Reich[24]. The new operation is nothing but a Schauta–Amreich operation prepared laparoscopically.

In the Schauta–Amreich operation assisted by laparoscopy, the paracervical ligaments are divided. In this technique, the paracervical ligament is divided during the laparoscopic step of the combined operation. After the lymphadenectomy has been achieved, the paravesical and pararectal spaces are opened and the ligament located in between is divided. As for performing the division, the endoGIA stapler (USSC) is used. If the instrument is introduced through the ipsilateral ancillary door, i.e. following the adequate axis, the division is made very close to the pelvic insertion of the ligament; the amount of removed parauterine tissue is very large. Two cartridges are usually enough; Schneider and co-workers[25] make the same very lateral division, while controlling (bipolar cauterization) and dividing each of the vessels which represent the vascular skeleton of the paracervical ligament.

Performing the Schauta–Amreich operation after laparoscopic preparation enables removal of parauterine tissues, which is more than can be obtained with the reference technique, while avoiding the paravaginal incision. However the morbidity is not decreased. This appears in all the published series[12,14,18,24–26]. From 1992 to 1994 we operated on 28 patients using this technique. The mean operating room time was 196 min. The rates of blood transfusion, visceral injuries, re-operation and persisting bladder dysfunction were 28.6%, 14.3%, 14.3% and 50%, respectively.

Schauta–Stoeckel operation assisted by laparoscopy

Another way to prepare the Schauta operation by laparoscopy is by making a 'lateral parametrial lymphadenectomy' with the laparoscope. After the laparoscopic cleaning out of the lateral route of the parametrium, one can perform, through the vaginal route, a modified radical hysterectomy. This Schauta–Stoeckel operation assisted by laparoscopy has the same radicality as the Schauta–Amreich operation while keeping the advantage of the less aggressive procedure. It involves two steps.

Laparoscopic step

The modified laparoscope-assisted vaginal radical hysterectomy starts with a laparoscopic pelvic dissection, to which a so-called parametrial or, better, a paracervical dissection is added, to ensure less radical parauterine tissue removal, achieved at the time of the forthcoming modified vaginal radical hysterectomy, does not lead to an increasing risk of pelvic side-wall recurrence. This lymphadenectomy is carried out while removing all the lymph node-bearing tissues located in the vasculo-nervous web making up the parauterine ligaments. One starts with the so-called deep obturator nodes, which are removed from front to back, until arriving at the origin of the obturator artery, i.e. at the level where the internal iliac vessels give rise to their ventral collaterals. Thus, the ventral aspect of the paracervical ligament is made free. In a second step, the pararectal space is opened while pushing, medially, the dorsal sheet of the broad ligament, to which the ureter is attached. It is just lateral and dorsal to the point where the ureter crosses the uterine artery that one has to enter the dry space which is made free up to the level of the pelvic floor, as was the paravesical space during the prior step. The lymph node-bearing tissues located at the contact of the posterior aspect of the internal iliac vessels, are removed. The paracervical lymphadenectomy (Figure 6) finishes with the cleaning out of the space located between the iliac vessels and the pelvic wall. The vessels are pushed medially. The cellulo-adipose tissues, lying between the external iliac vessels, and the psoas muscle, are retrieved. The obturator nerve is exposed and, then, followed from front to back. The space located cranial to the sacro-iliac join is opened

and emptied. At the end of the procedure, the obturator nerve is visible along its entire length at the same time as the sacrolumbar nerve, which runs parallel and caudal to the former, crosses the superior gluteal vessels, then disappears in the upper sciatic channel. Identification of this anatomical structure witnesses the radicality of the cellulectomy better than any lymph node count (Figure 7).

Transvaginal step (Figures 8–18)

In contrast, to the classic Stoeckel operation, the modified laparoscopic-assisted vaginal radical hysterectomy does not require the performance of the paravaginal incision (Stoeckel himself did not perform one but two, one on each side). The prior laparoscopic dissection relaxes the natural supports of the uterus and vagina and makes it easier to accomplish, even in nulliparous women, the successive (and rather complex) moves involved in the extended operations. A median episiotomy can be helpful for certain patients but the true paravaginal incision is not necessary.

Making the vaginal cuff is the first part of the operation. The separation of the upper third of the vagina is carried out while first creating a sort of internal prolapse of the vagina, which is obtained while putting on a circular line of a series of Köcher forceps and exerting on them a downwards traction (Figure 8). The incision is made on the external surface of the prolapsed cylinder (Figure 9). In order not to enter the deep sheet of the fold after having divided the superficial one, it is recommended that first an infiltration of saline (+ vasopressin) is made. The incision is made with a cold knife. As soon as the saline drop becomes apparent, the pressure on the blade is released. In fact it is only on the anterior and posterior vaginal walls that the incision has to be a full-thickness incision. In the postero-lateral parts (between the forceps put at 3 o'clock and 4 o'clock), the incision has to be limited to the vaginal skin. This detail is highly important. Making a deep incision on

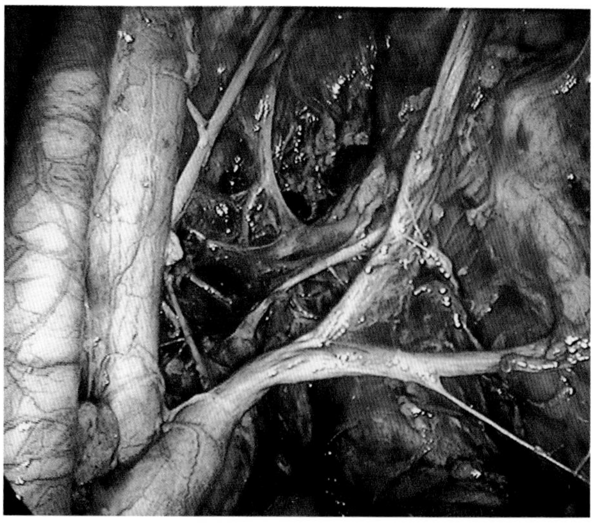

Figure 6 The pelvic side wall after parametrial dissection

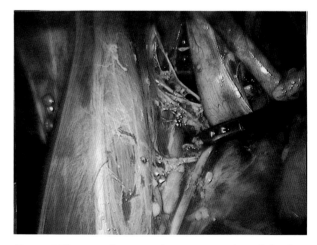

Figure 7 The space between the psoas muscle and the iliac vessels after parametrial dissection: the dorsal part of the obturator nerve and the lumbosciatic trunk are visible

the parts where the parauterine tissues are inserted on the vaginal fornices leads to an incomplete removal and increases the risk of local recurrence. Furthermore, maintaining the relationship between the vaginal cuff and its lateral supports makes the next steps easier (Figure 10).

Freeing the ventral aspect of the specimen to come is the second procedure of the operation. The dorsal aspect of the bladder floor and the ventral aspect of the specimen to come are separated by cellular tissue which is crossed by the ureters lateral to the cervix and cranial to the vaginal fornices. This tissue is denser at the level of the ureteral orifices and the bladder neck. Traction exerted on the vaginal cuff make this dense part appear as pseudo-aponeurosis and pseudoligaments whose division is the key for making free the ventral aspect of the specimen to come. The first step is the opening of the 'supravaginal septum' (Figure 11) which joins the bladder neck to the vagina on the midline. The pseudo-aponeurotic curtain is opened with the scissors handled perpendicular to the vagina until the moment the smooth cellular tissue of the vesicovaginal space appears (Figure 12). At this moment, the development of the space is achieved with the forefinger.

The management of the bladder pillars follows the aperture of the vesicovaginal space. Each of these pseudo-ligaments is made by a condensation of the pelvic cellular tissue located lateral and medial to the ureter at the point it joins the bladder floor. The tractions exerted on the vaginal cuff pull down the ureter (which takes a 'knee' shape) and makes the ligament denser at the same time. For identifying and, then, managing the bladder pillar one

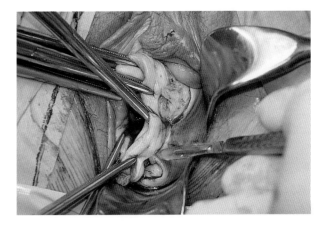

Figure 10 Lateral incision of the vaginal skin

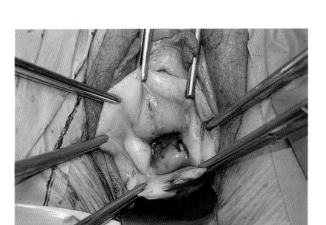

Figure 8 Kocher forceps making 'the vaginal prolapse'

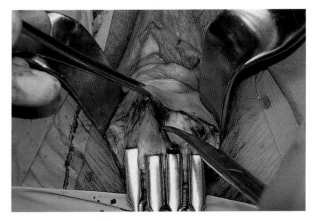

Figure 11 Dividing the 'supravaginal septum'

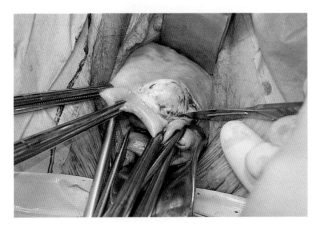

Figure 9 Incision of the three layers of the vagina

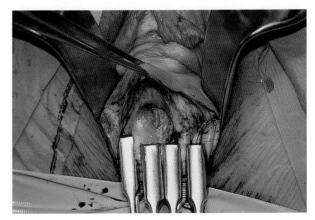

Figure 12 The vesicovaginal space

has, at first, to open the paravesical space, which is made by pulling on the vagina laterally, and entering the smooth space located at the contact of the deep aspect of the flap (Figure 13). A retractor being put in the paravesical space (Figure 14), the pseudoligament separating this space from the previously opened midline space is divided into two steps. The fibers located lateral to the ureter are divided first (Figure 15). The knee of the ureter being exposed (Figure 16), the medial fibers are divided, giving access to the 'para-isthmic window' where the arch of the uterine artery is lying. This window is located above the superior brim of the paracervical ligament, which is made sharp by the traction exerted downwards and contralaterally. This situation makes it easy, in the cases where the visual assessment is not informative, to find, by pressure of the forefinger, the place where the window is, i.e. the place where the uterine artery arrives in the operative field (Figure 17). The afferent branch of the arch is dissected laterally and the uterine artery is divided close to its origin. The two bladder pillars being divided successively, one moves to the next step of the operation.

Freeing the dorsal aspect of the specimen to come and the inferior rim of the paracervical ligament is much easier than managing the ventral aspect. The traction exerted by

the vaginal cuff being inverted, the pouch of Douglas is opened. Then, each of the recto-uterine peritoneal folds is divided, after having been separated from the dorsal surface of the paracervical ligament, i.e. after the pararectal space has been opened. This division gives access to the dorsal aspect of the para-isthmic window, which is identified by palpation. The forefinger which identifies the anatomical defect provides guidance for introducing the

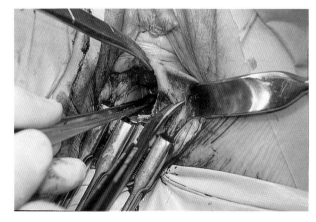

Figure 15 The lateral part of the pseudoligament is divided

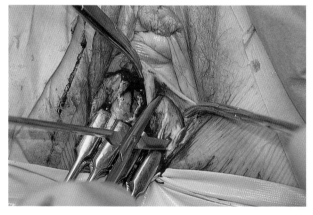

Figure 13 Opening the paravaginal space

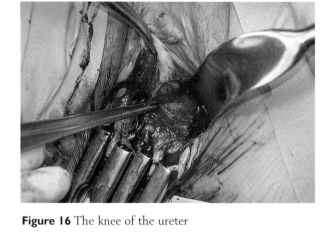

Figure 16 The knee of the ureter

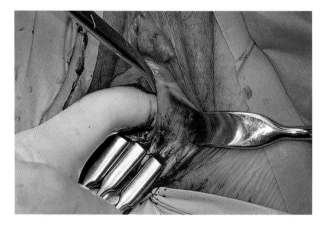

Figure 14 The 'click' maneuver to localize the ureter

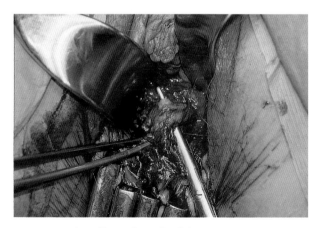

Figure 17 The afferent branch of the uterine artery

tip of a right-angle forceps, which is pushed ventrally at the same time as the traction exerted on the vaginal cuff is inverted. The tip of the instrument appears on the ventral aspect. The instrument is opened, which frees the superior brim of the paracervical ligament. Then, it is used as a means to push the specimen to come medially, in order to make freeing the inferior brim of the paracervical ligament, and dividing it, easier. A contralateral traction being exerted on the vaginal cuff, the superficial incision performed at the very beginning in the posterolateral part of the circular incision is deepened and the vagina is pushed into the incision, leaving a 1.5–2.0 cm space. A first clamp is put on the paracervical ligament A second clamp is placed, lateral to the first one, on which a centripetal attraction is exerted before the second clamp is closed in order to take the maximal amount of parauterine tissue. The second instrument is just at the contact of the knee of the ureter (Figure 18). If the length of the tissues taken between the two clamps appears too small, the ureter can be pushed more dorsally while cutting some more lateral fibers of the bladder pillar. Both cervical ligaments being divided, the retrieval of the specimen is made in the same way as in the simple vaginal hysterectomy. The successive steps of this retrieval will not be described nor will the different steps of the reconstruction.

During the years 1994 to 1999, we operated on 67 patients using the laparoscopically assisted Schauta–Stoeckel operation. The mean operating room time was 177 min. The rates of blood transfusion, visceral injuries, re-operation and persisting bladder dissection were 8.2%, 0%, 2.0% and 6.9%, respectively. From the surgical view point, the laparoscopically assisted Schauta–Stoeckel operation appears equivalent to the reference technique (if not better, but the differences are not statistically significant) and significantly better than the Schauta–Amreich operation, either performed with the paravaginal incision or without. On the other hand, while being less traumatic, the operation has the same curative value, as will be demonstrated in the following section.

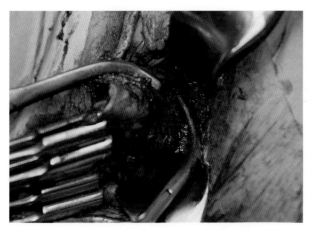

Figure 18 The clamps on the parauterine tissue

PLACE OF LAPAROSCOPIC SURGERY IN THE DIFFERENT PRESENTATIONS OF CERVICAL CANCER

As far as the place of laparoscopic surgery in the management of cervical cancer is concerned, two situations have to be distinguished. In early-stage cases (stage Ia2 and Ib1), laparoscopic surgery allows confirmation of the staging, at the same time as assisting radical surgery, in those cases where the staging procedure makes this surgery necessary. In advanced cases, the role of laparoscopic surgery is only carrying out the staging before choosing the therapy, in which laparoscopic surgery cannot play a direct role.

Early-stage cases

The first role of laparoscopic surgery in early-stage cervical cancer is dismissing those patients who are not suitable for radical surgery. Before undertaking the laparoscopic staging, one has to request imaging (MRI and CT scan) in order to identify those patients with obvious metastatic involvement. For these patients, laparoscopy is useless. As far as the other patients are concerned, laparoscopy can, from the very beginning, illustrate an unexpected bulky lymph node metastatic involvement. If debulking is likely to be feasible, it must be carried out. However, this debulking must be carried out with an open abdomen, even in those cases where it looks possible to perform it laparoscopically. For the other cases, a systematic dissection has to be undertaken and the nodes have to be sent to the laboratory where they will be either assessed after frozen sections or fixed, then embedded in paraffin before being assessed microscopically. The first option carries the advantage of a greater ease. The second includes higher safety while erasing the chances for false negatives. Whatever the elected solution, only the node-negative patients need to be kept for radical hysterectomy, which will be carried out either in the same session or in a second session scheduled in the following 10 days (a longer delay makes the surgery harder).

As far as radical surgery is concerned, two solutions can be offered: the purely laparoscopic radical hysterectomy and the laparoscopically assisted vaginal radical hysterectomy. The laparoscopic radical hysterectomy is potentially dangerous. On the other hand, the few data available are not convincing. As a matter of fact, in the only series[27] (including a rather long follow-up (8–80 months)), no recurrence was observed in 41 patients (12 stage Ia, 24 stage Ib and five stage II) which means that a bias of selection makes the data unacceptable. The laparoscopically assisted vaginal radical hysterectomy has more convincing data. In our series of 241 cases submitted to laparoscopically assisted VRH between December 1986 and December 1999 (47 stage Ia, 160 stage Ib1, 34 stage Ib2), the number of failures was, at the end-point (December 2000) 38 (14%), including 22 pelvic failures (9%) and 11 pelvic side-wall recurrences (5%). As far as the technique itself is concerned, the laparoscopically assisted Schauta–Stoeckel operation, whose surgical advantages have been pointed out in the preceding section, is also likely to offer the lowest risk of failures: no recurrence for the 32 patients stage Ia and Ib less than 2 cm in size, three failures for the 27 patients stage Ib 2 cm or more but less than 4 cm in size (11%), one failure for the eight patients stage Ib2 (12.5%). Interestingly, no pelvic side-wall recurrences were observed in the patients submitted to the laparoscopically assisted Schauta–Stoeckel operation.

Globally, the chances of cure appear, after laparoscopic management, to be equivalent to those offered by abdominal radical hysterectomy. However, they are not better. On the other hand, the quality-of-life issue and the cost-effectiveness, at the moment, have not been clearly assessed. The advantages of the laparoscopic surgery remain questionable. The only certainty concerns the conservative variant of the laparoscopically assisted radical hysterectomy, i.e. the radical trachelectomy[28] (Figure 19). In this operation, which is performed following the same technique, the uterine body, the tubes and the ovaries are left in place. As far as the risk of failure is concerned, no difference has been observed among the subpopulation of 71 patients submitted to radical trachelectomy, and the subpopulation of 170 patients submitted to radical hysterectomy. The 29 of the 38 patients who wanted to be, and were able to get, pregnant, succeeded. Among the 47 pregnancies they obtained, 27 finished with the birth of a normal living baby. Such a result cannot be obtained if the same operation is performed using laparotomy[29].

Advanced-stage cases

Advanced-stage cervical cancer includes bulky stage Ib (stage Ib2: more than 4 cm in size) and stage II. These cancers could be managed using primary radical surgery but most gynecologists/oncologists prefer to use radiotherapy (and concomitant chemotherapy). Stage III and IV cancers, with some exceptions, cannot be managed any other way. Surgery, in these presentations, has only an adjuvant role. It can be used systematically as 'intervention surgery' once the radiotherapy is completed and whatever the response to it. It can be reserved for those poor responders and carried out either after an intermediate assessment or after the completion of the primary treatment; in the cases where pelvic examination, imaging and/or biopsies show the response is not complete, intervention surgery is scheduled. A third option is waiting until the next check-up illustrates a recurrence. Laparoscopic surgery cannot be used either for performing this intervention surgery or assisting it, since the actinic alteration of the pelvic cellular tissue makes the laparoscopic dissection hazardous. In contrast, the laparoscopic staging surgery has definite interest for the different steps of the management.

Laparoscopic lymphadenectomy is helpful at the very beginning of the management of advanced-stage cases in order to assess the spread of the disease before undertaking the radiotherapy. Pelvic lymphadenectomy is of low interest because the pelvic side walls (and the pelvic lymph nodes) are inside the irradiated fields. Knowing the status of these nodes does not influence the management. On the other hand, if intervention surgery has to be performed, the alterations of the pelvic cellular tissues linked with the prior laparoscopic dissection (and the successive radiotherapy) make this surgery much more difficult. Aortic lymphadenectomy does not encompass this drawback and is more helpful. As a matter of fact, if the aortic nodes are involved, the management has to be changed and extended-field radiotherapy has to be administered. It is not certain that such a modification to the therapeutic tool actually saves many patients, especially in those cases where bulky metastases are present. However, it is certain that managing these patients without appealing to extended-field radiotherapy cannot cure them.

Laparoscopic aortic lymphadenectomy in advanced cases is nothing but a revival of staging laparotomy. This staging laparotomy encompassed a lot of inconvenient per- and postoperative complications, plus enhancement of the actinic complications because of postoperative adhesions limiting the mobility of the intestine and increasing the chances for actinic enteritis. In the GOG assay published in 1999[30], the rates of grade 3 actinic complications were 21% in the patients assigned to the intraperitoneal

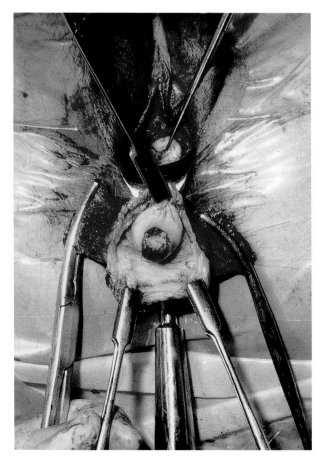

Figure 19 Specimen of radical trachelectomy

approach and 15.3% in the patients assigned to the extraperitoneal approach. Using the extraperitoneal left-side laparoscopic approach, the rate of intra- and peroperative complications was low (see preceding section). As far as the actinic complications are concerned, their rate was also very low: two cases of radiation enteritis only (2.7%) in the 48 patients that we gathered with Denis Querleu[21]. So far, the extraperitoneal left-side laparoscopic aortic lymphadenectomy, which has the same informative value as the staging laparotomy while not carrying the same costs (hospital stay and surgical complications) or risks (actinic complications), deserves to be used widely in the pretherapeutic work-up of advanced-stage cervical cancer.

Laparoscopic aortic lymphadenectomy recognizes another helpful indication in the pre-exenteration work-up. If a recurrence occurs in a patient who has not been submitted to aortic dissection prior to the primary treatment, and if the indication is to perform a pelvic exenteration, one knows that this operation, which carries a high risk and exposes the patient to troublesome sequelae, is contraindicated in the cases where the aortic nodes are involved because the chances for cure are very low. Rather than exposing this contraindication at the time the laparotomy has already been performed, one obtains a big advantage in exposing it by laparoscopic staging. In our experience[31], patients referred between April 1994 and June 1998 for recurrent cervical cancer confined to the pelvis according to the preoperative work-up (including normal CT scan) underwent a laparoscopic para-aortic assessment. All but one of the procedures were completely performed by laparoscopy. This patient was submitted to laparotomy for controlling a bleed from the right ovarian artery. Aortic nodes were not involved but pelvic debulking was impossible. Among the seven other patients, aortic lymph node metastases were in evidence in two patients who were not submitted to pelvic exenteration. Among the five patients with no para-aortic lymph node involvement who were submitted to the exenteration, one developed a liver metastasis 4 months after the surgery, one died with pelvic recurrence 16 months after surgery and three were still alive 2, 4 and 28 months after the surgery.

THE FUTURE: LAPAROSCOPIC ASSESSMENT OF THE SENTINEL NODE?

The concept of sentinel node assessment was born in 1992 at the time the urologist Cabanas proposed the replacement of the inguinofemoral dissection by the removal of the only node that was dyed after injection of blue dye close to the penile tumor that one had to manage. Such a policy enables avoidance of the heavy consequences that the inguinofemoral dissection carries, while not increasing the chance for inguinofemoral recurrence. The same argument is put forward in the management of breast cancer and vulvar cancer. The conditions for such a lightening of the management policy are, first that the identification of

the sentinel node is easy to perform and, second that the negative predictive value of the assessment of this node is 100% or close to 100% as far as the status of the other regional nodes is concerned. Another and very important question concerns the therapeutic value of the lymphadenectomy which will be dismissed on the pretext that, as the sentinel node is not involved, the other regional nodes are also not involved.

Identification of the sentinel node in cervical cancer seems, according to the literature, to be difficult. O'Boyle and co-workers[32] tried to obtain it while injecting blue dye into the cervix before an abdominal radical hysterectomy was performed. Among the 40 assessed areas (20 patients), sentinel nodes were identified in 15 cases only. Verheijen and colleagues[33] injected technetium 99m colloidal albumin and blue dye around the tumor. In six out of ten eligible women who had a Wertheim–Meigs operation for cervical cancer stage Ib, one or more sentinel nodes could be detected by scintigraphy prior to the surgery. The intraoperative gamma-probe detection was successful in eight of the ten women where the visual detection found sentinel nodes in only four. Kamprath and co-workers[34] used colloidal technetium in 16 of 18 patients in whom sentinel nodes were detected. A median of 2.1 pelvic sentinel nodes was found in 16 patients and a median of 1.4 para-aortic sentinel nodes was found in five patients. No false-negatives were registered by these authors; after systematic dissection no metastatic nodes were found if the sentinel nodes were not involved. However, the practical interest of such a statement is low. As a matter of fact, the only drawback of the systematic dissection is that it takes time; postoperative lymphedema is very rare, especially if no postoperative radiotherapy is given. Using laparotomy for identifying the sentinel node does not spare time. The same is true if laparoscopy is used, but the colloidal technetium technique leads in most of the cases to performance of an extended dissection.

The technique we propose differs from the others in that, first, we use the laparoscope, second, we do not use colloidal technetium but a blue dye, and, third, we do not look directly for the blue-dyed nodes but for the blue-dyed lymphatic channels which are followed from inside to outside and lead to the sentinel node which, in most of the cases, is unique. Between October 1998 and September 2000, we operated on 52 patients using this technique. One or more lymphatic channels were identified in 87% of the cases which led to one blue-dyed node in 95% of the cases and to two separate nodes in 5% of the cases. While being more selective than the colloidal technetium technique, this technique has the same safety. Among the 97 sentinel nodes which were assessed, 13 were involved and 82 were not. The systematic dissection performed after the sentinel node removal has never shown in these 82 cases that other regional nodes were involved. Another advantage of the technique we propose is that it actually spares time in most cases. As a matter of fact, the sentinel node in 82 of the 95 cases (86%) was located at the contact of the external vein, either medial to it or caudal to it (between it and the obturator nerve (Figure 20)) or cephalic to it (between it and the external iliac artery). In all these cases, the place where the sentinel node was lying was ventral to the origin of the uterine artery. This means that we were able to identify and remove it less than 10 min after the start of the dissection.

Following the data given here, it seems that the laparoscopic dissection undertaken after injection of a blue dye into the cervix can, in most of the cases, be very much shortened. However, it is not certain that dismissing the systematic dissection does not include a risk of enhancement of the rate of pelvic recurrences and, more precisely, of pelvic side-wall recurrences. In our 1986–1999 already quoted personal experience, the laparoscopically assisted vaginal radical hysterectomy, which was reserved for the patients with no pelvic node involvement, was performed without appealing to the parametrial lymphadenectomy (see section 'Schauta–Stoeckel operation assisted by laparoscopy') in 168 cases and with parametrial lymphadenectomy in 73 cases. The rates of pelvic recurrences were 15.5% and 5.3%, respectively. No pelvic side-wall recurrences were observed in the second population. That means that, by increasing the radicality of the dissection, one lessens the chances for recurrence, even in patients apparently free of lymph node metastasis. Such a phenomenon could be explained by the data of molecular biology, which show that cancer can be present even if not morphologically evident. From the practical view, it seems not to be sensible to renounce systematic lymphadenectomy even if the sentinel node is not involved, with the exception of the very early tumors (stage Ia and stage Ib less than 2 cm in size), in the management of which we have never observed recurrences whatever the technique of lymphadenectomy (176 cases).

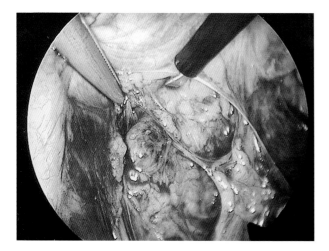

Figure 20 Main lymphatic channel and main lymphatic node (sentinel node) after injection of Patent Blue Violet in the cervix: the main lymphatic channel crosses the superior vesical artery and joins a node located alongside the podalic surface of the external vein

CONCLUSION: WARNING!

Laparoscopic surgery does not improve the outcomes in the management of cancer. Worse than that, this surgery can be deleterious if the rules of safety are not respected. It is mandatory to avoid direct manipulation of the tumor. Therefore, the place of laparoscopic surgery has to be restricted to staging and to assisting radical surgery. A careful preoperative work-up is necessary to dismiss those cases at risk. On the other hand, one has not to hesitate to convert to laparotomy if unexpected tumor bulk prevents the avoidance of direct manipulations. Actually, the advantage of laparoscopic surgery is only the lessening of surgical trauma while respecting better the forms and the functions. But that can lead, in the cases of early-stage cervical cancer in young patients, to surgery that makes possible the birth of normal babies. This result is worth the efforts of the gynecologic oncologists.

REFERENCES

1. Dargent D. A new future for Schauta's operation through pre-surgical retroperitoneal pelviscopy. *Eur J Gynecol Oncol* 1987;8:292–6
2. Whelan RL, Lee SW. Review of investigations regarding the etiology of port site tumor recurrence. *J Laparoendosc Adv Surg Tech A* 1999;9:1–16
3. Canis M, Botchorishvilli R, Wattiez A, *et al*. Cancer and laparoscopy, experimental studies: a review. *Eur J Obstet Gynecol Reprod Biol* 2000;91:1–9
4. Sonoda Y, Zerbe M, Barakat RR, *et al*. High incidence of positive peritoneal cytology in low-risk endometrial cancer treated by laparoscopically assisted vaginal hysterectomy (LAVH). Presented at *31st Annual Meeting of the SGO*, February, 2000, Abstr 21
5. Querleu D, Leblanc E, Castelain B. Laparoscopic pelvic lymphadenectomy. *Am J Obstet Gynecol* 1991;164:579–81
6. Childers JM, Hatch K, Surwit EA. The role of laparoscopic lymphadenectomy in the management of cervical carcinoma. *Gynecol Oncol* 1992;47:38–43
7. Childers JM, Brzechffa PR, Hatch KD, *et al*. Laparoscopically assisted surgical staging (LASS) of endometrial cancer. *Gynecol Oncol* 1993;51:33–8
8. Melendez TD, Childers JM, Nour M, *et al*. Laparoscopic staging of endometrial cancer: the learning experience. *J Lap Surg* 1997;1:45–9
9. Fowler JM, Carter JR, Carlson JW, *et al*. Lymph node yield from laparoscopic lymphadenectomy in cervical cancer: a comparative study. *Gynecol Oncol* 1993;51:187–92
10. Nezhat CR, Nezhat FR, Vurrel MO, *et al*. Laparoscopic radical hysterectomy and laparoscopically assisted vaginal radical hysterectomy with pelvic and paraaortic node dissection. *J Gynecol Surg* 1993;9:105–20

11. Spirtos NM, Schaert JB, Spirtos TW, *et al.* Laparoscopic bilateral pelvic and paraarotic lymph node sampling: an evolving technique. *Am J Obstet Gynecol* 1995;173:105–11

12. Hatch KD, Hallum AV, Nour M. New surgical approaches to treatment of cervical cancer. *J Natl Cancer Inst* 1996;21:71–5

13. Spirtos NM, Schlaerth JB, Gros GM, *et al.* Cost and quality of life analyses of surgery for early endometrial cancer: laparotomy versus laparoscopy. *Am J Obstet Gynecol* 1996;174:1795–9

14. Roy M, Plante M, Renaud MC, *et al.* Vaginal radical hysterectomy versus abdominal radical hysterectomy in the treatment of early stage cervical cancer. *Gynecol Oncol* 1996;62:336–9

15. Chu KK, Chang SD, Chen FP, *et al.* Laparoscopic surgical staging in cervical cancer – preliminary experience among Chinese. *Gynecol Oncol* 1997;64:49–53

16. Possover M, Krause N, Plaul K, *et al.* Laparoscopic para-aortic and pelvic lymphadenectomy: experience with 150 patients and review of the literature. *Gynecol Oncol* 1998;71:19–28

17. Yoon Soon Lee. Early experience with laparoscopic pelvic lymphadenectomy in women with gynecologic malignancy. *J Am Assoc Gynecol Laparosc* 1999;6:59–63

18. Lee CL, Huang KG, Wang HY, *et al.* New approach in laparoscopically assisted radical vaginal hysterectomy. *Int Surg* 1997;82:266–8

19. Fowler JM, Schlaerth J, Spirtos M. Laparoscopic retroperitoneal lymphadenectomy followed by laparotomy in women with cervical cancer. Society of Gynecologic Oncologist Abstract. *Gynecol Oncol* 1999

20. Querleu D. Laparoscopic para-aortic node sampling in gynecologic oncology: a primary experience. *Gynecol Oncol* 1993;49:24–9

21. Querleu D, Dargent D, Ansquer Y, *et al.* Extraperitoneal endosurgical aortic and common iliac dissection in the staging of bulky or advanced cervical carcinomas. *Cancer* 2000;88:1883–91

22. Dargent D, Ansquer Y, Mathevet P. Technical development and results of left extraperitoneal laparoscopic para-aortic lymphadenectomy for cervical cancer. *Gynecol Oncol* 2000;77:87–92

23. Dargent D, Mathevet P. Hysterectomie élargie laparoscopico vaginale. *J Gynecol Biol Reprod* 1992;21:709–10

24. Kadar N, Reich H. Laparoscopically assisted radical Schauta hysterectomy and bilateral laparoscopic pelvic lymphadenectomy for the treatment of bulky stage IB carcinoma of the cervix. *Gynecol Endosc* 1993;2:135–42

25. Schneider A, Possover M, Kamprath S, *et al.* Laparoscopy-assisted radical vaginal hysterectomy modified according to Schauta-Stoeckel. *Obstet Gynecol* 1996;88:1057–60

26. Dargent D. Radical vaginal hysterectomy in the primary management of invasive cervical cancer. In Rubin S, Hoskins W, eds. *Cervical Cancer and Preinvasive Neoplasia.* New York: Raven Press, 1996:142–8

27. Canis M, Dauplat J, Pomel C, *et al.* Laparoscopic radical hysterectomy for cervical cancer. Results about 41 cases. IGCS Abstract. *Int J Gynecol Cancer* 1997;7:3

28. Dargent D, Martin X, Sacchetoni A, *et al.* Laparoscopic vaginal trachelectomy: a treatment to preserve the fertility of cervical carcinoma patients. *Cancer* 2000;88:1877–82

29. Novak F. Radical abdominal subcorporeal extirpation of the cervix with bilateral pelvic lymph nodes dissection in cancer *in situ* of the cervix uteri. *Acta Med Yugoslavica* 1952;6:59–71

30. Weiser FB, Bundy BN, Hoskins WJ, *et al.* Extraperitoneal versus transperitoneal selective para-aortic lymphadenectomy in the treatment surgical staging of advanced cervical cancer (a GOG study). *Gynecol Oncol* 1999;33:283–9

31. Dargent D, Ansquer T, Mathevet P. Can laparoscopic paraaortic lymphadenectomy help to select patients with pelvic relapse of cervical cancer eligible for pelvic exenteration? *Gynecol Oncol* 1999;73:172

32. O'Boyle JD, Coleman RL, Bernstein SG, *et al.* Intraoperative lymphatic mapping in cervix cancer patients undergoing radical hysterectomy: a pilot study. *Gynecol Oncol* 1999;74:322

33. Verheijen RH, Pijpers R, Van Diest PJ, *et al.* Sentinel node detection in cervical cancer. *Obstet Gynecol* 2000;96:135–8

34. Kamprath S, Possover M, Schneider A. Laparoscopic sentinel node detection in patients with cervical cancer. *Gynecol Oncol* 2001;in press

Part 5
Complications

Ureteral and bladder injury during laparoscopic surgery

35

J. Donnez, P. Jadoul, F. Chantraine and M. Nisolle

The reported risks of laparoscopy include perforation of the bowel, bladder, uterus, or blood vessels, in addition to the risks of general anesthesia.

In the years since 1980, tubal sterilization has become the most frequent indication for laparoscopy. The main complications of laparoscopy are hemorrhage and perforation of the bladder and bowel by the Verres needle and trocar. Tubal sterilization by electrocoagulation carries some further specific risks, such as electrical burns and hemorrhage in the mesosalpinx. Reports of ureteral burn injuries during laparoscopic sterilization are rare[1-4].

URETERAL INJURIES

Ureteral injuries occurring during laparoscopy were documented in a review by Donnez and colleagues[5]. Table 1 summarizes the 15 cases of ureteral injury resulting from laparoscopy that are reported in the literature[6-10]. Four of these 15 cases were complications of laparoscopic sterilization procedures and seven were complications of laparoscopic treatment of endometriosis. Although the ureter may often be visualized through the peritoneum in the upper pelvis (Figure 1), it cannot be identified reliably in the area of the uterosacral ligaments. This is particularly true in the presence of diseases such as endometriosis. The presence of uterosacral ligaments that are thickened and nodular can induce a distortion of the normal anatomy of the ureter in this area.

Electrocoagulation has been used routinely in sterilization. It is erroneously assumed that bipolar coagulation is 'safe'; five reported ureteral injuries have occurred using this method. In addition to direct tissue damage, the electrical current may damage the vascular supply to the coagulated tissue.

Case 1

A 35-year-old woman presented with a 5-year history of severe dysmenorrhea. Physical examination demonstrated tenderness in the cul-de-sac consistent with endometriosis. Laparoscopy revealed stage I endometriosis. Black peritoneal lesions were present extensively on both uterosacral ligaments. CO_2 laser vaporization of the endometriotic implants was performed, as well as laser uterine nerve ablation (LUNA). Because of bleeding at the level of the left uterosacral ligament, unipolar electrocoagulation was used. The ureter was well visualized and was seen 1 cm from the site of coagulation.

On postoperative day 7, the patient presented with increasing abdominal pain, peritonitis, leukocytosis and fever (39.1°C). A computerized tomography (CT) scan revealed the presence of fluid in the retroperitoneal space (Figure 2). An intravenous pyelogram (IVP) revealed a urinoma on the left side of the pelvis. A JJ stent was inserted and removed 3 months later. No complications occurred.

Case 2

A 29-year-old patient was referred for evaluation of infertility and recurrent pelvic pain. One year previously, she had undergone laparoscopy for acute salpingitis treated by antibiotics. Postoperative hysterosalpingography revealed a

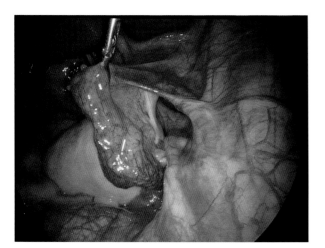

Figure 1 Ureter visualized through the peritoneum

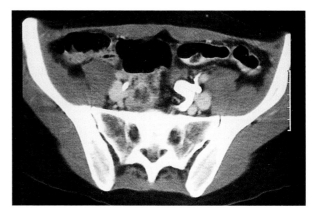

Figure 2 Computerized tomography scan: presence of contrast medium in the retroperitoneal space after pyelography

Table I Summary of the 15 cases of ureteral injury resulting from laparoscopy that are reported in the literature up to 1994

Case number*	Time of presentation	Indication for initial procedure	Treatment modality	Method of diagnosis	Treatment
1	7 days	endometriosis (LUNA)	CO_2 laser/unipolar coagulation	IVP–CT scan	retrograde stent (JJ)
2	7 days	salpingo-ovariolysis	CO_2 laser/bipolar coagulation	IVP	retrograde stent (JJ)
3[6]	48 h	endometriosis	unipolar coagulation	IVP	end-to-end anastomosis
4[6]	48 h	adhesions/endometriosis	unipolar coagulation	IVP	transverse uretero-ureterostomy
5[6]	24 h	uterosacral ligament transection	unipolar coagulation	repeat laparoscopy	transverse uretero-ureterostomy
6[6]	36 h	adhesions	bipolar coagulation	repeat laparoscopy	end-to-end anastomosis
7[6]	48 h	endometriosis	CO_2 laser/bipolar	IVP	percutaneous stent
8[3]	5 days	endometriosis	unipolar coagulation	IVP	transverse uretero-ureterostomy
9[2]	2 weeks	sterilization	bipolar coagulation	IVP	Boari flap
10[4]	unknown	endometriosis	unipolar coagulation	IVP	unknown
11[7]	3 weeks	sterilization	coagulation (not specified)	laparotomy	ilial interposition
12[8]	3 weeks	diagnostic laparoscopy	trocar injury (?)	IVP	end-to-end anastomosis
13[9]	5 days	adhesions	coagulation (not specified)	IVP	stent at laparotomy
14[1]	4 days	sterilization	bipolar coagulation	IVP, repeat	retrograde stent
15[10]	5 days	sterilization	bipolar coagulation	IVP	transverse uretero-ureterostomy

* Cases 1 and 2 are from the present study; other cases are from references indicated by superscript numbers. LUNA, laser uterine nerve ablation; IVP, intravenous pyelogram; CT, computerized tomography

bilateral hydrosalpinx and a laparoscopy for salpingostomy was proposed to the patient. At laparoscopy, the ovaries were found to be fixed to the broad ligament by very dense adhesions. During left ovariolysis, bleeding, encountered 1 cm beneath the ovary, was controlled with bipolar coagulation. The left ureter was clearly visible about 1.5 cm from the bleeding. Because a vein of the ovarian hilus was responsible for the bleeding, there was some difficulty in achieving complete hemostasis and numerous attempts were made before cessation of bleeding was accomplished. The patient was discharged the next day. Seven days later, she developed fever and peritonitis. An IVP revealed extravasation of urine in a left urinoma (Figure 3a and b). Retrograde stent placement was successful (Figure 4); a JJ stent was inserted for 3 months. Three months after

removal, IVP demonstrated a small ureteral stenosis (Figure 5a and b), which was successfully dilated by a retrograde stent with satisfactory outcome (Figure 6).

Time of presentation of symptoms

Ureteral injury was symptomatic soon after the procedures – between 24 h and 7 days – except in three cases, in which diagnosis was made 2–3 weeks after endoscopic surgery. In our two cases, the ureter was precisely visualized before coagulating the artery of the uterosacral ligament (case 1) or a venous blood vessel (case 2). In both cases, the distance between the ureter and the blood vessel was at least 1.5 cm. The time lapse between endoscopic surgery and the onset of symptoms was 7 days in both cases. We conclude that 7 days are required for the

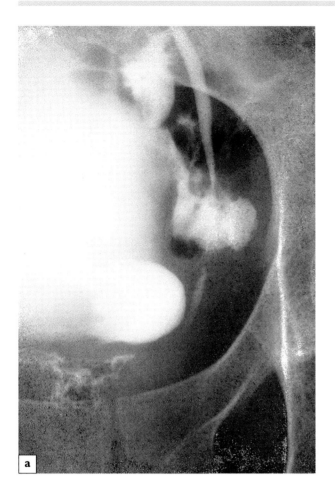

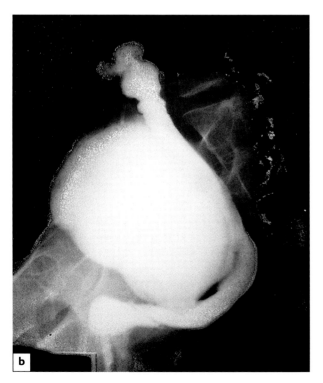

Figure 3 (a) Intravenous pyelogram revealing a urinoma; (b) extravasation of urine in a left urinoma after pyelography. The urinoma is clearly separated from the rectum

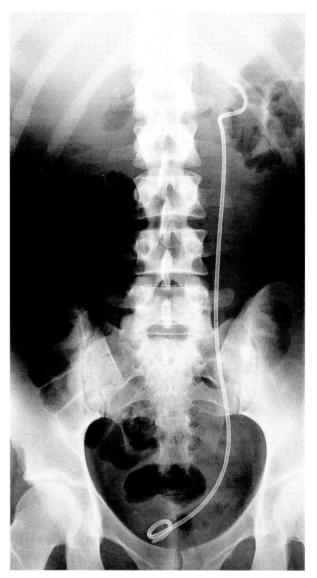

Figure 4 A JJ stent was inserted for 3 months

creation of a ureteral fistula when the cause is the propagation either of the current or of heat. In the review by Grainger and co-workers[6], the most common symptoms were abdominal pain with peritonitis, leukocytosis and fever.

Mode of diagnosis

The diagnosis of ureteral injury is usually made by IVP, which shows that the cause of the 'retroperitoneal mass' is a urinoma, and also demonstrates the site of a fistula. Our two cases were diagnosed by the presence of a pelvic mass confirmed by echography and CT scan.

Treatment

Among the reviewed cases, management consisted of exploratory laparotomy with one of the following procedures:

365

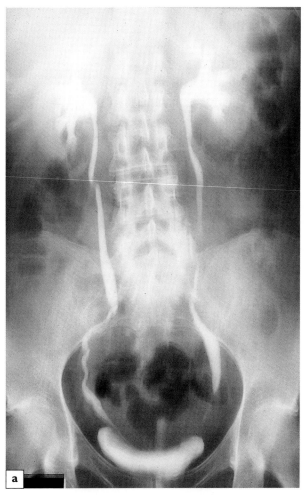
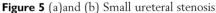
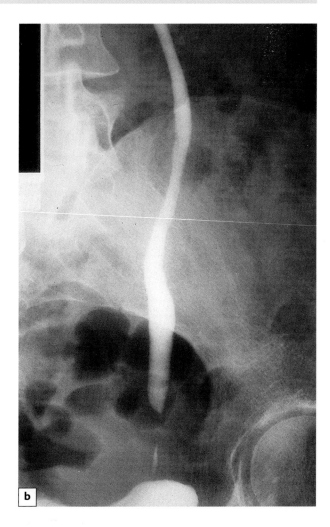

Figure 5 (a)and (b) Small ureteral stenosis

(1) Reimplantation of the ureter into the bladder (one case);

(2) Anastomosis of the damaged ureter (three cases);

(3) Transureteral ureterostomy (four cases);

(4) Interposition of an isoperistaltic loop of ileum between the ureter and the bladder (one case).

In our series, both patients avoided laparotomy for ureteral repair. The placement of a ureteral stent allowed drainage of urine, resolution of the pelvic urinoma and spontaneous healing of the injured site. The placement of these ureteral stents may be accomplished in a retrograde manner. If technically possible, this method of treatment is preferable in managing such types of ureteral injuries.

Several ureteral injuries occurred at the time of sterilization. These were most likely a result of the cautery forceps touching the side-wall during application of the current. It is unlikely that these injuries will occur as a result of 'arcing' of electrical energy, or from burning through the peritoneum by excess heat in the coagulated tissue after the sterilization is complete. Therefore, the tube must be grasped in the bipolar forceps and moved away from the side-wall before applying the current. Bleeding in the area of the uterosacral ligaments, whether it occurs at the time of uterosacral ligament transection or ablation of endometriosis, must be carefully controlled. The advent of laparoscopically applied surgical clips may provide a greater margin of safety when controlling bleeding in this area. Other techniques that can now be applied laparoscopically include suturing, endocoagulation and electrocoagulation. The best solution remains prevention, and an increase in aquadissection and dissection of the ureter before performing coagulation in the area of the uterosacral ligaments is suggested.

SECOND REVIEW: PERSONAL SERIES (1992–2000)

The incidence of this type of injury has grown during the last 5–10 years, because the number of operative laparoscopies for complicated surgical procedures has increased. This is due to new instruments used to perform, for example, hysterectomy or lymphadenectomy and the increasing number of gynecologic surgeons using these

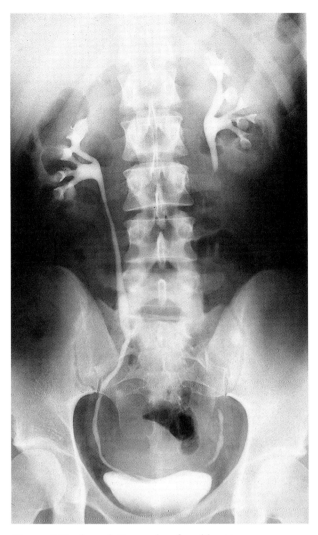

Figure 6 Final result 3 months after dilatation

techniques. Furthermore, the highest incidence of complications is noted in laparoscopic (assisted) hysterectomy; indeed, laparoscopic hysterectomies are associated with a 1% risk of ureteral injury[11].

In our department, from 1986 to 2000, we noted ten ureteral injuries in the more than 19 000 gynecologic laparoscopies performed. Lesions occurred with an incidence of 0.05%. The prevalence was 2/12 000 (0.16%) until 1992 and then 8/7000 (0.11%), i.e. 6.8 times higher than in the first series. In the literature, the incidence ranges from 0.12 to 0.25[11–13].

Ureteral injury is often not due to complete transection but frequently to thermal energy applied near the ureter causing tissue necrosis with subsequent stenosis and fistulas.

Diagnosis

Although only a hundred cases of ureteral injury in laparoscopy-related procedures have been reported in the literature, extreme care must be taken when dissecting

within the pelvis. In only two cases described in the literature was the diagnosis made intraoperatively[14,15]. In our series, one diagnosis of ureteral injury was made intraoperatively. Immediate retrograde JJ stenting was performed. If ureteral lesions are suspected intraoperatively, intravenous injection of indigo-carmine can help to detect the injury.

Usually, patients tend to present 48 h to 7 days postoperatively, with symptoms of abdominal pain, peritonitis, leukocytosis and fever. Flank tenderness or hematuria are rarely described. In some cases, an evaluation of abdominal fluid drainage, with measurement of urea and creatinine, may aid diagnosis. In a few rare cases, diagnosis was made 2 or 3 weeks after surgery. One of our patients presented with a ureterovesical fistula 3 weeks after surgery, causing a watery vaginal discharge. Clinical diagnosis was made with the discovery on examination.

In a recent review, delays ranging from 3 to 33 days to diagnosis were observed[16]. In our series, diagnosis was made, in one case, 2 months after surgery, when the patient presented with pyelonephritis. Repair was achieved by ureteral stenting. The presence of ascites and/or a pelvic mass is indicated by sonography, and the diagnosis is confirmed by intravenous pyelography, which reveals if the cause of the pelvic mass is a urinoma, and also demonstrates the site of a fistula. A CT scan can be helpful in some instances.

Management

Repair of ureteral injuries must be undertaken with the collaboration of a urologic surgeon. Percutaneous or cystoscopic techniques can probably be used to manage most such injuries. Exploratory laparoscopy and/or laparotomy can be employed for surgical repair in cases requiring end-to-end reanastomosis, reimplantation of the ureter into the bladder, transureteral ureterostomy and similar procedures. Some cases of primary repair of transected ureters by laparoscopy have been reported[17,18].

Often, if diagnosis is made postoperatively and the lesion is not too fibrotic, insertion of a ureteral stent can be attempted, as we suggested in 1994[5]. This stent allows drainage of urine, resolution of the pelvic urinoma, and spontaneous healing of the injured site. Placement of such ureteral stents may be accomplished in a retrograde manner. If technically possible, this method of treatment is preferable in managing such types of ureteral injuries.

In our series (Table 2), insertion of a JJ stent was successful in 70% (7/10) of cases.

Prevention

The ureter enters the pelvis at the pelvic brim, crossing over the common iliac artery and vein. It then runs posteriorly, crossing under the uterine artery and matching the level of the cervix. At this point, the ureter is 1–1.5 cm lateral and anterior to the uterosacral ligament. Unfortunately, direct visualization of the ureter can prove

Table 2 Personal series: summary of the ten cases of ureteral injury resulting from laparoscopy which occurred in our department

Case number	Time of presentation	Indication for initial procedure	Treatment modality	Method of diagnosis	Treatment
1 (1986)	7 days	endometriosis (LUNA)	monopolar coagulation	IVP-CT scan	retrograde stent (JJ)
2 (1987)	7 days	salpingo-ovariolysis, endometriosis	bipolar coagulation	IVP	retrograde stent (JJ)
3 (1992)	7 days	endometriosis (LUNA)	bipolar coagulation	IVP	retrograde stent (JJ)
4 (1994)	13 days	LAVH	extensive coagulation	IVP	uretero-ureterostomy (other hospital)
5 (1994)	8 days	LAVH	bipolar coagulation	IVP	retrograde stent (JJ)
6 (1998)	intraoperatively (observation of thermal damage)	LASH	bipolar coagulation	intraop	retrograde stent (JJ)
7 (1998)	2 months	LASH	extensive coagulation	IVP	retrograde stent (JJ)
8 (1999)	48 hours	retrovaginal adenomyotic nodule (> 4 cm)	dissection, CO_2 laser (transsection)	IVP	failed stenting nephrostomy spontaneous healing without surgery
9 (2000)	5 days	LH	bipolar coagulation	IVP–CT scan	retrograde stent (JJ)
10 (2000)	3 weeks	LASH	bipolar coagulation	IVP	failed stenting vesico-uretero implantation

IVP–CT, intravenous pyelogram – computerized tomography; LUNA, laser uterine nerve ablation; LAVH, laparoscopy-assisted vaginal hysterectomy; LASH, laparoscopy-assisted supracervical hysterectomy; LH, laparoscopic hysterectomy

difficult via pelviscopy. Although the ureter may be visualized through the peritoneum in the upper pelvis, it cannot be identified reliably in the area of the uterosacral ligaments. Identification is particularly difficult when endometriosis or pelvic adhesions are present. Although specific guidelines are not available to prevent this serious complication, the following general points should be considered.

(1) The operator must understand the anatomy of the pelvic ureter and appreciate its proximity to the cervix in cases of endometriosis or when performing LUNA or other risky surgery.

(2) Sometimes, dissection of the ureter may help avoid complications.

(3) In addition, some authors have advocated using hydrodissection or hydroprotection to protect retroperitoneal structures[19,20]. This technique involves making a small incision on the lateral parietal peritoneum and pumping fluid into the retroperitoneal space. Hydroprotection is particularly helpful when a laser is used in the procedure.

(4) In the case of laparoscopic hysterectomy (LH), ureteral and/or bladder damage occurs at a rate of 1.4%[21]. The technique of laparoscopic supracervical hysterectomy (LASH) appears to reduce the risk of such damage.

(5) A ureteral marker can be placed before starting the operative procedure or ureteral dissection. Some authors using an intra-operative stent or the trans-illumination technique may avoid ureteral injury[22,23]. This technique is, in our opinion, too aggressive for the ureter when compared to careful dissection.

(6) Electrocauterization must always be performed with strict visual control of the structures lying under and around the field of application.

(7) Bipolar coagulation is preferred to monopolar coagulation[24]. It is sometimes erroneously assumed that bipolar coagulation is 'completely safe'; in fact, it is safe only when the bipolar forceps are correctly positioned a sufficient distance from the ureter and used for a well-calculated coagulation time[25]. Longer

coagulation induces diffusion of thermal energy and the current may damage the vascular supply around the coagulated tissue, leading to delayed tissue necrosis[26,27].

(8) To prevent such problems, the surgeon must check the energy unit (i.e. isolation, return electrode, power setting), and ensure that it functions correctly. In many instances, burn injuries result from faults in the electrocoagulation equipment and its use. Faulty insulation of the cautery device may also cause burns[28].

(9) The use of a hyperfrequenced electrocautery unit with a low peak voltage of 600 V and a maximum output of 100 W is preferred to other high-energy (3000–8000 V), spark-gap generators[29,30].

BLADDER INJURIES

Injury to the bladder is rare. The incidence is not well known and ranges from 0.01 to 0.06% in recent large studies. In a review of the literature (from 1970 to 1996), the incidence of bladder injury during laparoscopic procedures ranged from 0.02 to 8.3%, depending on the type of institution and the surgeon's experience[31]. This complication occurs more frequently in cases of patients who have a history of Cesarean section or previous surgery, or whose bladder is not empty before surgery. The injury can happen during the installation phase (insertion of the insufflation needle or trocars) or during the operative procedure, by thermal injury (electrocoagulation, laser) and blunt dissection. A frequent and known cause of bladder injury is the second trocar insertion, with an incidence of approximately 1.6% of all laparoscopic procedures[32].

In our series of 900 LASH, the bladder was injured in four cases. Of these women, three had undergone two or three Cesarean sections. The bladder was laparoscopically repaired.

In our series of 12 000 laparoscopies (published in 1994)[5], three cases of such injury were reported: one was due to the second-puncture trocar and one to dilaceration during transabdominal myoma removal (Figure 7) and one to vesico-uterine space dissection during the vaginal approach in laparoscopy-assisted vaginal hysterectomy. The surgeon may see or suspect a bladder injury; in our series, cases 1 and 3 were suspected at the time of laparoscopy and immediately confirmed by the infusion of 500 ml of saline solution with methylene blue into the bladder by gravity drainage.

Mode of diagnosis

Urine may be seen in the pelvis, usually secondary to an extraperitoneal perforation or laceration. If an injury is suspected but no definitive urine is seen, two tests for diagnosis are possible. First, 5 ml of indigo-carmine or methylene blue can be administered intravenously. Another possibility is to inject methylene blue, diluted in 500 ml of saline solution, retrogradely through a urine catheter, so the bladder can be checked laparoscopically for leakage. Because the bladder is hidden within the true pelvis, injuries to the lateral and posterior wall may be missed visually. Therefore, if, after operation, bladder damage is suspected, a gravity cystogram should be performed immediately. Approximately 250 ml of contrast medium is infused into the bladder by gravity drainage and an X-ray film is obtained. If a rupture is seen, a catheter is inserted to allow gravity drainage, which starts immediately. Small bladder perforations may be seen on the lateral, oblique or drain-out films. Radiographically, intraperitoneal injuries will allow contrast medium to fill the cul-de-sac, outline loops of bowel, and extend along the pericolic gutter.

Suprapubic pain and fullness, with or without diminished urine output, may suggest bladder injury. If an intraperitoneal bladder injury has been missed, a dramatic increase in blood urea nitrogen (BUN), due to urinary contact with the peritoneum, is observed. The definitive diagnosis is made by cystography.

Thermal injuries to the bladder may not manifest themselves initially. Sudden hematuria, well into the postoperative period, may be a sign of thermal damage. A true perforation may not yet be present and, therefore, a negative cystogram may be misleading. Cystoscopy should be performed to identify any areas of devitalized tissue.

Treatment

There is a consensus that all large intraperitoneal bladder (> 1.5 cm) injuries should be repaired by laparoscopy at the time the diagnosis is made. In our first series[5], two cases of bladder injury, provoked by trocars, were managed with large-bore Foley catheter drainage for 10 days. Usually, the bladder will heal. A gravity cystogram is performed on day 8–10 and if no extravasation is noted, the catheter is removed.

In the case of bladder laceration, open surgery is required in order to identify the lesion clearly and to close the perforation carefully in two layers, using Vicryl 2-0. The peritoneal cavity is not drained but the space of Retzius is drained. In the case of bladder laceration in our first series, the diagnosis was made during the vaginal approach in laparoscopy-assisted vaginal hysterectomy. The closure of the laceration was performed vaginally, using 2-0 chromic catgut.

Management

The first rule in the treatment of a bladder injury is a 12–15-day drainage. In cases of small leaks (< 2 cm) or extraperitoneal damage, drainage may be sufficient. In other cases, immediate surgical repair is necessary. Prolonged manipulation of perforating instruments

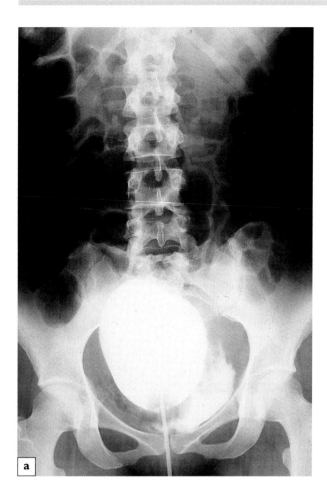

a

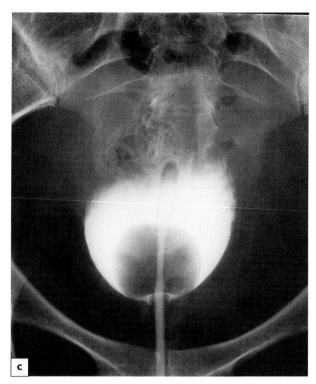

c

Figure 7 Cystography: (a) and (b) extravasation of contrast medium through the dilaceration site (2 days after the endoscopic procedure); (c) absence of extravasation after management with large-bore Foley catheter drainage (7 days later)

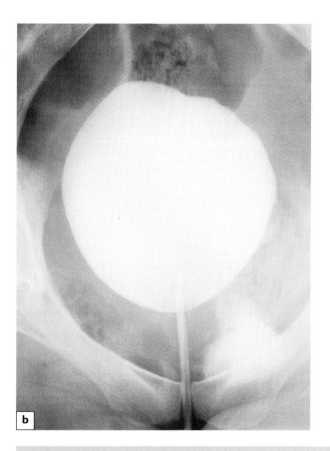

b

increases the degree of damage. If the damage is recognized intraoperatively, the trocar is left in place and by minilaparotomy, a purse-string (two- or three-layer closure) is immediately performed. Laparoscopic repair with a two-layer closure must be considered only by experienced laparoscopists. A patient managed in this way remained asymptomatic throughout a 1-year follow-up. If the damage is suspected intraoperatively without any demonstrable leak or intraperitoneal spillage, drainage and observation may be useful. In case of delayed diagnosis, bladder injuries are handled in the same way as other traumatic ruptures. Intraperitoneal leaks are repaired and drained. Prior to catheter removal, a cystogram can be performed. If the leak persists, drainage is prolonged up to 30 days prior to repeating the cystogram.

Prevention

The first step before inserting the suprapubic trocar is to check that the bladder is well catheterized. For short procedures, this can be an in-and-out catheterization. For longer procedures, a Foley catheter must be drained constantly in a sterile closed system. This may be very useful when the surgeon has frequently to replace the secondary trocar. After emptying the bladder, the second step to prevent trocar damage is visualization of the dome of the bladder when inserting the trocar. Patients who have had a previous Cesarean section, or who have undergone multiple pelvic surgery, could present with distortion in peritoneal bladder repair; thus, trocars have to be placed taking this anatomy into consideration. In difficult cases, the insertion site can be modified.

Conclusion

In case of bladder injury during laparoscopic hysterectomy, separate stitches (Vicryl 2-0) are usually easily placed by laparoscopy. Injuries to the urinary tract are rare, but exist in gynecologic laparoscopy. The incidence has increased during recent years because more and more operations are performed using a laparoscopic technique. Only perfect knowledge of one's trade (surgical technique and instruments) and knowledge of the pelvic anatomy can prevent complications in gynecologic laparoscopy which, nevertheless, also occur in experienced hands.

REFERENCES

1. Bauman H, Jaeger P, Huch A. Ureteral injury after laparoscopic tubal sterilization by bipolar electrocoagulation. *Obstet Gynecol* 1988;71:483–6

2. Stengel JN, Felderman ES, Zamora D. Ureteral injury: complication of laparoscopic sterilization. *Urology* 1974;4:341–2

3. Cheng YS. Ureteral injury resulting from laparoscopic fulguration of endometriotic implant. *Am J Obstet Gynecol* 1976;8:1045–6

4. Daly JW, Higgins KA. Injury to the ureter during gynecologic surgical procedures. *Surg Gynecol Obstet* 1988;167:19–22

5. Donnez J, Bassil S, Anaf V, et al. Ureteral and bladder injury during laparoscopic surgery. In Donnez J, Nisolle M, eds. *Atlas of Laser Operative Laparoscopy and Hysteroscopy*. Carnforth, UK: Parthenon Publishing Group, 1994:237–43

6. Grainger DA, Soderstrom RM, Schiff SF, et al. Ureteral injuries at laparoscopy: insights into diagnosis, management and prevention. *Obstet Gynecol* 1990;75:839–43

7. Irvin TT, Gligher JC, Scott JS. Injury to the ureter during laparoscopic tubal sterilization. *Arch Surg* 1975;110:1501–3

8. Schapira M, Dizerensh H, Essinger A, et al. Urinary ascites after gynecological laparoscopy. *Lancet* 1987;1:871–2

9. Winslow PH, Kreger R, Ebbesson B, et al. Conservative management of electrical burn injury of ureter secondary to laparoscopy. *Urology* 1986;27:60–2

10. teBrevil W, Boeminghaus F. Harnleitorlasion bei laparoskopistcher lubensterilisation. *Geburtshilfe Frauenheilkd* 1977;37:572–6

11. Härkki-Siren P, Sjörberg J, Kurki T. Major complications of laparoscopy: a follow-up Finnish study. *Obstet Gynecol* 1999;94:94

12. Chapron C, Querleu D, Bruhat MA. Surgical complications of diagnostic and operative gynaecological laparoscopy: a series of 29 966 cases. *Hum Reprod* 1998;13:867

13. Janse FW, Kapiteyn K, Trimbos-Kemper T. Complications of laparoscopy: a prospective multicenter observational study. *Br J Obstet Gynaecol* 1997;104:595

14. Lee CL, Huang KG, Lai YM, et al. Ureteral injury during laparoscopically assisted radical hysterectomy. *Hum Reprod* 1995;10:2047–9

15. Donnez J, Bassil S, Smets M, et al. LASH: laparoscopic supracervical (subtotal) hysterectomy. In Cusumano P, Deprest J, eds. *Advanced Gynecologic Laparoscopy*. Carnforth, UK: Parthenon Publishing Group, 1996:79–83

16. Oh BR, Kwon DD, Park KS, et al. Late presentation of ureteral injury after laparoscopic surgery. *Obstet Gynecol* 2000;95:337–9

17. Nezhat C, Nezhat F. Laparoscopic repair of ureter resected during operative laparoscopy. *Obstet Gynecol* 1992;80:543–4

18. Tulikangas PK, Goldberg JM, Gill IS. Laparoscopic repair of ureteral transection. *J Am Assoc Gynecol Laparosc* 2000;7:415–16

19. Donnez J, Nisolle M. Instrumentation and operational instructions. In Donnez J, Nisolle M, eds. *An Atlas of Laser Operative Laparoscopy and Hysteroscopy*. Carnforth, UK: Parthenon Publishing, 1994:21–4

20. Nezhat C, Nezhat FR. Safe laser endoscopic excision or vaporization of peritoneal endometriosis. *Fertil Steril* 1989;52:149–51

21. Harkki-Siren P, Sjoberg J, Tiitinen A. Urinary tract injuries after hysterectomy. *Obstet Gynecol* 1998;82:113–18

22. Lee CL, Huang KG, Wang CW, et al. New approaches in laparoscopically assisted radical vaginal hysterectomy. *Int Surg* 1997;82:266–8

23. Ben Hur H, Phipps JH. Laparoscopic hysterectomy. *J Am Assoc Gynecol Laparosc* 2000;7:103–6

24. Seiler JC, Gidwana G, Ballard L. Laparoscopic cauterization of endometriosis for fertility: an controlled study. *Fertil Steril* 1986;46:1098–100

25. Bauman H, Jaeger P, Huch A. Ureteral injury after laparoscopic tubal sterilization by bipolar electrocoagulation. *Obstet Gynecol* 1988;71:483–5

26. Schwimmer WB. Electrosurgical burn injuries during laparoscopy sterilization. Treatments and prevention. *Obstet Gynecol* 1974;44:526–30

27. Jaffe RH, Willis D, Bachem A. The effect of electric currents on the arteries. A histologic study. *Arch Pathol* 1929;7:244–52

28. Irvin TT, Goligher JC, Scott JS. Injury to the ureter during laparoscopic tubal sterilization. *Arch Surg* 1975;110:1501–3

29. Levinson CJ, Schwartz SF, Saltzstein CE. Complications of laparoscopic tubal sterilization: small bowel perforation. *Obstet Gynecol* 1973;41:253–6

30. Corsoin SL, Bolognese RJ. Electrosurgical hazards in laparoscopy. *J Am Med Assoc* 1974;927:1261

31. Ostrezenski A, Ostrezenska KM. Bladder injury during laparoscopic surgery. *Obstet Gynecol* 1988;55:175–80

32. Godfrey C, Wahle GR, Schilder JM, *et al.* Occult bladder injury during laparoscopy: report of two cases. *J Laparoendosc Adv Surg Tech A* 1999;9:341

Complications of laparoscopic surgery in gynecology

36

J. Donnez, F. Chantraine and M. Nisolle

INTRODUCTION

Over the last 20 years, laparoscopy has developed into a major tool in gynecologic surgery. Initially used as a diagnostic procedure in female infertility and for tubal sterilization, it now allows one to perform almost any surgery previously performed by laparotomy (including tubal and ovarian surgery, hysterectomy, lymphadenectomy). The advantages over laparotomy have been well documented (e.g. reduced postoperative pain, smaller surgical scars, shorter hospital stay, reduced costs). Even if laparoscopy is a relatively safe procedure, complications do occur.

The frequency of indications, the increasing number of surgeons using endoscopy, the introduction of new instruments (forceps, trocars, electrocoagulation, lasers) and the increasing number of major laparoscopic surgical procedures have given rise to new types of complications.

The larger reviews of laparoscopic complications reveal an overall complication rate of approximately 4/1000. A retrospective analysis of 32 205 laparoscopies in Finland between 1995 and 1996 shows a total complication rate of 4 per 1000; 0.6 per 1000 for diagnostic laparoscopy, 0.5 per 1000 for tubal sterilization and 12.6 per 1000 in operative surgery (treatment of endometriosis, ectopic pregnancy, adhesiolysis, ovarian cysts, myomectomy and hysterectomy)[1]. Data files from the National Patient Insurance Association and the Finnish Hospital Discharge Register were used. Seventy-five per cent (88 of 118) of major complications in operative laparoscopy occurred during hysterectomy. All major complications in operative laparoscopies increased, from 0 per 1000 in 1990 to 14 per 1000 in 1996, but part of this increase could be attributed to the increased proportion of laparoscopic hysterectomies. The author also mentioned that complications were more frequently encountered in local rather than university hospitals.

In a retrospective study of complications occurring during 29 966 laparoscopies in seven top French centers for laparoscopy, Chapron and colleagues[2] describe a complication rate of 4.64/1000 (1.84/1000 for diagnostic surgery, 0.84/1000 for minor surgery, 4.3/1000 for major surgery and 17.45/1000 for advanced surgery)[2]. The operative procedures were performed by top gynecologic surgeons and so the results cannot be generalized. The mortality rate observed in this study was 3.33 per 100 000 laparoscopies. Furthermore, one in three complications occurred while setting up for laparoscopy, and one in four was not diagnosed during the operation. Increased experi-

ence in laparoscopy by surgeons has had two consequences: a significant decrease in the rate of complications requiring laparotomy for those laparoscopic surgical procedures that are well defined, and a change in the way complications are treated, with a significant increase in the proportion of incidents treated by laparoscopy.

In a nationwide, prospective, multicenter, observational study of 25 764 laparoscopies in The Netherlands, where data were registered from 1 January to 31 December 1994 by 72 hospitals, the overall complication rate reached 5.7/1000, again correlated to the difficulty of the procedure[3]. The complication rates were 2.7/1000, 4.5/1000 and 17.9/1000 for diagnostic, sterilization and operative laparoscopies, respectively. In 57% of cases, the complication was caused by the surgical approach, while, in the other 43%, the technique was at fault. The most frequently observed complications were hemorrhage of the epigastric vein and intestinal injuries.

In these three analyses, the majority of complications occurred during hysterectomy.

In this chapter, technical and general surgical aspects of laparoscopic complications, their management and recommendations for prevention will be described.

Each laparoscopic procedure may be divided into two steps:

(1) The first step or 'blind step' includes the induction of the pneumoperitoneum and the installation of the laparoscope;

(2) The second step or 'visual step' includes the installation of the operating trocars and surgical procedures.

COMPLICATIONS OF THE FIRST STEP

Subcutaneous emphysema

Subcutaneous emphysema is reported to occur during laparoscopy at a rate between 0.4 and 2%[4,5]. This phenomenon results from improper positioning of the insufflation needle. The introduction of CO_2 into the preperitoneal space will allow its dissection up along the anterior chest wall, neck and face.

Diagnosis

The diagnosis is made by the palpation of the CO_2 bubbles under the skin.

Management

After introduction of the laparoscope, the suprapubic trocar must be inserted into the preperitoneal space, with the valve in the open position. The operator must then press the skin with his hands to push the CO_2 out of the preperitoneal space.

Prevention

It is not a major complication, but the distension of the preperitoneal space could occupy the operation area and thus make the exposure of organs more difficult. Furthermore, this iatrogenic emphysema may cause and/or increase postoperative pain and extend recovery time. Preventing this complication is easy, by respecting the technique of introducing the insufflation needle, and respecting the limits of the insufflating pressure.

Tests based on the negative intra-abdominal pressure may be helpful in cases of difficulties encountered when inducing the pneumoperitoneum to avoid this occurrence.

Besides preperitoneal insufflation, other risk factors for subcutaneous emphysema have been mentioned[6], namely, operative time greater than 200 minutes and use of six or more surgical ports.

Vascular injuries

We must distinguish 'major vascular injury' from 'minor vascular injury'. Major vascular injuries include lesions of the principal vessels, arteries and veins. Perforation of the aorta, vena cava, common right and left iliac arteries and veins, superior mesenteric and inferior epigastric vessels has been reported.

Major vascular injuries

In the Finnish study of 32 205 laparoscopies[1], four major vascular injuries occurred (0.12/1000), one to the aorta and three to the iliac vessels. Injuries were caused by a trocar in two patients, electrocoagulation in one, and laparoscopic scissors in one. All injuries were treated by laparotomy without further complications. Eight hemorrhages of smaller vessels (epigastric, mesenteric, uterine) were also reported (0.25/1000).

In 1997, Hulka and colleagues published a review of 14 911 laparoscopic hysterectomies and noted a major vascular injury rate of 1/1000[7]. Most of these complications were linked to the insertion of the Verres needle, but one case of fatal aortic injury at the time of skin incision was reported (Morrow, personal communication). Furthermore, in this study, most vessel injuries occurred with the use of large (> 10 mm) disposable pyramidal trocars.

In our series, we observed two cases of major vascular injury, both lesions of the vena cava. The lesions occurred at the time of the insertion of the Verres needle. Diagnosis

was made at the moment when the laparoscope was installed. A retroperitoneal hematoma was observed (Figure 1). Because it was a venous lesion, treatment was expectant with blood transfusion. Complete healing of the injury was achieved after spontaneous hematoma resorption.

Diagnosis

A vascular injury is suspected in the presence of one of these signs:

(1) Return of blood from the open insufflation needle;

(2) Sudden deterioration in blood pressure of a previously stable patient after needle or trocar insertion, especially if the positioning of the needle was difficult;

(3) The presence of an unexplained volume of blood in the peritoneal cavity, and if this blood reappears after aspiration[8];

(4) Dark color and increase in volume of the retroperitoneal space.

In over half of the cases reported in the literature[9–11], the diagnosis was made immediately and a laparotomy was performed. In other cases, the diagnosis was delayed (6–21 days) and, in one case[12], a patient had a 3-month-old laparoscopic lesion and was treated on suspicion of a ruptured aortic aneurysm. In another case, injury to the left common iliac artery and vein was recognized 3 h after the end of laparoscopic surgery. Intraperitoneal CO_2 pressure on the bleeding vessels and decreased venous return caused by the steep Trendelenburg position may explain the failure to recognize the injury during the laparoscopy itself. These factors can sometimes delay the diagnosis of venous injuries[13].

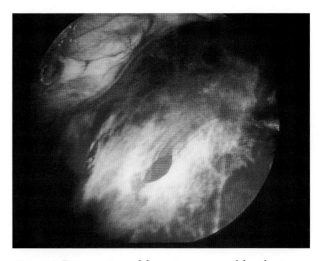

Figure 1 Retroperitoneal hematoma caused by the insertion of the Verres needle in the vena cava

Management

If vascular injury with the insufflation needle is strongly suspected, the needle is left in place to help mark the site of injury while an expeditious midline incision is made for laparotomy. A trocar injury of the major vessels is more serious and the measures described above must be applied. Usually, in the case of a major vessel injury, the retroperitoneal hematoma occupies all of the fields of view, and, once laparotomy is performed, the first priority is the compression of the aorta. This can be accomplished with the hand or with a vascular clamp and may reduce the bleeding until a vascular surgeon arrives. If vascular injury is not certain and blood pressure is stable, the insufflation needle is still left in place and the pneumoperitoneum can be achieved in another way. A 5-mm laparoscope is introduced through a suprapubic trocar. If bleeding is very minimal, endoscopic repair must be considered for small vessels, but laparotomy is necessary for major vessel injury. In cases of delayed symptoms, a computed tomograph and/or magnetic resonance image are helpful for diagnosis, and management is decided upon in collaboration with a vascular surgeon. Sometimes, in the case of small, venous injuries (insertion of the Verres needle, for example), expectant management with spontaneous blood resorption can be tried. An example is our patient presenting with a vena cava hematoma after Verres needle insertion. If the injury is a lesion of an artery, operative treatment is indicated because spontaneous healing of an active bleeding artery is almost impossible.

Prevention

The success of the prevention of such an injury depends on the surgeon's experience, knowledge of anatomy and understanding of the procedure. Important points to consider include the following.

Thin patients have the highest risk of vascular injury; the aorta may lie less than 3 cm below the skin in these women. Introduction of an insufflation needle or trocar must be done with due consideration of this anatomy.

The position of the tip of the needle must be checked before any mobilization. Many tests have been proposed for this; all depend on the principle of negative abdominal pressure.

In the case of malpositioning of the insufflation needle, it must be removed and the pneumoperitoneum reestablished. The manipulation of the needle, in an attempt to position it properly intra-abdominally, exposes the patient to a high risk of vascular injury. If blood returns from the open insufflation needle, the needle must be left fixed without any manipulation, because this may induce a wide laceration of the vascular wall.

Elevation of the abdominal wall is recommended prior to needle insertion. This will increase the distance over which the needle must travel to reach the major vessels[14].

This must be done manually; attempts to elevate the abdominal wall with towel clips merely give the illusion of safety. They elevate the skin or subcutaneous space only and do nothing to the peritoneum[15].

It is important to ensure that an adequate pneumoperitoneum is created, prior to inserting the trocar.

Both blunt trocars and disposable sharp trocars have been implicated in major vessel trauma[16,17]. The use of blunt needles and trocars increases the risk of vascular injury, because blunt instruments need increased force for insertion and this may cause the trocar to slip[18]. Disposable sharp trocars can also provoke vascular injuries because the introduction of this type of trocar does not need much pressure. For a surgeon who normally works with non-disposable trocars, it can be dangerous to introduce this sharp instrument into the abdomen. In the 1995 survey by the American Association of Gynecological Laparoscopists[7], the vast majority of vessel injuries occurred with disposable trocars. In another study[19], disposable trocars were associated with a higher but not statistically significant complication rate. Furthermore, disposable trocars were not cost-effective. Therefore, for the author, the more expensive disposable trocars are not recommended. So, clearly, sharp instruments and safety shields do not preclude significant injuries to large vessels. Moreover, the Food and Drug Administration of America requested manufacturers and distributors of shielded trocars to eliminate claims of increased safety because these indications give a false reassurance to the surgeon.

Introducing the laparoscope trocar without any pneumoperitoneum has been attempted by some authors[20–24]. They do not report any vascular injury from more than 10 000 laparoscopies. According to Nezhat and colleagues[25], direct trocar insertion reduces the risk of omental injuries and subcutaneous emphysema. We do not have any experience of this technique but it should be taken into consideration in difficult cases.

Minor vascular injury

Essentially, this concerns injury to the omentum or presacral vessels. In most cases, it is unlikely that this injury can induce acute shock and the management depends on the experience of the surgeon.

Diagnosis

Minor vascular injury is suspected when blood returns from the open insufflation needle, or when blood is present in the peritoneal cavity. In both cases, the blood pressure remains stable without shock. In the first case, the diagnosis can be made by visualization of the bleeding using a 5-mm suprapubic laparoscope introduced after the creation of a pneumoperitoneum in another site with another insufflation needle. In the second case, the bleeding is visualized when the laparoscope is introduced.

Management

Usually, the bleeding is controlled by bipolar coagulation or with laparoscopic suture. It is rare that the bleeding necessitates a laparotomy.

Prevention

The same preventive measures as for major vascular injury apply for minor vascular injury.

Gastrointestinal injury – stomach injury

Gastric perforation by the insufflation needle or the trocar is a rare occurrence. Its incidence was evaluated as 0.027% by Loffer and Pent[26]. In the literature, more than 30 cases have been reported[27–29].

Chapron and colleagues[30] analyzed 56 patients with 62 gastrointestinal injuries, found in the SFEG (French Society of Gynecological Endoscopy) complications register. One out of the 62 injuries involved the stomach (1.6%). Furthermore, in this study, one-third of the complications (32.2%) occurred during the installation phase of laparoscopy and 10.7% of gastrointestinal injuries were provoked by the pneumoperitoneum needle[30].

In our series, two cases of stomach perforation occurred during the installation phase. The first occurred with the Verres needle. Diagnosis was made at the moment of introduction of the laparoscope when the lesion was visualized during the routine control of the abdominal cavity. No further treatment was necessary because the lesion healed spontaneously. In the second case, a 5-mm trocar was inserted into the left upper quadrant while adhesions were suspected in the umbilical region. After introducing the telescope (4 mm), the stomach mucosa was visualized. The telescope was gently removed from the stomach and only a small red area without obvious perforation was noted on the surface of the stomach. The patient was treated for 5 days with prophylactic antibiotics and a stomach sound. No suture was necessary. The recovery was uneventful.

Diagnosis

The main sign of gastric perforation by the insufflation needle is the occurrence of bouts of eructation. Perforation with the trocar is diagnosed by visualization of the gastric mucosa.

Management

In cases of gastric perforation with the insufflation needle without any tearing, no further therapy is needed because its small diameter leaves no defect. In all other cases of such injury, suture of the stomach by laparotomy or laparoscopy must normally be performed. The patient in our series who presented with a stomach injury caused by

a 5-mm trocar was treated by medical therapy with broad-spectrum antibiotics and a nasogastric sound for 5 days. Food and fluid administration was forbidden during this time. The recovery was normal.

Prevention

The most common conditions which lead to gastric injury are distortion of the abdominal anatomy by previous surgery, difficult induction of anesthesia[26,28,31] and acrophagia[27]. In the presence of one of these conditions, some precautions are mandatory:

(1) Inserting a nasogastric or oropharyngeal tube after induction of anesthesia;

(2) Placing the patient in a 15° Trendelenburg position prior to insertion of the insufflation needle;

(3) Lifting the abdominal wall and respecting an angle of 45° with the skin of needle insertion;

(4) Ensuring that an adequate pneumoperitoneum is created to prevent injury to the stomach at the time of trocar insertion.

A stomach aspiration by inserting a nasogastric sound or tube should be performed systematically after induction of the anesthesia and before the insertion of any laparoscopic instrument. This technique is applied in every procedure by the anesthetists working in our operating theater.

Gastrointestinal injury – bowel injuries

Inadvertent traumatic perforation of the bowel is a well-recognized potential complication of laparoscopy. This complication has been reported to occur with an incidence of 0.06 to 0.30%[30,32,33]. Insertion of the insufflation needle and the initial trocar into the peritoneal cavity is the most common cause of bowel perforation[34,35]. Indeed, in our series, a small bowel perforation occurred when introducing the Verres needle. Diagnosis was made immediately because the gas pressure was not correct and a foul smell was detected. The needle was left in place and a 4-mm telescope was introduced into the left upper quadrant which confirmed the small bowel perforation. To treat this complication, the umbilical incision was enlarged (mini-laparotomy) and the bowel lesion was sutured. After observation for some days in hospital with broad-spectrum antibiotic cover, the patient was discharged and a normal recovery was observed.

Diagnosis

Injuries to the bowel can be treacherous because they may not be recognized at the time of surgery. Diagnosis is made immediately in the presence of stool on the tip of the needle or the trocar, if fecal material is seen in the abdominal cavity, if the surgeon notices a foul smell when introducing the laparoscope, if a hematoma is noticed on the bowel serosa, or if the laparoscope is introduced into the lumen of the intestine. In the review by Chapron and co-workers[30], diagnosis of gastrointestinal injuries was made during surgery in only 35.7% of cases and the mean time before diagnosis was 4 days (range 0–23). In cases of delayed diagnosis, especially with through-and-through perforation of the bowel, signs of peritonitis may be present postoperatively and the diagnosis is confirmed at laparotomy. A through-and-through injury to a loop of bowel may only be detected at the moment of surgery by removing the laparoscope under direct vision to catch a glimpse of the bowel lumen.

Management

The treatment of bowel injury will depend on etiology. Perforations with the insufflation needle without any laceration of the intestinal wall do not require any surgical repair, and a medical approach with broad-spectrum antibiotics may be sufficient. In the case of trocar perforation or wide laceration, surgical repair is mandatory and the method of repair depends on the instruments available and the proficiency of the laparoscopist. Laparotomy with suture repair is probably the preferred treatment for most laparoscopists. However, laparoscopic repair is possible providing the injury is not extensive and stool contamination of the abdominal cavity is limited. In cases of delayed diagnosis with peritonitis, laparotomy is still indicated.

Prevention

Certain predisposing factors, such as a dilated gastrointestinal tract or an atypical anatomical laceration secondary to adhesions will increase the risk of bowel injury. Attention must be paid in cases of patients with previous laparotomy, the use of blunt instruments, or patients with prior operation causing or describing adhesions.

The trocar insertion technique should be standardized; with the patient in a completely horizontal position, an angle of 45° with the skin must be respected when introducing the trocar. Premature Trendelenburg positioning does nothing to avoid bowel injuries. Exploration of the anterior abdominal wall with a syringe and needle to check for the presence of bowel adhesions is a helpful test in patients with previous laparotomy. After the pneumoperitoneum has been established, a 10-ml syringe containing 3 ml normal saline is connected to a short 18-gauge spinal needle, which is inserted through the umbilicus. If there is adequate peritoneal space to accommodate the trocar, gas bubbles will appear in the saline. The limits of the potential space can be further confined by gradually advancing the needle. In patients suspected of having subumbilical bowel adhesions, which might lead to injury even with the 'open' technique of Hasson[36], Soderstrom[37] insufflates with the Verres needle placed in the left upper quadrant and, after insufflation is accomplished, a 5-mm trocar

sleeve is inserted, again in the left upper quadrant. Through this trocar sleeve, a 4.5-mm telescope is inserted to view the subumbilical area before placing the laparoscope trocar under direct vision[38]. This technique is also used in our department for patients in whom we suspect subumbilical adhesions. Much attention has been paid to the disposable trocar, because of its sharp tip and spring-loaded safety shield[39]. Nevertheless, there have been no large-scale clinical trials to establish the advantage of single-use trocars[18].

Urinary tract injuries

Urinary tract injuries can also occur as a result of inadvertent instrument insertion. Essentially, this happens with an over-distended bladder because of a lack of catheterization before the procedure. The diagnosis is made when urine comes out of the insufflation needle; no surgical repair is required in this case. A small hole may require only Foley catheter drainage[40]. Such injuries are more likely to occur with suprapubic trocars and are discussed in Chapter 35.

COMPLICATIONS OF THE SECOND STEP

During the second step, complications could occur while inserting the secondary trocars or during the surgical procedures. Vascular, urinary or intestinal structures may be injured with the trocars or while performing electrosurgery, laser surgery or sharp dissection.

Injuries with secondary trocars

Major vascular injury or bowel injury is diagnosed and managed as described above. Epigastric vessel perforation and bladder injury are managed differently, as described further.

Epigastric vessel perforation by secondary trocars

Perforation of the inferior and/or superficial epigastric vessels is the most common complication encountered during laparoscopic surgery (Figure 2). The inferior epigastric artery extends from the external iliac artery and lies beneath the rectus muscle and above the peritoneum. The superficial epigastric artery extends from the femoral artery near the inguinal ring and courses medially over the rectus muscle toward the midline.

Diagnosis

If injured, these large vessels can produce a rapid and massive hemorrhage. One fatal injury to an epigastric vessel is described in the literature[41]. While an injured inferior epigastric artery creates retroperitoneal or intraperitoneal bleeding, superficial epigastric vessel

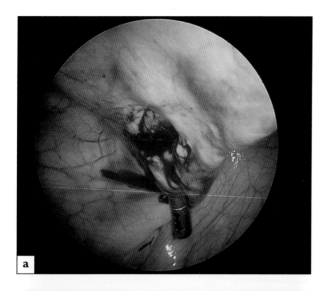

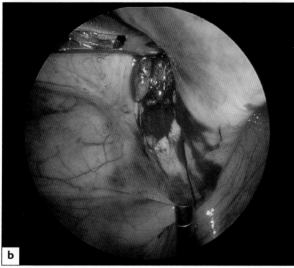

Figure 2 (a) and (b) Epigastric vessel perforation

damage induces intramuscular or subcutaneous bleeding. In most cases, blood spillage around the trocar sleeve announces the injury.

Management

An essential rule to bear in mind is that the sleeve cannot be removed, as it is the only mark of the vessel's location. In case of minimal bleeding and a small hematoma, no repair is required. Sometimes the bleeding can be extremely swift, and repair using several techniques might be necessary. Both ends of the transected vessel must be secured for an adequate hemostasis. Bipolar coagulation of the vessel through the peritoneum is the best and fastest way to ensure optimal hemostasis. This can be efficacious only when there is no hematoma in the field of view, making the vessel's identification impossible. Laparoscopic ligation of the vessel will achieve hemostasis. A large curved or straight needle can be passed through the

abdominal wall and into the abdomen. The needle is then passed back through the abdominal wall and tied outside the abdominal wall, cephaled and cauded to the sleeve. At the end of surgery, the ligature can be removed without any recurrence of bleeding. Another similar suture technique, using two sutures with straight needles, is described by Chatzipapas and Magos[42]. Hemostasis can also be achieved by simple compression. As soon as the swift bleeding is noticed around the sleeve, a number 12 Foley catheter is passed through the sleeve into the abdominal cavity[43]. The Foley balloon is inflated with fluid. The sleeve is pulled out and the Foley balloon is pulled up against the abdominal wall. The pressure maintained on the Foley balloon occludes the bleeding vessel. As soon as hemostasis is obtained, a second trocar is inserted and the operation can continue. In some rare cases, hemostasis cannot be achieved; the skin incision must be enlarged around the trocar sleeve and the vessel promptly secured by ligature.

Prevention

An injury to the superficial and/or inferior epigastric vessels may occur during any laparoscopy, but is more likely to happen under specific circumstances. Obese women, or patients who have undergone previous abdominal surgery, are prone to having an epigastric vessel obscured by the fat paniculus or by the incisional scar. Marret and colleagues[44], analyzing complications caused by trocars, observed that 70% of patients presenting with a complication had previous abdominal surgery and 50% of them were obese. Removing and replacing trocars of different sizes and/or trying repeatedly to place the second trocar increase the risk of such injury. During the laparoscopy, a security triangle should be visualized using the obliterated umbilical arteries as the lateral sides of the triangle and the dome of the bladder as the third side of the triangle. Secondary puncture trocars must be inserted within the margins of this triangle. The epigastric vessels rarely lie within the confines of this area. Sometimes, close laparoscopic inspection of the peritoneal side of the anterior abdominal wall allows the visualization of these vessels, so that the surgeon can choose a safe location to introduce the suprapubic trocar. Another technique is to localize the epigastric vessels by transillumination[45]. Superficial abdominal wall vessels may be located by transillumination in the majority of women of normal weight, but it is of less value in overweight and obese women. The deep (inferior) epigastric vessels cannot be effectively located by transillumination.

Bladder injury by secondary trocars

Bladder injuries are more common with secondary trocars and occur in approximately 1.6% of all laparoscopic procedures[46]. A lack of bladder catheterization is the main reason for such injuries. Although the bladder heals rapidly, intraoperative recognition of the injury is crucial because it facilitates management and postoperative recovery. Delay in the diagnosis can result in abdominal distension and azotemia, although ascites, urinoma and vesicocutaneous fistulas are sometimes encountered.

Diagnosis

Diagnosis is made intraoperatively by the recognition of the bladder muscularis separated by the trocar, or by urine spillage around the trocar sleeve. If a Foley catheter is left in place, the appearance of gas in the Foley bag or hematuria must be investigated. To detect and visualize the lesion, a contrast liquid (methylene blue) can be injected through the urinary catheter into the bladder. If the blue liquid is seen in the abdominal cavity at the laparoscopy, the injury is demonstrated. In every other case, the diagnosis is made postoperatively in the presence of hematuria, decreased urinary output, anuria, abdominal swelling or peritoneal signs. In the absence of infected urine, peritoneal signs rarely occur. A retrograde cystogram localizes the leak from the bladder and abdominal sonography confirms the presence of liquid in the abdominal cavity.

Management

The first rule in the treatment of a bladder injury is a 12–15-day drainage. In cases of small leaks (< 2 cm) or extraperitoneal damage, drainage may be sufficient. In other cases, immediate surgical repair is necessary. Prolonged manipulation of perforating instruments increases the degree of damage. If the damage is recognized intraoperatively, the trocar is left in place and a purse-string (two- or three-layer closure) is immediately performed by minilaparotomy[47,48]. Laparoscopic repair with a two-layer closure must be considered only by experienced laparoscopists. A patient managed in this way remained asymptomatic throughout a 1-year follow-up[49]. If the damage is suspected intraoperatively without any demonstrable leak or intraperitoneal spillage, drainage and observation may be useful[50]. In cases of delayed diagnosis, bladder injuries are handled in the same way as other traumatic ruptures. Intraperitoneal leaks are repaired and drained[50]. Prior to catheter removal, a cystogram may be performed. If the leak persists, drainage is prolonged up to 30 days prior to repeating the cystogram.

Prevention

The first step before inserting the suprapubic trocar is to check that the bladder is well catheterized. For short procedures, this can be an in-and-out catheterization. For longer procedures, a Foley catheter must be drained constantly in a sterile closed system. This may be very useful when the surgeon has to replace the secondary trocar often. After emptying the bladder, the second step to prevent trocar damage is the visualization of the dome of the bladder when inserting the trocar. Patients who have had a previous Cesarean section or who have undergone multiple pelvic surgery could present a distortion in peritoneal bladder repair; thus, trocars have to be placed taking this anatomy into consideration. In difficult cases, the insertion side can be modified.

Injuries during surgical procedures

A host of instruments have been developed for specific purposes during laparoscopic procedures. In addition to sharp and blunt dissection, performed by means of a laparoscope, there are special laser and electrosurgical devices specifically designed for laparoscopic application. It has been demonstrated that tissue damage can be caused up to 5 cm beyond the point of contact using monopolar electrosurgery[51], up to 5 mm for bipolar electrosurgery[52] and to 2.7 mm for the CO_2 laser[53]. Two major complications have been described when using these devices: bowel and ureteral injury.

Bowel injury during surgical procedures

Bowel perforation could occur during laparoscopic dissection. Besides occurrences directly related to dense adhesions and the dissection plane, complications could be induced by the use of a thermal energy device[35]. In 1993, 27 bowel traumas were described[54], which occurred during 17 531 laparoscopies (1.54/1000). Twenty of them occurred during adhesiolysis and the incidence was correlated to the procedure's difficulty.

Of Soderstrom's 66 bowel injuries, 60 were traumatic and six were due to electrocoagulation[55].

In our series of 1055 cases of rectovaginal adenomyotic nodules, rectal injury (incision from 1 to 3 cm) occurred in eight cases. The rectum was repaired by laparotomy in three cases and by posterior colpotomy in three cases. In all six cases, the postoperative phase was uneventful. In this series, a rectovaginal fistula occurred after laparoscopic resection of a rectovaginal adenomyotic nodule with suture of the vaginal dome by a vaginal approach and completed by a left salpingectomy (Figure 3). Two weeks after surgery, the patient mentioned loss of stools vaginally. Conservative treatment (antibiotics and a diet with no fiber) was applied for several weeks. Three months later, a control X-ray of the bowel with contrast injection confirmed complete healing. This lesion was probably due to a thermal injury.

In this series, one case of fecalis peritonitis occurred 10 days after adenomyotic nodule resection. A bowel enema (with gastrographine) revealed a large lateral defect 8–10 cm from the anal margin. A first treatment involving insertion of a drain through the vagina was insufficient. A laparotomy was carried out for peritoneal lavage and drainage, as well as to perform a colostomy (Figure 4).

379

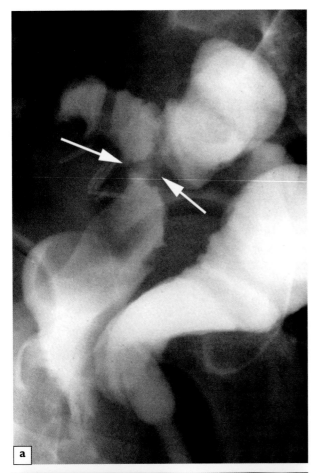

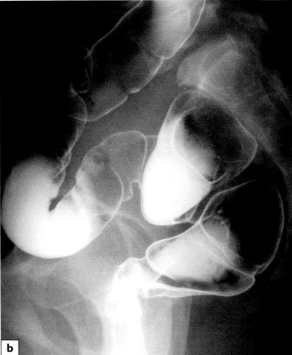

Figure 3 (a) Visualization of the rectovaginal fistula (arrows) by retrograde bowel contrast injection. The vagina is obviously filled by contrast medium; (b) control X-ray showing complete healing after conservative treatment for 3 months

Diagnosis

In the majority of cases, diagnosis is delayed and patients present with signs of peritonitis or bowel occlusion. Intraoperatively, diagnosis is made by the direct visualization of the damage.

Management

Management of perforations of the bowel is related to the site and the extent of damage, and to when the injury is discovered. For perforations by the laser beam or an electrosurgical device diagnosed intraoperatively, a laparotomy with resection of the necrotic zone is necessary. If the lesion is very small and if the patient has had a preoperative bowel preparation, repair by laparoscopic suture is possible for an experienced surgeon[56]. The bowel must be repaired with two- or three-layer sutures. This type of closure is appropriate only if the damage is limited and superficial. In the presence of a significant bowel lesion or peritonitis, a timely intraoperative consultation with the general surgeon is mandatory to decide how to handle the damage (Table 1).

Prevention

Laser surgery must be carried out by an experienced surgeon, with adequate instruments[57]. In addition, the laser should always be placed on stand-by mode when not used. Care must be taken when using monopolar electrosurgery to ensure that the patient's return plate is properly attached, the instruments are well insulated and the bowel is out of the field of energy application. With bipolar coagulation, the forceps must not come into contact with the bowel when activated or immediately after inactivation.

In our department, if difficult laparoscopic surgery (resection of a rectovaginal adenomyotic nodule, suspicion of numerous adhesions) is to be performed, the patient has a bowel preparation. In case of bowel lesions diagnosed during surgery, direct suture can be performed. This technique avoids the temporary colostomy that is normally indicated in this type of complication without a bowel preparation.

Ureteral injury during surgical procedures

Ureteral injuries are a major concern for the laparoscopic surgeon. Most injuries occur during dissection of the ovary adherent to the pelvic side wall, uterosacral transection (laser uterine nerve ablation), coagulation of the uterine vessels during hysterectomy, lymphadenectomy and coagulation or vaporization of endometriosis (see Chapter 35 on ureteral injury).

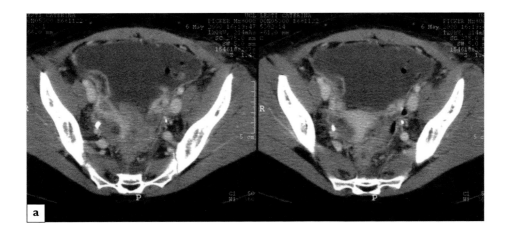

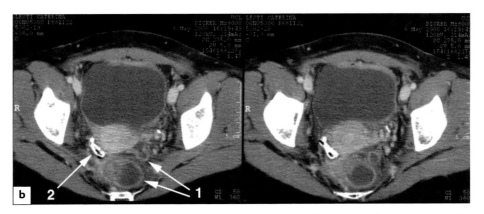

Figure 4 (a) Liquid collection in the abdominal cavity, 10 days after adenomyotic nodule resection. Diagnosis of fecalis peritonitis was made; (b) 1, a 3-cm collection in the left pararectal space; 2, vaginal drain

Table 1 Our series of 1125 laparoscopic resections of adenomyotic nodules: injuries due to nodule surgery and outcome

	Diagnosis	*Treatment*	*Outcome*
Rectal injuries (n = 8)	*intraoperative* (n = 6)	direct repair (n = 6)	complications (n = 0)
	postoperative (n = 2)		
	R-V fistula (n = 1)	conservative	spontaneous healing after 3 months
	R-V fistula with peritonitis (n = 1)	temporary colostomy	chronic R-V fistula requiring surgery and reanastomosis 3 months later
Ureteral injury (n = 1)	postoperative	failure of double J stent	nephrostomy and conservative treatment for 3 months followed by complete healing

R-V, rectovaginal

Diagnosis

When a ureteral injury is suspected intraoperatively, indigo carmine or methylene blue dye can be administered intravenously. Several minutes later, these products are excreted by the kidney and can be visualized in the abdominal cavity if a urinary tract injury has occurred.

Usually, diagnosis is missed intraoperatively and patients tend to present 48–72 h postoperatively with abdominal pain and peritonitis, leukocytosis and fever. Flank tenderness or hematuria are rarely described. Sometimes an evaluation of the drained abdominal fluid including levels of urea and creatinine is helpful. The presence of ascites and/or a pelvic mass is constant on sonography, and the diagnosis is confirmed by intravenous pyelography.

Management

The repair of ureteral injuries must be performed with the collaboration of the urological surgeon. Percutaneous or cystoscopic techniques can probably be used to manage most of such injuries[58]. Exploratory laparoscopy and/or laparotomy are used for surgical repair in cases of end-to-end reanastomosis, reimplantation of the ureter to the bladder, transureteral ureterostomy and other techniques[59].

Prevention

Unfortunately, direct visualization of the ureter is difficult at the time of pelviscopy. Although the ureter may be visualized through the peritoneum in the upper pelvis, it cannot be identified reliably in the area of the uterosacral ligaments. In case of hysterectomy, the technique of laparoscopic supracervical hysterectomy (LASH) appears to reduce the risk of ureteral injuries[60]. Specific guidelines are unavailable to prevent this serious complication. Several general points must be considered.

The operator must understand the anatomy of the pelvic ureter and appreciate its proximity to the cervix in cases of endometriosis or when performing LUNA or other high-risk procedures. Sometimes the dissection of the ureter may be helpful. Some have advocated using hydrodissection or hydroprotection to protect retroperitoneal structures[57,61]. This technique involves making a small incision on the lateral parietal peritoneum and inserting fluid into the retroperitoneal space. Hydroprotection is useful when using the laser.

Electrocauterization must always be done under strict visual control of the structures lying under and around the field of application. Bipolar coagulation is preferred over monopolar coagulation[58]. However, it is erroneously assumed that bipolar coagulation is completely safe; in fact, it is safe only when the bipolar forceps is correctly positioned without touching the ureter, and when an appropriate coagulation time is calculated[62,63]. A lengthy

coagulation induces a diffusion of thermal energy and the current may damage the vascular supply around the coagulated tissue leading to delayed tissue necrosis[64,65]. The operator must check the energy unit that he is using and ensure that it functions correctly. It appears that burn injuries are related to faults in the electrocoagulation equipment and its use. Faulty insulation of the cautery device may cause burns[66]. Also, the use of a hyperfrequency electrocautery unit is preferable to other high-energy, spark-gap-type generators[67,68].

Complications due to CO_2 gas insufflation

Venous air embolism is a complication in laparoscopy that can happen at any time during the surgical procedure. In gynecological procedures, venous air embolism is usually sudden and, therefore, it is crucial to detect it immediately. Any delay in exsufflation and treatment can prove to be fatal[69]. The incidence is very low; the reported figures vary from 1/63 000 to 1/7500[70,71].

Diagnosis

Clinical signs such as decreased blood pressure, tachycardia, arrhythmia and increasing central venous pressure come too late to be useful as warning signals. An easy and non-invasive way of embolism detection is measurement of end-tidal CO_2. As soon as the end-tidal CO_2 drops, abdominal pressure must be immediately reduced. If this maneuver is not followed by an increase in end-tidal CO_2 or if there is any sign of cardiovascular problems, venous air embolism must be considered to have occurred and appropriate measures must be taken.

Management

The patient should immediately be ventilated with 100% oxygen to prevent hypoxemia. The Trendelenburg position should be maintained and the pneumoperitoneum emptied. A large catheter must be inserted into the right atrium through the internal jugular vein to aspirate the gas. Any delay in exsufflation and treatment can prove fatal[69].

Prevention

Gynecological laparoscopy should only be performed by trained surgeons in the presence of experienced anesthetists and with adequate time available. Abdominal pressure should be closely observed. Use of continuous end-tidal CO_2 analyzers is required.

Incisional hernias

Herniation of the small bowel or the omentum through the trocar incision is a complication of laparoscopy well described in the literature. Sometimes, other organs can cause herniation. For example, tubal herniation after operative laparoscopy has been reported[72]. The risk increases with trocars > 10 mm in particular. In a retrospective study by the American Association of Gynecological Laparoscopists, 933 hernias were reported from an estimated 4 385 000 laparoscopic procedures (0.02%)[73]. Kadar and colleagues observed an incidence of 0.23% and 3.1% in using 10-mm and 12-mm trocars, respectively[74]. These data were confirmed by Nezhat and colleagues[75], who published an incidence of 0.2% (11 hernias in 5300 laparoscopies).

In our series of 18 500 laparoscopies, we encountered two cases of hernias, probably because we used 5-mm trocars and because peritoneal and fascial incisions were systematically closed with stitches.

In one case, incarceration of the transverse colon in the umbilical incision occurred. A 59-year-old woman was operated on for bilateral adnexectomy. The principal trocar was introduced three times because insertion was difficult. This provoked a wide laceration of the peritoneal hole. During the hospital stay, re-alimentation was difficult, the patient mentioned abdominal pain and fever was observed. At the computerized tomography scan (Figure 5), performed on day 5, an incarceration of an intestinal loop in the umbilical incision was diagnosed. Perforation of the transverse colon in very inflamed tissue was visualized during laparotomy performed with the general surgeon.

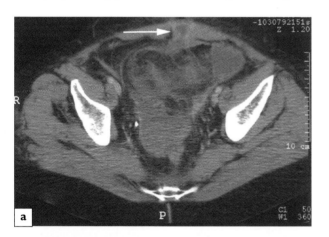

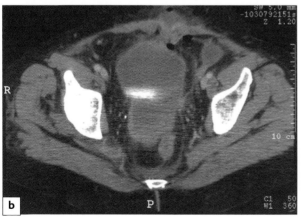

Figure 5 (a) and (b) Incarceration of the transverse colon in the umbilical incision

Temporary colostomy for 3 months was carried out and bowel resection was avoided.

Diagnosis

Mostly, hernias occur later than 1 week after surgery. However, some cases of early herniation in the postoperative phase are known. Indeed, if reversal of the general anesthesia is too early at the end of the surgical procedure, herniation can be precipitated by the coughing movements of the patient[76]. Symptoms of incisional hernia are (chronic) pain in the region where the trocar has been inserted and the classic symptoms of bowel obstruction (nausea, vomiting, pain).

Management

If incisional herniation is suspected, a laparoscopy must be performed to reduce the hernia. Sometimes, bowel resection is necessary if the tissue is necrotic.

Prevention

To avoid this kind of complication, suture in two layers (fascia, peritoneum and skin) is indicated in all cases of trocar incisions larger than 10 mm. In our department, we use a special technique to suture the aponeurosis and the peritoneum if the incision is > 10 mm. A special needle (Philipps needle) is introduced under laparoscopic control. To prevent any lesions when retracting the needle, the tip is then covered with a 5-mm trocar. The knot is tied outside the abdominal cavity. Many other suture techniques have been described[77,78].

The underlying fascia and peritoneum should be closed not only when using trocars of 10 mm or more, as previously suggested, but also when extensive manipulation is performed through a 5-mm trocar port, causing extension of the incision.

Rare complications reported in the literature

Diaphragm lesions

First, a case was reported of a patient presenting with a congenital diaphragmatic defect causing a complete right pneumothorax during operative laparoscopy[79]. The lesion was recognized and appropriately treated intraoperatively.

Another complication with a diaphragmatic injury occurred in our department in a 25-year-old woman presenting with endometriotic lesions in the pelvis and at the diaphragm. In treating these lesions by CO_2 laser vaporization, perforation (3 mm) of the fibrotic part of the diaphragm occurred. The operation was stopped immediately and a moderate right pneumothorax was diagnosed. Spontaneous healing without any drainage was observed after a few days (Donnez, unpublished results).

Spleen laceration after laparoscopic surgery

Salpingoplasty was performed on a 31-year-old woman to correct bilateral hydrosalpinges. Nine hours after the operation, an emergency exploratory laparotomy was performed due to massive abdominal bleeding. The cause was a small tear in the inferior splenic tail. The etiology of this laceration is uncertain. Many complications of laparoscopy are physiologic, and this one might have occurred while establishing pneumoperitoneum. Distortion and stretching of small vascular adhesions of the spleen with the abdominal wall may also have played a role[80].

Bowel subocclusion by suture of the umbilical incision

One week after a laparoscopic procedure, a patient presented to the accident and emergency department with signs of subocclusion of the bowel (loss of appetite, abdominal pain) without any sign of peritonitis. At diagnostic laparoscopy (hysteroscope in the left upper quadrant), performed to confirm a bowel lesion, we observed that the small bowel was incarcerated in the umbilical incision. After cutting the suture points, the bowel spontaneously fell into the abdominal cavity. No signs of necrosis were observed and no suture of the bowel was necessary. Reintroduction of food started 2 days after surgery and recovery was straightforward. This complication was probably due to anesthesia which was reversed too fast, as the patient was coughing while the surgeon was suturing.

DISCUSSION

The increased use of laparoscopy as a therapeutic method necessitates a reappraisal of the risk involved. Complications frequently described include injuries to the large and small bowel, uterus, bladder, ureters and blood vessels. These risks, in addition to the risk of general anesthesia, have been increased by the addition of new devices and instruments for operative laparoscopy. Each complication has a specific etiology that is usually preventable or treatable if recognized in time. Usually complications of the first (blind) step and second (visual) step are recognized intraoperatively and treated, with a simple postoperative recovery. Complications of surgical procedures, specifically thermal injuries, are diagnosed postoperatively.

This is still a major problem with operative laparoscopy because delayed diagnosis worsens the prognosis and increases morbidity. Also, this type of injury often requires repair by laparotomy. The exact percentage of laparoscopic complications is unknown. In Table 2, data of different studies are summarized. The complication rate requiring laparotomy varied from 0.14 to 0.33%. The likelihood of laparotomy being required was directly related to the degree of complexity of the laparoscopic surgical

Table 2 Frequency of complications of laparoscopic surgery necessitating laparotomy

Reference	n	Laparotomy n	/1000
Henry-Suchet *et al.*[81]	9 662	14	1.4
Von Theobald *et al.*[82]	1 429	3	2.0
Peterson *et al.*[83]	36 928	96	2.6
Bruhat *et al.*[†]	7 604	21	2.8
Chapron *et al.*[2]	29 966	96	3.2
Jansen *et al.*[3]	25 764	84	3.3
Donnez and Nisolle*[§]	18 500	32	1.7

* Including cases in which the rectal perforation was closed by posterior colpotomy; [†]personal communication; [§]present series

procedure and to the experience of the surgeon. Intestinal or ureteral injuries represented more than 60% of complications requiring laparotomy and, in more than 50% of these cases, the diagnosis was delayed. Major vessel injury or bladder injury occurred more commonly with trocars. Bowel and ureteral injury occurrences were more frequently caused by surgical procedures, and complications with thermal energy represented about 40% of these cases. According to data now available, there are numerous possible complications directly related to surgical laparoscopy. However, major complications are relatively rare when there are no technical complications. The rate of complications of the surgical procedure itself does not seem to be higher than that occurring during surgery by laparotomy.

In conclusion, with thousands of gynecological operative laparoscopies and hysteroscopies having been performed around the world, it has been shown that both procedures are extremely safe and effective. However, the possibility of complications must be kept in mind. Understanding these complications and how to assess them is the only way to avoid them in the future. Gynecological surgeons are now dealing with a host of new instruments and devices. As well as knowledge of the anatomy, knowledge of the new instrumentation is recommended. For this purpose, the following are required:

(1) Didactic lectures on both laparoscopic and hysteroscopic procedures and their complications;

(2) Hands-on experience with live laboratory animals;

(3) Preceptorship with experienced operators, or special residency training.

Respecting these conditions will enhance endoscopic surgery results and minimize the rate of complications.

REFERENCES

1. Härkki-Siren P, Sjöberg J, Kurki T. Major complications of laparoscopy: a follow-up Finnish study. *Obstet Gynecol* 1999;94:94

2. Chapron C, Querleu D, Bruhat M-A, *et al.* Surgical complications of diagnostic and operative gynaecological laparoscopy: a series of 29 966 cases. *Hum Reprod* 1998;13:867

3. Jansen FW, Kapiteyn K, Trimbos-Kemper T, *et al.* Complications of laparoscopy: a prospective multicentre observational study. *Br J Obstet Gynaecol* 1997;104:595

4. Kalhan SB, Reaney JA. Pneumomediastinum and subcutaneous emphysema during laparoscopy. *Cleve Clin J Med* 1990;57:639

5. Vasquez JM, Demarque AM, Diamond MP. Vascular complications of laparoscopic surgery. *J Am Assoc Gynecol Laparosc* 1994;1:163

6. Murdock CM, Wolff AJ, Van Geem T. Risk factors for hypercapnia, subcutaneous emphysema, pneumothorax and pneumomediastinum during laparoscopy. *Obstet Gynecol* 2000;95:704–9

7. Hulka JF, Levy BS, Parker WH, *et al.* Laparoscopic-assisted vaginal hysterectomy: AAGL 1995 membership survey. *J Am Assoc Gynecol Laparosc* 1997;4:167

8. Lynn CS, Katz RA, Ross JP. Aortic perforation sustained at laparoscopy. *J Reprod Med* 1982;27:217

9. Rust M, Buquoy F, Bonke S. Retroperitoneale Gefässverletztung bei gynäkologischen Laparoskopien. *Anästh Intensivether Notfallmed* 1980;15:356

10. Heinrich P, Jahn R, Neumann A. Iatrogene Gefässchaden im Beckenbereich. *Zentralbl Gynäkol* 1985;107:432

11. Erkrath KD, Weiler G, Adebahr G. Zur Aortenverletzung bei Laparoskopie in der Gynäkolgie. *Geburtshilfe Frauenheilkd* 1979;39:687

12. Bisler H, Sinde J, Alemany J, *et al.* Verletzungen der grossen Gefässe bei gynäkologischen Laparoskopien. *Geburtshilfe Frauenheilkd* 1980;40:553

13. Leron E, Piura B, Ohana E, *et al.* Delayed recognition of major vascular injury during laparoscopy. *Eur J Obstet Gynecol Reprod Biol* 1998;79:91

14. Bergqvist D, Bergqvist A. Vascular injuries during gynecologic surgery. *Acta Obstet Gynecol Scand* 1987;66:19

15. Corson SL. Major vessel injury during laparoscopy. *Am J Obstet Gynecol* 1980;138:589

16. McDonald PT, Rich NM, Collins GJ, *et al.* Vascular trauma secondary to diagnostic and therapeutic procedures: laparoscopy. *Am J Surg* 1978;135:651

17. Shin CS. Vascular injury secondary to laparoscopy. *N Y State J Med* 1982;82:935

18. Oshinsky GS, Smith AD. Laparoscopic needles and trocars: an overview of designs and complications. *J Laparoendosc Surg* 1992;2:117

19. Ransom SB, McNeeley SG, White C, *et al.* A cost-effectiveness evaluation of laparoscopic disposable versus nondisposable infraumbilical cannulas. *J Am Assoc Gynecol Laparosc* 1996;4:25

20. Dingfelder JR. Direct laparoscope trocar insertion without prior pneumoperitoneum. *J Reprod Med* 1978;21:45

21. Saidi MH. Direct laparoscopy without prior pneumoperitoneum. *J Reprod Med* 1986;31:684

22. Copeland C, Wing R, Hulka JF. Direct trocar insertion at laparoscopy: an evaluation. *Obstet Gynecol* 1983;62:655

23. Borgatta L, Gruss L, Barad D, *et al.* Direct trocar insertion versus Verres needle use for laparoscopic sterilization. *J Reprod Med* 1990;35:891

24. Woolcott R. The safety of laparoscopy performed by direct trocar insertion and carbon dioxide insufflation under vision. *Aust NZ J Obstet Gynaecol* 1997;37:216

25. Nezhat FR, Silfen SL, Evans D, *et al.* Comparison of direct insertion of disposable and standard reusable laparoscopic trocars and previous pneumoperitoneum with Veress needle. *Obstet Gynecol* 1991;78:148

26. Loffer FD, Pent D. Indications, contraindications and complications of laparoscopy. *Obstet Gynecol Surg* 1975;30:407

27. Endler GC, Moghissi KS. Gastric perforation during pelvic laparoscopy. *Obstet Gynecol* 1976;47(Suppl):40S

28. Edgerton WD. Laparoscopy in the community hospital: safety, performance, control. *J Reprod Med* 1974;12:239

29. Hirt PS, Morris R. Gastric bleeding secondary to laparoscopy in a patient with salpingitis. *Obstet Gynecol* 1982;59:655

30. Chapron C, Pierre F, Harchaoui Y, *et al.* Gastrointestinal injuries during gynaecological laparoscopy. *Hum Reprod* 1999;14:333

31. Gautier G, Péchinot M, Galloux Y, *et al.* Eructation révélatrice d'une perforation gastrique accidentelle lors de la création du pneumopéritoine pour chirurgie laparoscopique. Rôle contributif de l'anestésiste. *Ann Fr Anesth Réanim* 2000;19:67

32. Birns MT. Inadvertent instrumental perforation of the colon during laparoscopy: nonsurgical repair. *Gastrointest Endosc* 1989;35:54

33. Levy BS, Soderstrom RM, Dail DH. Bowel injuries during laparoscopy, gross anatomy and histology. *J Reprod Med* 1985;30:168

34. El-Banna M, Abdel-Atty M, El-Meteini M, *et al.* Management of laparoscopic-related bowel injuries. *Surg Endosc* 2000;14:779

35. Krebs HB. Intestinal injury in gynecologic surgery: a ten year experience. *Obstet Gynecol* 1986;155:509

36. Hasson HM. Open laparoscopy: a report of 150 cases. *J Reprod Med* 1974;12:234–8

385

37. Soderstrom RM. Bowel injury litigation after laparoscopy. *J Am Assoc Gynecol Laparosc* 1993;1: 74–7

38. Howard FM, El Minawi AM, DeLoach VE. Direct laparoscopic cannula insertion at the left upper quadrant. *J Am Assoc Gynecol Laparosc* 1997;4:595

39. Corson SL, Batzer FR, Gocial B, *et al*. Measurement of the force necessary for laparoscopic trocar entry. *J Reprod Med* 1989;34:282

40. Evans MR, Hulbert CJ, Reddy KP. Complications of laparoscopy. *Semin Urol* 1992;10:164

41. Norestgaard A, Bodily K, Osborne R, *et al*. Major vascular injury during gynecologic laparoscopy. *Am J Surg* 1995;169:543

42. Chatzipapas IK, Magos AL. A simple technique of securing inferior epigastric vessels and repairing the rectus sheath at laparoscopic surgery. *Obstet Gynecol* 1997;90:304

43. Aharoni A, Condea A, Leibovitz Z, *et al*. A comparative study of Foley catheter and suturing to control trocar-induced abdominal wall haemorrhage. *Gynaecol Endosc* 1997;6:31

44. Marret H, Pierre F, Chapron C, *et al*. Complications de la coelioscopie occasionnées par les trocards. *J Gynecol Obstet Biol Reprod* 1997;26:405

45. Quint EH, Wang FL, Hurd WW. Laparoscopic transilumination for the location of anterior abdominal wall blood vessels. *J Laparoendosc Surg* 1996;6:167

46. Godfrey C, Wahle GR, Schilder JM, *et al*. Occult bladder injury during laparoscopy: report of two cases. *J Laparoendosc Adv Surg Tech A* 1999;9:341

47. De Cherney AH. Laparoscopy with unexpected viscus penetration. In Nichols DH, ed. *Clinical Problems, Injuries and Complications of Gynecologic Surgery*. Baltimore: Wiliams and Wilkins, 1988:63

48. Peters PC. Intraperitoneal rupture of the bladder. *Urol Clin N Am* 1989;16:279

49. Reich H, McGlynn F. Laparoscopic repair of bladder injury. *Obstet Gynecol* 1990;76:909

50. Corriere JN Jr, Sandler CM. Management of extraperitoneal bladder rupture. *Urol Clin N Am* 1989;16:275

51. Wheeles CR. Thermal gastrointestinal injuries. In Philips JM, ed. *Laparoscopy*. Baltimore: Williams and Wilkins, 1977:231–5

52. Hulka JF, Peterson HB, Phillips JM, *et al*. Operative laparoscopy: AAGL 1991 membership survey. *J Reprod Med* 1991;28:569

53. Martin DC. Tissue effects of lasers. *Sem Reprod Endocrinol* 1991;9:127

54. Querleu D, Chevallier L, Chapron C, *et al*. Complications of gynaecological endoscopic surgery. A French multicenter collaborative study. *Gynaecol Endosc* 1993;2:3

55. Soderstrom RM. Bowel injury litigation after laparoscopy. *J Am Assoc Gynecol Laparosc* 1993;1:74

56. Renault B, Elhage A, Querleu D. Bowel complications in gynecologic laparoscopic surgery and their immediate repair without laparotomy. Four cases. *J Gynecol Obstet Biol Reprod* 1996;25:360

57. Donnez J. Instrumentation and operational instructions. In Donnez J, ed. *Laser Operative Laparoscopy and Hysteroscopy*. Leuven: Nauwelaerts Printing, 1989:15

58. Seiler JC, Gidwana G, Ballard L. Laparoscopic cauterization of endometriosis for fertility. A controlled study. *Fertil Steril* 1986;46:1098

59. Tulikangas PK, Golberg JM, Gill IS. Laparoscopic repair of ureteral transection. *J Am Assoc Gynecol Laparosc* 2000;7:415

60. Donnez J, Bassil S, Smets M, *et al*. LASH: laparoscopic supracervical (subtotal) hysterectomy. In Cusumano P, Deprest J, eds. *Advanced Gynecologic Laparoscopy*. Carnforth, UK: Parthenon Publishing Group, 1996:79

61. Nezhat C, Nezhat FR. Safe laser endoscopic excision or vaporisation of peritoneal endometriosis. *Fertil Steril* 1989;52:149

62. Bauman H, Jaeger P, Huch A. Ureteral injury after laparoscopic tubal sterilization by bipolar electro-coagulation. *Obstet Gynecol* 1988;71:483

63. Grainger DA, Soderstrom RM, Schiff SF, *et al*. Ureteral injuries at laparoscopy: insights into diagnosis, management and prevention. *Obstet Gynecol* 1990;75:839

64. Schwimmer WB. Electrosurgical burn injuries during laparoscopy sterilization. Treatment and prevention. *Obstet Gynecol* 1974;44:526

65. Jaffe RH, Willis D, Bachem A. The effect of electric currents on the arteries. A histologic study. *Arch Pathol* 1929;7:244

66. Irvin TT, Goligher LC, Scott JS. Injury to the ureter during laparoscopic tubal sterilization. *Arch Surg* 1975;110:1501

67. Levinson CJ, Schwartz SF, Saltzstein EC. Complication of laparoscopic tubal sterilization: small bowel perforation. *Obstet Gynecol* 1973;41:253

68. Corson SL, Bolognese RJ. Electrosurgical hazards in laparoscopy. *J Am Med Assoc* 1974;927:1261

69. Servais D, Althoff H. Fatal carbon dioxide embolism as a complication of endoscopic intervention. *Chirurg* 1998;69:773

70. Wadhwa RK, McKenzie R, Wadhwa SR, *et al*. Gas embolism during laparoscopy. *Anesthesiology* 1978;48:74–6

71. Yacoub OF, Cardona I, Coveler LA, *et al*. Carbon dioxide embolism during laparoscopy. *Anesthesiology* 1982;57:533–5

72. Chatman DL. Incarcerated tubal herniation, an unusual complication of operative laparoscopy and an odd cause of pelvic pain. *J Am Assoc Gynecol Laparosc* 2000;7:159–60

73. Montz FJ, Holschneider CH, Munro MG. Incisional hernia following laparoscopy: a survey of the American Association of Gynecologic Laparoscopists. *Obstet Gynecol* 1994;84:881–4

74. Kadar N, Reich H, Liu CY, *et al*. Incisional hernias after major laparoscopic gynecologic procedures. *Am J Obstet Gynecol* 1993;168:1493–5

75. Nezhat C, Nezhat F, Seidman DS, *et al*. Incisional hernias after operative laparoscopy. *J Laparoendosc Adv Surg Tech A* 1997;7:111–15

76. Leung TY, Yuen PM. Small bowel herniation through subumbilical port site following laparoscopic surgery at the time of reversal of anethesia. *Gynecol Obstet Invest* 2000;49:209–10

77. Goldrath MH, Phillips E. A method of closing laparoscopy port incisions using a modified Verres Needle. *J Am Assoc Gynecol Laparosc* 1996;3:287–90

78. Stringer NH, Levy ES, Kezmoh MP, *et al*. New closure technique for laterale operative laparoscopic trocar sites. A report of 80 closures. *Surg Endosc* 1995;9:838–40

79. Childers JM, Caplinger P. Spontaneous pneumothorax during operative laparoscopy secondary to congenital diaphragmatic defects. A case report. *J Reprod Med* 1995;40:151–3

80. Chang MY, Shiau CS, Chang CL, *et al*. Spleen laceration, a rare complication of laparoscopy. *J Am Assoc Gynecol Laparosc* 2000;7:269–72

81. Henry-Suchet J, Tort-Grumbach J, Loysel F. Complications des coelioscopies colligées par le Club Gynéco-informatique en 1980–1982. *Contr Fertil Sex* 1984;12:901

82. Von Theobald P, Marie G, Herlicoviez M, *et al*. Morbidité et mortalité de la coelioscopie: étude rétrospective d'une série de 1429 cas. *Rev Fr Gynecol Obstet* 1990;85:611

83. Peterson HB, Hulka JF, Phillips JM. American Association of Gynecologic Laparoscopists 1988: Membership survey on operative laparoscopy. *J Reprod Med* 1990;35:587

SECTION II
Operative hysteroscopy

37

Instrumentation for hysteroscopy

J. Donnez and M. Nisolle

Carbon dioxide is used as a gas medium. It is a product of the endogenous respiratory chain, has very good optical qualities and has no influence on the course of the illness in the case of inflammatory or malignant processes. Lindemann reports on a multicenter study with 185 000 CO_2 hysteroscopies with no serious complications. In order to be able to guarantee this safety rate, however, great care must be taken to restrict the flow rate to < 100 ml/min. In rare case reports on CO_2 embolisms, it could not be clearly explained in retrospect whether it had really been a CO_2 embolism or, rather, another phenomenon, such as an air embolism (see also Chapter 50). No CO_2 embolisms have been reported up to the time of writing in non-anesthetized patients. A special hysteroflator must be used for the application of CO_2. It works with a maximum rate of 100 ml/min. When the preselected pressure has been reached, any further gas inflow automatically ceases. Using a laparoflator for a hysteroscopy is strictly forbidden because it permits far higher flow rates and, thus, within a very short space of time a lethal CO_2 embolism could occur.

DISTENSION MEDIUM

Either a liquid or gas medium can be used to distend the uterine cavity. In the case of liquid media, there is a distinction between aqueous solutions, such as 5% glucose solution, physiological saline solution, or Ringer (lactate) solution, and solutions with low viscosity, such as sorbitol/mannitol solution (Purisole) or 1.5% glycine solution (glycocol), and solutions with high viscosity such as 32% dextran (Hyskon®). Sorbitol/mannitol and glycine solutions are only used in surgical hysteroscopy, as they are electrolyte-free. Hyskon was used for a while, especially in the United States, but should now no longer be used for hysteroscopy due to its high-risk profile. Liquids create different optical conditions, due to their refractive index, which is different from that of air. Aqueous solutions become murky quicker than a viscous solution, through being mixed with blood and mucus. This, however, does not pose a problem, provided that irrigation (through the cervix, the Fallopian tube or with a continuous flow system) is possible.

An aqueous isotonic solution, such as 0.9% saline or Ringer solution, is used for outpatient diagnostic hysteroscopy. An ordinary manually operated pressure cuff is pumped up to 80–120 mmHg and supplies the pressure for distending the cavity.

SET OF INSTRUMENTS FOR OPERATIVE HYSTEROSCOPY

In contrast to the diagnostic hysteroscopy, which can be performed in general practice, surgical hysteroscopy is restricted to the operating room. The operation may be performed under general anesthetic or local/regional anesthesia, on an outpatient basis, or with a short stay in hospital. We subdivide surgical hysteroscopies into mechanical, laser and electrosurgical procedures, depending on the energy mode, each of these requiring an appropriate set of instruments.

Mechanical procedures

In this surgical technique, we use a hysteroscopic sheath which is slid over the telescope. Through this sheath, small, rigid, semi-rigid, or flexible instruments can be used, as well as the distension medium.

Equipment includes: grasping forceps to remove polyps after the resection (Figure 1); scissors for dissecting septum, adhesions, or the base of the polyps; and biopsy forceps for optically controlled biopsy collection.

The traditional rigid diagnostic hysteroscope consists of a 30°-telescope (Figure 2) with 4-mm diameter, integrated fiberoptic light transmission and an outer sheath for distension medium inflow.

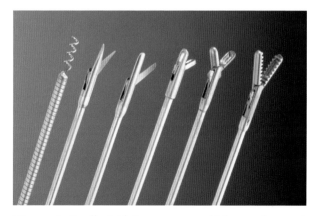

Figure 1 Small rigid instruments which can be used through a hysteroscopic sheath

Modern miniature hysteroscopes have a 25°- or 30°-telescope with 2.7–3-mm diameter, integrated fiberoptic light transmission and a sheath diameter between 3.5 and 4 mm (Figure 3). This allows direct access to the uterine cavity in almost all cases and is associated with significantly fewer complaints in comparison with 5-mm instruments. The field of view and brightness are reduced in these hysteroscopes, due to the smaller diameter of the telescope, and this can cause occasional difficulties in a large, bleeding uterine cavity.

Some manufacturers offer hysteroscopes which allow the optional use of an additional inner sheath that is inserted into the outer sheath (Figure 4). By assembling both sheaths, it is possible to create a continuous flow system which can be used for controlled irrigation of the uterine cavity (Figures 5 and 6). The entire outer diameter can then be extended to 4.5–5 mm.

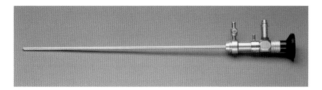

Figure 2 Rigid hysteroscope (telescope and sheath)

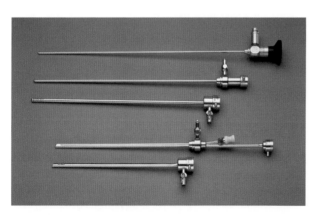

Figure 3 Karl Storz hysteroscope, Bettocchi type with rod lens telescope (diameter 2.9 mm), single-flow sheath (diameter 3.7 mm) and an optional assembly of a continuous flow system through use of the 5-mm outer sheath

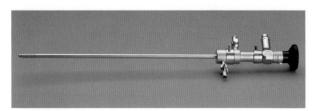

Figure 4 Karl Storz hysteroscope, Bettocchi type: continuous flow hysteroscope, outer diameter 5 mm

Resectoscope (Figures 7 and 8)

The resectoscope is an instrument borrowed from urology, where it has been used for transurethral prostate resection and the removal of biopsy specimens from the bladder wall. It has a 0°-, 12°- or 30°-rod lens telescope with integrated fiberoptic light transmission.

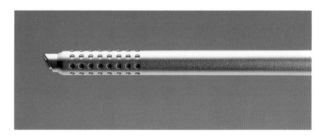

Figure 5 Karl Storz hysteroscope, Bettocchi type: close-up with 3.7-mm and 5-mm outer sheath system

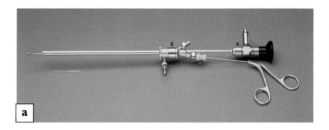

a

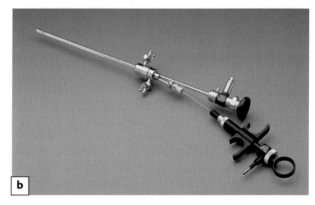

b

Figure 6 (a) and (b) Instruments, telescope and sheath

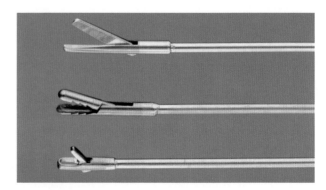

Figure 7 Close-up view of the instrument tips

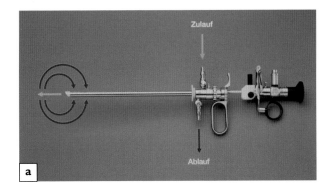

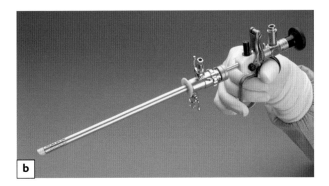

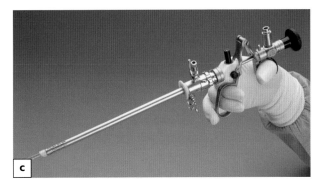

Figure 8 (a) – (c) Hysteroscopy and resection: the resectoscope is an instrument borrowed from urology

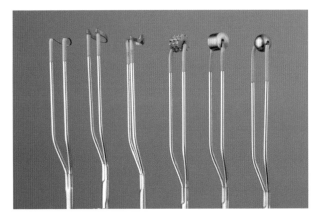

Figure 9 Different working elements from the resectoscope: from left to right, resection loop 90°; resection loop 45°; rollerball; dissection needle; vaporization electrode; rollerball

Working elements (Figure 9)

Various elements, such as resection loops, rollerballs, roller cylinders, dissection needles and vaporization electrodes, are available as working elements. The loop is used in myoma, polyp and endometrial resections. Rollerballs and roller cylinders are applied during endometrial destruction by means of coagulation technology. The vaporization electrode is generally an oblong electrode with three or four relatively small recesses, equally distanced. It is operated with a very high-performance cutting current.

High-frequency generator

The resectoscope is operated with monopolar current, supplied from a standard surgical high-frequency generator. There is an option of electrosurgical cutting and coagulation. In order to avoid thermal damage of adjacent organs, the lowest necessary power setting is recommended. The use of modern high-frequency generators, with automatic voltage control, seems favorable.

38

Hysterosonography

J. Squifflet, W. Abdul-Nour, M. Nisolle and J. Donnez

INTRODUCTION

Hysterosonography is a technique first described in 1988 by Deichert and colleagues[1]; it uses saline solution as contrast medium for evaluation of the uterine cavity during transvaginal ultrasonography. Before performing this examination, the patient must be asked about her gynecological history, number of pregnancies, previous history of pelvic inflammatory disease, sexually transmitted diseases, pelvic surgery, Cesarean section, etc. A classic gynecological examination has to be performed first with a Papanicolaou smear and vaginal examination to evaluate the size of the uterus and the inclination of the axis of the uterus, to determine whether there is anteversion or retroversion. A colposcopy with cervix visualization serves to predict and to estimate the feasibility of the examination and the catheter size that will be necessary.

Transvaginal ultrasonographic examination is then performed in which the size of the uterus is measured, as well as the thickness of the endometrium; the adnexa are checked to exclude pathologies such as hydrosalpinx or, even worse, suspicion of adnexal neoplasia.

Most echographists experience some difficulty in evaluating the endometrium in obese patients, in whom the endometrium is along the same axis as the vaginal probe, or who have increased thickness of the endometrial mucosa just before the menses. All of these conditions make the detection and correct diagnosis of uterine pathology difficult in terms of screening for or excluding certain pathologies.

TECHNIQUE

Saline infusion sonohysterography (SIS) is performed via a catheter placed inside the cervical os (female catheter CH10 or CH12, manufactured by Maersk Medical a/s DK 3390) (Figure 1).

A speculum is placed, disinfection performed, and the cervix may be secured by grasping the anterior lip with a Pozzi tenaculum (one-tooth tenaculum forceps). Traction is applied to align the cervical canal and uterine cavity, or to introduce the catheter more easily in case of cervical stenosis.

A catheter fixed onto a fully sterile saline solution syringe is introduced through the cervical canal. It is important to avoid and remove any bubbles in the syringe before introducing it because they could produce some echogenic disturbances. The Pozzi forceps are removed. A

transvaginal ultrasound probe is introduced after speculum removal. The uterus is surveyed in the sagittal and transverse planes. An adequate SIS visualizes all parts of the uterus from the cervix to the uterine fundus (Figure 2). Usually, only a few milliliters of saline solution are needed to evaluate the uterine cavity. In case of cervical fluid reflux, different-sized catheters may be used, or a Foley catheter could be placed in the cervical canal. All of these catheters are cheap and there is no need to use more expensive devices to achieve a good evaluation with this technique.

This examination does not require expensive material as required in outpatient hysteroscopy. Pain rating also shows that this examination is less uncomfortable than hysterosalpingography and hysteroscopy. Irradiation is not used. In case of suspicion of uterine pathology, for example when one is not sure if the small echogenic structure observed is a blood clot or otherwise, the same investigation may be proposed some days later. This technique could be a useful follow-up for patients who are at high risk of intrauterine pathologies. Good visualization of the intramural part of myomas may be achieved to evaluate the correct size of this pathology, and, if uterine submucosal fibroids are to be removed hysteroscopically, one could correctly evaluate the thickness of the myometrium behind the fibroids (myometrium security between fibroids and the serosa). The correct differential diagnosis between a polyp and a fibroid may sometimes be difficult but the use of Doppler ultrasound could give a better diagnosis. The Doppler view shows vascular flux in the

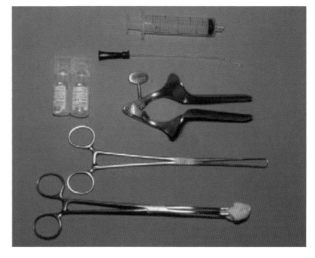

Figure 1 Equipment

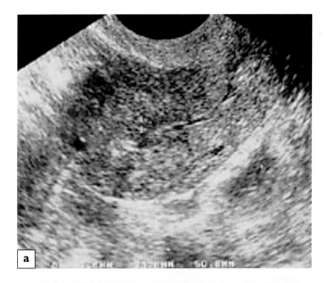

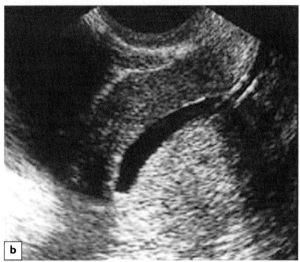

Figure 2 (a) Transvaginal sonography provides a sagittal view of the uterus; (b) with saline infusion sonohysterography, after saline infusion, the endometrium appears normal, without pathology

pellicles of polyps, while fibroids usually have a pedicle that is more heterogeneous and with peripheral vascularity.

Certain problems could occur, however. Sometimes, SIS may be impossible to perform because of cervical stenosis, but, in experienced hands, this technique has been carried out in more than 98% of women. In most cases, it takes no longer than 3–5 min.

There have been no reported cases of infection, although, in our series, one woman developed pelvic inflammatory disease after SIS; however, she had undergone hysterosalpingography some days earlier. We do not prescribe antibiotics routinely. In case of suspected pelvic inflammatory disease or hydrosalpinx, hysterosonography is not performed.

The possibility has been questioned of retrograde seeding of adenocarcinoma cells in cases of intrauterine

neoplasia. Alcazar and colleagues[2] observed one case out of 14 in which malignant cells were present in the spilled fluid after SIS in a case of endometrial carcinoma. This observation has already been previously reported after diagnostic D & C or after hysterosalpingography and does not appear to have any worse impact on the prognosis (in this pathology) of the neoplasia. In the case of cervical incompetence, such as reflux, a Foley catheter could be used.

Indications

Saline infusion sonohysterography is indicated in the following situations:

(1) Infertility investigation of uterine malformations, submucosal fibroids, polyps or synechiae;

(2) Menorrhagia unsuccessfully treated with medication (Figures 3–5);

(3) Metrorrhagia (Figure 6);

(4) Follow-up of endometrial tissue at high risk of neoplasia, such as in patients with high blood pressure or diabetes, tamoxifen-treated patients or the obese (Figure 7);

(5) Endometrial thickness > 5 mm in menopausal women (Figure 8);

(6) Poor imaging quality arising from the aspect axis or echogenicity of the endometrium.

Transvaginal sonography can be an accurate diagnostic tool in evaluating women with abnormal vaginal bleeding. Endometrial thickness can be measured and the ovulatory and hormonal status observed. Transvaginal sonography can detect endometrial thickening and heterogenicity and suggest possible masses; however, it is not as useful in determining the exact location of the masses. Saline infusion sonohysterography could enhance visualization of the endometrial lining and possible intracavitary masses.

Contraindications

Saline infusion sonohysterography should not be used in women with:

(1) Pelvic inflammatory disease;

(2) Positive pregnancy test;

(3) Suspect endometrial neoplasia.

RESULTS

Sonohysterography is a highly sensitive, specific and accurate screening procedure for evaluation of the uterine cavity in abnormal uterine bleeding (menorrhagia or metrorrhagia). Chittacharoen and colleagues[3] have observed a specificity of 83%, a sensitivity of 97%, a positive predictive value of 97%, and a negative predictive value of 83% in a study in which SIS was compared with pathological findings in 52 women (mean age 41 years, range 29–58 years). Adenocarcinomas were excluded and SIS correctly diagnosed two-thirds of the cases of endometrial hyperplasia. Clevenger-Hoeft and co-workers[4] observed that premenopausal women with abnormal bleeding had a higher prevalence of polyps (43%), intracavitary myomas (21%) and intramural myomas (58%) than premenopausal women without abnormal bleeding (respectively, 10, 1 and 13%). It is necessary that uterine pathologies are diagnosed and, therefore, if a patient presents with abnormal bleeding, she must undergo the most thorough investigation in order to treat her correctly. We suggest that women with multifocal or sessile lesions should undergo a guided biopsy procedure (hysteroscopy) and that polyps of benign appearance should also be removed to control bleeding and eliminate the risk of intraepithelial neoplasia, especially in older women.

In 1998, Schwarzler and colleagues[5] evaluated the use of transvaginal sonography, sonohysterography and diagnostic hysteroscopy for the preparatory assessment of the uterine cavity. The endpoints were uterine abnormalities detected by operative hysteroscopy and histology. More than 100 patients with abnormal uterine bleeding were recruited. Uterine abnormalities were present in 53% of cases. The overall sensitivity of transvaginal sonography improved after sonohysterography (from 67 to 87%) and the specificity from 89 to 91%. The positive predictive value increased from 88 to 92% and the negative predictive value from 71 to 86%. The use of SIS also improved the quality of information about the localization and size of polyps and submucosal fibroids.

The use of saline infusion to enhance visualization of the endometrium increased the diagnostic accuracy of transvaginal sonography, and also provided some additional information. Thus, SIS is a simple, non-invasive and effective tool which may be used in the evaluation of patients, instead of diagnostic hysteroscopy.

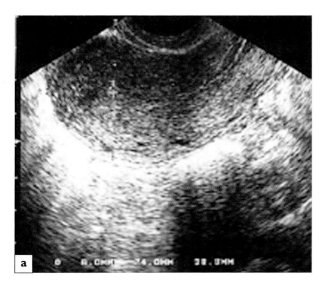

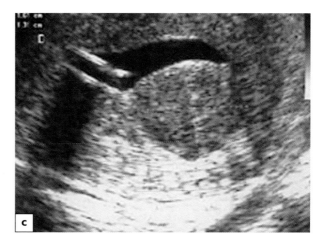

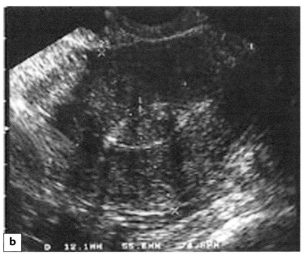

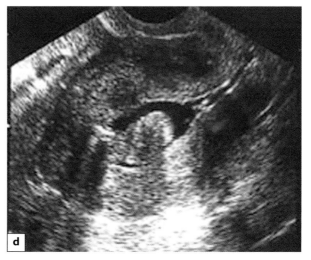

Figure 3 A 40-year-old patient with menorrhagia. Transvaginal sonography shows (a) sagittal view of the endometrium of 6-mm thickness; and (b) endometrial thickness with a small focus at 12 mm; (c) and (d) saline infusion sonohysterography gives visualization of a polyp

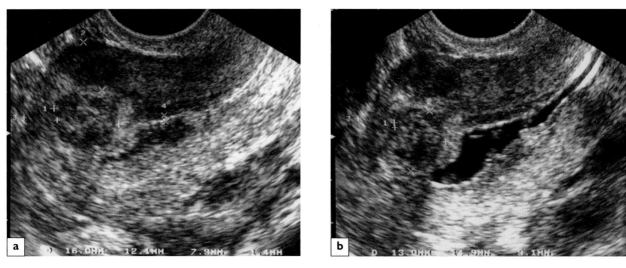

Figure 4 A 40-year-old patient with menorrhagia. (a) Transvaginal sonography, sagittal view, shows a normal endometrium and an intramural myoma of 16 mm; (b) the deformation of the endometrium by the myoma is visualized with saline infusion sonohysterography. Saline infusion sonohysterography shows that a part of the myoma is submucosal and could be removed by hysteroscopy

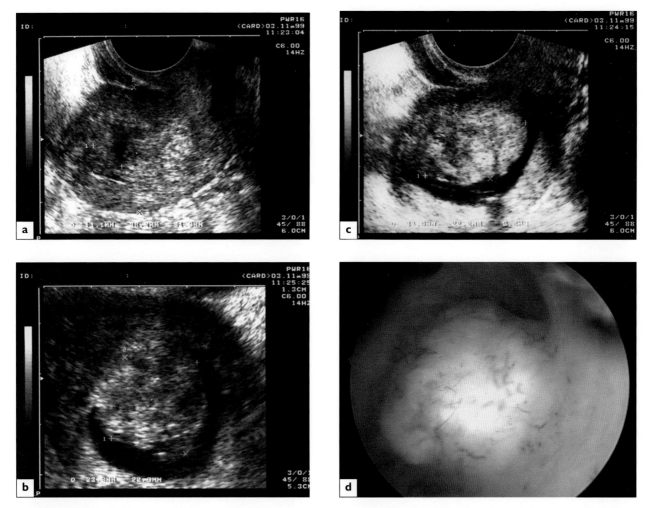

Figure 5 A 40-year-old patient with menorrhagia. (a) Transvaginal sonography, sagittal view, shows the normal uterine size, and suspicion of a mass effect inside the uterus with irregular limits; (b) and (c) saline infusion sonohysterography provides visualization of a pure submucosal myoma of 22 × 22 mm; (d) hysteroscopic view (note atrophic endometrium due to GnRH agonist treatment)

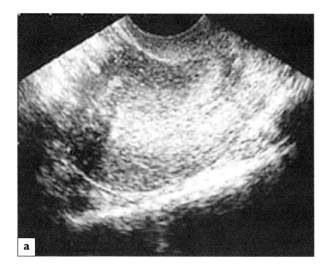

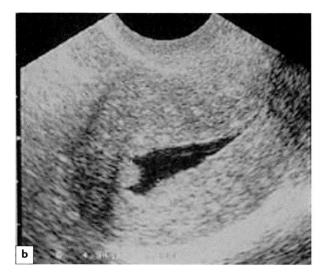

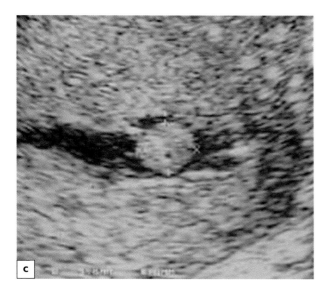

Figure 6 A 45-year-old patient with metrorrhagia. (a) Transvaginal sonography shows a normal appearance and thickness of the endometrium; (b) and (c) saline infusion sonohysterography provides visualization of a small fundal polyp

INFERTILITY AND *IN VITRO* FERTILIZATION

Soares and co-workers[6] evaluated the diagnostic accuracy of sonohysterography in uterine cavity diseases in infertile patients. Each patient underwent SIS, conventional transvaginal sonography, hysterosalpingography and hysteroscopy.

Sonohysterography was, in general, the most accurate test. Its diagnostic accuracy was markedly superior for polypoid lesions and endometrial hyperplasia, and in total agreement with the gold standard. In the diagnosis of intrauterine adhesions, SIS had limited accuracy, with a high false-negative diagnostic rate.

Gronlund and colleagues[7] confirmed that sonohysterography is a simple, fast, well-tolerated and accurate method of investigating the uterine cavity in patients with metrorrhagia or infertility. However, we believe that, before any attempt at *in vitro* fertilization (IVF) is made, an outpatient hysteroscopy should be performed because, in our opinion, hysteroscopy remains the gold standard.

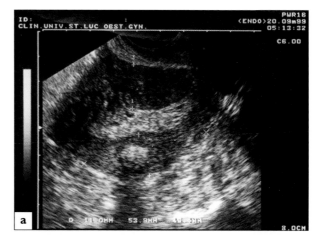

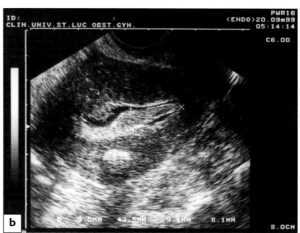

Figure 7 A 60-year-old patient taking tamoxifen. (a) Transvaginal sonography: endometrial thickness of 11 mm; (b) saline infusion sonohysterography shows two polyps, anterior 8 mm and posterior 9 × 20 mm (note atrophic endometrium)

399

Hysterosalpingography is an alternative to hysteroscopy in some units but involves ionizing radiation and referral to a radiology department. However, 10–35% of women with a normal cavity at hysterosalpingography have abnormal hysteroscopic findings. Magnetic resonance imaging is accurate in the diagnosis of congenital uterine abnormalities, but its disadvantages include its high cost and limited availability.

In the study by Ayida and colleagues[8], which compared SIS to office hysteroscopy, SIS had an 87.5% sensitivity and 100% specificity (SIS was less able to discover uterine adhesions and small endometrial pathologies). Due to the high cost, and, in some countries, the limited accessibility of IVF, it may be better, from the cost/benefit point of view, to propose hysteroscopy before an IVF attempt.

PERIMENOPAUSAL BLEEDING OR SCREENING

Cohen and colleagues[9] proposed carrying out sonohysterography to detect intrauterine pathology before initiating hormone replacement therapy, because an endometrial thickness of less than or equal to 5 mm, measured by transvaginal sonography, excludes hyperplasia but does not eliminate other intrauterine pathologies that may be discovered by sonohysterography.

POSTMENOPAUSAL BLEEDING

The endometrium in patients who are receiving hormone replacement therapy undergoes sequential changes, and cyclic bleeding occurs that is similar to the cyclic bleeding of the premenopausal endometrium. However, if other cyclic bleeding occurs, evaluation for hyperplasia, polyps or carcinoma must be performed (Figure 8).

For abnormal postmenopausal bleeding, O'Connell and co-workers[10] proposed sonohysterography combined with endometrial biopsy. The combination of these reliable office tools correlated positively with the surgical findings (> 95% of the time), with a sensitivity and specificity of 94% and 96%, respectively. More than 100 patients were enrolled and SIS and endometrial biopsies were compared with fractional curettage with hysteroscopy. The conclusions were that SIS plus endometrial biopsy had a high specificity and predictive value and that SIS increased the sensitivity for detection of intraluminal masses and was superior to routine vaginal probes in diagnosing intrauterine lesions in patients with postmenopausal bleeding.

However, Twu and Chen[11] studied women aged 50 years or over who presented with postmenopausal bleeding and underwent either D & C or endometrial biopsy. They followed all the patients who experienced 77 cases of recurrent postmenopausal bleeding in the following 5 years, and in whom an initial diagnosis of benign tissue was

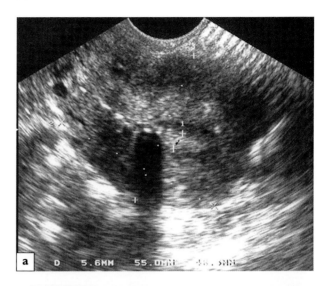

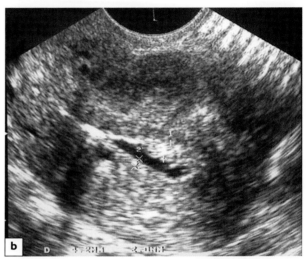

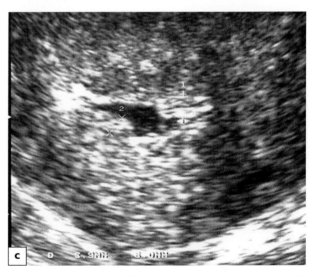

Figure 8 A 55-year-old patient with metrorrhagia. (a) Transvaginal sonography shows normal uterine size, and an endometrial thickness of maximum 5 mm but irregular; (b) and (c) saline infusion sonohysterography reveals irregular endometrium and pathological findings of adenocarcinoma

made. After another D & C or endometrial biopsy, more than 20% of the patients were found to have endometrial cancer or complex endometrial hyperplasia. Patients aged over 65 years had a higher risk than others. For this reason, in order to have the most accurate test to exclude endometrial pathology in patients with postmenopausal bleeding, we always propose hysteroscopy with biopsy. If this examination is normal, transvaginal sonography may be proposed to exclude benign tumors or ovarian cancer.

MONITORING ASYMPTOMATIC POSTMENOPAUSAL BREAST CANCER PATIENTS TAKING TAMOXIFEN

In asymptomatic postmenopausal patients with breast cancer who are taking tamoxifen, endometrial thickness is evaluated by transvaginal ultrasonography (Figure 7). If the thickness is more than 7–8 mm or irregular, or there is some doubt as to the measurement, then SIS is performed at the same time (Figure 9). In the case of intracavitary pathology, office hysteroscopy with biopsy is proposed to confirm the pathology or, in the case of neoplasia, to evaluate the spread of the disease (whether the spread is to less than or more than half the uterine cavity or there is cervi-

cal invasion). If the intracavitary pathology seems to be benign, a hysteroscopic resection of the endometrial pathology is carried out under general or epidural anesthesia. In cases of neoplasia, a hysterectomy with bilateral salpingo-ovariectomy is carried out.

SUMMARY

Sonohysterography is superior to unenhanced transvaginal sonography[12,13]. SIS is recommended as a minimally invasive tool in the assessment of endometrial changes in asymptomatic, postmenopausal breast cancer patients on long-term tamoxifen therapy with a thickened endometrium or inadequately visualized endometrial echo on transvaginal sonography. In cases of metrorrhagia, we always prefer to perform office hysteroscopy with biopsy. There is a place for screening and follow-up of endometrial pathology in patients taking tamoxifen if they have other risk factors, such as high blood pressure, obesity, diabetes or previous history of endometrial pathology before taking tamoxifen[14].

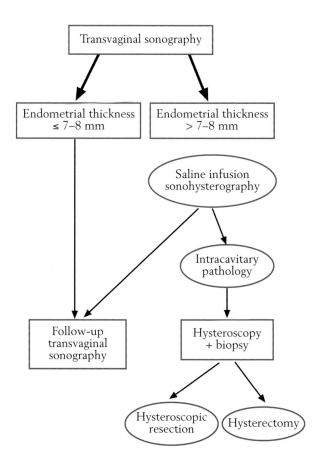

Figure 9 Evaluation of postmenopausal patients treated with tamoxifen

REFERENCES

1. Deichert U, van de Sandt M, Lauth G, et al. Transvaginal contrast hysterosonography. A new diagnostic procedure for the differentiation of intrauterine and myometrial findings. *Geburtshilfe Frauenheilkd* 1988;48:835–44

2. Alcazar JL, Errasti T, Zornoza A. Saline infusion sonohysterography in endometrial cancer: assessment of malignant cells dissemination risk. *Acta Obstet Gynecol Scand* 2000;79:321–2

3. Chittacharoen A, Theppisai U, Linasmita V, et al. Sonohysterography in the diagnosis of abnormal uterine bleeding. *J Obstet Gynecol Res* 2000;26:277–81

4. Clevenger-Hoeft M, Syrop CH, Stovall DW, et al. Sonohysterography in premenopausal women with and without abnormal bleeding. *Obstet Gynecol* 1999;94:516–20

5. Schwarzler P, Concin H, Bosch H, et al. An evaluation of sonohysterography and diagnostic hysteroscopy for the assessment of intrauterine pathology. *Ultrasound Obstet Gynecol* 1998;11: 337–42

6. Soares SR, Barbosa dos Reis MM, Camargos AF. Diagnostic accuracy of sonohysterography, transvaginal sonography, and hysterosalpingography in patients with uterine cavity diseases. *Fertil Steril* 2000;73:406–11

7. Gronlund L, Hertz J, Helm P, et al. Transvaginal sonohysterography and hysteroscopy in the evaluation of female infertility, habitual abortion or metr-

orrhagia. A comparative study. *Acta Obstet Gynecol Scand* 1999;78:415–18

8. Ayida G, Chamberlain P, Barlow D, *et al.* Uterine cavity assessment prior to *in vitro* fertilization: comparison of transvaginal scanning, saline contrast hysterosonography and hysteroscopy. *Ultrasound Obstet Gynecol* 1997;10:59–62

9. Cohen MA, Sauer MV, Keltz M, *et al.* Utilizing routine sonohysterography to detect intrauterine pathology before initiating hormone replacement therapy. *Menopause* 1999;6:68–70

10. O'Connell LP, Fries MH, Zeringue E, *et al.* Triage of abnormal postmenopausal bleeding: a comparison of endometrial biopsy and transvaginal sonohysterography versus fractional curettage with hysteroscopy. *Am J Obstet Gynecol* 1998;178:956–61

11. Twu NF, Chen SS. Five-year follow-up of patients with recurrent postmenopausal bleeding. *Chung Hua I Hsueh Tsa Chih (Taipei)* 2000;63:628–33

12. Elhelw B, Ghorab MN, Farrag SH. Saline sonohysterography for monitoring asymptomatic postmenopausal breast cancer patients taking tamoxifen. *Int J Gynecol Obstet* 1999;67:81–6

13. Cohen I, Beyth Y, Tepper R. The role of ultrasound in the detection of endometrial pathologies in asymptomatic postmenopausal breast cancer patients with tamoxifen treatment. *Obstet Gynecol* 1998;53:429–38

14. Berlière M, Smets M, Galant C, *et al.* Identifying risk factors for the development of atypical endometrial lesions while on tamoxifen is easier than understanding oncogenic mechanisms. *Am J Obstet Gynecol* 2001;in press

Hysteroscopy in the diagnosis of specific disorders

39

J. Donnez, M. Nisolle, M. Smets and J. Squifflet

A wide variety of conditions can be diagnosed hysteroscopically, and hysteroscopy has become a diagnostic gold standard against which other methods are assessed. Conditions amenable to hysteroscopic diagnosis include abnormal uterine bleeding, infertility and recurrent abortion, uterine and cervical cancer, location of intrauterine devices, complicated abortion and fetal examination. Physiological studies are also possible.

INFERTILITY

Hysteroscopy is becoming an important tool in the evaluation of infertility in women[1]. Evaluation of the endometrial cavity by either hysterosalpingography or hysteroscopy should be performed early. Hysteroscopic abnormalities are common in infertile patients; intrauterine abnormalities have been detected in 19–62% of infertile women in some studies[2]. Abnormal findings include intrauterine synechiae, Müllerian fusion defects (arcuate, septate or bicornuate uterus), endometrial polyps and submucous myomas.

Müllerian anomalies

Müllerian anomalies may be associated with normal fertility, infertility or recurrent abortion. The extent of the anomaly can range from complete agenesis of the Müllerian system to minimal deformities of the uterine form. Diagnosis usually requires combined hysteroscopy and laparoscopy. The presence of a uterine filling defect at hysterosalpingography or at hysteroscopy should be further evaluated by laparoscopy. The defect may represent a uterine septum (Figure 1), a bicornuate uterus or a submucous myoma. Rudimentary uterine horns, another form of Müllerian anomaly, can be detected laparoscopically and their relationship with the main cavity evaluated hysteroscopically.

Intrauterine synechiae

Traumatic intrauterine adhesions (Asherman's syndrome) (Figure 2) usually result from manipulation of the endometrial cavity following pregnancy. Curettage performed postpartum or following an abortion may cause scarring and synechiae secondary to the destruction of the basal layer of the endometrium. Patients may present with hypomenorrhea, amenorrhea, infertility or spontaneous pregnancy loss. Recurrent abortion and abnormalities of

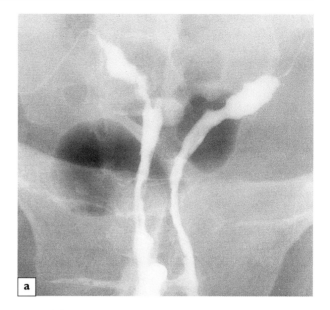

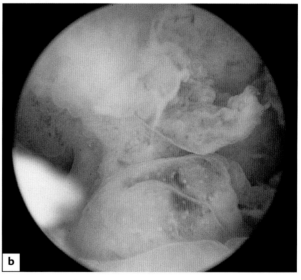

Figure 1 Müllerian anomalies: (a) hysterography reveals the presence of a complete uterine septum. Note the presence of fistula between the two cervical canals and of endometrial polyps; (b) hysteroscopy confirms the diagnosis of both septum and polyps

implantation and placental development have also been described in association with this condition.

Intrauterine synechiae can be diagnosed by hysterosalpingography or hysteroscopy. The hysterosalpingogram shows a small, fragmented and distorted uterine cavity. The hysteroscopic image consists of pale endometrial patches

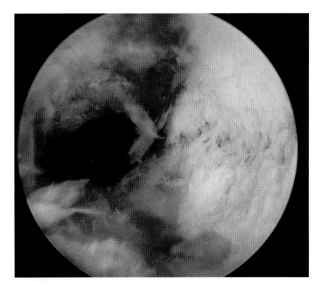

Figure 2 Intrauterine adhesions

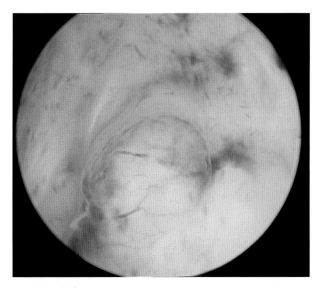

Figure 3 Submucous myoma

and fibrotic strands, crossing the endometrial cavity. The adhesions are paler than the surrounding endometrium.

A hysteroscopic diagnosis of intrauterine adhesions is essential, as the disease can be missed or mistakenly diagnosed by hysterosalpingography. Hysteroscopy also permits a better assessment of the extent of the adhesions, an important factor in determining therapy and prognosis.

Submucous myomas

Uterine myomas can be found in a variety of locations. Those protruding into the uterine lumen are a common cause of abnormal uterine bleeding and may lead to infertility. Submucous myomas cause infertility by a variety of mechanisms related to embryo implantation. They can also cause preterm or dysfunctional labor. Submucous myomas are suspected in patients with enlarged uteri and those in whom filling defects are detected by hysterosalpingography. The hysterosalpingographic suspicion of the lesions should be confirmed by hysteroscopy. At hysteroscopy, the tumor is seen to protrude into the uterine cavity (Figure 3) and is covered with pale endometrium. Submucous myomas can be distinguished from endometrial polyps. In addition to providing definitive diagnosis, hysteroscopy can reveal more accurately the localization of the tumor and permit a better assessment of its size. The degree of intramural involvement cannot be determined.

Tubal disease

Involvement and occlusion of the intramural portion of the Fallopian tubes may be detected hysteroscopically. The significance of these lesions and their relationship to infertility has not been clearly established. Transuterine evaluation of tubal status prior to tuboplasty has been recommended[3]. The value of this method is debatable, however,

as it is difficult to perform and the same information can be obtained by a simple hysterosalpingogram.

Endometritis

Endometritis is a potential cause of infertility and recurrent pregnancy loss.

Sperm migration test

Hysteroscopy has been used to assess the survival of spermatozoa in the upper genital tract. Using a CO_2 hysteroscope, spermatozoa are obtained from the uterine cavity and the tubal ostia following intercourse and their motility is assessed.

Gamete intrafallopian transfer and zygote intrafallopian transfer

Because the hysteroscope provides an excellent means of delivering instrumentation or substances to the Fallopian tubes from the uterine side, several techniques of intratubal manipulation have been attempted, such as tubal insemination and the postcoital test. More recently, hysteroscopy has been used with the techniques of gamete intrafallopian transfer (GIFT) and zygote intrafallopian transfer (ZIFT) to transfer the gametes or the zygote into the Fallopian tubes from the uterine side, rather than from the fimbriated end by laparoscopy or minilaparotomy.

It is possible that, with experience and simplification of the outpatient hysteroscopy, this may become a routine study for candidates for *in vitro* fertilization to evaluate the maturity or dysmaturity of the endometrium and predict the likelihood of implantation[4]. Furthermore, the transfer of the early embryo could be accomplished under visual control.

404

Abortion

In cases of abortion, hysteroscopy is useful to check the presence or absence of trophoblastic tissue (Figure 4). Echography, computerized tomography, magnetic resonance imaging and hysteroscopy can help in the diagnosis of a suspected hydatidiform mole (Figure 5).

ABNORMAL UTERINE BLEEDING

The common causes of abnormal uterine bleeding differ with age. In the early pubertal years, abnormal bleeding is usually dysfunctional and is only rarely associated with an organic lesion. Dysfunctional bleeding often responds favorably to hormonal manipulation, and hysteroscopy is not usually needed. On occasion, however, persistent or severe bleeding may signal uterine pathology, such as endometrial polyps (Figure 6), myomas or adenomyosis

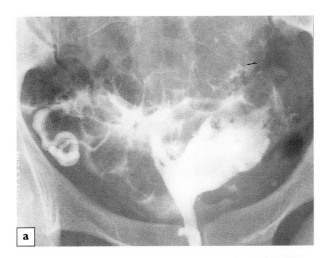

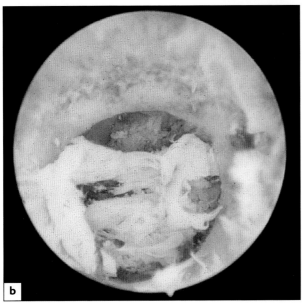

Figure 4 Uterine septum with residual trophoblastic tissue in the left horn. (a) Hysterography; (b) hysteroscopy

(Figure 7). In the reproductive years, pregnancy-related complications are the most common cause of abnormal bleeding. Hysteroscopy is of value in some patients with retained products of conception following a spontaneous or induced abortion, which can be difficult to locate by dilatation and curettage. Uterine myomas and endometrial and cervical polyps are also a common cause of abnormal bleeding in this age group. Polyps tend to move with the flow of the distension medium, whereas submucous myomas, which may have a similar appearance, do not. Evaluation should consist of endometrial sampling, hysterosalpingography and hysteroscopy.

In postmenopausal women with abnormal uterine bleeding, uterine and cervical neoplasia must be excluded. Hysteroscopy can serve as an adjunct to other diagnostic methods in patients in whom abnormal bleeding persists. Atrophic endometrium, another common cause of bleeding in this age group, can easily be diagnosed at hysteroscopy. Endometrial polyps can sometimes also be detected in these patients.

Historically, dilatation and curettage (D & C) has been used as a diagnostic and, often, therapeutic tool. The diagnostic accuracy of D & C has been scrutinized in efforts to determine the sensitivity and specificity of the technique. The advantages of the hysteroscope in the evaluation of abnormal uterine bleeding include, most notably, the ability to see lesions and to evaluate the endometrial cavity more objectively[5]. Indeed, comparisons have been made between the results of hysteroscopically directed biopsy and D & C in treating patients. Valle[5], Mohr[6] and Gimpelson[7] all concluded that panoramic hysteroscopy, especially with directed biopsy, is superior to D & C in patients with uterine bleeding. Alternatively, Goldrath and Sherman combined outpatient panoramic hysteroscopy with suction curettage and suggested the superiority of this technique to D & C in terms of diagnostic accuracy, cost, safety and convenience[8].

Endometrial and cervical cancer

Hysteroscopy for abnormal bleeding can detect suspicious areas in the uterus and the cervix. The hysteroscopic appearance of endometrial carcinoma consists of exophytic or endophytic lesions. Polypoid or whitish areas may indicate necrosis within the tumor. The concern about cancer spread secondary to the hysteroscopic procedure has been addressed by various authors, and no evidence for its occurrence has been found[9,10]. Hysteroscopic examination has been found to be reliable, particularly when difficulties are encountered in assigning the tumor to stage I or II.

The instrument may also be used in detecting premalignant endometrial lesions, such as polypoid or adenomatous lesions with dystrophic or dyplastic hyperplasia. The microhysteroscope can be of great value in detecting such early changes in patients with a known high risk of endometrial cancer, such as diabetics and obese individuals. Hysteroscopy can also provide an excellent view of the cervical canal and can thus be used in the diagnosis of cervical neoplasia[11].

Assessing the extent of involvement

Joelsson and co-workers in 1971 used hysteroscopy to try to distinguish cervical infiltration by tumors[12]. Clearly, if a tumor is seen growing within the endocervix, the endocervix is involved. However, the diagnosis of stage II carcinoma of the endometrium should be based on the histological contiguity of the endometrial carcinoma to normal cervical tissue (glands and stroma). This is not difficult if cervical glands or even the cervical squamous epithelium are contiguous to the cancer. However, this may be difficult if there is only stromal tissue with cancer or if there is only cancer and no cervical tissue at all. To make a diagnosis of stage II endometrial cancer in both these cases, the specimen must come from the endocervix. Such a biopsy requires experience rather than direct visualization of the biopsy site because the small cup of even the Storz instrument will not yield sufficiently deep tissue. The most tantalizing aspect of this problem is that the more anaplastic adenocarcinomas and serous uterine papillary tumors may infiltrate the stroma of the endocervix, but the endocervical canal may look quite normal. A deep endocervical biopsy may be better than the hysteroscope for detecting such cases of endometrial cancer. In patients with super-

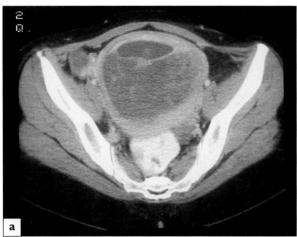
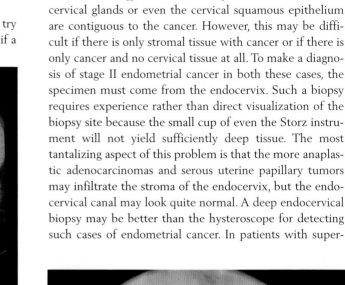
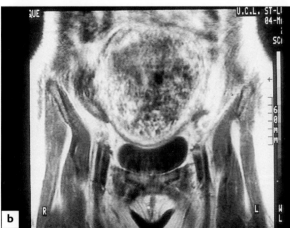
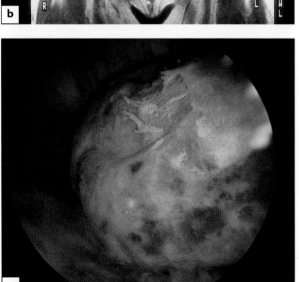
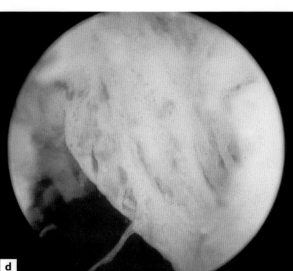
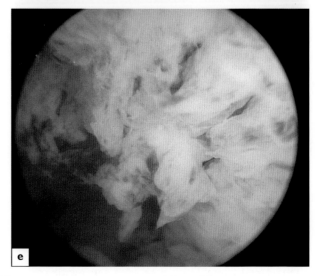

Figure 5 Hydatidiform mole: (a) computerized tomography; (b) magnetic resonance imaging; (c) – (e) hysteroscopy

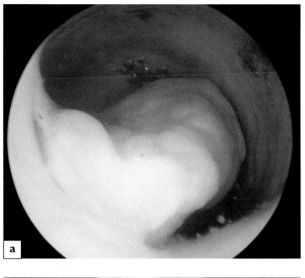

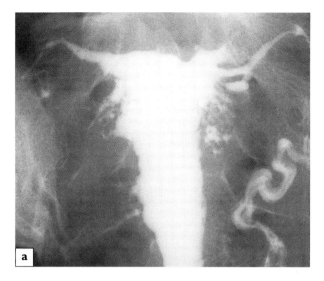

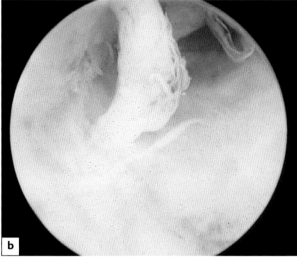

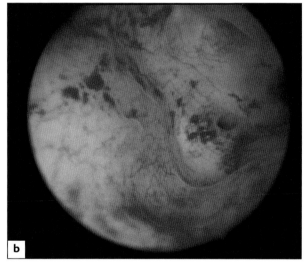

Figure 6 (a) Small endometrial polyp in the left uterine horn; (b) larger polypoid structure

Figure 7 Adenomyosis: (a) hysterography; (b) hysteroscopy reveals holes in the uterine cavity

ficial infiltration of the upper endocervix by endometrial cancer, hysteroscopy will certainly provide a precise topographic description of the lesion. The final diagnosis, however, still needs to be histological. Furthermore, such early superficial spread to the endocervix probably carries no worse a prognosis than a stage I lesion. Deep cervical infiltration is a danger signal for deep myometrial invasion and lymph node involvement[13].

The danger of tumor cell dissemination by the Hyskon or saline solution or even by the flow of CO_2 into the uterine veins is probably not great. Data from hysterographies showed that there was no greater frequency of metastases among patients who had undergone hysterography than among those who had not[9].

INTRAUTERINE FOREIGN BODIES

Until recently, foreign bodies within the uterine cavity were not uncommon. The most common offender is still the intrauterine device (IUD), which often becomes misplaced, making retrieval desirable. Several papers have described the usefulness of hysteroscopy in locating displaced IUDs[14–16].

Four patients with retained intrauterine fetal bones examined hysteroscopically have been described[17]. The bones were removed with hysteroscopic instruments in all patients. Other uncommon uses of the hysteroscopic approach include the removal of a Heyman capsule[18] and the broken tip of a plastic suction curette[19].

REFERENCES

1. Taylor PJ. Correlations in infertility: symptomatology, hysterosalpingography and hysteroscopy. *J Reprod Med* 1983;8:339

2. Lindemann HJ. Hysteroscopy for the diagnosis of intrauterine causes of sterility. *Proceedings of the 8th*

World Congress on Fertility and Sterility, Kyoto, Japan, October, 1971

3. Quinones GR, Alvarado DA, Aznar RR. Tubal catheterization: applications of a new technique. *Am J Obstet Gynecol* 1974;114:674

4. Bordt J, Belkien L, Vancaillie T, *et al*. Ergebnisse diagnosticher Hysteroskopien in einem IVF/ET Program. *Geburtschilfe Frauenheilkd* 1984;44:813

5. Valle RF. Hysteroscopic evaluation of patients with abnormal uterine bleeding. *Surg Gynecol Obstet* 1981;153:521

6. Mohr JW. Hysteroscopy as a diagnostic tool in postmenopausal bleeding. In Philips JM, ed. *Endoscopy in Gynecology*. Downey, CA: American Association of Gynecologic Laparoscopists, 1978:347

7. Gimpelson RJ. Panoramic hysteroscopy with directed biopsies vs. dilatation and curettage for accurate diagnosis. *J Reprod. Med* 1984;29:575

8. Goldrath MH, Sherman AI. Office hysteroscopy and suction curettage: can we eliminate the hospital diagnostic dilatation and curettage. *Am J Obstet Gynecol* 1984;152:220

9. Johnson JE. Hysterography and diagnostic curettage in carcinoma of the uterine body. *Acta Radiol* 1973;326(Suppl 1):1

10. Sugimoto O. Hysteroscopic diagnosis of endometrial carcinoma: a report of fifty-three cases examined at the Women's Clinic of Kyoto University Hospital. *Am J Obstet Gynecol* 1975;121:105

11. Hamou J. Microhysteroscopy: a new procedure and its original applications in gynecology. *J Reprod Med* 1981;26:375

12. Joelsson I, Levine RU, Moberger G. Hysteroscopy as an adjunct in determining the extent of carcinoma of the endometrium. *Am J Obstet Gynecol* 1971;111:696

13. Anderson B. Hysterography and hysteroscopy in endometrial cancer. In Sciara JJ, Buchsbaum HJ, eds. *Gynecology and Obstetrics*. New York: Harper & Row, 1980:850–5

14. Siegler AM, Kemmann E. Location and removal of misplaced or embedded intrauterine devices by hysteroscopy. *J Reprod Med* 1976;16:139

15. Taylor PJ, Comming DC. Hysteroscopy in 100 patients. *Fertil Steril* 1979;31:301

16. Valle RF, Sciarra JJ, Freeman DW. Hysteroscopic removal of intrauterine devices with missing filaments. *Obstet Gynecol* 1977;49:55

17. Chervenak FA, Amin HK, Neuwirth RS. Symptomatic intrauterine retention of fetal bones. *Obstet Gynecol* 1982;59:585

18. Zipkin B, Rosenfeld DL. Hysteroscopic removal of a Heyman radium capsule. *J Reprod Med* 1979;22:133

19. Sciarra JJ, Valle RF. Hysteroscopy: a clinical experience with 320 patients. *Am J Obstet Gynecol* 1977;127:340

Müllerian duct anomalies

M. Nisolle and J. Donnez

40

Three main principles govern the practical approach to malformations of the genital tract:

(1) The Müllerian and Wolffian ducts are so closely linked embryologically that gross malformations of the uterus and vagina are commonly associated with congenital anomalies of the kidney and ureter.

(2) The development of the gonad is separate from that of the ducts. Normal and functional ovaries are therefore usually present when the vagina, uterus and Fallopian tubes are absent or malformed.

(3) Müllerian duct anomalies are usually not associated with anomalies in the sex chromosome make-up of the individual.

EMBRYOLOGY

Gonadal development will not be examined in this chapter, which is limited to Müllerian and Wolffian duct development.

Late in the fifth or sixth week of embryonic life, at the level of the third thoracic somite, a precise area of the celomic epithelium invaginates at several points on the lateral surface of the urogenital ridge, and coalesces to form a tube, termed the Müllerian or paramesonephric duct (Figure 1a). The duct extends caudally to the urogenital ridge, immediately lateral to the Wolffian duct. The paired Müllerian ducts give rise to the Fallopian tubes, uterus, cervix and upper vagina. For proper Müllerian duct migration to occur, it is essential that the Wolffian duct is present[1].

Each Müllerian duct, guided by the respective Wolffian duct, migrates and develops independently of the other, and one usually descends ahead of the other. Defects in the development of the Wolffian duct lead to Müllerian anomalies. At first lateral to the Wolffian ducts, the Müllerian ducts cross over to lie medial to them as they enter the pelvis. By the end of the seventh week of embryonic life, the Müllerian ducts fuse to form a single structure between the two Wolffian ducts. The two Müllerian ducts penetrate the posterior wall of the urogenital sinus, between the orifices of the Wolffian ducts, on a mound called Müller's tubercle. It is important that the point where the tip of the Müllerian duct abuts on the posterior wall of the urogenital sinus is within the patch of mesoderm inserted into the wall of the sinus by the Wolffian

ducts. This point defines the site of the future vaginal orifice, the hymenal membrane (Figure 1b).

Two solid epithelial evaginations (sinovaginal bulbs) grow posteriorly from Müller's tubercle to meet the two solid tips of the fused Müllerian ducts. This epithelial proliferation of sinovaginal bulbs and the caudal ends of the Müllerian ducts form the solid vaginal plate (Figure 2a). The vaginal plate and the adjoining Müllerian ducts

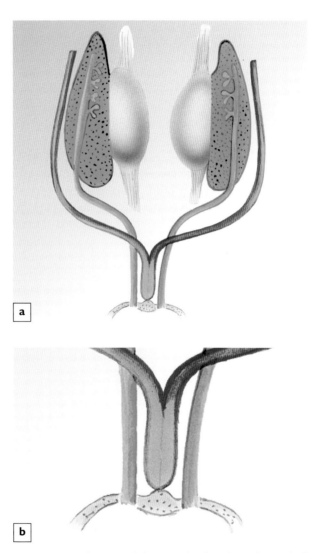

Figure I (a) The genital ducts in the female at the end of the second month of development. Note the Müllerian tubercle and the formation of the uterine canal; Müllerian ducts (orange), urogenital sinus (yellow); (b) higher power detail of the genital ducts in the female at the end of the second month of development

elongate, canalize, and migrate from pelvic to perineal locations. At the same time the urogenital sinus exstrophies into the vestibule, the urethra elongates and the plate canalizes (Figure 2b). The hymen remains as a membrane between the urogenital sinus and the canalized vaginal plate. The vaginal plate is first seen distinctly when the embryo is about 60–75 mm long, and its formation is complete at about 140 mm. Finally, when the cells of the plate desquamate, the vaginal lumen is formed[2] (Figure 2c).

Felix[3] and Frazer[4] believed that canalization occurred in the bulbar and vaginal components of the plate and that the hymen demarcated the junction between the Müllerian and urogenital structures. In 1933, Koff[5] proposed that the sinovaginal bulbs formed the entire plate, that the plate canalized predominantly in a caudocranial direction giving rise to the hymen, and that the hymen and the caudal fifth of the vagina were formed from the plate and were therefore of urogenital sinus origin.

Witschi[6] believed that the hymen was formed from sinus and Müllerian epithelia with lateral contributions from the Wolffian ducts. He histologically identified Wolffian duct structures in the walls of the vaginal plate down to the urogenital sinus.

Frazer[4] observed the termination of the Wolffian ducts between the two layers of the hymen and the Müllerian contribution to the length of the vagina. These observations support the findings of Witschi: first, that the hymen marks the junction of the canalized vaginal bulbs of the urogenital sinus and the Müllerian ducts at the introitus, and second, that the Wolffian duct itself guides and mediates the caudal migration of the vaginal plate from pelvis to perineum. Having guided the Müllerian ducts to their destination and participated in the development of the vaginal plate, the Wolffian ducts become atrophic.

As early as the end of the first trimester[7], there is a mesenchymal thickening around that portion of the fused Müllerian duct that is destined to become the endocervix. This mesenchymal thickening includes the Wolffian ducts, so that remnants of the latter, which persist into adulthood, are found within the body of the cervix. At all other levels of the genital canal, remnants of the Wolffian ducts are external to the wall of the adult Müllerian derivative.

Smooth muscle appears in the walls of the genital canal between 18 and 20 weeks, and, by approximately 24 weeks, the muscular portion of the uterine wall is well developed[7]. Vaginal, uterine and tubal muscular walls develop around the Müllerian duct alone, so that the Wolffian duct remnants are external to the true wall of the canal.

Cervical glands appear at about 15 weeks and rudimentary endometrial glands by 19 weeks, but the endometrium is not well developed even at term in most infants.

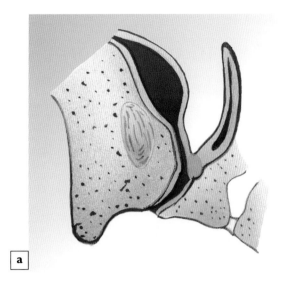

a

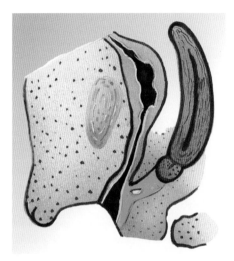

b

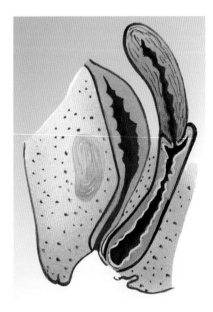

c

Figure 2 Sagittal section showing the formation of the uterus and vagina during development

CLINICAL AND PATHOLOGICAL IMPLICATIONS OF THE EMBRYOLOGIC DEVELOPMENT

The genital ducts and external genitalia develop as a result of hormones circulating *in utero*[8]. A non-steroidal compound, termed Müllerian-inhibiting factor (MIF), secreted by the fetal testes, inhibits the development of the Müllerian ducts and potentiates the development of the Wolffian ducts. The fetal testes also secrete androgens that stimulate the development of the external genitalia, as well as the central nervous system. If the fetal gonads are ovaries, MIF is not produced, and therefore the Müllerian ducts develop and the Wolffian ducts regress. In the absence of androgens, the indifferent external genitalia differentiate in a female direction.

Other congenital abnormalities, unrelated to the action of hormones, arise from a faulty morphogenesis and result in genital tract malformations, such as accessory tubal orifices, bicornuate uterus, or vaginal septa. These anomalies result from the lack of fusion of the Müllerian ducts or a lack of degeneration of the solid vaginal plate. Urinary tract abnormalities are also frequently associated with Müllerian duct anomalies. Improper development of the Wolffian ducts results in failure of proper migration of the Müllerian ducts. Thus, the urinary tract anomaly is primary, and the genital tract anomaly is secondary[1]. Patients who are found to have Müllerian duct-related abnormalities should, therefore, undergo an intravenous pyelogram, performed in order to assess the status of the urinary tract.

The anatomical abnormalities induced by *in utero* diethylstilbestrol exposure can be understood on the basis of the embryological development of both the lower and upper genital tracts[9–11]. Diethylstilbestrol inhibits the development of the vaginal plate, resulting in the Müllerian duct component of the vagina being lower in the adult canal than is normally the case. This results in the presence of columnar, Müllerian-type epithelium as far down the vagina as the hymenal ring in extreme cases. Diethylstilbestrol also disorganizes the stromal differentiation, which is responsible for the overall structure of the cervix, uterus and tubes. This accounts for the gross structural anomalies of the cervix, such as the cervical collar, pseudopolyp and hood, as well as the uterine deformities that may be encountered, such as the T-shaped endometrial cavity (Figure 3).

CLASSIFICATION OF MÜLLERIAN DUCT ANOMALIES

Müllerian duct anomalies can be classified into those of development and those of fusion (Table 1).

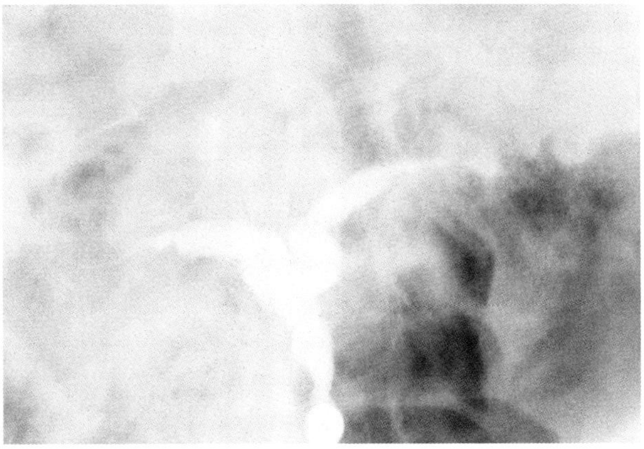

Figure 3 *In utero* diethylstilbestrol exposure: T-shaped endometrial cavity

Table 1 Classification of Müllerian duct anomalies

Development anomalies
Absence of both Müllerian ducts
Absence of one Müllerian duct
Incomplete development of both Müllerian ducts
Incomplete development of one Müllerian duct
Fusion anomalies
(1) Lateral fusion anomalies
arcuate uterus
uterus subseptus and uterus septus
uterus bicornis
uterus didelphys
septate and subseptate vagina
(2) Vertical fusion anomalies
cervical atresia
vaginal atresia
transverse vaginal septum

Development anomalies

Absence of both Müllerian ducts

Complete failure of development of the Müllerian ducts results in an absence of the Fallopian tubes, uterus and most of the vagina. In such cases, the vulva is likely to be normal and there may be a depression of variable depth representing the lower (urogenital sinus) part of the vagina. It is usual to find such a depression covered with a normal hymen[12,13] (Figure 4).

The Mayer–Rokitansky–Küster–Hauser syndrome affects one in every 4000–5000 females and is the second most common cause of primary infertility after gonadal dysgenesis. Although familial aggregates have been described, the defect usually appears sporadically[14].

Absence of one Müllerian duct

Absence of one Müllerian duct (Figure 5) results in a unicornuate uterus with only one Fallopian tube. The cervix and vagina may be normal in appearance and function, but they strictly represent only one half of the fully developed organs. A true unicornuate uterus is rare and is usually associated with an absence or gross malformation of the renal tract on the side of the missing Müllerian duct.

Incomplete development of both Müllerian ducts

Poorly formed ducts of full length result in hypoplasia of the whole genital tract. Incomplete development some-

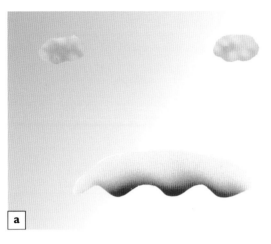

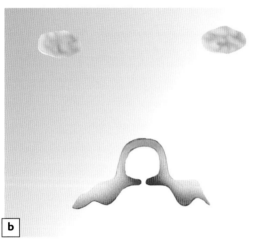

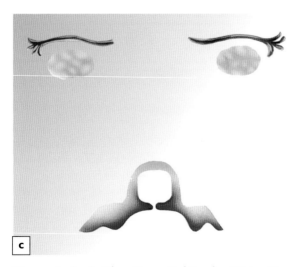

Figure 4 (a–c) The Mayer–Rokitansky–Küster–Hauser syndrome: development of internal genital tract

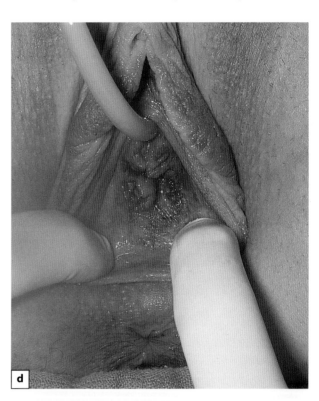

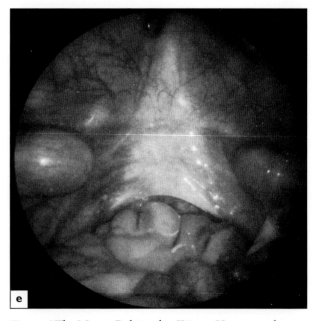

Figure 4 The Mayer–Rokitansky–Küster–Hauser syndrome: (d) external genital tract; (e) laparoscopic view

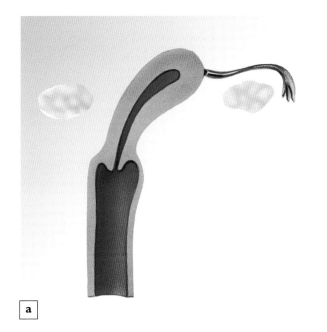

a

times affects the lower parts of the ducts only. Thus, well-formed abdominal ostia may be associated with hypoplasia or absence of the remainder of the tubes, of the uterus and of the vagina (Figure 4). It is possible for the tubes and uterus to be present and the vagina absent, rudimentary, or imperforate. The converse is not true because the ducts grow downwards; a well-formed uterus is never associated with absence of Fallopian tubes.

Incomplete development of one Müllerian duct

Incomplete development of one Müllerian duct (Figure 6) gives rise to the more common apparent unicornuate malformation; this is distinguished by the discovery of a Fallopian tube and round ligament, rudimentary though they may be, on the affected side. In this condition, two kidneys are usually present although, occasionally, the one on the affected side may also be hypoplastic and not apparent on intravenous pyelography.

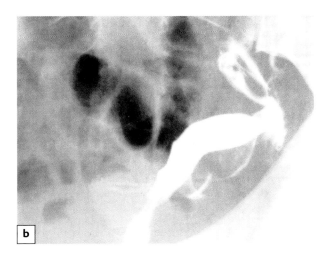

b

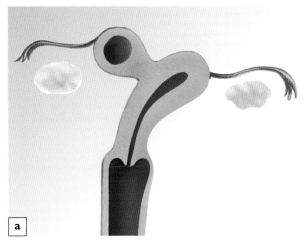

a

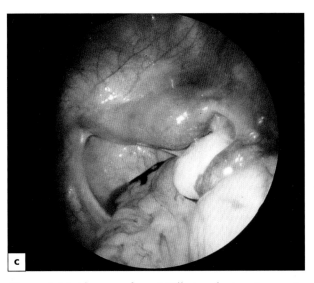

c

Figure 5 (a) Absence of one Müllerian duct: unicornuate uterus; (b) view on hysterography; (c) view on laparoscopy

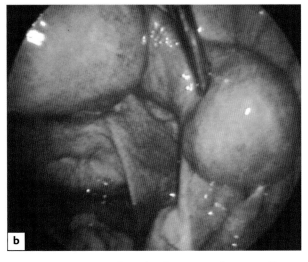

b

Figure 6 (a) Incomplete development of one Müllerian duct; (b) laparoscopic view. The rudimentary horn is visible on the right side

Fusion anomalies

Lateral fusion anomalies

The anomalies result from a failure of lateral fusion of the two Müllerian ducts, a condition which may be obstructive or non-obstructive. Failure of fusion of the Müllerian ducts occurs in varying degrees. If minor degrees affecting uterine shape are taken into consideration, this type of malformation is extremely common. The different nomenclatures and classifications of the resulting deformities are confusing.

(1) *Arcuate uterus* (Figure 7a). This is a flat-topped uterus in which the fundal bulge has not developed after fusion of the ducts.

(2) *Uterus subseptus and uterus septus* (Figure 7b). The uterus is outwardly normal but contains a complete or incomplete septum, which reflects a failure in the breakdown of the walls between the two ducts. The cervical canal may be single or double, and the vagina whole or septate.

(3) *Uterus bicornis* (Figure 7c). In this condition only the lower parts of the ducts fuse, leaving the cornua

separate. The cervix and vagina may be single or double.

(4) *Uterus didelphys* (Figure 7d). If the two Müllerian ducts remain separate, the two halves of the uterus remain distinct and each has its own cervix. Some distinguish between uterus didelphys and uterus pseudodidelphys according to the degree of separation between the two ducts.

(5) *Septate and subseptate vagina* (Figure 8). A sagittal septum with a crescentic lower edge may be present in the upper vagina or throughout its length. It can occur alone or in conjunction with a septate or bicornuate condition of the uterus, and may have one or two cervices opening into it. This condition arises either because late fusion of the Müllerian ducts gives rise to two Müllerian tubercles, or because of a failure of proper canalization of the two sinovaginal bulbs.

In some cases, the hemivagina is not patent, taking the form of a blind vaginal pouch. The obstructed hemivagina is associated with either a functioning double uterus or a degenerate remnant of the paramesonephric duct. This uterine remnant is lined with ciliated columnar cells with

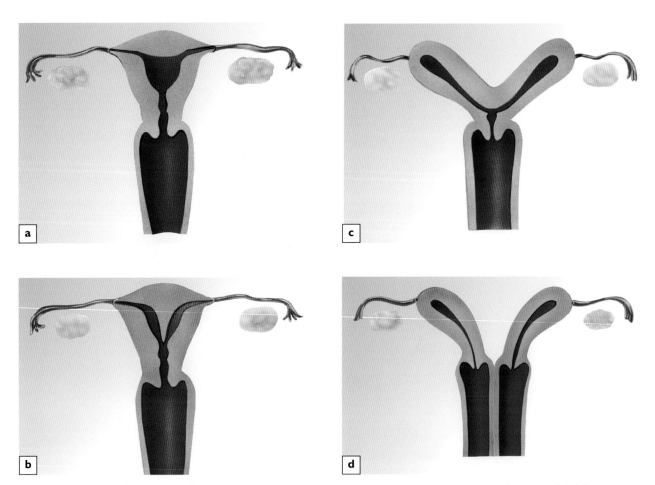

Figure 7 (a) Lateral fusion anomalies: (a) arcuate uterus; (b) uterus septus; (c) uterus bicornis; (d) uterus didelphys

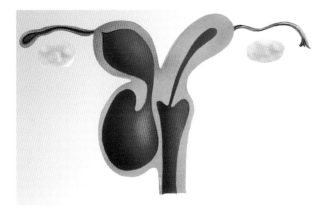

Figure 8 Septate vagina. The obstructed hemivagina is associated with a functioning double uterus

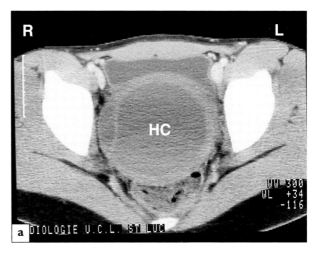

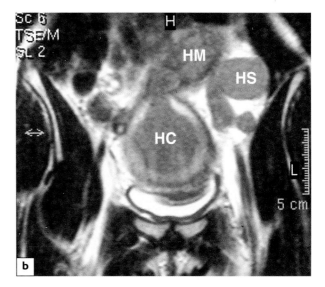

occasional papillary projections. It may also contain patches of endometrial and/or glandular epithelium that produce a mucoid and/or menstrual discharge. At the time of puberty, the absence of the lower part of the hemivagina is responsible for the development of hematocolpos while the opposite hemivagina is patent. Diagnosis is usually facilitated by computerized tomography scan (Figure 9) which reveals not only a hematocolpos but also hematometria and hematosalpinx. In childhood, an obstructed hemivagina is usually asymptomatic unless distended by mucus. In this case, a simple incision and resection of the vaginal septum will allow continued drainage. With menstruation, the resulting hematocolpos may be evacuated after a complete resection of the septum. Obstructed hemivagina and a double uterus are almost always associated with ipsilateral renal agenesis[15,16].

Vertical fusion anomalies – incomplete canalization

The Müllerian buds have solid tips behind which canalization takes place progressively. The Müllerian and sinovaginal bulb tissue which forms the vagina is also lumenless at first. Failure to canalize results in either solid organs or membranes of varying thickness obstructing the genital canal. Thus a rudimentary uterus sometimes lacks a cavity and the vagina may be represented by an uncanalized column of tissue. Atresia may affect only one Müllerian duct, so that one horn of a bicornuate uterus may fail to communicate with the cervical canal, or one half of a septate vagina may be a closed cavity. Unilateral hematocolpos, mucocolpos and pyocolpos are not common.

(1) *Cervical atresia* (Figure 10). Congenital atresia of the cervix of an otherwise normal uterus or of a bicornuate uterus is rare. When it does occur, a reasonably normal vagina is invariably present. It is more common to encounter apparent cervical atresia in association with an absence of the lower vagina.

(2) *Vaginal atresia – transverse vaginal septum*. Disorders of vertical fusion result from defects in the union

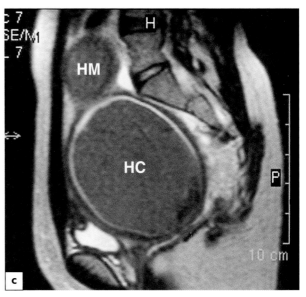

Figure 9 (a) Computerized tomograph of the completely obstructed hemivagina; (b) and (c) note the presence of hematocolpos (HC), hematometria (HM) and hematosalpinx (HS)

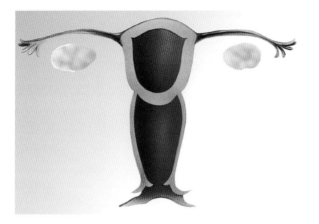

Figure 10 Cervical atresia

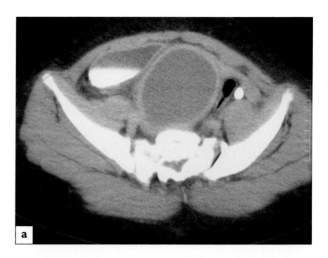

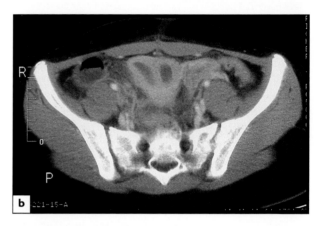

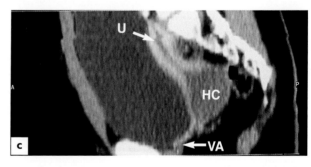

Figure 11 (a) Computerized tomography reveals the hematocolpos; (b) it has been found to be associated with uterine septum; (c) magnetic resonance imaging reveals partial vaginal atresia (VA), hematocolpos (HC) and the uterus (U)

between the downward progressing Müllerian tubercles and the up-growing derivative of the urogenital sinus. Similar defects may also occur secondary to a failure in the canalization of the solid vaginal tube, either because of abnormal proliferation of paravaginal mesoderm or because of some form of intrauterine infection. Partial vaginal atresia is usually diagnosed in young patients at the time of puberty. Indeed, an absence of the lower part of the vagina is responsible for the development of hematocolpos. Progressive distension of the upper part of the vagina causes hypogastric pain and, in cases of very large hematocolpos (> 500 ml), dysuria or urinary retention may be associated. Vulvar and rectal examinations allow us to make the diagnosis of vaginal atresia. A computerized tomography scan or magnetic resonance image reveals the hematocolpos, associated or not with a uterine malformation (uterus septus) (Figure 11).

Transverse vaginal septae are relatively rare, affecting approximately one in every 80 000 females. The septum consists of a central fibromuscular plate or ring of varying thickness (Figure 12). When the obstruction is complete, the outer surface is covered with stratified squamous epithelium, while the inner aspect is composed of glandular columnar epithelium. The interruption can occur at any level of the vagina, and may be multiple. The middle and lower zones of the vagina may be imperforate over a length of 0.5–6.0 cm. More frequently, the vagina is obstructed by a thinner membrane situated in the vagina, just above the hymen. Transverse vaginal septae usually go unnoticed in children unless a mucocolpos has developed or vaginal patency is tested. A rim of hymenal tissue will help distinguish the low transverse septa from an imperforate hymen. Distension of the septum as seen vaginally will depend on its thickness and location. As in the imperforate hymen, the vulva may be very engorged and swollen.

Obstruction of menstrual flow and subsequent endometriosis may result in infertility. In a study of 15 teenage patients with pelvic pain and endometriosis, six (40%) were found to have obstructive anomalies of the genitalia[17]. Goldstein and colleagues reported endometriosis in 52% of 140 adolescents evaluated laparoscopically for pelvic pain[18]. Of these cases, only 50% of patients had obstructive uterine anomalies.

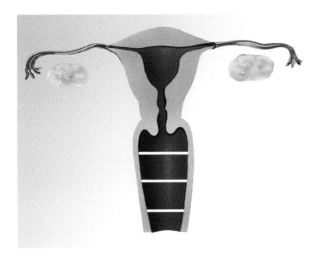

Figure 12 Transverse vaginal septum showing three types: high transverse vaginal septum; transverse septum of the middle third of the vagina; transverse septum of the lower third of the vagina

REFERENCES

1. Marshall FF, Beisel DS. The association of uterine anomalies. *Obstet Gynecol* 1978;51:559
2. O'Rahilly R. The development of the vagina in the human. *Birth Defects* 1977;13:123–36
3. Felix W. The development of the urogenital organs. In Keibel F, Mall FP, eds. *Manual of Human Embryology*. Philadelphia: Lippincott, 1912:979
4. Frazer JE. *A Manual of Embryology: The Development of the Human Body*. London: Baillière Tindall, 1931:431–40
5. Koff AK. Development of the vagina in the human fetus. *Contrib Embryol Carneg Inst* 1933;24:61–91
6. Witschi E. Embryogenesis of the adrenal and the reproductive glands. *Rec Prog Horm Res* 1951;6:1
7. O'Rahilly R. The embryology and anatomy of the uterus. In Norris H, Hertig A, eds. *The Uterus*. Baltimore: Williams-Wilkins, 1973
8. Jost A. Embryonic sexual differentiation (morphology, physiology, abnormalities). In Jones H Jr, Scott WW, eds. *Hermaphroditism, Genital Anomalies and Related Endocrine Disorders*, 2nd edn. Baltimore: Williams Wilkins, 1971:16
9. Kaufman RH, Adam E, Binder GL, Gerthoffer E. Upper genital tract changes and pregnancy outcome in offspring exposed *in utero* to diethylstilbestrol. *Am J Obstet Gynecol* 1980;137:299
10. Robboy SJ. A hypothetic mechanism of diethylstilbestrol (DES)-induced anomalies in exposed progeny. *Hum Pathol* 1983;14:831
11. Robboy SJ, Taguchi O, Cunha GR. Normal development of the human female reproductive tract and alterations resulting from experimental exposure to diethylstilbestrol. *Hum Pathol* 1982;13:190
12. Nisolle M, Donnez J. Malformations and maldevelopments of the Müllerian ducts. In Donnez J, ed. *Laser Operative Laparoscopy and Hysteroscopy*. Leuven: Nauwelaerts, 1989:231–48
13. Nisolle M, Donnez J. Vaginoplasty using amniotic membranes in cases of vaginal agenesis or after vaginectomy. *J Endosc Surg* 1992;8:25–30
14. Carson SA, Simpson JL, Malinak LR, *et al*. Heritable aspects of uterine anomalies II. Genetic analysis of müllerian aplasia. *Fertil Steril* 1983;40:86
15. Woolf RB, Allen WM. Concomitant malformations. *Obstet Gynecol* 1953;2:236
16. Fekete CN, Nisolle M. Anomalies de fusion ou d'accolement des canaux de Müller. *Revue médico-Chirurgicale de l'Hôpital des Enfants Malades*. Paris, 1988:1
17. Schifrin BS, Erez S, Moore JG. Teenage endometriosis. *Am J Obstet Gynecol* 1973;116:973
18. Goldstein DP, Decholnoky C, Emans SJ, Leventhal JM. Laparoscopy in the diagnosis and management of the pelvic pain in adolescents. *J Reprod Med Obstet Gynecol* 1980;24:251

Vaginoplasty in cases of vaginal agenesis

41

M. Nisolle and J. Donnez

Malformations of the vagina are an uncommon but serious problem. Their severity ranges from complete vaginal agenesis (Figure 1), with or without a functional uterus, to vaginal shortening.

The treatment of certain gynecological malignancies, such as vaginal adenocarcinoma or severe vaginal dysplasia induced by diethylstilbestrol, requires vaginectomy, which makes coitus impossible. In some instances, radical hysterectomy for severe cervical dysplasia is accompanied by vaginectomy because of associated vaginal dysplasia. Vaginal construction or reconstruction has become well established as a method of permitting or restoring sexual function, and a variety of procedures have been described. The most popular method involves the lining of a surgically created space either with a partial thickness skin graft[1] or with amnion[2-11].

In 1934, Brindeau used human amnion to construct a vagina in a patient with Müllerian agenesis[2]. Between 1939 and 1947, Burger[3] used amnion more extensively for the same purpose. In 1973, Trelford and colleagues[4-6] successfully used fetal amnion to reconstruct the vagina during anterior exenteration. We report our experience with the use of amniotic membranes to line artificially constructed vaginas. Amniotic membranes were obtained immediately postpartum from an HIV- and HB$_s$-seronegative patient who had delivered 3–6 h before the vaginoplasty. She was afebrile and her membranes had been ruptured for less than 6 h. Delivery was vaginal in all cases. Elective Cesarean section was not a condition for use of the membranes.

Membranes were rinsed in sterile saline solution to remove all the blood and stored at 4°C in saline without antibiotics. Amnion was not stripped from the chorion before use.

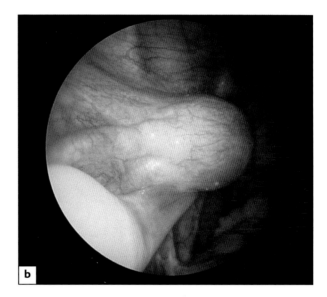

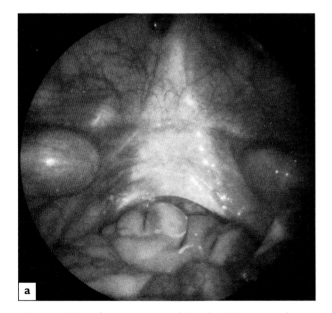

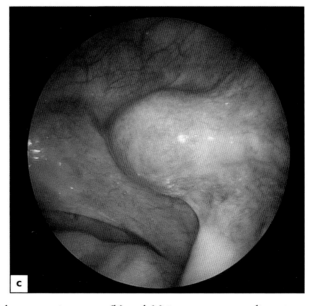

Figure 1 Vaginal agenesis in Rokitansky–Hauser syndrome: (a) laparoscopic aspect; (b) and (c) in some cases, rudimentary horns are visible

419

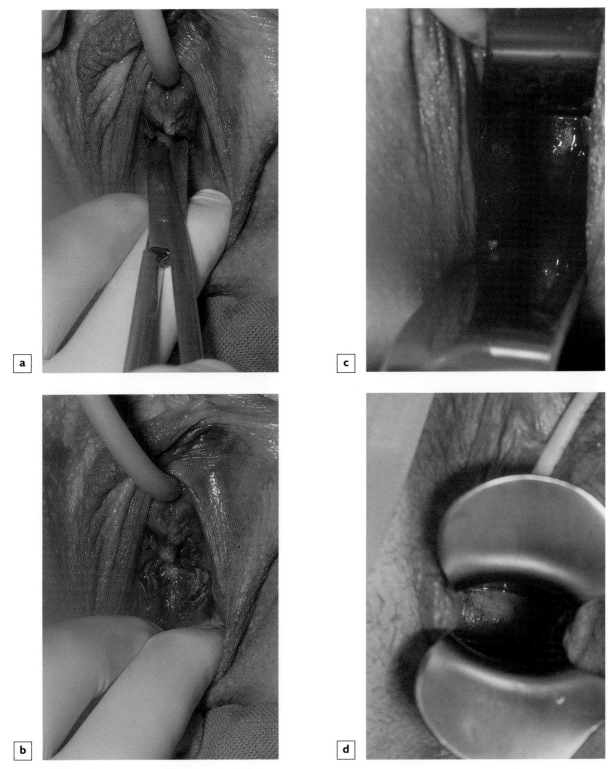

Figure 2 (a)–(d) Dissection of the vesico-rectal space

SURGICAL PROCEDURE

Under general anesthesia, the patient is placed in the lithotomy position and vaginal dissection is performed (Figure 2). A vaginal pouch is created by blunt dissection, with the help of scissors (Figure 2a and b). At the same time, a laparoscopy is performed to confirm the diagnosis and

check the blunt dissection. When hemostasis has been achieved (Figure 2c and d), a rigid vaginal mold (Figure 3a) is selected, just large enough to ensure firm application of the amniotic membranes, with which it is covered (Figure 4a). The labia majora are approximated with silk sutures to keep the mold in place (Figure 4b). Laparoscopy is not necessary for the dissection, but, when performed to

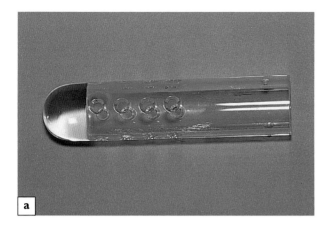

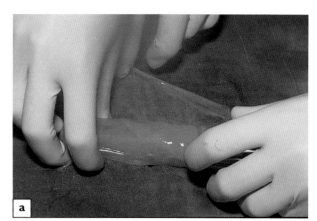

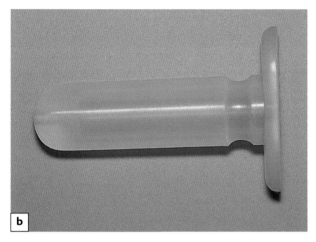

Figure 3 (a) Rigid vaginal mold (diameter 3.5 cm, length 10 cm). The holes allow the drainage of vaginal exudates. Two small holes allow the mold to be fixed; (b) non-rigid mold (diameter 3.5 cm, length 10 cm). This mold can be introduced and removed very easily by the patient

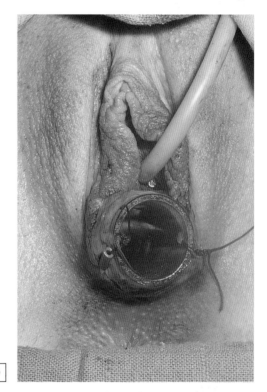

Figure 4 (a) A rigid mold is wrapped in amniotic membranes; (b) the rigid mold is introduced into the vaginal pouch and fixed to the skin

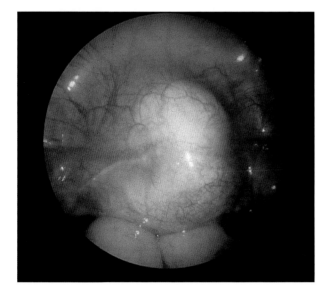

Figure 5 Laparoscopic view after blunt dissection and introduction of a rigid mold

ascertain the diagnosis, it permits the visualization of the top of the mold between the bladder and the rectum (Figure 5). A Foley catheter is inserted before the blunt dissection and left in place for 48 h. Two rudimentary horns are sometimes clearly visible at the time of laparoscopy (Figure 6). When the patient is suffering from pelvic pain and dysmenorrhea, echography often reveals small areas of hematometria. In this case, during the same procedure, both rudimentary horns are removed laparoscopically.

Electrocoagulation of the isthmic portion of the Fallopian tube, the utero-ovarian ligament and the uterine artery is subsequently performed (Figure 6). The uterine

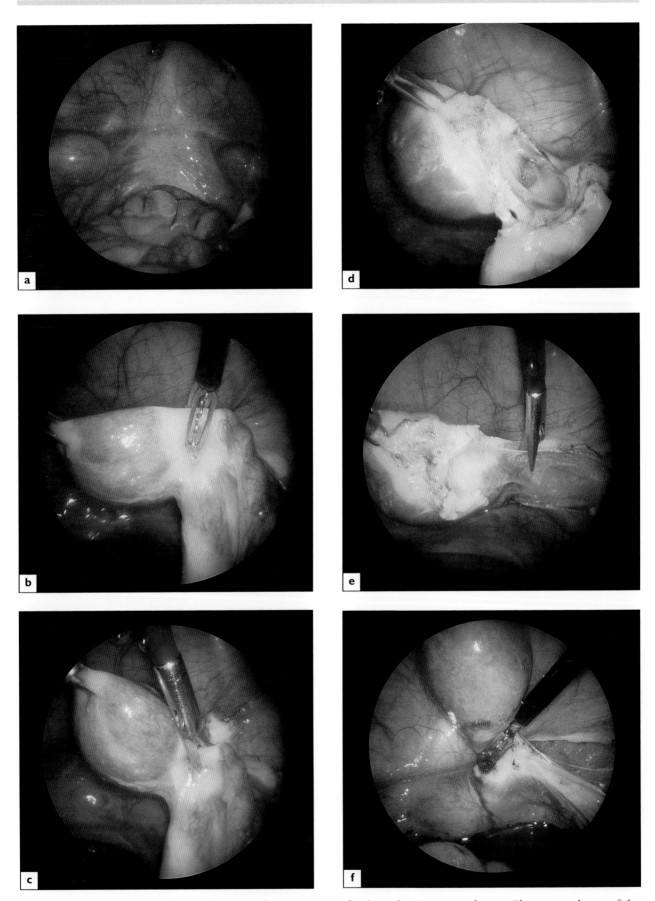

Figure 6 Laparoscopic view of two rudimentary horns in a case of Rokitansky–Hauser syndrome. Electrocoagulation of the isthmic portion of the Fallopian tube, the utero-ovarian ligament and the artery *(continued on next page)*

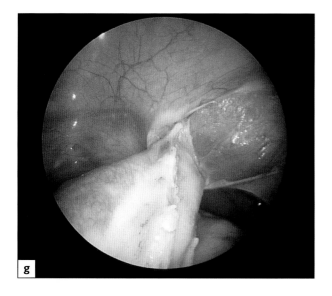

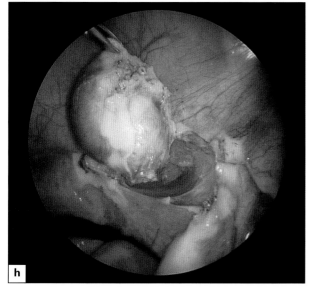

Figure 6 *Continued*

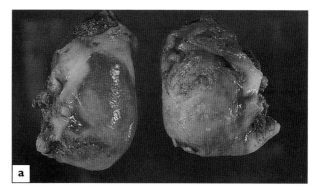

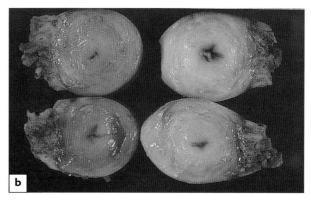

Figure 7 Macroscopic view of the removed rudimentary horns: (a) external view; (b) transection reveals the presence of collected blood

PATIENTS AND RESULTS

Between 1986 and 1992, amniotic membranes were used in 11 patients (aged 14–59 years) undergoing vaginoplasty for vaginal agenesis. None of them had undergone an anterior vaginoplasty. All patients found the mold uncomfortable postoperatively, but all were mobile and required mild analgesia only for the mold change on day 7. Routine urinary catheter insertion was performed in all cases for 48 h. All patients received prophylactic antibiotics, penicillin and metronidazole. No patients developed a urinary tract infection. At the mold change, the amniotic membranes could be seen as a distinct layer applied to the vaginal wall. At the end of 7 days, the vaginal tunnel was covered with a smooth lining, with extensive but small areas of congestion.

By the fourth week postoperatively, healthy pink vaginal epithelium was visible with, in some cases, only small areas of granulation tissue. Initial epithelialization was excellent. At the end of 8 weeks, the vagina was found to be well formed and was of normal depth and caliber. There was no exudate, adhesions, drying, or scarring. Constant use of the mold produced no inflammatory reaction or formation of granuloma in unmarried patients.

The rectum was not entered in any patient during vaginal dissection.

All patients were reviewed at 2 weeks and at 1 month postoperatively and then at monthly intervals. Vaginal

horns are then easily removed, either through the pouch of Douglas or transabdominally, with the help of a forceps. The macroscopic view after transection of the horn (Figure 7) reveals blood in the rudimentary uterine cavity. The entire procedure is completed in 20 min. All patients receive antibiotics for 6–7 days postoperatively.

The mold is removed under light sedation 7 days later, and the newly constructed vagina is inspected and cleaned. The amniotic membranes are found to be adherent to the vagina. A flexible mold (Figure 3b) is then inserted and the patient discharged the following day, having been advised to refrain from sexual activity for an additional 2 weeks and to use the mold at night during this period. Dienoestrol cream is used as a lubricant. The patient is then encouraged to have sexual intercourse. All patients are reviewed at 2 weeks and 1 month postoperatively and then at monthly intervals.

smears at 8 weeks postoperatively showed numerous squamous epithelial cells. In all but one patient with vaginal agenesis, epithelialization was complete, as proved by biopsy, which showed early epithelialization (at weeks 4–6) and mature vaginal epithelium by the end of 8–10 weeks (Figure 8). In one patient, granulation tissue was found: this patient had not used vaginal estrogen cream.

The anatomic and functional results are summarized in Table 1. The length of the vagina varied from 7 to 8 cm. All patients had greatly improved vaginal length and capacity as a result of this treatment. Excellent results were achieved in all cases. The vaginal tissue remained supple, with no evidence of fibrous tissue formation. Chronic granulation tissue was not observed and vaginal shrinkage did not occur.

Since 1992, the same technique of vaginoplasty has been performed in 18 patients. Very recently, we used a new product, Surgisis™ Enhanced Strength (Cook, Brussels, Belgium), in order to avoid the application of human tissue with the potential risk of viral transmission in young women (Figure 9). Small intestinal submucosa (SIS) is a new biomaterial for replacement and repair of damaged tissue. It does not contain cells because it is extracted from the porcine small intestine in a manner that removes all cells because it is extracted from the porcine small intestine in a manner that removes all cells, but leaves the complex matrix intact. The manufacturing process has been validated to ensure that any virus that might be present in source animals is completely inactivated. The cells of adjacent tissue invade the SIS material. Progressively, capillary growth and progressive degradation of the SIS material should be observed. This new tissue graft has already been used in animal surgery by several authors and it looks to be encouraging for use in human surgery[12,13].

Vesico-rectal dissection is performed as previously described, but, instead of applying amniotic membranes to the rigid mold, two pieces of Surgisis are sutured with four

Table 1 Postoperative functional results after vaginoplasty for vaginal agenesis due to Rokitansky–Küster–Hauser syndrome (*n* = 11). From Nisolle and Donnez[11]

Vaginal length (cm)		
Preoperative	Postoperative	Functional results
1	7	+++*
1	7	+++
1	7	+++
1	8	+++
1	7	+++
1	7	+++
1	7	+++
1	7	+++
1	7	+++*
1	7	+++
3	8	+++

* No sexual intercourse; only the mold was used; +++ normal vaginal capacity

stitches of Vicryl-1/0 to the lateral side of the newly created vaginal pouch.

More than 7 days are required for the development of the new vaginal epithelium. Two weeks after surgery, the Surgisis is no longer recognizable and granulation tissue is observed. Long-term follow-up and large series of procedures are needed to confirm the results with this new product. This technique (using Surgisis) has also been applied in one case of partial vaginal atresia. Blunt dissection allowed us to locate the hematocolpos and, after its drainage, a small mold and one piece of Surgisis were used to facilitate epithelialization of the lower part of the vagina.

The final result is directly related to the motivation of the patient and her postoperative use of the mold. No long-term complications have been observed so far: follow-up extends from 3 months to 5 years.

DISCUSSION

Various treatments have been described for vaginal agenesis. Frank[14] reported graduated vaginal dilatation but this technique has given good results in less than 50% of patients. Williams[15] described the method of a turned-in labial flap. Although the procedure required no graft, no satisfactory results were reported. The vaginal axis was often badly placed and difficulties with micturition and repeated urinary tract infections were observed.

Creating a tunnel for congenital absence of the vagina is a step common to all surgical procedures. The need for the use of a graft, and the best tissue to use (skin, intestine, or amnion) are debatable. The use of cecal or sigmoid

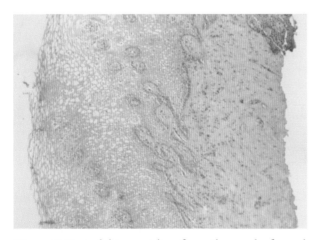

Figure 8 Vaginal biopsy taken from the newly formed vaginal cavity 8 weeks after surgery (Gomori's trichrome; x 25) shows mature vaginal epithelium

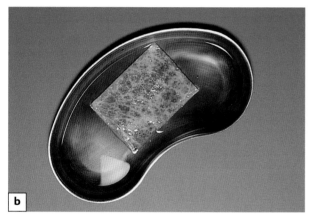

Figure 9 (a) A 10 x 7 cm piece of small intestine submucosa (SIS); (b) Surgisis® (Cook) has been placed in Rifocine® solution for 2–3 min before being sutured to the newly created vaginal pouch

bowel segments was reported by Baldwin in 1904[16]. Although some authors claimed good results, this method is a major surgical procedure with significant morbidity and mortality. Turner-Warwick and Kirby[17] have recently reported successful reconstruction of the vagina with colocecum, with no serious surgical complication. However, profuse secretions, persistent unpleasant odor and ulceration of the mucosal surface could be major side-effects.

Wharton[18] devised an operation based on the remarkable regenerative potential of granulation tissue in the vaginal canal. To keep the space patent, a condom-covered mold was used. McIndoe and Bannister[1] modified Wharton's operation by the additional step of transplanting a split-thickness skin graft into the newly formed vaginal cavity, held in place by a vaginal mold. Great variations in success rate, a high incidence of postoperative infection, necrosis of the skin graft and scarring make this technique less acceptable. The patient also suffers considerable discomfort from the donor skin site, which may remain visible.

Myocutaneous flaps have been used by several surgeons. The gracilis myocutaneous flap has become very

popular in recent years[19–22], but a serious disadvantage is the precarious vascularity of the flaps. In McCraw's series of 22 patients[23], six suffered catastrophic loss of the flap. The rectus abdominis flap is another popular flap, but creates a large abdominal donor site defect[24] and requires a long operative procedure. The neurovascular pudendal thigh flap procedure can be used reliably to reconstruct the vagina[25]. All flap techniques, however, are reported to suffer from an unacceptable failure rate due to partial flap loss and necrosis. Such dissections also cause major scars and can only be indicated for vaginal reconstruction after pelvectomy for pelvic cancer, when subsequent irradiation must be carried out.

In order to overcome these difficulties, amnion alone, with the clean mesenchymal surface placed towards the host, has been used by several surgeons[2–6,9]. Dino and co-workers[26] suggested sterilization of amniotic membranes. Trelford and colleagues[4–7] found that membranes stored at 4°C in 0.5% normal saline with antibiotics were sterile at the end of 48 h. In our study[11], amniotic membranes were taken immediately postpartum (< 6 h). Saline solution with antibiotics was never used. Membranes were only rinsed in sterile physiological solution (NaCl 0.9%).

Faulk and colleagues[27] have demonstrated microscopic evidence of new vessel formation and suggested that an angiogenic factor is produced by amnion. There is no problem with immune rejection because amnion does not express histocompatibility antigens and Akle and associates[28] found no evidence of tissue rejection when amnion was implanted subcutaneously in volunteers.

Tancer and co-workers[8], Dhall[9] and Ashworth and colleagues[10] have reported the successful use of amnion as a graft in vaginoplasties. Removal of the more antigenic chorion has been suggested to contribute to the successful use of the amnion. In the study of Nisolle and Donnez[11], however, the amnion was not stripped from the chorion. Our results showed the vagina to be well formed and of normal depth and caliber. There was no problem of immune rejection. Sexual intercourse was reported to be satisfactory in all cases. Vaginal smears and vaginal biopsy specimens were taken at follow-up visits. Vaginal epithelium was present by 8–10 weeks.

In conclusion, amniotic membranes are readily available, easily stored and inexpensive, and can be used without a sterilization procedure as a graft for vaginal reconstruction. The amniotic membranes adhere firmly, protect the underlying granulation and facilitate epithelialization. The use of a new tissue graft (Surgisis) appears to be without risk of viral transmission. Hospitalization is considerably reduced and major skin defects occurring after myocutaneous flap reconstruction are avoided. No postoperative dilatation is needed once normal sexual intercourse is resumed.

REFERENCES

1. McIndoe AH, Bannister JE. An operation for the cure of congenital absence of the vagina. *J Obstet Gynaecol Br Emp* 1938;45:490

2. Brindeau A. Creation d'un vagin artificiel à l'aide des membranes ovulaires d'un oeuf à terme. *Gynecol Obstet* 1934;29:385

3. Burger K. Weitere Erfahrungen über die kunstliche Scheidenbildung mit Eihäuten. *Zentralbl Gynäkol* 1947;69:1153

4. Trelford JD, Hanson FW, Anderson DG. Amniotic membrane as a living surgical dressing in human patients. *Oncology* 1973;28:358

5. Trelford JD, Anderson D, Hanson F, *et al.* Amniotic membrane used for radical vulvectomies. *Obstet Gynecol Observ* 1973;12:1

6. Trelford JD, Hanson FW, Anderson DS. The feasibility of making an artificial vagina at the time of anterior exenteration. *Oncology* 1973;28:398

7. Trelford-Sauder M, Telford JD, Matolo NM. Replacement of the peritoneum with amnion following pelvic exenteration. *Surg Gynecol Obstet* 1977;145:699

8. Tancer ML, Katz M, Veridiano NP. Vaginal epithelialization with human amnion. *Obstet Gynecol* 1979;54:345

9. Dhall K. Amnion graft for treatment of congenital absence of the vagina. *Br J Obstet Gynaecol* 1984;91:279

10. Ashworth MF, Morton KE, Dewhurst J, *et al.* Vaginoplasty using amnion. *Obstet Gynecol* 1986;67:443

11. Nisolle M, Donnez J. Vaginoplasty using amniotic membranes in cases of vaginal agenesis or after vaginectomy. *J Gynecol Surg* 1992;8:25–30

12. Badylak SF, Kropp B, McPherson T, *et al.* Small intestinal submucosa: a rapidly resorbed bioscaffold for augmentation cystoplasty in a dog model. *Tissue Engineering* 1998;4:379–87

13. Kropp BP, Ludlow JK, Spicer D, *et al.* Rabbit urethral regeneration using small intestinal submucosa onlay grafts. *Urology* 1998;52:138–42

14. Frank RT. The formation of an artificial vagina without operation. *Am J Obstet Gynecol* 1938;35:1053

15. Williams EA. Congenital absence of the vagina – a simple operation for its relief. *J Obstet Gynaecol Br Commonw* 1964;71:511

16. Baldwin JF. The formation of an artificial vagina by intestinal transplantation. *Ann Surg* 1904;40:398

17. Turner-Warwick R, Kirby RS. The construction and reconstruction of the vagina with the colocecum. *Surg Gynecol Obstet* 1990;170:132

18. Wharton LR. A simple method of constructing a vagina. *Ann Surg* 1938;107:842

19. Heath PM, Woods JE, Podratz KC, *et al.* Gracilis myocutaneous vaginal reconstruction. *Mayo Clin Proc* 1984;59:21

20. Lagasse LD, Berman ML, Watring WG, *et al.* (1978). The gynecologic oncology patient: restoration of function and prevention of disability. In McGowan L, ed. *Gynecologic Oncology.* New York: Appleton-Century-Crofts, 1978:398

21. Lacey PM, Morrow CP. Myocutaneous vaginal reconstruction. In Morrow CP, Smart GE, eds. *Gynecologic Oncology.* Berlin: Springer-Verlag, 1986:255

22. Wheeless CR. Vulvar-vaginal reconstruction. In Coppleson M, ed. *Gynecologic Oncology: Fundamental Principles and Clinical Practice.* Edinburgh: Churchill Livingstone, 1981;2:933

23. McCraw JB, Massey FM, Shanklin KD, *et al.* Vaginal reconstruction with gracilis myocutaneous flaps. *Plast Reconstr Surg* 1976;58:176

24. Gordon RT, Thomas GD. Vaginal and pelvic reconstruction with distally based rectus abdominis myocutaneous flaps. *Plast Reconstr Surg* 1988;81:71

25. Wee TK, Joseph VT. A new technique of vaginal reconstruction using neurovascular pudendal-thigh flaps: a preliminary report. *Plast Reconstr Surg* 1989;83:701

26. Dino BR, Eufemio GG, De Villa MS. Human amnion: the establishment of an amnion bank and its practical applications in surgery. *J Philippine Med Assoc* 1966;42:357

27. Faulk WP, Matthews R, Stevens PJ, *et al.* Human amnion as an adjunct in wound healing. *Lancet* 1980;1:1156

28. Akle CA, Adinolfi M, Welsh KI, *et al.* Immunogenicity of human amniotic epithelial cells after transplantation into volunteers. *Lancet* 1980;2:1003

Müllerian fusion defects: septoplasty and hemihysterectomy of the rudimentary horns

42

M. Nisolle and J. Donnez

The endoscopic technique for the management of uterine septa was first proposed in 1970 by Edström and Fernström[1] but the method has only become widely used in recent years.

In the past, whenever a patient presented with a Müllerian fusion defect that was thought to be the cause of recurrent pregnancy loss, a Jones, Strassman, or Tompkins procedure would be performed by laparotomy. These procedures required lengthy anesthesia and surgery could be complicated by infection or hemorrhage, necessitating antibiotic treatment and blood transfusions. Also, because the full thickness of the uterine fundus was surgically damaged during the procedure, the patient would require Cesarean section for future deliveries. Some women became infertile as a result of adhesions or tubal occlusion, developing secondary to the procedure itself.

Many Müllerian fusion defects are amenable to hysteroscopic treatment. Several different procedures have been adopted, with more or less similar results. The basic concept involves the transcervical observation of the uterine septum by means of hysteroscopy, followed by its resection[2-5]. The use of an operative hysteroscope allows the passage of surgical instruments.

UTERINE SEPTUM: PARTIAL AND COMPLETE

Prevalence and diagnosis

Uterine septum is the most common Müllerian fusion defect. Its incidence in the general population is estimated to be 1.8%[6].

Between 1986 and 1996 in our department, 170 patients underwent a hysteroscopic septoplasty with the help of the neodymium : yttrium–aluminum–garnet (Nd : YAG) laser (Table 1)[7]. In 83% of cases (141/170), the uterine septum was partial (Figure 1) and, in 17% of cases (29/170), the uterine septum was complete with cervical duplication. A vaginal septum was noted in 15 cases (9%). The diagnosis of a complete uterine septum may be delayed, particularly if a vaginal septum is associated[8]. Indeed, the vaginal septum can easily be misdiagnosed by gynecological examination, and at hysterosalpingography the uterus may appear to be unicornuate, except if there is a fistula between the two uterine cavities (Figure 2). However, in the absence of a vaginal septum, the diagnosis is simple because two distinct external cervical orifices are clearly visible. The opacification through these

Table 1 Hysteroscopic septoplasty in 170 patients (1986–1996)

	Number of cases	
Partial uterine septum	141	(83%)
Complete uterine septum	29	(17%)
no vaginal septum	14	(8%)
vaginal septum	15	(9%)
Nd : YAG laser septoplasty		
in two steps (1986–93)	10	
in one step (1994–96)	19	

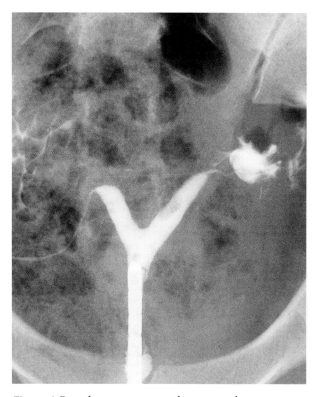

Figure 1 Partial uterine septum: hysterography

two orifices allows the diagnosis of a septate uterus with cervical duplication.

The traditional liquid distension medium used to be dextran 70 or a solution of 5% dextrose; however, glycine is now preferred by most authors. This medium is not viscous, permits a clear visual field and is not a conductor of electricity. If electricity is not used, saline or Ringer's lactate can be employed. These are well tolerated when

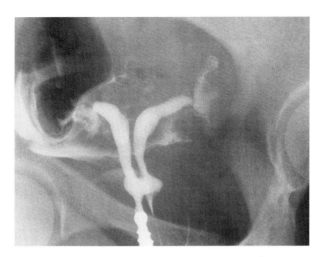

Figure 2 Complete uterine septum (uterocervical septum) with a fistula between the two uterine cavities

absorbed into the system and represent an advantage of the laser.

Instruments

Various instruments can be used for the resection of the septum: miniature scissors or semi-rigid miniature scissors which permit the required pressure but are small enough to pass through the hysteroscopic operating sheath and along the cervical canal with no difficulty or risk. The blades can be opened wide enough to allow resection of even thick septa. Other surgeons prefer to use the resectoscope[9–11]. High-frequency electric sources are advised for safety reasons.

The resectoscope has several advantages: it is inexpensive and readily available in most operating rooms, as well as being simple to operate and highly efficient at removing the septum. Finally, others have suggested the use of lasers for this type of hysteroscopic surgery[12–14].

Argon, krypton, KTP/532 and Nd : YAG lasers have all been successfully employed in the resection of uterine septa. However, certain limiting factors must be taken into consideration. First, hyskon should not be used because caramelization can prove troublesome and may damage the laser fiber, resulting in delay while fibers are replaced or repaired. Second, the surgeon must be thoroughly acquainted with the physics of the particular laser being used. Third, only bare fibers should be used: CO_2-conducting fibers may cause bubbling of the medium which may lead to gas embolism, cardiovascular compromise and even death.

The Nd : YAG laser uses a solid-state rig (garnet) in which the neodymium atoms play the active lasing role. The energy is supplied by a flashlight lamp which illuminates the rod. Both are housed in a container called the resonator. The resonator is ellipsoid and its inner surface is coated with a highly reflective material. The lamp and the rod are placed at the two focal points of the ellipsoid. The

light emitted by the lamp is reflected by the internal coating of the resonator and is collected, almost in its entirety, by the rod positioned at the opposite focal point.

In contrast to the CO_2 laser, the beams of the Nd : YAG laser propagate well through commercially available glass fibers, very much like visible light. The propagation is effected by a chain of internal reflections occurring at the boundaries of the glass fiber. Hence, the delivery devices used in Nd : YAG lasers are a variety of fibers (see below) equipped with a connector that attaches to the output port of the laser system.

Manufacturers offer Nd : YAG laser units featuring different maximum powers, from 40 to 100 Watts. Nd : YAG laser systems are composed of:

(1) A laser head or resonator;

(2) A power supply, which furnishes the flashlight lamp with the necessary electrical energy;

(3) A closed-circuit water-cooling system, further chilled by a radiator which removes excess heat from the resonator;

(4) A control system, based on a microcomputer;

(5) A helium–neon laser tube;

(6) An output-port optical assembly to which the external glass fiber is attached.

The accessories offered with Nd : YAG systems are almost exclusively fibers. They fall into two categories:

(1) Non-contact fibers, whose distal end is flat and highly polished. They operate at a short distance from the tissue, in order to create deep coagulation. A well-known example of their use is in the treatment of superficial bladder tumors, where the fibers are inserted through a cystoscope. Non-contact fibers have no incision capability. These fibers are usually reusable. However, after a limited number of surgical procedures, they must be repolished with the aid of a special polishing kit.

(2) Contact fibers, featuring a sharpened sculpted conical tip. The laser radiation is concentrated at the very narrow tip and the fiber functions like a hot knife, capable of performing fine incisions when in contact with the tissue. Moreover, the tapered fiber prevents the rays from progressing forwards, while enabling their exit through the sides of the tip. The end result is that the forward penetration is reduced, much as in the case of the CO_2 laser. The side radiation, on the other hand, produces a hemostatic effect on the lateral surfaces of the wedge created by the incision. Contact fibers are used in a variety of configurations for freehand and endoscopic applications. They feature different shapes (conical, hemispherical) and different diameters (400, 600, 800 and 100 µm). They are offered as disposable, single-use, sterilized fibers.

Recently, new types of fibers have been introduced onto the market. These fibers possess a polished distal face which is inclined with respect to the fiber axis. This angle enables the fiber to emit the laser beam at right angles to its long axis. Employed transurethrally, these fibers are used to treat benign prostatic hypertrophy by coagulating the adenoma. Another type of fiber, emanating lateral diffusive radiation from an elongated segment located at its distal end, is used for interstitial laser thermotherapy of benign and malignant lesions.

Partial uterine septum

With the help of the 'bare fiber', the surgeon begins the resection of the septum (Figure 3), continuing until it has been resected almost flush with the surrounding endometrium. Regardless of the type of medium employed, the surgeon must be able to see the right and left cornual regions completely and keep the septum in view at all times. Concurrent laparoscopy at the time of hysteroscopic resection is recommended to confirm the diagnosis but is not mandatory if the diagnosis has previously been confirmed.

The septum is cut using the 'touch technique' (Figure 3a and b). The hysteroscope with the laser fiber is advanced and melts away the septum, while visual contact

is maintained with the right and left uterine ostia. The mean time of hysteroscopic resection is < 15 min. The risk of fluid overload is therefore minimal.

The most delicate part of the procedure is probably deciding exactly when the resection is sufficient, and when continuing would cause damage to the myometrium and immediate complications, such as perforation, or more delayed complications, such as uterine rupture during

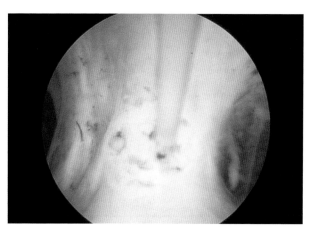

Figure 3 (a) Resection of the uterine septum is carried out with the help of the Nd : YAG laser

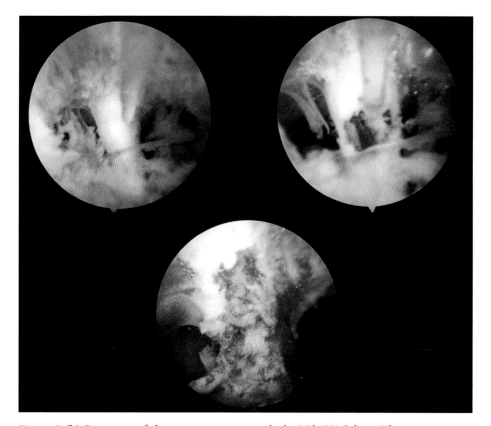

Figure 3 (b) Resection of the uterine septum with the Nd : YAG laser. The septum is cut using the touch technique. The hysteroscope with the laser fiber is advanced and the septum is melted away by simply advancing the bare fiber

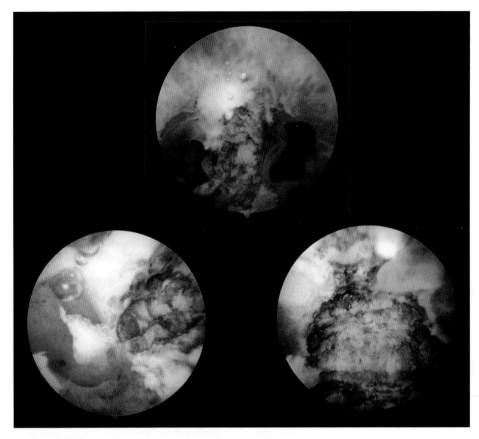

Figure 3 (c) Resection of the uterine septum with the Nd : YAG laser. Resection is stopped when the area between the tubal ostia is a line

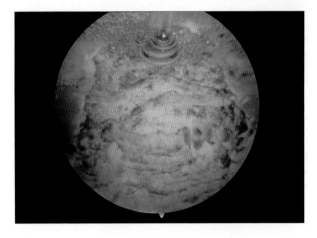

Figure 3 (d) Resection of the uterine septum with the Nd : YAG laser; final view

pregnancy. Almost all surgeons stop resection when the area between the tubal ostia is a line (Figure 3c and d). Simultaneous laparoscopic control is extremely useful for this purpose, especially for beginners. Querleu and associates[15] use echography to distinguish the septum from the myometrium, and thus the decision to stop the resection is easily made.

Complete uterine septum

For many years, only partial septal defects were treated hysteroscopically and wide (> 2 cm) or complete septal defects were corrected via an abdominal metroplasty. Donnez and co-workers[13,14,16], however, described a method that allows even complete septal defects to be managed hysteroscopically (Figures 4 and 5a and b). Rock and colleagues[17] proposed the use of the resectoscope for the lysis of a complete uterine septum by means of a new method which makes it possible to leave the cervical septum intact, thus avoiding any subsequent cervical incompetence. To treat a complete uterine septum, they describe a one-stage method where the other cervical os is occluded with the balloon of a Foley catheter, in order to prevent loss of the distending medium. They believe that it is better not to remove the cervical canal, since this might lead to subsequent cervical incompetence. We do not agree with this hypothesis, and all complete uterine septa are removed using the following surgical procedure, previously performed in two steps, but now in one.

In some cases, not only may a double cervical canal be observed, but a vaginal sagittal septum may also be present in the upper vagina or throughout its length (Figure 6a). First, the vaginal septum (if present) is resected using a CO_2 laser or unipolar coagulation (Figure 6b). Both

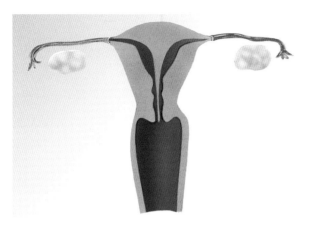

Figure 4 Complete uterine septum dividing the uterine cavity and cervix into two parts

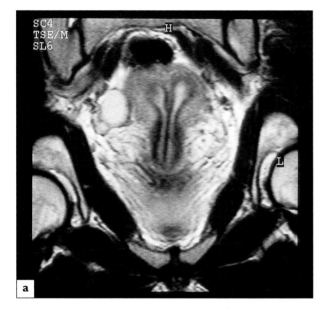

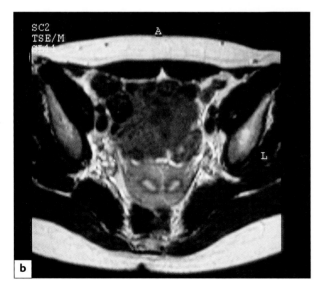

Figure 5 Magnetic resonance imaging clearly shows the presence of (a) a complete uterine septum and (b) two separate cervices

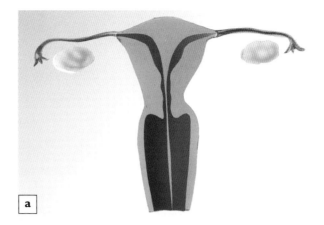

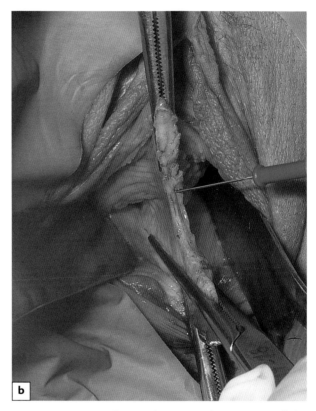

Figure 6 (a) Vaginal sagittal septum; (b) resection of the vaginal septum using unipolar coagulation

cervices are dilated (Figure 7a) and the cervical septum is then incised with scissors (Figure 7b) or with a CO_2 laser connected to a colposcope, until the lower portion of the uterine septum is seen. After section of the cervical septum, the external cervical os appears completely normal (Figure 7c). In the past, the second step was performed 2 months after the first operation. Now, however, Nd : YAG laser resection of the uterine septum is carried out during the same procedure. The hysteroscope is advanced while visual contact is maintained with the right and left uterine ostia. Because the septum is poorly vascularized, bleeding is usually minimal. When this procedure was carried out in two steps, hysterosalpingography demonstrated the presence of a normal, single cervical

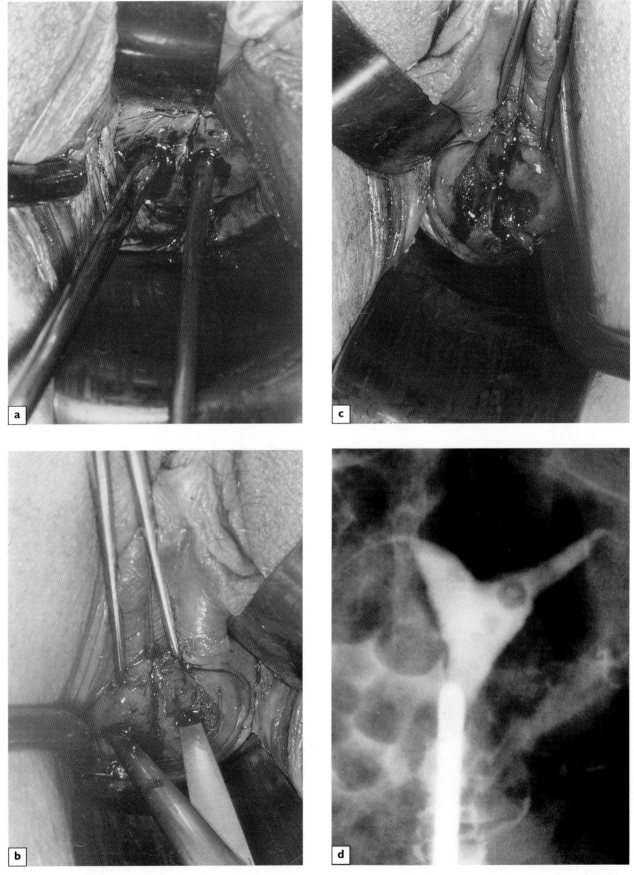

Figure 7 (a) Dilatation of both cervical canals; (b) the cervical septum is incised with scissors; (c) the external cervical os is completely normal; (d) postoperative hysterography: the morphology of the uterine cavity resembles an arcuate uterus

canal 2 months after the first step and a normal uterine cavity 2 months after the second step. Nowadays, all cases of complete uterine septa with or without a vaginal septum are managed in one step.

A double cervix and septate vagina with a normal uterus is an unusual Müllerian anomaly, inconsistent with the current understanding of Müllerian development[18,19]. In such cases, the vaginal septum and the cervical septum can be removed as previously described.

Pre- and postoperative management

Following excision of very wide septa, the surgeon's vision may be obscured by pieces of resected tissue and, at times, by uterine bleeding. The Nd : YAG laser produces no debris and carries a reduced risk of bleeding. Several authors have suggested preoperative treatment with danazol or luteinizing hormone releasing hormone (LHRH) agonists; others[11] inject a solution of pitressin into the cervix. Neither pitressin nor hormone administration is required with laser therapy.

Although preoperative hormonal therapy causes atrophy of the endometrium and reduces vascularization and intraoperative bleeding, it also reduces the depth of the myometrium and therefore increases the risk of perforation and/or myometrial damage. It is suggested that surgery be performed immediately after the end of menstrual bleeding. Postoperatively, a broad-spectrum antibiotic is administered for 3–4 days.

In order to avoid the risk of synechiae, an intrauterine device (IUD, Multiload®) is inserted into the uterine cavity. Hormone replacement therapy with estrogens (100–200 µg of ethinylestradiol) and progestogens (5–15 mg lynestrenol) is given for 3 months. De Cherney and co-workers, however, use neither hormone replacement therapy nor IUDs[9]. Formerly, Perino and associates[20] both administered estrogens and medroxyprogesterone and inserted IUDs, but they have recently abandoned these measures and now administer no postoperative therapy. Hamou[11] performs a hysteroscopic procedure 1 month after surgery in order to separate synechiae, if necessary.

Almost all authors agree that a follow-up examination should be performed 1–2 months after the operation, irrespective of the postoperative management. Inspection can be made either by means of hysterosalpingography or hysteroscopy. Hamou performs a hysteroscopic inspection 1 month after resection of the septum; in his opinion, this is early enough to prevent the development of synechiae.

In our department, the postoperative morphology of the uterine cavity is systematically evaluated 4 months after the resection. One month after the removal of the IUD, a hysterosalpingography is carried out; the morphology of the uterine cavity almost always resembles an arcuate uterus (Figure 7d). Indeed, it is preferable not to resect the septum too much, but to leave a sufficient depth of myometrium at the top of the uterus. Hysteroscopy was performed in a first series[16] to confirm that re-epithelialization of the resected endometrial area had occurred. Nowadays, this procedure is not performed systematically.

Results and complications

De Cherney and associates[9] reported the successful use of the urological resectoscope in 72 women, with a term pregnancy rate of 89%. The full-term pregnancy rate reported in various studies ranges from 81% to 89%. Table 2 shows the results of hysteroplasty from the literature, with a pregnancy rate of 86%[3,9,10,21–23].

Operative hysteroscopy is a safe and effective method for the management of uterine septa that are associated with recurrent pregnancy loss, and it makes future vaginal delivery possible. In one of our series of 17 complete uterine septa, 10 out of 17 women became pregnant and no signs of cervical incompetence were observed[8]. Prophylactic cerclage was never performed after resection of a complete cervical and uterine septum. Following hysteroscopic metroplasty, Cesarean section should be performed only for obstetric reasons.

In our series, intraoperative and postoperative complications were encountered in only three cases (1.8%). Classic intraoperative complications, such as fluid overload, hemorrhage, or perforation, could result from the

Table 2 Results of hysteroscopic treatment for uterine septum. From Donnez and Nisolle[7]

Authors	Patients treated	Pregnancies	Pregnancies > 1st trimester		Miscarriages	
Corson & Batzer 1986[10]	18	17	14	(82.3%)	3	(17.6%)
de Cherney et al. 1986[9]	72	72	64	(89%)	8	(11%)
Fayez 1986[21]	19	16	14	(87.5%)	2	(12.5%)
Valle & Sciarra 1986[3]	12	13	11	(84.6%)	2	(15.4%)
March 1987[22]	66	63	55	(87.3%)	8	(12.7%)
Blanc et al. 1994[23]	45	31	25	(81%)	6	(19.3%)
Total	232	212	183	(86%)	29	(13.7%)

hysteroscopic procedure itself. In our series of 170 patients, no fluid overload or hemorrhage was encountered and a perforation was noted in only one case. This was due to the fact that the patient had already undergone a uterine septum resection a few months before, which was considered to be insufficient. The postoperative hysterosalpingography revealed a persistent uterine septum which needed to be resected a second time. Upon diagnosis of the perforation, laparoscopy enabled us to exclude serious complications such as bowel damage or hemorrhage. In 1996, Fedele and colleagues[24] suggested that a remaining uterine septum of less than 1 cm after hysteroscopic metroplasty does not impair reproductive outcome and therefore does not require a second hysteroscopic surgical procedure.

A postoperative complication which was encountered in another hospital was uterine rupture during delivery. This occurred in two cases of twin pregnancy in which the deliveries were very long, taking more than 24 h. The patients finally delivered by emergency Cesarean section. The babies lived and the myometrium was sutured in each case. In both cases, the rupture occurred at the fundus of the uterus. Obviously, in normal conditions, the delivery can be performed vaginally following a uterine septum resection, but, in the case of multiple pregnancies, Cesarean section should be considered.

NON-COMMUNICATING RUDIMENTARY HORNS

Pregnancy in a non-communicating rudimentary horn (Figure 8a and b) is uncommon and usually results in abortion or uterine rupture. At hysterography, a hemi-uterus is diagnosed; indeed, the non-communicating rudimentary horn is not opacified. Pregnancies in a non-communicating rudimentary horn are due to transmigration of sperm into the Fallopian tube of the affected horn. Most complications occur within the first 20 weeks, the most severe being uterine rupture and maternal death. Raman and colleagues[25] recently described a 17-week pregnancy occurring in a rudimentary horn, treated by laparotomy and excision. In order to avoid maternal complications, we systematically perform excision of the rudimentary horn. A laparoscopic hemihysterectomy can easily be carried out using the same techniques as for laparoscopic hysterectomy.

In rare cases, such non-communicating rudimentary horns can lead to dysmenorrhea and should then be laparoscopically removed (Figure 9).

A Foley catheter is inserted during surgery to empty the bladder. Four laparoscopic puncture sites including the umbilicus are used: 10-mm umbilical, 5-mm right, 5-mm medial and 5-mm left lower quadrant sites.

These are located just above the pubic hairline and lateral incisions are made next to the deep epigastric vessels. A cannula is placed in the single cervix for appro-

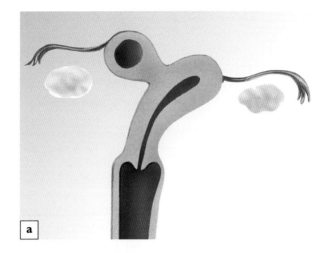

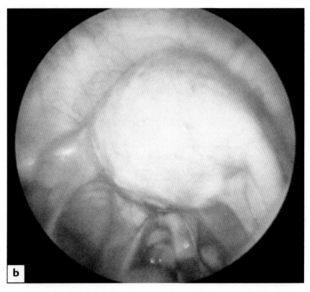

Figure 8 (a) Non-communicating rudimentary horn; (b) laparoscopic view of left non-communicating rudimentary horn

priate uterine mobilization. Bipolar forceps are used to compress and desiccate the fibrous tissue between the horns (Figure 9a). The tissue is then cut with scissors and with a CO_2 laser. Bipolar coagulation is used to coagulate the pedicle. Scissor division is carried out close to the line of desiccation to ensure that a compressed pedicle remains. The mesosalpinx is then cut (Figure 9b). If necessary, the peritoneum of the vesico-uterine space is grasped and elevated with forceps, while the scissors dissect the vesico-uterine space. Aquadissection may be used to separate the leaves of the broad ligament, distending the vesico-uterine space and defining the tendinous attachments of the bladder in this area, which are coagulated and cut. The tube of the affected horn is then removed (Figure 9c).

The external tubal vessel is identified and exposed by applying traction to the adnex with opposite forceps. The dissection of the two horns is performed as follows. If there is true separation of the two horns, the fibrous tissue is

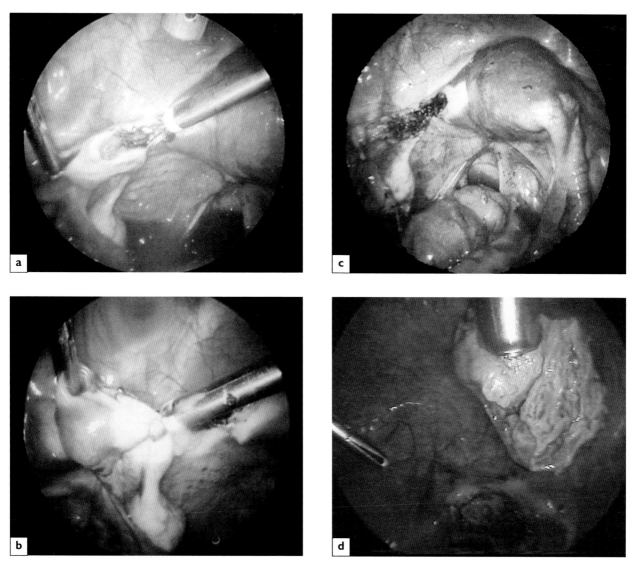

Figure 9 (a) Coagulation and section of fibrous tissue separating two horns; (b) coagulation and section of the mesosalpinx and the tube; (c) final view; (d) removal of the horn with the help of the Steiner morcellator

coagulated with bipolar coagulation and then cut with scissors or with the CO_2 laser. If there is no external separation of the two horns, the dissection is more difficult; after coagulation, the myometrium must be cut in order to allow the removal of the rudimentary horn. For this purpose, bipolar coagulation and the CO_2 laser or the Nd : YAG laser fiber can be used to achieve coagulation and resection of the myometrium.

In the past, the rudimentary horn was removed either through the trocar of the laparoscope, or through a posterior colpotomy in cases of larger rudimentary horns.

Nowadays, removal of large rudimentary horns is carried out with the help of a morcellator (Steiner morcellator) (Figure 9d) (Storz, Tuttlingen, Germany) previously described for the removal of the uterus in laparoscopic supracervical hysterectomy[26].

This procedure has been successfully performed in our department on 14 women up to 1996. Of the eight who

desired pregnancy, six became pregnant and had a normal vaginal delivery (> 36 weeks), except one woman on whom Cesarean section was performed for fetal reasons.

REFERENCES

1. Edström K, Fernström I. The diagnostic possibilities of a modified hysteroscopic technique. *Acta Obstet Gynecol Scand* 1970;49:327

2. Chervenak FA, Neuwirth RS. Hysteroscopic resection of the uterine septum. *Am J Obstet Gynecol* 1981;141:351

3. Valle RF, Sciarra JJ. Hysteroscopic resection of the septate uterus. *Obstet Gynecol* 1986;67:253

4. Valle RF. Hysteroscopic treatment of partial and complete uterine septum. *Int J Fertil* 1996;41: 310–15

5. Gallinat A. Endometrial ablation using the Nd-YAG laser in CO_2 hysteroscopy. In Leuken RP, Gallinat A, eds. *Endoscopic Surgery in Gynecology*. Berlin: Demeter Verlag GmbH, 1993:109–16

6. Ashton D, Amin HK, Richart RM, Neuwirth RS. The incidence of symptomatic uterine anomalies in women undergoing transcervical tubal sterilization. *Obstet Gynecol* 1988;72:28–30

7. Donnez J, Nisolle M. Endoscopic laser treatment of uterine malformations. *Hum Reprod* 1997;12: 1381–7

8. Nisolle M, Donnez J. Letter to the Editor. *Fertil Steril* 1995;63:934–5

9. De Cherney AH, Russel LJB, Graebe RA, *et al*. Resectoscopic management of Müllerian defects. *Fertil Steril* 1986;45:726

10. Corson SL, Batzer FR. CO_2 uterine distension for hysteroscopic septal incision. *J Reprod Med* 1986;31: 710

11. Hamou J. Electroresection of fibroids. In Sutton C, Diamond M, eds. *Endoscopic Surgery for Gynaecologists*. London: Saunders, 1993:327–30

12. Daniell JF, Osher S, Miller W. Hysteroscopic resection of uterine septa with visible light laser energy. *Colpos Gynecol Laser Surg* 1987;3:217

13. Nisolle M, Donnez J. Müllerian fusion defects: septoplasty and hemihysterectomy of the rudimentary horns. In Donnez J, Nisolle M, eds. *An Atlas of Laser Operative Laparoscopy and Hysteroscopy*. Carnforth, UK: Parthenon Publishing, 1994:295–304

14. Nisolle M, Donnez J. Endoscopic treatment of uterine malformations. *Gynecol Endoscop* 1996;5:155–60

15. Querleu D, Brasme TL, Parmentier D. Ultrasoundguided transcervical metroplasty. *Fertil Steril* 1990; 54:995–8

16. Donnez J, Nisolle M. Operative laser hysteroscopy in Müllerian fusion defects and uterine adhesions. In Donnez J, ed. *Laser Operative Laparoscopy and Hysteroscopy*. Leuven: Nauwelaerts Printing, 1989:249–61

17. Rock JA, Murphy AA, Cooper WH. Resectoscopic technique for the lysis of a class V complete uterine septum. *Fertil Steril* 1987;48:495

18. Candiani M, Busacca M, Natale A, Sambruni I. Bicervical uterus and septate vagina: report of a previously undescribed Müllerian anomaly. *Hum Reprod* 1996;11:218–19

19. Goldberg JM, Falcone T. Double cervix and vagina with a normal uterus: an unusual Müllerian anomaly. *Hum Reprod* 1996;11:1350–1

20. Perino A, Mencaglia L, Hamou J, Cittadini E. Hysteroscopy for metroplasty of uterine septa: report of 24 cases. *Fertil Steril* 1987;48:321

21. Fayez JA. Comparison between abdominal and hysteroscopic metroplasty. *Obstet Gynecol* 1986;70: 399–406

22. March CM, Israel R. Hysteroscopic management of recurrent abortion caused by the septate uterus. *Am J Obstet Gynecol* 1987;156:834–42

23. Blanc B, d'Ercole C, Gaiato ML, Boubli L. Le traitement endoscopique des cloisons utérines. *J Gynecol Obstet Biol Reprod* 1994;23:596–601

24. Fedele L, Bianchi S, Marchini M, *et al*. Residual uterine septum of less than 1 cm after hysteroscopic metroplasty does not impair reproductive outcome. *Hum Reprod* 1996;11:727–9

25. Raman S, Tai C, Neom HS. Non-communicating rudimentary horn pregnancy. *J Gynecol Surg* 1993;9: 59–62

26. Donnez J, Nisolle M. Laparoscopic supracervical (subtotal) hysterectomy (LASH). *J Gynecol Surg* 1993;9:91–4

43

Fetal endoscopy

C. Hubinont

INTRODUCTION

The first fetal endoscopic visualization was reported in 1954, using a 10-mm hysteroscope in early pregnancy[1]. In the 1970s, before the development of real-time ultrasound, fetoscopy was used for prenatal diagnosis and therapy despite a limited optical system[2-5]. In the 1980s, the fetoscopic approach was progressively replaced by percutaneous ultrasound guidance techniques as the resolution of modern equipment improved. Finally, it was abandoned until the early 1990s.

Thanks to technological progress in the size, field of view and image quality of fiberoptic endoscopes, Quintero and colleagues[6] described a new approach with a 21-gauge trocar introduced transabdominally even during the first trimester of pregnancy, for early prenatal diagnosis and for some specific therapeutic alternatives.

A review of fetal endoscopy diagnostic and surgical applications is discussed in this chapter.

TECHNIQUES

The types of fetal endoscopy reported in the literature (embryoscopy and fetoscopy) relate more to the gestational age at which the procedure is performed than to the route used (either transabdominal or transcervical).

Embryoscopy

Embryoscopy (between weeks 8 and 12) was first performed using transcervical introduction of the endoscope into the extraembryonic celom[7,8]. The material used was a rigid 1.7 fiber endoscope in a 2-mm sheath, equipped with a side channel for saline infusion. The technique was improved using smaller size endoscopes (20-gauge needle and 0.7-mm endoscope) and a safer transabdominal route (Figure 1). It was reported in the literature under the name of transabdominal thin-gauge embryofetoscopy or TGEF[6]. In our experience as well as that of others's[9] (Figure 2), a semi-rigid 1-mm diameter endoscope (ART 11510, Karl Storz, Tuttlingen, Germany) introduced in an 18-gauge trocar can be used transabdominally as early as 10 weeks' gestation and, in most of the cases, provides a clear view of the fetus (Figures 3–5).

Fetoscopy

Fetoscopy (from the second to the third trimester) has been reported previously[1-5]. The first endoscopes used for this purpose had a large diameter of up to 6.8 mm. Their applications included both diagnostic (Figure 6) and therapeutic aspects. However, with improvements in ultrasound, their use in diagnosis has decreased while their role

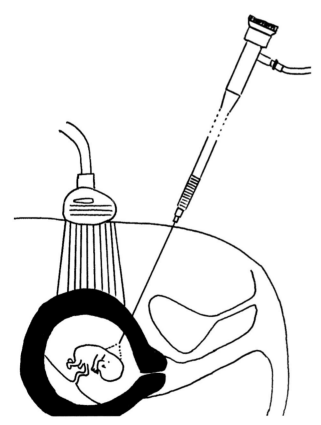

Figure 1 Fetoscopy technique

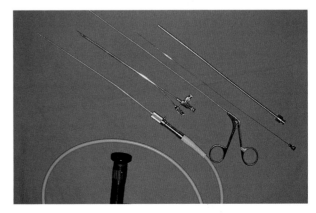

Figure 2 Fetoscopic equipment

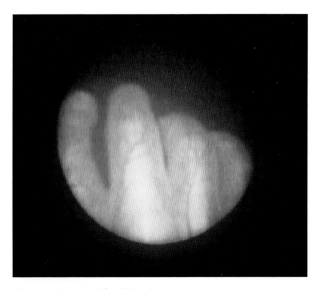

Figure 3 Normal fetal hand

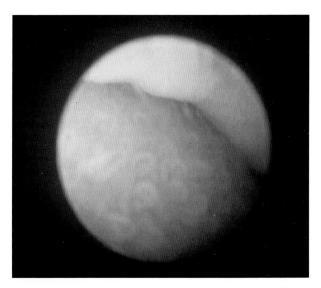

Figure 6 Third-trimester fetoscopy showing a normal fetal upper lip without cleft and, below, the tongue

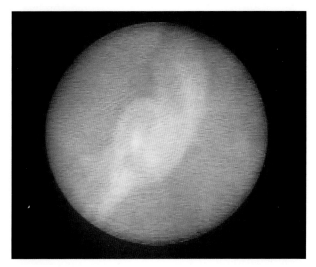

Figure 4 Umbilical cord and vessels

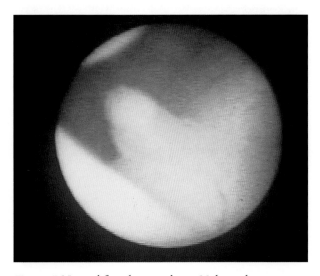

Figure 5 Normal female genitalia at 11th week

as a tool for fetal surgery has emerged during the last decade.

Ultrasound guidance is necessary for both routes in order to avoid the placenta and to rule out any unknown multiple pregnancy or miscarriage. In case of bleeding, saline or Ringer's lactate may be amnioinfused in order to improve the fetal view[6]. The use of CO_2 could induce acidosis and should be avoided[10]. Glycine, used safely in animal models, may be a potential alternative[11]. The procedure can be performed on an outpatient basis under local or locoregional anesthesia. Anti-D prophylaxis should be administered to Rhesus-negative patients. Antibiotics are given routinely in case of transcervical procedures[7].

INDICATIONS

Primary diagnostic endoscopy

Prenatal diagnosis by fetal endoscopy should be offered in three distinct clinical conditions.

Suspicion of a first-trimester abnormality

As early endovaginal ultrasound is now able to diagnose major congenital anomalies[12] and as amniocentesis is indicated for aneuploidy diagnosis, fetoscopy may be performed to confirm rapidly the final diagnosis. Fetoscopy may also be performed prior to dilatation and curettage for fetal anomaly in order to exclude an unsuspected polymalformative syndrome. We previously reported two cases of conjoined twins in which combined ultrasound and endoscopy enabled us to confirm the diagnosis and allowed early termination of the pregnancies[13] (Figure 7). Several cases of first-trimester anomalies confirmed by fetoscopy have been reported, such as multiple amniotic band syndrome[14] and omphalocele[15]. Suspicion of neural tube defects in the presence of increased alpha-fetoprotein and a non-contributive ultrasound was also excluded by fetoscopy[8].

Patients at risk of polymalformative syndromes

Polymalformative syndromes affecting at least the face and/or the limb extremities are listed in Table 1. In patients with genetic syndromes transmitted with either recessive or dominant inheritance, fetoscopic diagnosis may be performed at an earlier gestational age than ultrasound. Among hand anomalies, mono-, a-, syn-, brachy-, campo-, clino- and polydactylism (Figure 8) may be diagnosed. A week-10 prenatal diagnosis of polydactylism associated with recurrent Meckel–Gruber syndrome has been reported[16]. Smith–Lemli–Opitz type II syndrome[17] and Ellis van Creveld syndrome[6] were both diagnosed at the 11th week in the presence of polydactylism. Gross facial anomalies such as cleft lip, anophthalmia and ear aplasia may be confirmed by fetoscopy as early as the 10th week, as reported in a prenatal diagnosis of Fraser cryptophthalmos syndrome[18]. Robert's syndrome was excluded at 12 weeks as no gross facial and limb malformations were

seen[19]. Albinism was also diagnosed by fetoscopic view of fetal hair color[20]. The presence of club foot may also be diagnosed by fetoscopy (Figure 9).

Early fetal tissue sampling

Evans and colleagues[21] reported two cases of endoscopically assisted fetal muscle biopsy performed for prenatal diagnosis of Duchenne muscular dystrophy. Endoscopic guidance allowed an earlier gestational age diagnosis with an accurate site of biopsy. First-trimester umbilical vessel sampling was reported using transabdominal fetoscopy between 8 and 12 weeks[22]. Directed skin biopsies in order to diagnose rare genodermatoses, such as junctional epidermolysis bullosa[23] or trichothiodystrophy[24], have been recently reported.

Secondary therapeutic endoscopy

Endoscopic fetoplacental surgery is now recognized as an effective alternative therapy in severe twin-to-twin transfusion syndrome (TTTS) and umbilical cord ligation in abnormal twin pregnancy. Some other experimental applications, such as obstructive uropathy and congenital diaphragmatic hernia, have also been reported. For these indications, a larger diameter sheath (> 2 mm) and parallel ports should be employed in order to use graspers, scissors, knots pushers and laser fibers. Fetal endoscopic surgery (Fetendo) requires ethical consideration about its related risks and potential benefits for the fetus (Figure 10).

Twin-to-twin syndrome

TTTS is a severe complication of monochorionic diamniotic twin pregnancy with an incidence ranging from 2 to 35%[25,26]. The pathophysiological mechanism is an unbalanced intertwin hemodynamic flow at the level of some type of placental vascular anastomoses[25–27]. The

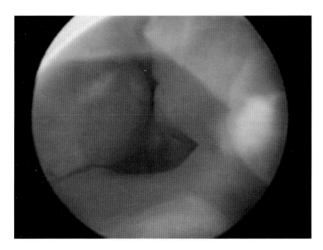

Figure 7 Thoraco-omphalopagus conjoined twins

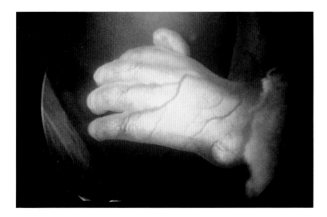

Figure 8 Hexadactylism

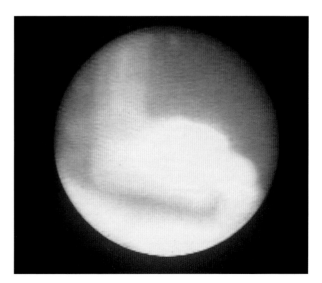

Figure 9 Club foot associated with neural tube defect

439

Table I Polymalformative syndromes and teratogenic embryopathy

---

Polymalformative syndromes associated with facial anomalies

Antley–Bixler (midfacial hypoplasia, dysplastic ear, radiohumeral synostosis) (AR)

EEC (ectodermic dysplasia, syndactyly, cleft lip) (AD)

Fraser cryptophthalmos (hidden eyes, syndactyly, renal, genital anomalies) (AR)

Frontonasal dysplasia sequence (unknown)

Hay–Wells (cleft lip, ectodermal dysplasia) (AD)

Majewsky short rib–polydactyly type II (cleft lip, polysyndactyly) (AR)

Meckel–Gruber (encephalocele, polydactyly, kidney dysplasia) (AR)

Mohr or orofacialdigital (OFD) type II (bilateral feet and hand polysyndactyly, partial
  cleft) (AR)

Neu Laxova (clino-, syndactyly, cleft lip, exophthalmos, microcephaly) (AR)

Orofacialdigital (OFD) type I (partial cleft, clino-, syn-, polydactyly) (X-linked
  dominant)

Popliteal pterygium or faciogenitopopliteal (cleft lip, genital dysplasia, popliteal
  web)(AD)

Roberts–SC phocomelia (midfacial defect, pseudothalidomide hypomelia) (AR)

Treacher–Collins (malar hypoplasia, ear dystrophy) (AD)

Van der Woude (lip pit, cleft lip) (AD)

Polymalformative syndromes including limb anomalies

Apert (syndactyly, cleft palate, craniosynostosis) (AD)

Baller–Gerold (radial and thumb aplasia or hypoplasia, craniosynostosis) (AR)

Barbet–Biedl (clino-, syn-, polydactyly, obesity, retinal pigmentation) (AR)

Carpenter (syn-, brachy-, polydactyly, acrocephaly) (AR)

Catel–Manzke (index hyperphalangy, cleft palate) (sporadic)

Cerebrocostomandibular (clinodactyly of fifth finger, pterygium colli, micrognathia)(AR)

CHILD (unilateral hypomelia, cardiac defect) (X-linked)

Coffin–Siris (hypoplastic fifth finger, hypoplastic toenails, coarse facies) (AR ?)

Ellis–van Creveld chondroectodermal dysplasia (polydactyly, nail hypoplasia) (AR)

Escobar (multiple pterygia, cleft palate, campto-, syndactyly)(AR)

---

continued

preferential blood transfer from one twin to the other is responsible for the polyhydramnios and plethoric aspect of the recipient twin. The donor twin is generally growth-retarded and has oligohydramnios with a typical aspect of 'stuck twin'[28,29]. In the absence of treatment, the mortality rate of severe TTTS in the pre-viable period reaches 100%[30,31] due to recipient cardiac failure responsible for hydrops and intrauterine fetal death (IUFD)[11,12]. The surviving twin is also at risk of IUFD or, when surviving, may have severe sequelae. Another cause of fetal morbidity in TTTS is the high incidence of preterm labor due to polyhydramnios. It is associated with an increased risk of late miscarriage, severe prematurity and its neonatal sequelae[34].

Given this high fetal mortality rate, TTTS should be treated; medical therapies such as digoxin[35] and indomethacin[36] have been reported to have poor results.

Invasive therapies are now currently offered, including serial amniodrainage[37–41], endoscopic selective coagulation of placental anastomoses[42–44] and interfetal septum amniotomy[45–48]. Selective feticide with endoscopic clamping of the umbilical cord is an alternative when the survival of both twins is not attainable[49,50].

Endoscopic coagulation of placental anastomoses. This technique (Figures 11 and 12) was first reported by the groups of de Lia and Ville[42,43]. The rationale of this therapy is to interrupt the anastomotic blood flow and then to offer a causal treatment[44]. It is often combined with amniodrainage, which may increase its efficacy. Recently, in a series of 67 cases, 82% delivered with an overall survival rate of 69%[42]. Moreover, in a study comparing laser treatment with amniodrainage, Hecher and colleagues reported similar survival rates of 51% versus 61% but a lower inci-

Table I *Continued* Polymalformative syndromes and teratogenic embryopathy

Fg syndrome (clino-, campto, syndactyly, face dysmorphy) (X-linked)

Golaby–Rosen (polydactyly) (X-linked)

Grebe (distal limb deficiency, polydactyly) (AR)

Greig cephalopolysyndactyly (frontal bossing, feet and hand polydactyly) (AD)

Holt–Oram (distal limb hypoplasia, syndactyly, heart defect) (AD)

Levy–Hollister (syn-, clino-absent thumb and radius) (AD)

Miller (postaxial limb deficiency, syndactyly, facial dysmorphy) (AR)

Multiple synostosis (synphalangism, clino-, brachydactyly, face dysplasia) (AD)

Nager syndrome (radial limb hypoplasia, mandibular hypoplasia, ear defects) (?)

Oculodentodigital (microphthalmos, campto-, syndactyly, finger aplasia) (AD)

Otopalatodigital (OPD) type II (face dysmorphy, syn-, polydactyly) (X-linked)

Poland (hand syn-, oligodactyly, thoracic defect) (?)

Rothmund–Thomson (poikiloderma, cataract, absent thumb, syndactyly, club feet) (AR)

Saldino–Noonan or short rib polydactyly type I (syn-, polydactyly, cardiac defect) (AR)

Smith–Lemli–Opitz (syn-, polydactyly, microcephaly, genital anomalies) (AR)

TAR or radial aplasia thrombocytopenia (bilateral radial aplasia) (AR)

Taybi (otopalatodigital (OPD) type I (broad digits, short nails, cleft palate) (X-linked)

Townes–Brocks (hypoplastic fingers, clinodactyly fifth finger)

Teratogenic agent embryopathy

Aminopterin/methotrexate (facial hypoplasia, syndactyly, talipes)

Herpes zoster or fetal varicella (limb hypoplasia, skin scars)

Hydantoin (cleft lip, syndactyly, distal limb hypoplasia)

Retinoic acid (facial dysmorphy, cleft palate, micro- or aniotia, cardiopathy, neural tube defect)

Trimethadione (cleft lip, cardiopathy)

Valproate (cleft lip, midface hypoplasia, neural tube defect)

Warfarin (nasal hypoplasia, limb hypoplasia)

AR, autosomal recessive; AD, autosomal dominant; ?, unknown inheritance

dence of intrauterine demise and neonatal ultrasound brain anomalies in the laser-treated group[44]. The procedure is generally performed percutaneously[43,44] but some cases of anterior placenta required laparotomy for an easier approach[42]. Recently, a selective procedure using ultrasound and endoscopic criteria for pathological anastomoses has been reported[51,52].

Controversy about the technique as well as the potential maternal risk should be resolved by a prospective randomized trial of TTTS treatment with alternative therapy.

Septostomy. This technique, involving intentional rupture of the intertwin septum, was reported by our team following one case of unintentional septostomy which led to an improvement in TTTS[45], and also by Saade and co-workers[46]. Recently, other cases of septostomy have been reported with differing outcomes[47,53] and a prospective randomized trial is now in progress. A possible mechanism

for the therapeutic effect of septostomy could be the equilibration of amniotic fluid between the two sacs, associated with a correction of the unbalanced flow, mainly in the donor umbilical vessels and on the placental surface[54]. The involvement of amniotic fluid pressure changes has been suggested but a recent paper, based on only two cases, reports a similarly increased pressure in both sacs[55]. In the donor twin, the filling of the amniotic sac may decrease cord compression mainly when there is a velamentous insertion, a common finding in TTTS[56]. Another argument for the therapeutic effect of septostomy is the role of the intertwin septum in TTTS, as it is rare in monoamniotic twin pregnancies despite the presence of numerous placental anastomoses[57].

Technically, septostomy could be performed by fetoscopic neodymium : yttrium–aluminum–garnet (Nd-YAG) laser fulguration alone or associated with placental anastomoses coagulation (Figures 13–15). However, in our latest cases, it was performed under ultrasound guidance by

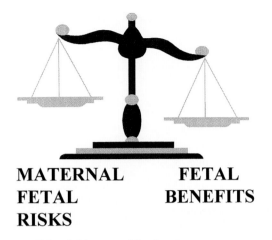

Figure 10 Ethical dilemma of fetal endoscopy

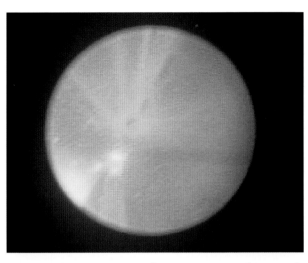

Figure 13 Fetoscopic view of an intertwin membrane with laser-operated coagulation

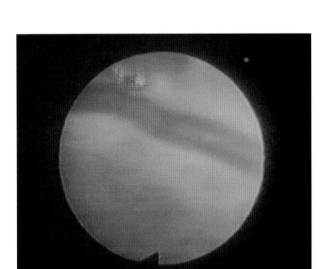

Figure 11 Endoscopic view of placental anastomoses in twin-to-twin transfusion syndrome (pre-laser coagulation)

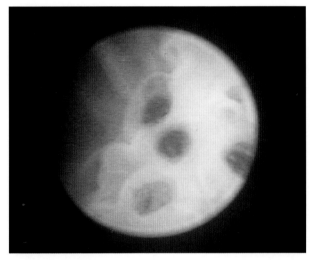

Figure 14 Fetoscopic view of an intertwin membrane with several laser shots

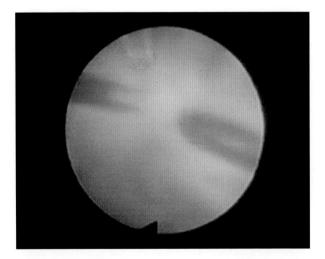

Figure 12 Endoscopic view of placental anastomoses in twin-to-twin transfusion syndrome (post-laser coagulation)

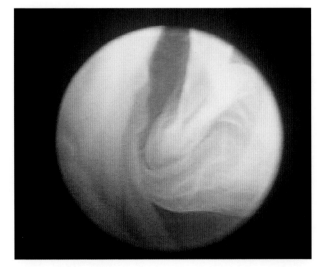

Figure 15 Fetoscopic view of an intertwin membrane rupture following laser-operated coagulation

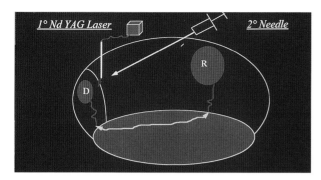

Figure 16 Septostomy techniques

Table 2 Survival rate of fetuses with twin-to-twin transfusion syndrome (TTTS) treated by septostomy

	Hubinont, et al.[48] (n = 7)	Saade, et al.[46] (n = 9)
Second-trimester TTTS	7	5
Third-trimester TTTS	0	4
Intrauterine death	5	3
Neonatal death	1	0
Alive and well	8	15
Survival rate (%)	57	83

intentional needling of the intertwin membrane, as shown in Figure 16. Table 2 shows the combined results of the two pioneer centers using this technique, with a mean survival rate of 65%[46,48,58]. The results of fetal hemodynamics (mainly umbilical artery Doppler) reported by our group and others[46,48] are associated with increased donor urine production. This factor has been reported to be associated with a better survival rate[59].

The main specific risk associated with amniotomy is the iatrogenic creation of pseudomonoamniotic twin pregnancy with cord entanglement[60]. However, this may be reduced by performing a small hole, as in twin pregnancy transeptal diagnostic amniocentesis[61]. Another potential risk associated with septostomy is the presence of membrane flaps which may induce amniotic band syndrome[62] and further compromising fetoscopic procedures such as cord ligation.

Cord occlusion in abnormal twin pregnancy

In cases of acardiac twin pregnancy or in monochorionic multiple pregnancy with a compromised twin, selective feticide may be an ethically acceptable option aiming to improve the outcome of the healthy co-twin. As KCl injec-

tion cannot be used because of placental anastomosis, fetoscopic cord obliteration may be offered as a safe alternative for the surviving twin. It may be performed either by cord ligation using two or three ports[49,50] (Figures 17–20) or by a recently described single-port technique using bipolar coagulation forceps[63]. This cord occlusion technique aims to decrease the morbidity and mortality of the surviving twin. In terms of results, a recent review of the literature on cord ligation in 23 cases reported a 71% survival rate but a 40% rate of preterm prelabor rupture of the membranes[50].

Obstructive uropathies

Fetal lower urinary tract obstruction, such as that of posterior urethral valve, is associated with a risk of chronic renal failure, oligohydramnios and pulmonary hypoplasia[64]. In utero therapy is offered in these pregnancies, either by open fetal surgery[64] or, more often, by percutaneous ultrasound-guided vesicoamniotic shunt[65]. The high morbidity associated with open surgery and the displacement or obstruction of the catheter recently opened the door to a third therapeutic alternative: percutaneous fetal cystoscopy with laser fulguration of the urethral valve[66]. This procedure improves the diagnosis (visualization of thickened bladder neck, dilated proximal urethra, ureteral orifices) and can exclude other abnormalities such as urethral atresia or persistent cloaca. However, the survival rate and the urological outcome should be studied in a larger series before being routinely applied[67].

Congenital diaphragmatic hernia

This abnormality is associated with a risk of severe pulmonary hypoplasia and a high neonatal mortality rate[68]. Prenatal surgery based on animal studies involves performing a fetal tracheal occlusion, either by an open procedure[69] or, more recently, by fetoscopy[70]. This can prevent abnormal lung fluid dynamics and enhances lung growth. Preliminary results suggest that this procedure increases the survival rate at birth. However, long-term follow-up will be required to confirm the fetal benefits of this new approach.

Myelomeningocele

This neural tube defect with a prevalence of five cases for every 10 000 births is associated with various degrees of paraplegia, neurogenic sphincter dysfunction and severe mental retardation in the presence of associated hydrocephaly[71]. A recent paper reported four second-trimester cases of myelomeningocele who underwent endoscopic coverage of the defect with a maternal skin graft[72]. Only two of them survived at birth and these remaining two had a satisfactory neurological outcome. Even if the technique is feasible and seems attractive, randomization and long-term follow-up are needed.

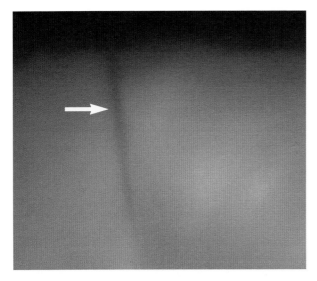

Figure 17 Fetoscopically operated cord ligation in abnormal monochorionic twin pregnancy: looping of the cord by a black-colored suture (arrow)

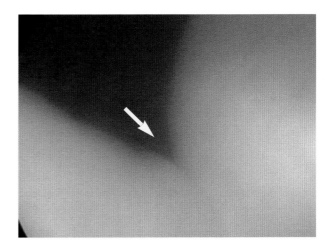

Figure 19 Fetoscopically operated cord ligation in abnormal monochorionic twin pregnancy: cord with the knot (arrow)

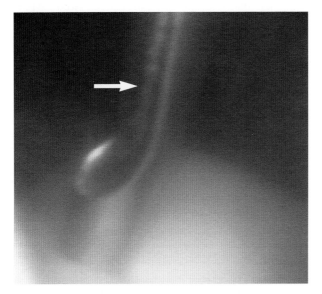

Figure 18 Fetoscopically operated cord ligation in abnormal monochorionic twin pregnancy: the knot is tied by using a knot pusher (arrow)

Sacrococcygeal teratoma

This rare tumor is generally treated surgically at birth but, in some cases, large tumors associated with substantial blood sequestration may induce high output heart failure and fetal hydrops with a poor prognosis. Several fetal surgical approaches have been reported including *ex utero* surgery[73], endoscopic laser coagulation[74], cystic decompression by needling[75] and, in our department, a trial of thermocoagulation of the feeding vessels using a needle-size device introduced transabdominally under ultrasound guidance (unpublished data).

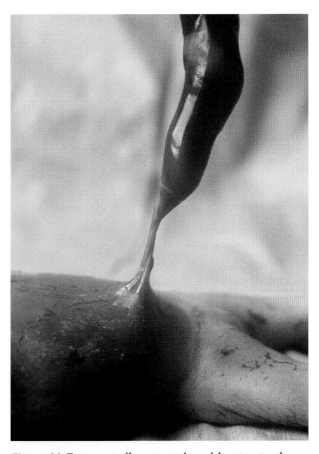

Figure 20 Fetoscopically operated cord ligation in abnormal monochorionic twin pregnancy: postmortem aspect of cord ligation

Fetal cardiac surgery

Fetal catheterization has been successfully performed in sheep[76] and could be a potential approach to treat fetal heart block using a pacemaker as well as performing valvuloplasty in cases of severe vessel stenosis.

RISKS, SAFETY AND COMPLICATIONS

Before performing a fetoscopy, both the risks and potential benefits should be clearly explained to the patient. Potential risks for maternal and/or fetal injury have been previously reported[6-8]: fetal loss is the most common complication, with an incidence between 3%[5,6] and 9%[8]. In diagnostic fetoscopy, premature rupture of the membranes occurs in approximately 5–7% of cases[6]. It may reach 10% in a group of therapeutic endoscopy (TTTS treated by laser coagulation)[43] and even 30% in fetoscopic cord ligation[50]. This amniotic fluid leakage may be avoided by reducing trocar size, the number of ports and perhaps by using a gelatin sponge[77] or a collagen plug[78], as demonstrated in animal models. The risk of fetal eye injury by endoscopic white light has been excluded in the fetal lamb and rat models[79,80].

Quintero reported a failure rate of 16% in diagnostic endoscopy, mainly due to early gestation (5th and 6th week), obesity and severely retroverted uterus[6]. Maternal risks are not negligible, including hemorrhage (one case in our experience, unpublished data), chorioamnionitis, pulmonary embolism and potential amniotic embolism[81].

CONTRAINDICATIONS

Fetal endoscopy should not be performed in pregnant patients with active bleeding, suspicion of premature rupture of the membranes and intrauterine infection[6,8,81].

CONCLUSIONS

Fetoscopy is now a well-established tool in fetal medicine. Embryofetoscopy allows confirmation of first-trimester prenatal diagnosis of structural anomalies affecting mainly the face and/or limb extremities. It can confirm early ultrasound diagnosis prior to dilatation and curettage, allowing in some cases, genetic counselling. Early tissue sampling is feasible in early gestation. Minimally invasive fetal surgery by endoscopy is used in specific fetal conditions such as TTTS and fetal cord ligation. It will have a greater therapeutic role in the future with both technical improvements in the equipment and prevention of complications. Several indications have been reviewed in this chapter and others are still under animal investigation, such as cleft lip repair[82]. Ethical considerations relating to the balance of risks and benefits should always be kept in mind and not be underestimated.

Future developments, such as access to embryos for either stem cell injection to treat some immunological disorders *in utero*[83] or gene therapy[84], will be among the challenges in fetal therapy for the new millennium.

REFERENCES

1. Westin B. Hysteroscopy in early pregnancy. *Lancet* 1954;2:872
2. Kan YW, Valenti C, Guidotti R, *et al*. Fetal blood sampling *in utero*. *Lancet* 1974;1:79–80
3. Rodeck CH, Campbell S. Sampling pure fetal blood by fetoscopy in the second trimester of pregnancy. *Br Med J* 1978;2:728–30
4. Valenti C. Endoamnioscopy and fetal biopsy: a new technique. *Am J Obstet Gynecol* 1972;114:561–4
5. Rodeck CH. Fetoscopy guided by real-time ultrasound for pure fetal blood samples, fetal skin samples and examination of the fetus *in utero*. *Br J Obstet Gynaecol* 1980;87:449–56
6. Quintero RA, Puder KS, Cotton DB. Embryoscopy and fetoscopy. *Obstet Gynecol Clin North Am* 1993;3:563–81
7. Dumez Y, Oury JF, Duchetel F. Embryoscopy and congenital malformations. In *Proceedings of the International Conference on Chorionic Villus Sampling and Early Prenatal Diagnosis*, Athens, Greece, 1988
8. Reece EA, Homko C, Goldstein I, *et al*. Toward fetal therapy using needle embryoscopy. *Ultrasound Obstet Gynecol* 1995;5:281–5
9. Ville Y, Bernard JP, Multon O, *et al*. Transabdominal fetoscopy in fetal anomalies diagnosed by ultrasound in the first trimester of pregnancy. *Ultrasound Obstet Gynecol* 1996;8:11–15
10. Luks FI, Deprest J, Marcus M, *et al*. Carbon dioxide pneumoamnios causes acidosis in fetal lamb. *Fetal Diagn Ther* 1994;9:105–9
11. Ford WDA, Cool JC, Byard R, *et al*. Glycine as a potential window for minimal access fetal surgery. *Fetal Diagn Ther* 1997;12:145–8
12. Cullen MT, Green J, Whetham J, *et al*. Transvaginal ultrasonographic detection of congenital anomalies in the first trimester. *Am J Obstet Gynecol* 1990;163:466–76
13. Hubinont C, Kollmann P, Bernard P, *et al*. First trimester diagnosis of conjoined twins by means of ultrasound and embryoscopy. *Fetal Diagn Ther* 1997;12:185–7
14. Schwarzler P, Moscoso G, Senat MV, *et al*. The cobweb syndrome: first trimester sonographic diagnosis, multiple amniotic bands confirmed by fetoscopy and pathological examination. *Hum Reprod* 1998;13:2966–9
15. Reece EA, Rotmensch S, Whetham J, *et al*. Embryoscopy: a closer look at first trimester diagnosis and treatment. *Am J Obstet Gynecol* 1992;166:775–80
16. Quintero RA, Abuhamad A, Hobbins JC, *et al*. Transabdominal thin-gauge embryofetoscopy: a technique for early prenatal diagnosis and its use in the diagnosis of a case of Meckel–Gruber syndrome. *Am J Obstet Gynecol* 1993;168:1552–7

17. Hobbins JC, Jones OW, Gottesfeld S, *et al.* Transvaginal ultrasonography and transabdominal embryoscopy in the first trimester diagnosis of Smith–Lemli–Opitz syndrome type II. *Am J Obstet Gynecol* 1994;171:546–9

18. Kabra M, Gulati S, Ghosh M, *et al.* Fraser Cryptophthalmos syndrome. *Indian J Pediatr* 2000;67:775–8

19. Reece EA, Homko CJ, Koch S, *et al.* First trimester needle embryoscopy and prenatal diagnosis. *Fetal Diagn Ther* 1997;12:136–9

20. Wu Y, Sun N, Wang F. Antenatal diagnosis of albinism fetuses by fetoscopy. *Chung Hua Fu Chan Ko Tsa Chih* 1998;33:482–3

21. Evans MI, Quintero RA, King M, *et al.* Endoscopically assisted ultrasound guided fetal muscle biopsy. *Fetal Diagn Ther* 1995;10:167–72

22. Reece EA, Goldstein I, Chatwani A, *et al.* Transabdominal needle embryofetoscopy: a new technique paving the way for early fetal therapy. *Obstet Gynecol* 1994;84:634–6

23. Seubert DE, Feldman B, Krivchenia EL, *et al.* Molecular and fetal tissue biopsy capabilities are needed to do prenatal diagnosis of junctional epidermolysis bullosa: fetal biopsy using a 1mm microendoscope. *Fetal Diagn Ther* 2000;15:89–92

24. Quintero RA, Morales WJ, Gilbert Barness E, *et al.* In utero diagnosis of trichothiodystrophy by endoscopically fetal eyebrow biopsy. *Fetal Diagn Ther* 2000;15:152–5

25. Urig MA, Clewell WH, Elliott JP. Twin-twin transfusion syndrome. *Am J Obstet Gynecol* 1990;163:1522–6

26. Weiner CP, Ludomirski A. Diagnosis, pathophysiology and treatment of chronic twin to twin transfusion syndrome. *Fetal Diagn Ther* 1994;9:283–90

27. Radestad A, Thomassen AA. Acute polyhydramnios in twin pregnancy. A retrospective study with special reference to therapeutic amniocentesis. *Acta Obstet Gynaecol Scand* 1990;69:297–300

28. Mahony BS, Petty CN, Nyberg DA, *et al.* The stuck twin phenomenon. *Am J Obstet Gynecol* 1990;163:1513–21

29. Reisner DP, Mahoney BS, Petty CN, *et al.* Stuck twin syndrome: outcome in 37 consecutive cases. *Am J Obstet Gynecol* 1993;169:991–5

30. Bernischke K, Kim CK. Multiple pregnancy. *N Engl J Med* 1973;288:1276–80

31. Weir PE, Raten GJ, Beisher NA. Acute polyhydramnios – a complication of monozygous pregnancy. *Br J Obstet Gynaecol* 1979;86:846–53

32. Fusi L, McParland P, Fisk NM, *et al.* Acute twin-twin transfusion: a possible mechanism for brain-damaged survivors after intrauterine death of a monochorionic twin. *Obstet Gynecol* 1991;78:517–20

33. Bajoria R, Wee LY, Answar S, *et al.* Outcome of twin pregnancies complicated by intrauterine death in relation to vascular anatomy of the monochorionicity. *Hum Reprod* 1999;14:2214–30

34. Dickinson JE, Evans SF. Obstetric and perinatal outcomes from the Australian and New Zealand twin-twin transfusion syndrome registry. *Am J Obstet Gynecol* 2000;182:706–12

35. De Lia JR, Emery MG, Sheator SA, *et al.* Twin transfusion syndrome: successful *in utero* treatment with digoxin. *Int J Obstet Gynecol* 1985;23:197–201

36. Ash K, Harman CR, Gritter H. TRAP sequence successful outcome with indomethacin. *Obstet Gynecol* 1990;76:960–2

37. Elliott JP, Urig MA, Clewell WH. Aggressive therapeutic amniocentesis for the treatment of twin–twin transfusion syndrome. *Obstet Gynecol* 1991;77:537–40

38. Saunders NJ, Snijders RJM, Nicolaides KH. Therapeutic amniocentesis in TTTS appearing in the second trimester of pregnancy. *Am J Obstet Gynecol* 1992;166:820–4

39. Dennis LG, Winkler CL. Twin to twin transfusion syndrome: aggressive amniocentesis. *Am J Obstet Gynecol* 1997;177:342–7

40. Fesslova V, Villa L, Nava S, *et al.* Fetal and neonatal echographic findings in twin-twin transfusion syndrome. *Am J Obstet Gynecol* 1998;179:1056–62

41. Gary D, Lysikievicz A, Mays J, *et al.* Intraamniotic pressure reduction in twin-twin transfusion syndrome. *J Perinatol* 1998;18:284–6

42. De Lia JE, Kuhlmann RS, Lopez KP. Treating previable twin-twin transfusion syndrome with fetoscopic laser surgery: outcomes following the learning curve. *J Perinat Med* 1999;27:61–7

43. Ville Y, Hecher K, Gagnon A, *et al.* Endoscopic laser coagulation in the management of severe twin-twin transfusion syndrome. *Br J Obstet Gynaecol* 1998;105:446–53

44. Hecher K, Plath H, Bregenzer T, *et al.* Endoscopic laser surgery versus serial amniocenteses in the treatment of severe twin twin transfusion syndrome. *Am J Obstet Gynecol* 1999;180:717–24

45. Hubinont C, Bernard P, Mwebesa W, *et al.* Nd : YAG laser and needle disruption of the interfetal septum: a possible therapy in severe twin-twin transfusion syndrome. *J Gynecol Surg* 1996;12:183–9

46. Saade GR, Belfort MA, Berry DA, *et al.* Amniotic septostomy for the treatment of twin oligohydramnios–polyhydramnios sequence. *Fetal Diagn Ther* 1998;13:86–93

47. Pistorius LR, Howarth GR. Failure of amniotic septostomy in the management of 3 subsequent cases of severe previable twin twin transfusion syndrome. *Fetal Diagn Ther* 1999;14:337–40

48. Hubinont C, Bernard P, Pirot N, *et al.* Twin to twin transfusion syndrome: treatment by amniodrainage and septostomy. *Eur J Obstet Gynecol Reprod Biol* 2000;92:141–5

49. Hubinont C, Donnez J. Possible indications for cord ligation: endoscopy. In *The Uterus Throughout the Woman's Life*. Proceedings of the 4th Congress of the European Society for Gynaecological Endoscopy. Bologne: Monduzzi Editore, 1995

50. Deprest JA, Van Ballaer PP, Evrard VA, *et al.* Experience with fetoscopic cord ligation. *Eur J Obstet Gynecol Reprod Biol* 1998;81:157–64

51. Quintero RA, Comas C, Bornick PW, *et al.* Selective versus non selective laser photocoagulation of placental vessels in twin to twin transfusion syndrome. *Ultrasound Obstet Gynecol* 2000;16:230–6

52. Thilaganathan B, Gloeb DJ, Sairam S, *et al.* Sonoendoscopic delineation of the placental vascular equator prior to selective fetoscopic laser ablation in twin to twin transfusion syndrome. *Ultrasound Obstet Gynecol* 2000;16:226–9

53. Suzuki S, Ishikawa G, Sawa R, *et al.* Iatrogenic monoamniotic twin gestation with progressive twin twin transfusion syndrome. *Fetal Diagn Ther* 1999;14:98–101

54. Fisk NM, Tannirandorm Y, Nicolini U, *et al.* Amniotic pressure in disorders of amniotic fluid volume. *Obstet Gynecol* 1990;76:210–14

55. Hartung J, Chaoui R, Bollmann R. Amniotic fluid pressure in both cavities of twin-to-twin transfusion syndrome: a vote against septostomy. *Fetal Diagn Ther* 2000;15:79–82

56. Fries M, Goldstein RB, Kilpatrick SJ, *et al.* The role of velamentous cord insertion in the etiology of twin twin transfusion syndrome. *Obstet Gynecol* 1993;81:569–74

57. Tessen JA, Zlatnik FJ. Monoamniotic twins: a retrospective controlled study. *Obstet Gynecol* 1991;77:832–4

58. Hubinont C, Bernard P. Syndrome transfuseur-transfusé: prise en charge par amnioreduction itérative et amniotomie. *Med Foetal Echo Gynécol* 1999;38:18–21

59. Trespidi L, Boschetto C, Caravelli E, *et al.* Serial amniocentesis in the management of twin-twin transfusion syndrome: when is it valuable? *Fetal Diagn Ther* 1997;12:15–20

60. Cook TL, Shaughnessy R. Iatrogenic creation of a monoamniotic twin gestation in severe twin-twin transfusion syndrome. *J Ultrasound Med* 1997;16:853–5

61. Van Vugt JM, Nieuwint A, Van Geijn HP. Single needle insertion: an alternative technique for early second trimester genetic twin amniocentesis. *Fetal Diagn Ther* 1995;10:178–81

62. Deprest J, Van Schoubroeck D, Evrard V, *et al.* Chirurgie endoscopique intrautérine: invasion minimale pour le foetus? *Gunaïkeia* 1996;1:3115–19

63. Yesidaglar N, Zikulnig L, Gratacos E, *et al.* Bipolar coagulation with small diameter forceps in animal models for *in utero* cord obliteration. *Hum Reprod* 2000;15:865–8

64. Harrison M. *Atlas of Fetal Surgery*, Part II. New York: Chapman & Hall, 1996:63–79

65. Goldbus MS, Filly RA, Callen PW, *et al.* Fetal urinary tract obstruction: management and selection for treatment. *Semin Perinatol* 1985;9:91–101

66. Quintero RA, Hume R, Smith C, *et al.* Percutaneous fetal cystoscopy and endoscopic fulguration of posterior urethral valves. *Am J Obstet Gynecol* 1995;172:206–9

67. Quintero RA, Morales WJ, Allen MH, *et al.* Fetal hydrolaparoscopy and endoscopic cystotomy in complicated cases of lower urinary tract obstruction. *Am J Obstet Gynecol* 2000;183:324–30

68. Adzick NS, Nance ML. Pediatric surgery. Part two. *N Engl J Med* 2000;342:1726–32

69. Harrison M. *Atlas of Fetal Surgery*, Part II. New York: Chapman & Hall, 1996:93–145

70. Harrison MR, Mychaliska GB, Albanese CT, *et al.* Correction of congenital diaphragmatic hernia *in utero*: those with poor prognosis (liver herniation and low lung to head ratio) could be saved by fetoscopic temporary tracheal occlusion. *J Pediatr Surg* 1998;33:1017–22

71. Steinbok P, Irvine B, Cochrane DD, *et al.* Long term outcome and complications in children born with meningomyelocoele. *Childs Nerv Syst* 1992;8:92–6

72. Bruner JP, Richards O, Tulipan NB, *et al.* Endoscopic coverage of fetal myelomeningocoele *in utero*. *Am J Obstet Gynecol* 1999;180:153–8

73. Chiba T, Albanese CT, Jennings RW, *et al.* In utero repair of rectal atresia after complete resection of sacrococcygeal teratoma. *Fetal Diagn Ther* 2000;15:187–90

74. Hecher K, Hackelloer BJ. Intrauterine endoscopic laser surgery for fetal sacrococcygeal teratoma. *Lancet* 1996;347:470–2

75. Garcia AM, Morgan WM, Bruner JP. *In utero* decompression of a cystic grade IV sacrococcygeal teratoma. *Fetal Diagn Ther* 1998;13:305–8

76. Kohl T, Stumper D, Witteler R, *et al.* Fetoscopic direct fetal cardiac access in sheep: an important experimental milestone along the route to human fetal cardiac interintervention. *Circulation* 2000;102:1602–4

77. Luks FI, Deprest JA, Peers KHE, *et al.* Gelatin sponge plug to seal fetoscopy port sites: technique in ovine and primate models. *Am J Obstet Gynecol* 1999;181:995–6

78. Gratacos E, Wu J, Yesildaglar N, *et al.* Successful sealing of fetoscopic access sites with collagen plug in a rabbit model. *Am J Obstet Gynecol* 2000;182:142–6

79. Deprest J, Luks F, Peers KHE, *et al.* Natural protective mechanisms against endoscopic white-light

injury in the fetal lamb eye. *Obstet Gynecol* 1999;94:124–7

80. Bonnett ML, Quintero RA, Carreno C, *et al.* Effect of endoscopic white light on the developing rat retina. *Fetal Diagn Ther* 1997;12:76–80

81. Gratacos E, Deprest J. Current experience with fetoscopy and the euro fetus registry for fetoscopic procedures. *Eur J Obstet Gynecol Reprod Biol* 2000;92:151–9

82. Harrison M. Fetal surgery. *Am J Obstet Gynecol* 1996;174:1255–64

83. Cowan MJ, Goldbus MS. *In utero* hematopoietic stem cell transplants for inherited diseases. *Am J Pediatr Hematol Oncol* 1994;16:35–42

84. Yang EY, Cass DL, Sylvester KG, *et al.* Fetal gene therapy: efficacy, toxicity and immunologic effects of early gestation recombinant adenovirus. *J Pediatr Surg* 1999;34:235–41

Hysteroscopic lysis of intrauterine adhesions (Asherman's syndrome)

44

J. Donnez and M. Nisolle

Intrauterine adhesions have been related to recurrent abortion, sterility and menstrual disorders. Relief from adhesions has been associated with pregnancy rates of 50% and the disappearance of menstrual disorders in more than 75% of cases.

In 1948, Asherman described 'amenorrhea traumatica' as amenorrhea secondary to intrauterine adhesions, following a curettage for incomplete or missed abortion and postpartum hemorrhage[1]. The term 'Asherman's syndrome' is used to describe this condition.

ETIOPATHOGENESIS

Infection (endometritis) rarely causes adhesions, except in cases of tuberculous endometritis. Most frequently (> 90%) intrauterine adhesions develop after a curettage[2]. The most important factor in the development of intrauterine adhesions is traumatic curettage or manipulation of the endometrium during the postpartum or postabortal period. The denudation of the basalis layer and exposure of the muscularis layer produce adhesions by coaptation between the opposing uterine walls.

DIAGNOSIS AND CLASSIFICATION

Dilatation and curettage are not of diagnostic value for intrauterine adhesions. In amenorrheic women with a biphasic basal body temperature curve, failure of the progesterone challenge test to cause withdrawal bleeding may suggest the diagnosis, if the patient has a medical history of postpartum or postabortal curettage.

Hysterosalpingography is the most accurate screening method in the diagnosis of intrauterine adhesions[3]. Adhesions are suggested by radiographic filling defects. Hysteroscopy confirms the presence of intrauterine adhesions and allows definitive surgical treatment. Although adhesions can be diagnosed by hysterosalpingography or hysteroscopy, both are necessary to confirm their presence and their location.

There are many classifications of adhesions based on histology, hysterography, symptomatology and hysteroscopy. To be able to compare the results of treatment and to determine the therapeutic regimen, the adhesions should be classified from the hysteroscopic and hysterosalpingographic findings according to the IUA classification of the European Society of Hysteroscopy (ESH)[4]. We use our own classification (Table 1)[3], essentially based

on the location of the intrauterine adhesions. We consider location to be one of the most important prognostic factors in determining the postoperative pregnancy rate. Degree I adhesions are central (Figures 1 and 2) and are classified as thin or filmy adhesions and myofibrous adhesions. Degree II adhesions are marginal (Figures 3 and 4). Degree III adhesions are revealed by the absence of the uterine cavity at hysterography (Figure 5).

Valle and Sciarra[5] classified intrauterine adhesions as mild, moderate and severe, based on the degree of intrauterine involvement on hysterosalpingography and the extent and type of adhesions found on hysteroscopy. Mild adhesions are defined as filmy adhesions composed of basalis endometrial tissue, producing partial or complete uterine cavity occlusion; moderate adhesions are fibromuscular, characteristically thick and still covered with endometrium; severe adhesions are composed of connective tissue only[6].

The American Fertility Society[7] has proposed a classification of intrauterine adhesions based on the findings at hysterosalpingography and hysteroscopy and the correlation with menstrual patterns.

Table I Classification according to the location and the aspect of the adhesions[3]

Degree	Location
I	Central adhesions (bridge-like adhesions)
	(a) thin or filmy adhesions (endometrial adhesions)
	(b) myofibrous or connective adhesions
II	Marginal adhesions (always myofibrous or connective)
	(a) ledge-like projections
	(b) obliteration of one horn
III	Uterine cavity 'absent' on hysterosalpingography
	(a) occlusion of the internal os (upper cavity normal) (pseudo-Asherman's syndrome)
	(b) extensive coaptation of the uterine walls (absence of uterine cavity) (true Asherman's syndrome)

449

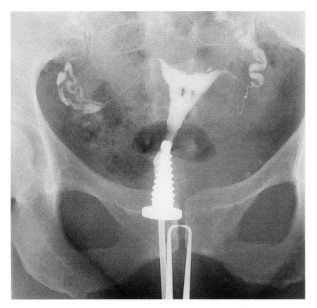

Figure 1 Intrauterine adhesions: degree Ia central adhesions (bridge-like adhesions)

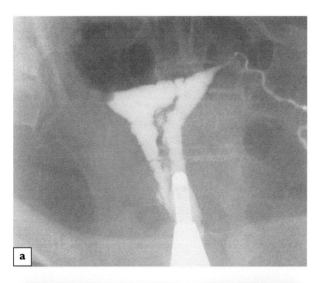

Figure 2 (a) and (b) Intrauterine adhesion, degree Ib myofibrous central adhesions

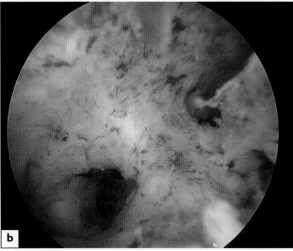

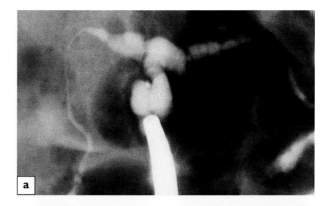

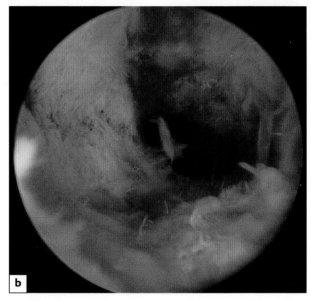

Figure 3 (a) and (b) Intrauterine adhesion, degree IIa marginal adhesions (always myofibrous or connective adhesions)

TREATMENT AND RESULTS

Hysterotomies for the division of adhesions and other blind transcervical manipulations are only of historical interest. Blind division of intrauterine adhesions by dilatation does not provide accurate and precise treatment.

Thin or filmy endometrial adhesions are often removed easily by pushing with the tip of the hysteroscopic sheath. Myofibrous or connective adhesions require a synechiotomy. The surgical treatment of intrauterine adhesions thus consists of dividing the adhesions mechanically, or using electrosurgery and/or fiberoptic lasers. The gynecological resectoscope with a modified knife electrode has been used to divide adhesions electrosurgically. Fiberoptic lasers, such as the argon, krypton (KTP) 532, and neodymium : yttrium–aluminum–garnet (Nd : YAG) laser with sculptured or extruded fibers, have also been used.

In our series, the Nd : YAG laser was used to remove endometrial adhesions, even when they were multiple and fibrous. Degree I and Ib adhesions were easily cut by the laser fiber (Figure 6). Combined laparoscopy and

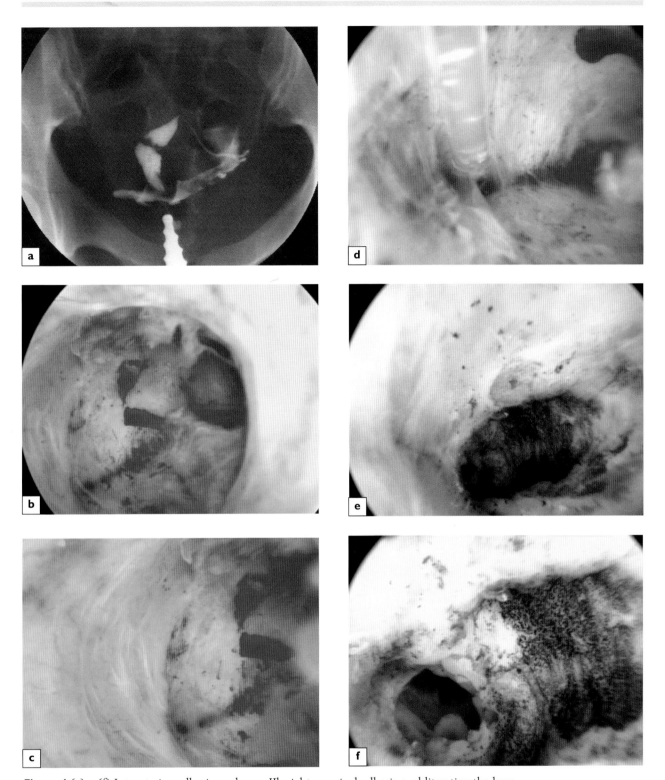

Figure 4 (a) – (f) Intrauterine adhesions, degree IIb right marginal adhesion, obliterating the horn

hysteroscopy can be used, if indicated, to decrease the risk of uterine perforation.

The lateral, back and front scattering of KTP and Nd : YAG laser beams may decrease the viability of the surrounding healthy endometrium. When the adhesions partially occlude the uterine cavity (degree Ib), their division is simple: they are divided in the middle, the remain-

ing stumps retract, and the uterine cavity distends, permitting a panoramic view (Figure 6). Marginal or lateral adhesions (degree IIa and b), particularly if they are extensive and fibromuscular or composed of connective tissue, may be difficult to divide (Figure 7). The Nd : YAG laser may not be a good tool for treatment of this type of adhesion. More severe adhesions may even develop, due to the

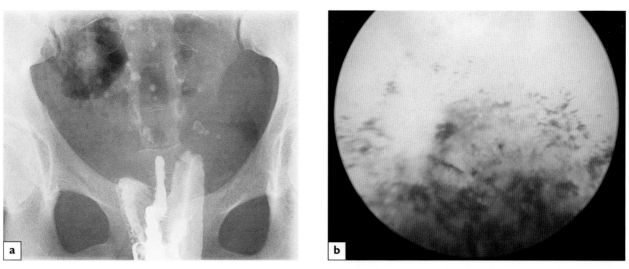

Figure 5 (a) and (b) Intrauterine adhesion, degree III. The cervical canal is visible. The uterine cavity is 'absent'. Only preoperative evaluation permits the differentiation of pseudo-Asherman's syndrome

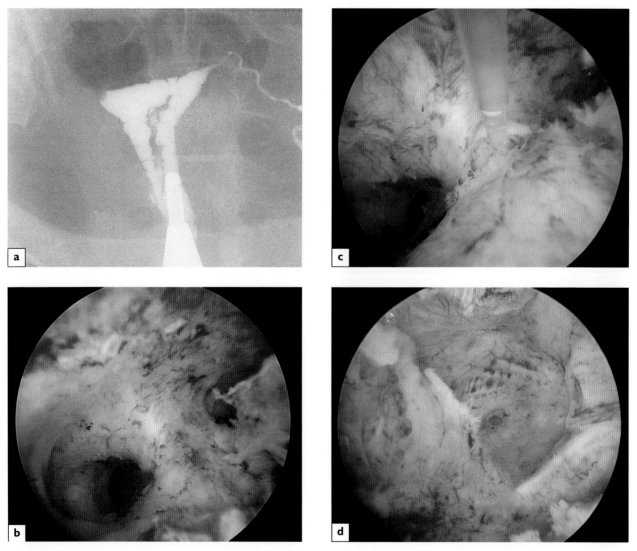

Figure 6 Intrauterine adhesion, degree Ib: (a) hysterosalpingography determines the location; (b) hysteroscopy determines the type (connective tissue); (c) the adhesion is divided with the help of the laser (Nd : YAG) fiber; (d) final view: the fundus of the uterine cavity (with tubal ostium)

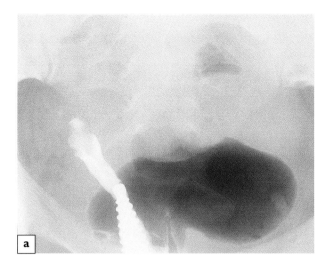

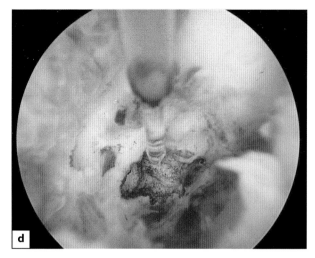

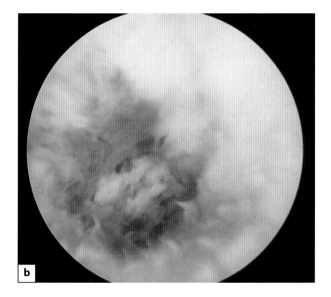

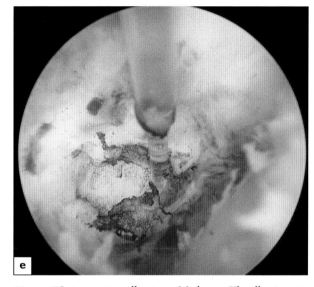

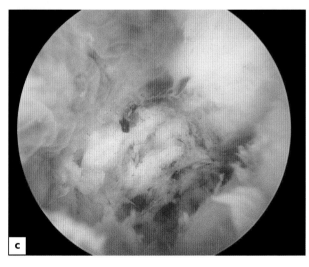

Figure 7 Intrauterine adhesions: (a) degree IIb adhesions in a unicornuate uterus; (b) and (c) the area of connective tissue appears white and fibrotic; (d) and (e) synechiotomy

scattering of the laser, decreasing the viability of the surrounding healthy myometrium.

For uterine adhesions of degree III (Figure 8), hysteroscopic observation of the uterine cavity should begin at the internal cervical os; if the adhesions extend to that area, their selective division begins there. As the adhesions are divided and the uterine cavity opens, the hysteroscope is advanced to the fundal area, and both uterotubal ostia are visualized. Sometimes, increased pressure in the uterine cavity, obtained by increasing the inflow pressure, can facilitate the dissection by distending the uterine cavity. Although the plane of dissection is better exposed, this procedure can lead to excessive fluid intravasation if prolonged.

Low viscosity fluids are frequently chosen for operative hysteroscopy because of their ability to remove debris and cleanse the uterine cavity, even in the presence of slight uterine bleeding. Normal saline and Ringer's lactate are excellent media to distend the uterine cavity when treating intrauterine adhesions with hysteroscopic scissors or with the Nd : YAG laser. Care must be taken to avoid

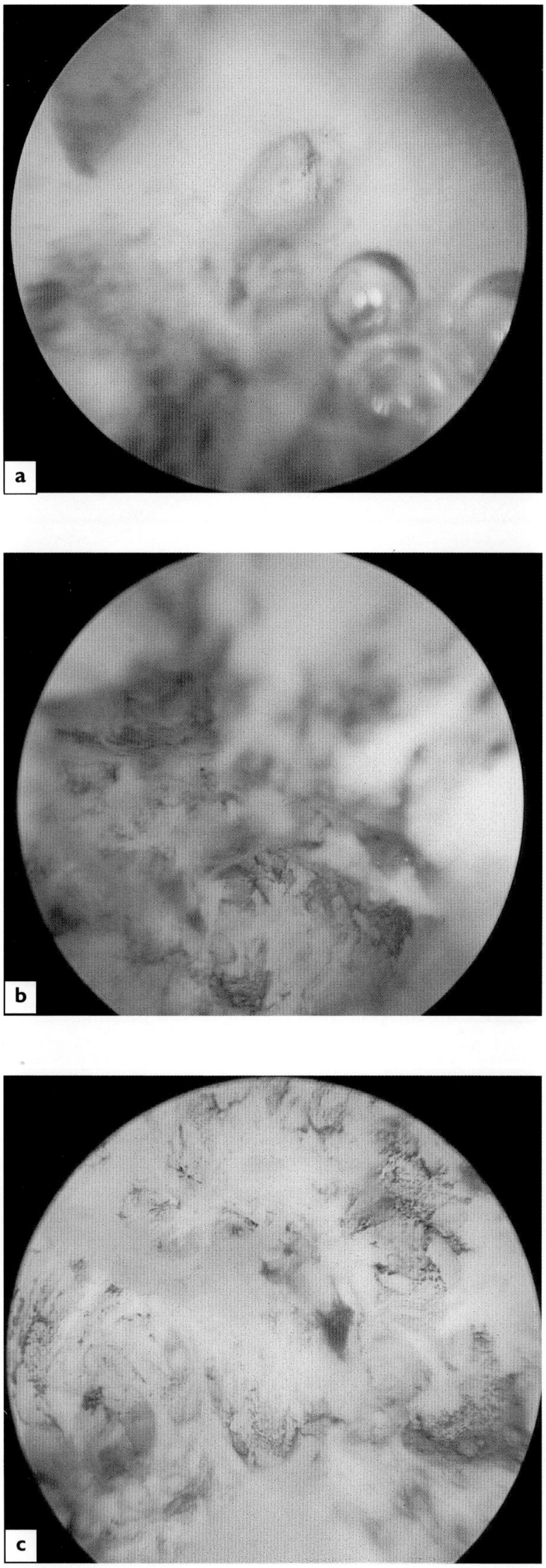

Figure 8 Asherman's syndrome: (a) uterine cavity absent; (b) synechiotomy; (c) rugged aspect of uterine cavity at the end of the procedure

solutions containing electrolytes while using electrocoagulation, to control the volume of fluids not accounted for, and to prevent excessive fluid intravasation, particularly when using fluids without electrolytes. Intrauterine adhesions of the moderate and severe type require extensive dissection, increasing the risk of excessive intravasation.

Prophylactic antibiotics are given 1 h prior to hysteroscopic treatment and for 2–3 days postoperatively, when a splint is left in the uterine cavity. We have not found a second hysteroscopy to be of any particular value. A second therapeutic hysteroscopy is performed only if hysterosalpingography demonstrates residual adhesions.

The subsequent insertion of an intrauterine device (IUD) and hormonal treatment have been associated with increasing success rates. In our department, estrogen and progestogen replacement therapy is initiated after surgery for 3 months (ethinylestradiol 100 μg/day and lynestrenol 10 mg/day for 6 weeks). The doses are doubled for the following 6 weeks.

SUCCESS RATE

In collective series (Table 2), success rates of 74–94% have been obtained[7]. It is very difficult to compare different series because the results have not been evaluated according to the degree of severity. In a review[7], the pregnancy rate was 60.5%, and 80% of those pregnancies reached term.

In our series of 74 patients treated for intrauterine synechiae, eight patients were amenorrheic with an absent uterine cavity at hysterography. Four were classified as degree IIIa, and four as degree IIIb. Surgery was successfully performed in group IIIa, with a pregnancy rate of 100%. In group IIIb, however, adhesions recurred; a second-look hysteroscopy showed only a tunnel-shaped uterine cavity with an absence of healthy endometrium. Hysterosalpingography, carried out 3 months after surgery, confirmed the presence of adhesions; some were more severe than the initial adhesions.

CONCLUSION

The hysteroscopic treatment of intrauterine adhesions restored normal menstruation in more than 80% of treated patients[7]. The results in terms of normal menses and pregnancy rates are excellent for those with adhesions of degrees Ia, Ib, IIa and IIIa. Degree IIb and IIIb adhesions tended to recur and to be more severe in six out of ten women, and no pregnancy occurred in this group.

Patients treated for moderate or severe adhesions should be considered at risk during delivery. Following delivery, care must be taken to make an early diagnosis of any abnormalities, such as placenta accreta or percreta[5].

Table 2 Hysteroscopic lysis of intrauterine adhesions

Reference	Number of patients	Technique	Normal menses		Pregnancy		Term pregnancy	
			n	%	n	%	n	%
8	27	scissors alongside hysteroscope	20	74	14	51.8	13	48.1
4	36	scissors/biopsy forceps	34	94.4	17	62.9	12	44.4
5	187	flexible/semi-rigid/ rigid scissors	167	89.3	143	76.4	114	79.7

REFERENCES

1. Asherman JG. Amenorrhoea traumatica (atretica). *J Obstet Gynaecol Br Emp* 1948;55:23–30
2. Schenker JG, Margalioth EJ. Intrauterine adhesions; an updated appraisal. *Fertil Steril* 1982;37:593
3. Donnez J, Nisolle, M. Operative laser hysteroscopy in Müllerian fusion defects and uterine adhesions. In Donnez J, ed. *Operative Laser Laparoscopy and Hysteroscopy*. Leuven, Belgium: Nauwelaerts Printing, 1989:249–61
4. Wamsteker K. Hysteroscopy in the management of abnormal uterine bleeding in 199 patients. In Siegler AM, Lindemann HI, eds. *Hysteroscopy, Principles and Practice*. Philadelphia: JB Lippincott, 1984:128–31
5. Valle RF, Sciarra JJ. Intrauterine adhesions: hysteroscopic diagnosis classification treatment and reproductive outcome. *Am J Obstet Gynecol* 1988;158:1459–70
6. Valle R. Lysis of intrauterine adhesions (Asherman's syndrome). In Sutton C, Diamond M, eds. *Endoscopic Surgery for Gynecologists*. London: Saunders, 1993:338
7. American Fertility Society. The American Fertility Society classifications of adnexal adhesions, distal tubal occlusion, tubal occlusion secondary to tubal ligation, tubal pregnancies, Müllerian anomalies and intrauterine adhesion. *Fertil Steril* 1988;49:944–55
8. Neuwirth RS, Hussein AR, Schiffman BM, *et al*. Hysteroscopic resection of intrauterine scars using a new technique. *Obstet Gynecol* 1982;60:111–13

45

Endometrial laser intrauterine thermo-therapy

J. Donnez, R. Polet, R. Rabinovitz, J. Squifflet and M. Nisolle

Excessive menstrual bleeding (menorrhagia) affects approximately 22% of the female population[1]. The ELITT™ (endometrial laser intrauterine thermal therapy) procedure, pioneered by Donnez[2,3], offers an inherently safe and simple alternative, providing controlled and effective treatment of the entire endometrium. In contrast to traditional endometrial ablation with the neodymium : yttrium–aluminum–garnet (Nd : YAG) laser, the ELITT procedure requires neither intensive training nor hysteroscopic control, and it is far less risky, as the power used per unit area is 1000 times lower.

Although the precise level of bleeding which determines menorrhagia is difficult to pinpoint, its manifestations are very tangible. Anemia, fatigue, irritability, depression and discomfort result in a general deterioration in the quality of life for the menorrhagic patient. In some cases, blood loss may be severe enough to warrant blood transfusions and periods of hospitalization.

Medication is typically the first-order treatment to control the physical and physiological effects of menorrhagia. Drugs, however, are ineffective in many cases, and often introduce unwanted side-effects. Curettage, which has been routinely employed in the past, is no longer considered to be therapeutically valid. In the 1980s, endometrial ablation was performed using various methods including electrosurgery[4] and laser[5]. These techniques require hysteroscopic control and general or epidural anesthesia, and are dependent on skill level, but are less traumatic than hysterectomy, which is too often considered to be the only current 'sure cure' for menorrhagia[6,7]. They are also less traumatic because they do not require a hospitalization of several days and recuperation of several weeks. While effective, the potential drawbacks and side-effects of these treatment modalities often deter many women from seeking therapy until the condition becomes critical.

Hysteroscopic ablation modalities[8–11], such as balloon technology, are less traumatic and offer shorter treatment and recovery times. However, these methods require direct contact with the endometrium and are, therefore, unable to access the entire endometrium, resulting in uncontrolled results with low amenorrhea rates of 15–35%.

THE ELITT™ PROCEDURE AND THE GYNELASER™ LASER SYSTEM

The ELITT procedure employs a laser light to destroy the endometrium by thermal therapy, increasing the temperature of the endometrium to induce coagulation. Unlike other global ablation modalities, ELITT does not require direct contact with the endometrium to induce coagulation. The laser light is diffused inside the uterine cavity in all directions, reaching the entire uterine cavity, including inaccessible areas such as the cornua. The 830-nm wavelength laser light penetrates the uterine wall to a precise depth, and it is absorbed by the hemoglobin. The absorbed light is then transformed to heat; it warms the endometrium and causes controlled coagulation. The inherent light scattering inside the endometrium positively contributes to the uniformity of the light distribution and the resultant coagulation.

The GyneLase system used in the ELITT procedure is manufactured by ESC Sharplan and is composed of a compact tabletop 20-W, 830-nm diode laser and a disposable handset, as shown in Figure 1.

The system simultaneously emits laser beams through three separate parallel channels. Each channel delivers equal laser power at any time, covering the laser beam to the target through an optical fiber.

The idea of the handset was conceived by J. Donnez and preliminary results with this design were published in 1995[2] and 1996[3]. The handset (Figure 1) includes three

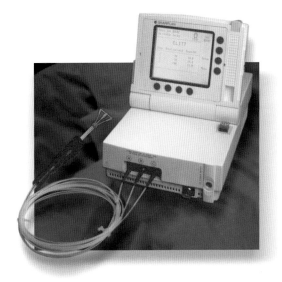

Figure I The GyneLase™ laser system and the disposable handset (ESC Sharplan, Needham, Massachusetts, USA). The disposable handset consists of three integrated optical light diffusers designed to conform to the shape of the uterus

proprietary optical light diffusers that are designed to transmit laser light in all directions to effect the destruction of the endometrial tissue in the fundus and cornua, away from the cervical opening. On each side, diffusers of the handset can be manipulated individually by the operator to conform to the shape of the uterine cavity. The portion of the handset that is inserted into the uterus and makes contact with the tissue is made of Teflon material which is biocompatible, transmits the laser light, and does not adhere to the tissue. The cross-section of the folded handset has the elliptical equivalent of a 6-mm diameter. The proximal ends of the three optical fibers are connected to the laser unit by three SMA 905 fiber connectors.

The 830-nm diode laser is preset for 7 min, delivering the pre-programmed lasing parameters for the treatment: 20 W during the first 90 s, 18 W during the next 90 s, and 16 W during the final 240 s, yielding a total energy of 7020 J, at an average power density of less than 1 W/cm^2 per diffuser.

The endocervical canal is dilated to 7 mm, and the light diffuser handpiece is inserted into the uterus. The operator advances the distal end of the handpiece (Figure 2) to the fundus, and adjusts the side diffusers, forming a butterfly-wing contour which conforms to the shape of the intrauterine cavity (Figure 3). The laser is then activated for a 7-min pre-programmed cycle (Figure 4) which automatically terminates at the end of the cycle (Figure 5). No

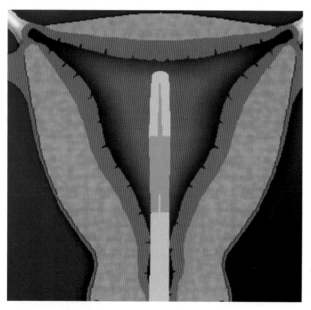

Figure 2 Simulation showing the ELITT™ procedure: handset insertion

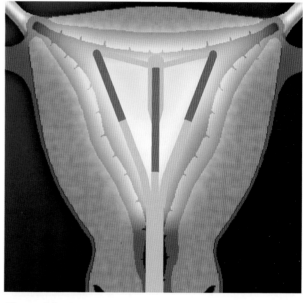

Figure 4 Lasing

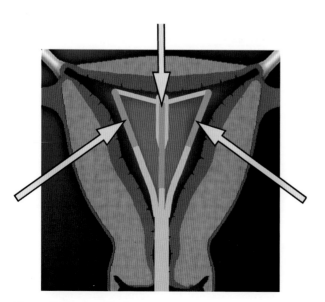

Figure 3 Handset deployment

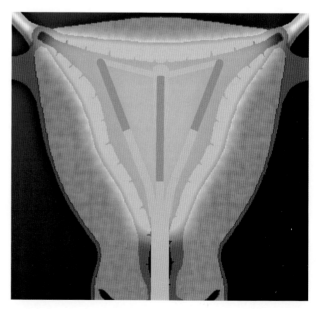

Figure 5 Endometrial coagulation

user setting or handset maneuvering is required. The extended wings are then refolded and the handpiece is removed from the uterus. The handset insertion, manipulation and treatment were performed blindly in our study. Following the handpiece removal, all cases were hysteroscopically evaluated for clinical procedures.

SELECTION CRITERIA

Candidates for ELITT were required to meet the following selection criteria:

(1) Candidates for endometrial ablation due to excessive bleeding;

(2) Absence of both pregnancy or desire for future fertility;

(3) Age range from 30 to 49 years;

(4) Non-menopausal status;

(5) Endometrial biopsy and normal Papanicolaou tests clear of (pre)malignancy;

(6) Uterine cavity sound measurement between 5 and 10 cm;

(7) Uterine cavity free of any irregularity, as evidenced by ultrasound and diagnostic hysteroscopy;

(8) No evidence of any documented gynecological uterine disorder.

The patients ranged in age from 31 to 49 years, with an average age of 42 ± 4.6 years SD.

EVALUATION OF MENSTRUAL BLEEDING

Menses status was documented using a subjective diary based on the pictorial chart method described by Higham and colleagues[12]. Study inclusion required a minimum score of 150. Menses status was defined categorically as follows: complete absence of uterine bleeding as amenorrhea; scores between 1 and 10 as spotting; between 11 and 30 as hypomenorrhea; between 31 and 100 as eumenorrhea; and above 100 as menorrhagia.

Each menstrual blood loss chart (MBLC) is a record of a single menstrual cycle that reflects the length and severity of uterine bleeding. Both the quantity and saturation of sanitary protection indicate the severity of bleeding on a daily basis. Additionally, patients were asked to rank their level of satisfaction with the ELITT at the 6-month follow-up, with five options ranging from the highest score of 'most satisfied' to the lowest of 'disappointed'.

All patients received two depots of slow-release gonadotropin releasing hormone (GnRH) agonist approximately 4 weeks prior to the procedure, and then again at the time of the procedure. Laminaria was inserted during the evening prior to the procedure to facilitate cervical dilatation. Patients were anesthetized either generally, regionally or locally, depending on their preference.

Immediately pre-ELITT, the uterus was sounded and dilated. Once inserted and in position, the handset was kept stationary throughout the treatment.

RESULTS

The surgical procedure was easily performed in the 100 patients included in the present study.

No perforation of the uterus or intraoperative complications occurred. Suspicion of incorrect positioning of the device can arise from an unusual resistance to deploying the fibers and when there is a discrepancy between the uterine length measured by the probe and the depth of insertion of the system, as reported by the graduated scale along the central rod of the device. In all cases, this risk is further limited by the use of cervical laminaria or by the use of oral prostaglandins the night before the procedure.

Of the 100 cases, 60% were carried out under general anesthesia, 21% under local anesthesia (paracervical block) supplemented with intravenous conscious sedation, 17% under epidural and 2% under conscious sedation only. All patients were given a dose of antibiotics prophylactically. All patients had 6- and 12-month follow-up results. After 12 months, the amenorrhea rate was 71% and the amenorrhea + severe hypomenorrhea rate (< one pad per day) was 91% (Table 1). The bleeding status is shown in Figure 6.

Most patients reported mild to severe cramping pain post-procedure, rarely continuing beyond the first day of treatment.

Of the 100 patients with 6- and 12-month Satisfaction Level Questionnaire scores, 87% were 'most satisfied' (highest score), 12% were 'satisfied' and one patient was 'not satisfied'. Although the Higham score was still high, it must be stressed that this patient had a score which was 88% lower than the pretreatment score. None of the patients were 'indifferent' or 'disappointed'.

Well-treated cornua reduce the risk of recurrence. This was proved histologically by NADPH staining tests, which showed destruction of the superficial layers to a depth of 4.5 mm in all regions analyzed[3] (Figure 7).

Table I Follow-up at 6 and 12 months

Bleeding status (n = 100)	6 months (%)	12 months (%)
Amenorrhea	69	71
Spotting (< 1 pad per day)	21	20
Hypomenorrhea	5	5
Eumenorrhea	4	2
Menorrhagia	1	2

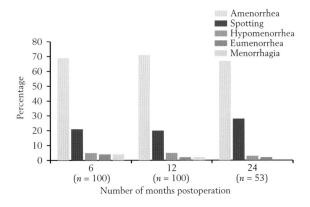

Figure 6 Menses status of patients at 6 months and 12 months after the ELITT™ procedure

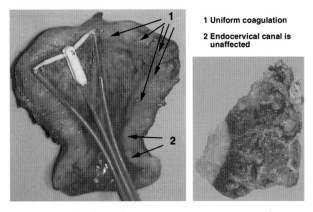

1 Uniform coagulation

2 Endocervical canal is unaffected

Figure 7 Histologically, NADPH staining tests demonstrate that the superficial layers were destroyed to a depth of 4.5 mm in all regions

Nevertheless, two patients suffered dysmenorrhea caused by cornual hematometra (less than 1-cm diameter) after exhibiting amenorrhea for more than 6 months. They underwent subtotal hysterectomies, one at 9 months, the other at 14 months post-procedure.

DISCUSSION

Menorrhagia frequently occurs, even in the absence of intrauterine organic lesions. Because dilatation and curettage often fail and hysterectomy may be associated with a 40% morbidity rate and a mortality rate close to 1%, other surgical techniques have been developed. In 1983, DeCherney and Polan[4] first described resection of the endometrium and Goldrath[5] described ablation of the endometrium with the YAG laser. Thermal uterine balloon therapy[8–11] was developed more recently in an attempt to simplify the ablative procedure. The amenorrhea rate after 12 months (Table 2) with this technique was low, varying from 15 to 25%. Recently (in 1995 and 1996), we described an intrauterine device using Nd : YAG

laser energy. We describe the GyneLase connected to a diode (wavelength 830 nm) laser in two recent papers[13,14].

The ELITT procedure is the ultimate simplified version of endometrial laser ablation (ELA). ELITT differs from ELA in several aspects. First, ELITT is a completely blind procedure whereas ELA is hysteroscopically guided, therefore requiring surgical experience, time and material; its concept is close to the blind insertion of a contraceptive intrauterine device. Because no distending medium is used, no risk of fluid overload exists. Second, the ITT quartz fibers diffuse the thermal radiation circumferentially, over a distance of 3–4 cm; it no longer needs to be dragged along the wall of the uterine cavity. Combined together in an inverted triangular configuration, the radiation spectrum covers the area of a normal-shaped uterine cavity. Third, the laser source itself has changed: the diode laser has replaced the Nd : YAG laser. It is less expensive, less cumbersome and its shoebox size makes it easily transportable.

Histology tests have demonstrated that the ELITT procedure destroys the entire endometrium and an additional 1–3.5 mm of the adjacent myometrium. A minimum of 67% of the uterine wall remains intact, leaving a sufficiently large safety buffer zone[15]. Additionally, due to the design of the handset, the endocervical canal also remains untouched.

The ELITT procedure was designed to treat dysfunctional uterine bleeding and refractory menorrhagia in normal-shaped uterine cavities in patients with no further desire for childbearing. Because menorrhagia is a very subjective complaint, we used a validated score defined by Higham and colleagues[12] to select patients with objective menorrhagia, with a score of more than 150 equivalent to blood loss of more than 80 ml.

Respecting the indications and contraindications is the cornerstone of the short- and long-term success of this procedure. Patient history must exclude past endometrial destruction procedures as they affect the size, shape and rigidity of the uterus. On vaginal examination, the uterus must be less than 7 weeks and the uterine depth must be within 5–10 cm. A larger uterine cavity would not allow the device to cover the whole endometrium; moreover, data on the transhysteroscopic destruction of the endometrium have clearly demonstrated that long-term results are poorer with larger cavities[15,16]. On the other hand, smaller cavities would force the base of the fibers to extrude from the endometrial cavity and burn the endocervical canal, with a risk of subsequent hematometra.

Normality of shape and size is sought by endovaginal echography, hysteroscopy and/or hysterography, and endometrial biopsy. Hysteroscopy excludes congenital malformations of the uterus, submucous fibroids, endometrial polyps and synechiae; it gives indications on the possibility of dealing with adenomyosis. Endometrial biopsy excludes endometrial neoplasia and endometrial hyperplasia; this latter condition is believed to be responsible for

Table 2 Amenorrhea rates after endometrial resection or ablation

Reference	Technique	Number	Amenorrhea rate (%) 6 months	≥ 12 months
Sorensen et al.[18]	electrosurgery	60	25	24
Yin et al.[19]	electrosurgery	127	18	ND
Chullapram et al.[20]	electrosurgery	142	ND	25
Baggish and Sze[21]	YAG laser and/ or electrosurgery	568	ND	58
Donnez et al. (Aztec group)[17]	electrosurgery	358	40* 26**	42* 26**
Martyn and Allan[22]	electrosurgery	301	ND	41
Garry et al.[23]	YAG laser	600	ND	28.9
Meyer et al.[8]	thermal balloon roller	125 114		15.2 27.2
Amso et al.[9]	thermal balloon	300	14	15
Donnez et al.[13]	ELITT	78	68	63
Donnez et al.[14]	ELITT	100	69	71

*GnRH agonist given preoperatively; ** no GnRH agonist given before surgery; ND, not done

cases of endometrial neoplasia development following endometrial resection.

The device and the technique are safe: the fibers are solid and do not break. Their integrity is checked prior to the procedure by introducing them into the power meter included in the laser source. Breakage during laser emission should not be feared. Insertion is blind and follows dilatation of the cervix up to Hegar 8; in case of difficulty or doubt, the correct intrauterine positioning and opening of the fibers can be checked by echography. When all the data are pooled, the risk of perforation is seen to be very limited: insertion of contraceptive intrauterine devices (IUDs), for example, is associated with a perforation risk of 0–8.7%. In our series, the rate of perforation was 0%.

Thermal damage to the viscera with a correctly inserted device is not possible. The mathematical model on which this allegation is based demonstrates that the temperature on the serosa cannot rise significantly because of the heat sink effect of the uterus. *In vivo*, temperatures were measured on the serosa during laser emission and no significant variation was observed[3]. Indeed, microelectrodes positioned 2–3 mm below the serosa failed to demonstrate any elevation of temperature, which remained constant during the entire procedure.

The use of GnRH agonists before ablation was considered beneficial because of their well-known effects on the uterus and the clinical data obtained from the techniques of endometrial resection and laser ablation[17]. They shrink the cavity and allow a tighter fit of the device; they thin the endometrium and reduce the arterial blood perfusion (which lowers the heat sink effect of the uterus).

The procedure can be performed under local anesthesia, using a paracervical block technique and intravenous sedation, in patients who wish it and who have shown a good tolerance to hysteroscopy. Painful hysteroscopy probably indicates the possibility of painful ELITT as, like others, we believe it reflects fairly the pain threshold of the patient. Cervical dilatation, device insertion and opening of the device are painless. Mild to moderate lower abdominal cramps are felt while lasing and use of non-steroidal anti-inflammatory drugs helps to make the early postoperative hours more comfortable.

The results of this series are analyzed in terms of the amenorrhea rate, incontestably the most objective indicator of therapeutic success. The impressive amenorrhea rate observed (69% at 6 months and 71% at 12 months) is believed to be the result of the excellent access to the tubal cornua obtained with the device. Indeed, when compared with the data published in the literature (Table 2), the amenorrhea rate after ELITT is higher than the amenorrhea rate achieved after endometrial resection (25–42%) or intrauterine thermal balloon therapy (15–27%). When the amenorrhea and severe hypomenorrhea, defined as less than one pad/day were considered, rates of 90% (6 months' follow-up) and 91% (12 months' follow-up) were observed.

In conclusion, the ELITT procedure is a new, revolutionary technique, which is very safe and offers an excellent alternative to hysterectomy in the management of dysfunctional uterine bleeding.

REFERENCES

1. Hallberg L, Hogdahl A, Nilsson L, *et al.* Menstrual blood loss – a population study. *Acta Obstet Gynecol Scand* 1966;45:320–51
2. Donnez J, Polet R, Mathieu PE, *et al.* Endometrial laser interstitial hyperthermy: a potential modality for endometrial ablation. *Obstet Gynecol* 1996;87:459–64
3. Donnez J, Polet R, Mathieu PE, *et al.* Nd : YAG laser ITT Multifiber Device (the Donnez Device): endometrial ablation by interstitial hyperthermia. In Donnez J, Nisolle M, eds. *Atlas of Laser Operative Laparoscopy and Hysteroscopy*. Carnforth, UK: Parthenon Publishing 1995:353–9
4. DeCherney AH, Polan ML. Hysteroscopic management of intrauterine lesions and intractable uterine bleeding. *Obstet Gynecol* 1983;61:392–7
5. Goldrath MH. Hysteroscopic endometrial ablation. *Obstet Gynecol Clin North Am* 1995;22:559–72
6. Basterday CL, Grimes DA, Riggs JA. Hysterectomy in the United States. *Obstet Gynecol* 1983;62:203–12
7. Carlson KJ, Nichols DH, Schiff I. Indications for hysterectomy. *N Engl J Med* 1993;83:792–6
8. Meyer WR, Walsh BA, Grainger DA, *et al.* Thermal balloon and rollerball ablation to treat menorrhagia: a multicenter comparison. *Obstet Gynecol* 1998;92:98–103
9. Amso NA, Stabinsky SA, McFaul P, *et al.* Uterine thermal balloon therapy for the treatment of menorrhagia: the first 300 patients from a multi-centre study. *Br J Obstet Gynaecol* 1998;105:517–23
10. Dequesne J, Galliant A, Garza-Leal JG, *et al.* Thermoregulated radiofrequency endometrial ablation. *Int J Fertil* 1997;42:311–18
11. Friberg B, Joergensen C, Ahlgren M. Endometrial thermal coagulation – degree of uterine fibrosis predicts treatment outcome. *Gynecol Obstet Invest* 1998;45;54–7
12. Higham JM, O'Brien PMS, Shaw RW. Assessment of menstrual blood using a pictorial chart. *Br J Obstet Gynaecol* 1990;97:734–9
13. Donnez J, Polet R, Squifflet J, *et al.* Endometrial laser intrauterine thermo-therapy (ELITT™): a revolutionary new approach to the elimination of menorrhagia. *Curr Opin Obstet Gynecol* 1999;11:363–70
14. Donnez J, Polet R, Rabinovitz R, *et al.* Endometrial laser intrauterine thermo-therapy: the first series of 100 patients observed for 1 year. *Fertil Steril* 2000;74:791–6
15. Donnez J, Polet R, Smets M, *et al.* Hysteroscopic myomectomy. *Curr Opin Obstet Gynecol* 1995;7:311–16
16. Donnez J, Gillerot S, Bougonjon D, *et al.* Nd-YAG laser hysteroscopy in large submucous fibroids. *Fertil Steril* 1990;54:999–1003
17. Donnez J, Vilos G, Gannon M, *et al.* Goserelin acetate (Zoladex) plus endometrial ablation for dysfunctional uterine bleeding: a large-randomized, double-blind study. *Fertil Steril* 1997;68:29–36
18. Sorensen SS, Colov NP, Veserslev LO. Pre-and post-operative therapy with GnRH agonist for endometrial resection. A prospective, randomized study. *Acta Obstet Gynecol Scand* 1997;76:340–4
19. Yin CS, Wei RY, Chao TC, *et al.* Hysteroscopic endometrial ablation without endometrial preparation. *Int J Gynecol Obstet* 1998;62:167–72
20. Chullapram T, Song JY, Fraser IS. Medium-term follow-up of women with menorrhagia treated by rollberball endometrial ablation. *Obstet Gynecol* 1996;88:71–6
21. Baggish MS, Sze EH. Endometrial ablation: a series of 568 patients treated over a 11-year period. *Am J Obstet Gynecol* 1996;174:908–13
22. Martyn P, Allan B. Long term follow-up of endometrial ablation. *J Am Assoc Gynecol Laparosc* 1998;5:115–18
23. Garry R, Shelley-Jones D, Mooney P, *et al.* Six hundred endometrial laser ablation. *Obstet Gynecol* 1995;85:24–9

46

Endometrial resection

B.J. van Herendael

INTRODUCTION

Sixty-four per cent of women are confronted with episodes of abnormal uterine bleeding (AUB)[1]. Menorrhagia is a specific type of bleeding episode. Often women do bleed so heavily that they find themselves at the wrong side of a vicious circle leading to a state of ferriprive anemia. Medication most often is not an acceptable long-term solution[2], neither is a hysterectomy. Although hysterectomy is often proposed as a 'hygienic' and definitive solution, there are numerous reports on morbidity[3] and recently on sexual and psychological dysfunction and costs[4]. Although hysterectomy is still the most widespread solution for all types of AUB problems, it should be used only after thorough investigation and thorough explanation with the patient and her partner.

Local medical therapy (a progestin-loaded intrauterine contraceptive device) can only be successful if the uterine cavity is anatomically perfect and if the patient is disciplined enough to submit herself to checks at regular intervals.

Hysteroscopic endometrial resection is a conservative solution. The endometrial lining is resected to a layer just above the myometrium. An endothelial layer then replaces the endometrium. The consequence is that the blood flow is reduced dramatically in over 80% of patients. Hysteroscopic endometrial resection is in competition with other endometrial ablation techniques, such as laser endometrial ablation under hysteroscopic control, balloon endometrial ablation, hydro-ablation of the endometrium, ultrasound endometrial ablation, bipolar- and cryo-endometrial ablation, and the latest diode laser endometrial ablation[5].

The advantages of the hysteroscopic electrical loop endometrial resection are twofold. First, it is a technique under visual observation – an advantage it shares with rollerball electrical ablation, laser ablation and even hydro-ablation. The second, and main, advantage is the possibility of collecting samples for pathology. In the literature, we do find reports of missed endometrial carcinomas picked up by the pathologist after examining the resected specimen[6]. The disadvantage of the technique is the high risk of complications, although these risks should not be exaggerated[7]. The mechanical complication of perforation is not what is meant here. Perforation is a hazard with all mechanical probes introduced into the uterine cavity, from simple Hegar dilators to very sophisticated instruments.

The most feared complication is the risk of circulatory overload with distension medium (transurethral resection of prostate). This risk is shared with hysteroscopic rollerball ablation and hysteroscopic laser endometrial ablation. This implies that hysteroscopic transcervical endometrial resection (TCER) requires more training than most techniques mentioned[8].

INSTRUMENTS

A passive resectoscope is used[9]. The normal diameter is 26 French. A passive scope means that the active element, the loop, is retracted into the inner sleeve and has to be brought out by the operator before starting the resection and will retract towards the final lens of the scope when left.

All resections should be carried out with a through-flow instrument. Through flow means that there are two sleeves, an inner sleeve carrying the distension medium towards the uterine cavity and an outer sleeve for aspiration of the medium out of the cavity.

Electrical cutting current (undamped current) is the current of choice even for coagulation; here we hold the loop at a small distance over the bleeding vessel and create a spark to coagulate the vessel. The lower voltage of the cutting current is less likely to cause problems. Energy should be supplied if possible by a variable output generator. The endometrial lining is not homogeneous, implying that different intensities are necessary to obtain an optimal result. The authors use 120 Watts for pure cutting and 80 Watts for coagulation.

Distension should be obtained with a pump mechanism that allows for variable settings for both the inflow and the intracavity pressure. The maximum intracavity pressure is set between the systolic and diastolic blood pressures of the patient. In doing this, we avoid infusing the distension medium into the patient throughout the whole cardiac cycle. Too low a pressure would cause the blood to mix with the distension medium and obscure the view and too high a pressure would cause a continuous flow of distension medium into the circulation of the patient. Aspiration into a collecting system allows us to have an idea of the amount of medium retrieved and, hence, be able to calculate the loss of distension medium. Classical endometrial resection is carried out in a non-ionic distension medium so as not to disperse the current. Glycine® 1% is the most commonly used distension medium in the low-viscosity media, mainly because of its low cost. We recommend the use of the same distension medium as the urologists in the institution. The most common complication is fluid overload, the classical TURP syndrome, just as in urology.

TECHNIQUE

An endometrial resection should never be performed if the resection is not preceded by a diagnostic hysteroscopy with tissue sampling or, at least, a curettage.

It must be borne in mind by the hysteroscopic surgeon that this is a very conservative technique and that this technique should, therefore, only be performed in patients with no underlying uterine disease such as adenomyosis.

If an overt endometrial carcinoma is found, or even a carcinoma *in situ*, the patient should be treated as an oncology patient with major ablative surgery. If hyperplasia is found, recent reports bring us to believe that there could be a place for conservative treatment. Further follow-up is, however, necessary before the treatment of hyperplasia by hysteroscopic resection of the endometrium can be considered as routine.

There is the question of pretreatment of the endometrium. In comparison with laser endometrial ablation, no special pretreatment is necessary but TCER is easier and takes less operative time if the endometrium is between 3 and 5 mm in height. All classical pretreatments can be used or the resection can be planned in the early follicular phase or an aspiration curettage with a 4–5-mm cannula can be performed to reduce the height.

Step one

The cervix is grasped with a valselum at the 11 o'clock position and is dilated up to Hegar 10 or 11, 33–35 French, corresponding to 11–12 mm. The dilatation up to this Hegar diameter is necessary to bring the scope easily into the uterine cavity and to easily remove it.

Step two

The resectoscope is brought into the uterine cavity under direct vision.

Step three

The uterine cavity is inspected.

Step four

The loop is brought into contact with the mid-portion of the fundal area. Resection is begun by bringing the loop towards the lens of the scope. The loop should be embedded into the endometrium as far as necessary. The depth has to be judged by visual appreciation of the different linings of the uterine wall and should stop when the striated alignment of the myometrial musculature becomes visible. The first furrow is the most important because this will set the depth for the whole of the resection.

The loop is brought into contact with the endometrium in the fundal area (Figure 1). Unipolar electricity, undamped, is activated. The first furrow is excised so that the endometrium is cut out to a depth just into the myometrium (Figure 2). If all the glandular buds are not excised in their totality a careful excision of 1 or 2 mm is performed over the first (Figure 3). This process is repeated until all the glandular buds are excised and we see the striated appearance of the layer above the myometrium can be seen (Figure 4).

Step five

The rest of the cavity is now treated. This can be performed in different sequences. Some surgeons proceed clockwise, others anticlockwise. I prefer to proceed first left and then right from the first furrow until I complete the resection of the posterior part of the uterus. The loop is half embedded into and half out of the furrow so that the depth of the resection is easy to ascertain (Figure 5). Once the posterior side is completed, the lateral and anterior sides are tackled (Figure 6). The anterior side is always slightly more difficult as the bubbles, caused by the heating of the distension medium by the electrical current, tend to collect in this area. It therefore becomes necessary to aspirate these bubbles at regular intervals (Figures 7 and 8). If necessary, the depth should be corrected until there are no glandular buds left (Figure 9). The resection is carried out to within 1 cm of the isthmus, a so-called incomplete resection. The complete resection continues down to the cervical canal. The percentage of amenorrhea is higher with the last technique.

Step six

The fundal and corneal areas are now treated (Figures 10–13). The fundal area can be treated with the loop by bringing the loop sideways over the fundal area. The corneal areas can also be treated with the loop. If the loop is too large for the cornua, a small ball can be used to coagulate these areas.

Step seven

The chips of tissue are grasped between the loop and the final lens of the resectoscope and brought out of the cavity (Figure 14).

Step eight

A last inspection of the uterine cavity is performed (Figure 15). If bleeding vessels are spotted, these are now coagulated. It can be useful to reduce the distension pressure in order to see the bleeding points (Figure 16).

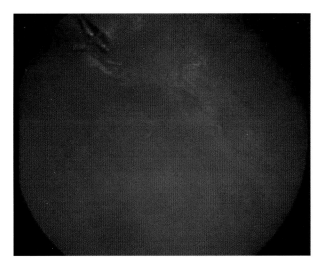

Figure 1 The loop is brought into contact with the endometrium in the fundal area

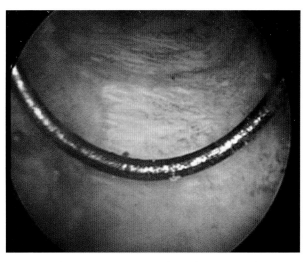

Figure 4 The process is repeated until the striated appearance of the layer above the myometrium is visible

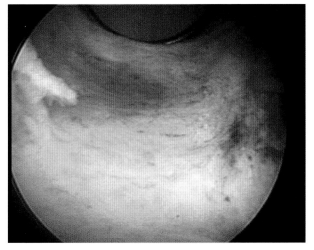

Figure 2 Excision of the first furrow

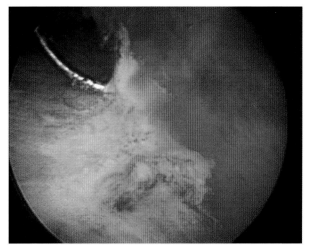

Figure 5 The loop is only half embedded in the endometrium so that the lowest part of the loop is at the level of the deepest passage of the previous furrow

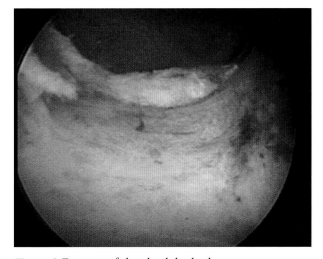

Figure 3 Excision of the glandular buds

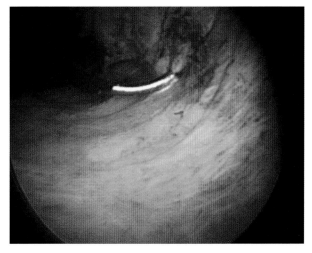

Figure 6 At the side walls, the loop is even less embedded so as to follow the curvature of the walls

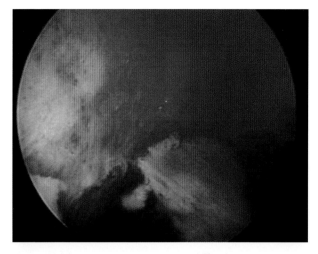

Figure 7 The anterior part is more difficult to treat as the tissue tend to fall towards the scope and the bubbles gendered by heating the distension medium make vision difficult. These bubbles must be aspirated

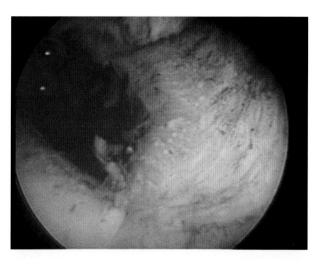

Figure 10 The tubal ostium, seen in the middle of the picture, is often difficult to treat with the classical resector loop

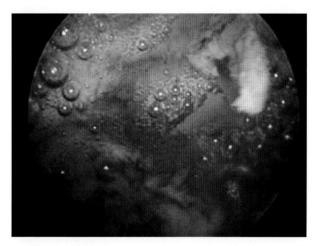

Figure 8 Example of the bubbles created by heating the distension medium

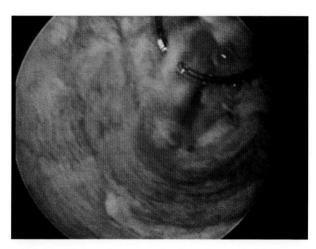

Figure 11 The combination of a deep-lying tubal ostium, a large resector loop and the bubbles makes it difficult to excise the osteal region precisely

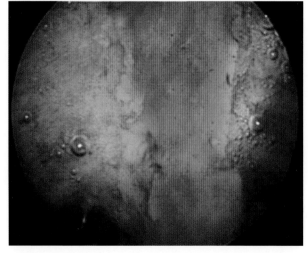

Figure 9 The circle is now completed and the treatment of the fundal area can start

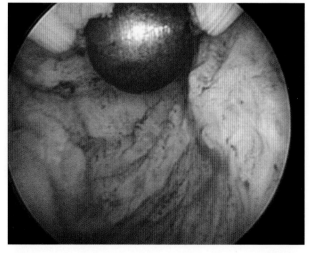

Figure 12 A small rollerball electrode can be useful in the treatment of these areas

466

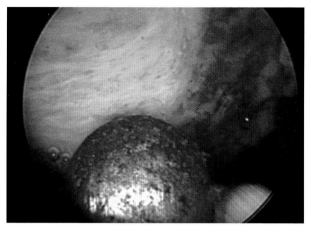

Figure 13 The rollerball electrode can also be used to treat the lower part of the resection in the cervix where deep resection is often dangerous as larger vessels can be opened inadvertently

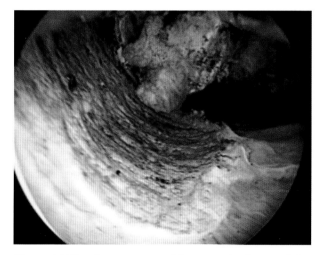

Figure 14 The chips are grasped between the loop and the final lens and brought out of the uterine cavity

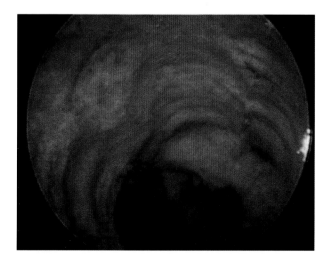

Figure 15 General view at the end of the resection

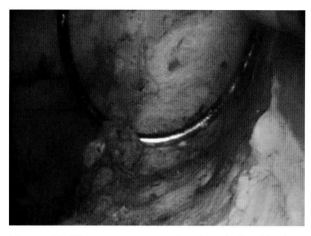

Figure 16 The pressure is reduced and the bleeding becomes visible so that the terminal part of the vessel can be coagulated

Management of the tissue chips

If the uterus is large enough, the chips of tissue should be 'parked' in the fundal area awaiting their removal at the end of the resection. If the uterus is small, resected chips should be brought out whenever they interfere with good visibility.

CONCLUSIONS

Provided the uterine cavity is of a reasonable size, authors have suggested resection of 10 cm. TCER is a well-documented technique that should be used as a first approach in patients with menorrhagia provided there are no other pathological conditions in the uterine wall or the endometrium. Most common problems or failures are caused by adenomyosis. This could be the reason why large uteri do worse than their normal counterparts, as often there is the presence of adenomyosis alongside the myomas in these uteri.

If there are polyps in the uterine cavity, these should be treated during the same session (Figures 17 and 18). The outcome is the same as that for classical TCER.

If myomas are treated at the same time, the results seem slightly worse in the long-term follow-up. Our own long-term follow-up study (unpublished data) revealed that, after 5 years, 92% of the patients were still satisfied with the TCER and 96% would have the intervention again.

An alternative for the unipolar high-frequency resection in Glycine® distension medium is the bipolar ablation in normal saline solution (Figures 19–21). It has to be said that fluid overload of the patient with normal saline has exactly the same consequences as overload with Glycine® except for the pharmacological effects of Glycine® that do not occur with normal saline. Ablation does not allow for pathological examination.

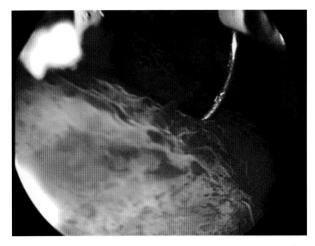

Figure 17 A polyp is removed at the same time as the endometrial resection

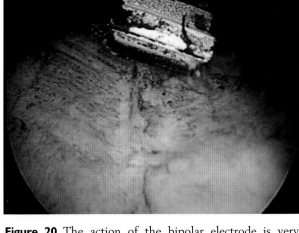

Figure 20 The action of the bipolar electrode is very powerful. The anatomical landmarks of the ablation are clearly visible. Note the different form of the electrode

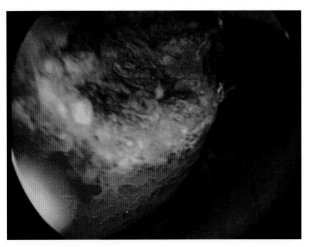

Figure 18 Note the glandular structure of the inside of the resected polyp

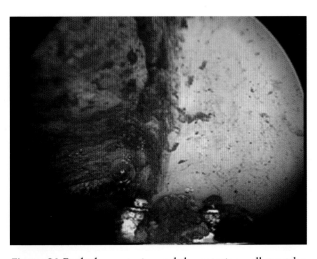

Figure 21 Both the posterior and the anterior wall must be treated. The bipolar electrodes are easier to manipulate than the classical resector loop

REFERENCES

1. Grainger DA, DeCherney AH. Hysteroscopic management of uterine bleeding. *Baillieres Clin Obstet Gynaecol* 1989;3:403–14

2. Wood C. Alternative treatment. *Baillieres Clin Obstet Gynaecol* 1995;9:373–97

3. Goldenberg M, Sivan E, Bider D, *et al.* Endometrial resection versus abdominal hysterectomy for menorrhagia. Correlated sample analysis. *J Reprod Med* 1996;41:333–6

4. Brumsted JR, Blackman JA, Badger GJ, *et al.* Hysteroscopy versus hysterectomy for the treatment of abnormal uterine bleeding: a comparison of cost. *Feril Steril* 1996;65:310–16

5. Donnez J, Polet R, Mathieu P-E, *et al.* Nd : YAG laser ITT multifiber device (the Donnez device): endometrial ablation by interstitial hyperthermia. In Donnez

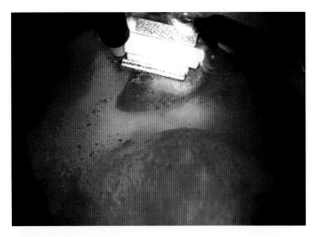

Figure 19 The electrode is brought in contact with the fundal area. Note that the visibility with normal saline is as good as with Glycine® when a through-flow resectoscope is used

J, Nisolle M, eds. *An Atlas of Laser Operative Laparoscopy and Hysteroscopy*. Carnforth, UK: The Parthenon Publishing Group, 1994:353–9

6. Mencaglia L. Hysteroscopy and adenocarcinoma. *Obstet Gynecol Clin North Am* 1995;22:573–9

7. Bhattacharya S, Cameron IM, Mollison J, *et al*. Admission-discharge policies for hysteroscopic surgery; a randomised comparison of day case with in-patient admission. *Eur J Obstet Gynecol Reprod Biol* 1998;78:81–4

8. van Herendael BJ. Hazard and dangers of operative hysteroscopy. In Sutton C, Diamond M, eds. *Endoscopic Surgery for Gynaecologists*. London: WB Saunders, 1998:118–25

9. van Herendael BJ. Instrumentation in hysteroscopy. *Obstet Gynecol Clin North Am* 1995;22:391–408

Second-generation technologies for endometrial ablation

47

G.A. Vilos

Menorrhagia from benign causes is a very common problem in women of reproductive age. Hysteroscopic endometrial ablation was introduced in the 1980s as an alternative to hysterectomy in women who failed medical management. Second-generation technologies, sometimes called global endometrial ablation, were introduced in the 1990s as easier, possibly safer, and equally effective alternatives to hysteroscopic ablation. Several devices have been introduced, some of which are still undergoing feasibility and/or comparative clinical trials. These devices include: three hot water intrauterine balloons, two intrauterine free saline circulating solutions, one multielectrode electrocoagulating balloon, one three-dimensional bipolar electrocoagulating system, one using microwaves, one diode fiber laser and at least three cryoprobes.

All these devices require less operator skill and no irrigant/distending solutions, except for the free circulating saline devices. All require some kind of thermal energy, such as heat or cold, to destroy the endometrium. Although all devices are promising and have produced impressive preliminary results, the long-term efficacy, complication rates and/or cost–benefit ratio have not been established.

This chapter describes these devices in the order in which they appeared chronologically and presents peer-reviewed publications and completed, but as yet unpublished, comparative randomized clinical trials with at least 12 months of follow-up. It is left to the readers to assess the evidence and reach their own conclusions and preferences. Criteria in choosing any of the devices should include:

(1) Maximum safety;

(2) User friendliness;

(3) Treatment time;

(4) Menstrual reduction rates;

(5) Avoidance of further treatment, such as medications, repeat surgery or hysterectomy;

(6) Costs of treatment compared to the first-generation ablation treatments and/or hysterectomy.

ENDOMETRIAL ABLATION

Endometrial ablation is the destruction or elimination of the endometrium by coagulation, freezing or resection, offered as an alternative to hysterectomy to those patients with dysfunctional uterine bleeding (DUB) and benign pathology who are unable or unwilling to tolerate traditional therapies. DUB is defined as menstrual blood loss greater than 80 ml per cycle, occurring in the absence of anatomic lesions in the pelvis or systemic diseases. DUB can be the result of both ovulatory and anovulatory abnormalities. The consequences of DUB are excessive menstrual blood loss (menorrhagia, hypermenorrhea) which is often a serious, embarrassing and debilitating condition for many women, adversely affecting their quality of life, and together with uterine fibroids account for up to 75% of all hysterectomies performed worldwide[1,2].

Patient assessment

The diagnostic approach to abnormal uterine bleeding should include, ascertaining whether there is anatomic pathology present, determining whether there is benign or (pre)malignant disease, and determining whether there is an underlying medical cause which could be treated.

Patient counselling

(1) Patients should be made aware that amenorrhea cannot be guaranteed. If patients wish or expect amenorrhea, they should be advised against endometrial ablation and rather consider a hysterectomy.

(2) Although the menstrual reduction rates are reported to be between 85 and 95%, the amenorrhea rate is between 15 and 50% depending on multiple factors, such as the technology used, the experience of the surgeon and the presence of pathology such as myomas and/or adenomyosis.

(3) It has been shown that the satisfaction rate following endometrial ablation is 80–90%.

(4) Approximately 15–25% of patients will require a second surgical procedure, such as repeat endometrial ablation and/or hysterectomy. Repeat endometrial ablation is performed in approximately 2–15% of patients and it may result in a higher complication rate, such as uterine perforation and/or excessive bleeding, than the first ablation. Up to 20% of patients will have a subsequent hysterectomy for pain, abnormal bleeding, or both. A higher prevalence of adenomyosis is usually found in the hysterectomy specimens[3,4].

The patient work-up

(1) A complete history, physical and pelvic examination;

(2) Papanicolaou smear;

(3) Complete blood count, coagulation profile, thyroid function;

(4) Sonography/saline sonohysterography (SIS) to assess uterine size, shape, endometrial thickness and presence of fibroids or polyps;

(5) Endometrial sampling (office biopsy, dilatation and curettage (D&C), hysteroscopic biopsy).

Indications for endometrial ablation

(1) Disabling uterine bleeding;

(2) Failed traditional therapies;

(3) Poor surgical risk for hysterectomy;

(4) Preservation of the uterus.

Relative contraindications

(1) Simple endometrial hyperplasia;

(2) Dysmenorrhea/chronic pelvic pain;

(3) Premenstrual syndrome (PMS);

(4) Multiple fibroids;

(5) Enlarged uterus (more than 12-cm cavity);

(6) Uterine prolapse.

Absolute contraindications

(1) Genital (pre)malignancy (cervical, uterine, tubal, ovarian);

(2) Women wishing to preserve their fertility;

(3) Women expecting amenorrhea;

(4) Acute pelvic inflammatory disease (PID).

Preparation prior to ablation

Assessment prior to endometrial ablation must include endometrial biopsy or D&C, or hysteroscopic evaluation with endometrial biopsies to exclude neoplasia. Sterilization must be discussed and documented[3]. Following ablation of the endometrium, intrauterine and ectopic pregnancies have been reported[5].

A thin endometrium is easier to coagulate, freeze or resect, may be associated with fewer intrauterine/postoperative complications and improves menstrual outcomes. Surgery may be more efficient and effective when performed in the immediate post-menstrual phase or following mechanical removal of the endometrium by sharp or suction curettage. Pharmacologic agents, such as oral contraceptives, progestins and danazol, have been proven to be effective in thinning the endometrium but one must bear in mind that progestins may decidualize the endometrium, resulting in hypervascularity and stromal edema which might impede the energy used for ablation[6]. Gonadotropin releasing hormone (GnRH) agonists have been shown to be very effective in thinning the endometrium and facilitate surgery by shortening operating time, reducing fluid absorption and improving menstrual outcome[4,7–11].

Photocoagulation of the endometrium (Nd : YAG laser)

The patient is prepped and draped under appropriate anesthesia (usually general). The uterus is distended with a sterile liquid solution and the endometrium is photocoagulated with the neodymium : yttrium–aluminum–garnet (Nd : YAG) laser fiber by direct contact[12] or by blanching the endometrium[13]. It requires expensive equipment (Nd : YAG laser system and fibers), and, for this reason, it has been the least frequently used technique. Because it destroys the endometrium, by direct contact or the blanching method, it is imperative to have a preoperative endometrial sample to exclude neoplasia. It has the lowest rate of complications, such as excessive bleeding, perforation, visceral burns and emergency interventions[14].

Electrocoagulation/resection of the endometrium

The patient is prepped and draped as for laser photocoagulation. The uterus is distended with an electrolyte-free sterile solution (glycine, sorbitol, dextrose, etc.) and the endometrium is coagulated, or resected, using an electrode connected to a high-frequency electrosurgical generator[3].

The overall effect of endometrial ablation (Nd : YAG laser or high-frequency energy) is amenorrhea (15–50%), hypomenorrhea (30–50%) and no change in menses (8–10%)[15,16]. The long-term outcome of endometrial ablation has been reviewed recently by Martyn[17]. Life-table analyses of up to 6.5 years have shown high satisfaction rates of approximately 85%. Surgical retreatment rates are approximately 20% for hysterectomy and 10% for repeat endometrial ablation. Patients undergoing surgery after the age of 40 years appear to have a better outcome[16,17].

Complications

Complications specific to endometrial ablation include[14–16,18]:

(1) Fluid overload (0.4–1.5%);

(2) Hemorrhage (0.2–1.0%);

(3) Uterine perforation (0.8–1.5%);

(4) Visceral injury (0.1–0.3%);

(5) Infection and septicemia (0.4–1.0%);

(6) Recurrence of abnormal bleeding (8–10%);

(7) Death (0.2 per 1000);

(8) Unintended pregnancy (both ectopic and intrauterine, estimated 0.3%);

(9) Burns to the genital tract and viscera[19–21];

(10) Laparotomy for visceral damage after uterine perforation and hysterectomy for uncontrolled bleeding.

Although hysteroscopic endometrial ablation is effective, and is associated with reduced morbidity, mortality, hospitalization and convalescence compared to hysterectomy[18], it requires additional training and surgical expertise, excessive non-physiological solutions to distend the uterus, and energy sources with their inherent hazards and complications[19–21]. Its general use has, therefore, been reluctantly accepted because many surgeons find the procedure and the energy sources intimidating.

Second-generation endometrial ablation technologies, sometimes called global endometrial ablation, were introduced in the mid-1990s to overcome these concerns and potential problems. Several devices and techniques have been investigated and introduced in the last decade. These devices are described in chronological order as they appeared in the gynecological field and not in order of importance or of the author's preferences. An attempt is made to present all these devices in an unbiased manner and describe their efficacy and safety only by the available peer-reviewed publications consisting of both Grade A evidence (randomized controlled trials) and Grade B evidence (well-conducted clinical cohort studies but not randomized). Available data from prospective randomized comparative clinical trials with at least 12 months of follow-up, but that are, as yet, unpublished, will be presented briefly. Reviews of these technologies have been published by Cooper and Erickson[22], Vilos[23] and the Middlesbrough Consensus Document[16].

HOT WATER BALLOON ENDOMETRIAL ABLATION

Thermachoice® I

The thermal balloon catheter was designed by Dr Bob Neuwirth of New York and described in 1994[24]. Preliminary results on 18 patients were published in 1994 by Singer and colleagues[25]. The first pilot study on 30 patients was performed in June/July 1994 when the pressure and duration of treatment were established by Vilos and co-workers[26].

The Thermachoice I system (Gynecare, Menlo Park, CA, USA) consists of a 16 cm long × 5 mm diameter catheter, with a latex balloon attached to its distal end, housing a heating element and two temperature sensors. The other end allows for inflation of the balloon and connects to a controller unit that monitors and controls preset intraballoon temperature, pressure and duration of treatment. The balloon catheter is first tested for leaks and the system is primed by inflating it with 30 ml of 5% dextrose in water (5 D/W) and deflating it to 200 mmHg negative pressure to remove any air. Subsequently, the balloon is inserted transcervically without hysteroscopic visualization. The balloon is inflated slowly to a pressure of 180 mmHg pressure. The heater is then activated and the intraballoon solution temperature is maintained at an even 87°C ± 2°C. An effective therapy has been determined to be 8 min long.

The results from a prospective Canadian Clinical Trial by Vilos and co-workers[27], an International Clinical Trial by Amso and colleagues[28], and a Food and Drug Administration (FDA)-approved US study comparing the Thermachoice with the rollerball[29,30] are consistent. The efficacy of the Thermachoice is equivalent to that of the rollerball hysteroscopic endometrial ablation, with an overall menstrual score reduction of 85.5% versus 92% and patient satisfaction of 86% versus 87% in the Thermachoice and rollerball groups, respectively. Furthermore, the treatment time is significantly reduced (per cent less than 30 min) in the balloon (71%) versus rollerball (29%) and the hysterectomy rates at 1 and 3 years of follow-up were 1% and 3% versus 3% and 9%, respectively[16,29,30]. The safety, efficacy and cost savings of the Thermachoice I have also been reported by other investigators[31–42].

It requires skills equivalent to those used in the insertion of an intrauterine device. It is simple, safe and effective, with no serious complications reported to date in over 100 000 cases performed world-wide. A significant number of selected patients can be treated without general anesthesia.

It is a blind procedure (not done under hysteroscopic visualization). However, the balloon will not be pressurized if it is not contained within the uterine cavity. It can only be used when a normal uterine cavity is present and it should not be used in the presence of fibroids, polyps, intrauterine adhesions or septa.

Thermachoice® II (Circulating Fluid Silicon Balloon)

Thermachoice® II (Gynecare, Menlo Park, CA, USA) is similar to Thermachoice I except that the balloon is made of silicone and it contains an impeller to agitate the fluid (Figure 1). It is tested for leaks and purged of any air as per Thermachoice I. The silicone balloon and the < 5 mm diameter catheter are inserted into the uterus. The balloon is then filled with sterile 5 D/W until the pressure reaches

180 mmHg. Once the pressure is confirmed to be stable by waiting for at least 30 s, the heater and the impeller are activated.

The heating element and the impeller fan inside the balloon raise the temperature to 87°C (186°F) and evenly circulate the fluid for 8 min during the therapy cycle. The controller continuously monitors and displays intrauterine pressure, regulates fluid temperature and controls therapy time throughout the procedure. The heating element automatically deactivates if preset parameters are exceeded. When the controller signals that treatment is completed, the balloon is deflated and the catheter is withdrawn and discarded.

Grainger and co-workers (unpublished) demonstrated in extirpated human uteri that the depth of tissue necrosis was consistent to a depth of 4 mm of myometrium except the cornua which extended only for 1 mm into the myometrium. Furthermore, the endomyometrial necrosis was more uniform and deeper throughout the uterine cavity compared to that obtained with Thermachoice I.

Clinical trial of Thermachoice II (July 1998–June 2000)

The effect of two pre-ablation endometrial thinning modalities on the efficacy of the new Thermachoice system was evaluated by Vilos and colleagues with a randomized clinical trial starting in July 1998. A secondary objective compared the rate of improvement in post-ablation bleeding of the suction curettage group, to previous studies of the passive-circulation (Thermachoice I) system, which used the same pretreatment regimen.

Qualified patients were randomized to one of two treatments for preoperative endometrial thinning: a 3-min suction curettage or 1 month of GnRH agonist administration (goserelin 3.6 mg intramuscularly; Astra-Zeneca, Mississauga, Canada). Uterine bleeding was documented by menstrual diary scores at baseline, 3 months, 6 months and 1 year.

One hundred and five patients with menorrhagia of benign etiology were randomized and 102 patients were treated. Pre- and post-procedure evaluations were conducted by the patients and the physician, to assess the degree of bleeding. Inclusion criteria required a patient's Higham menstrual score of > 150 1 to 2 months prior to treatment and the preoperative mean baseline scores were 407 and 392 in the GnRH agonist and suction curettage groups, respectively.

No safety issues related to the device were noted. Silicone balloon material appears to perform similarly to the previous latex balloon design, as observed by post-ablation hysteroscopy. The postoperative Higham scores at 6 and 12 months consistently showed a reduction of menstrual blood loss up to 90%, with mean scores of 25 versus 32 in the GnRH agonist and suction curettage groups, respectively. Patient satisfaction was reported to be up to 90–95% in both groups. The postoperative Higham score of Thermachoice I was 65 and reduction of menstrual bleeding was 84% in historical controls.

Advantages of Thermachoice II

The advantages of Thermachoice II are the following:

(1) Catheter comparable to the size of pipelle;

(2) Minimizes the need for cervical dilatation;

(3) Allows treatment of latex-sensitive patients;

(4) Provides more uniform distribution of heated fluid;

(5) Provides more uniform and deeper necrosis of tissue;

(6) Provides up to 90% reduction in menstrual bleeding;

(7) Provides up to 95% patient satisfaction.

Cavaterm™ hot water balloon

The Cavaterm™ hot water balloon (Wallsten Medical SA, Morges, Switzerland) consists of a disposable silicone balloon catheter (outside diameter 8 mm), in which a heating element is integrated, and a battery-operated controller (Figure 2). The balloon is filled with 1.5% glycine solution to a pressure of 180 mmHg. The liquid is

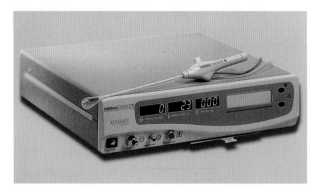

Figure 1 Thermachoice® II Uterine Balloon Therapy System (Gynecare, Menlo Park, CA, USA)

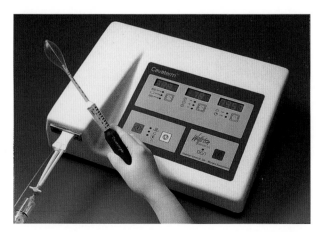

Figure 2 Cavaterm hot water balloon (Wallsten Medical SA, Morges, Switzerland)

vigorously circulated inside the balloon by pump, with oscillating pressure to ensure even heat transfer to the endomyometrium. The mean balloon temperature is 71°C and the treatment is completed after 15 min[43,44].

From the available published studies of patient cohorts and the company's brochure, there are 311 patients who have been treated with the Cavaterm system. At 12–60 months of follow-up, 92–96% of patients reported significant reduction in blood loss with a satisfaction rate of up to 95%. No major complications have been reported[43–53] and 23 (7.4%) hysterectomies have been performed.

The Cavaterm system appears to give results identical to Nd : YAG laser therapy and is currently undergoing comparative clinical trials against the Nd : YAG laser in the United Kingdom, and against the rollerball in North America.

The advantages and disadvantages of the Cavaterm system are similar to the Thermachoice I and II, except that the catheter diameter is 8 mm, requiring cervical dilatation up to 9 mm. No serious complications have been reported in over 8000 cases performed world-wide to date.

VESTA MULTIELECTRODE BALLOON

The concept was conceived by Theirry Vancaillie and the system consists of a handset for introduction of an electrode balloon, a controller to monitor and distribute the electrical energy and a Valleylab Force 2 electrosurgical generator, set to supply pure cut mode current at 45 W (Valleylab, Boulder, CO, USA)[54,55]. The silicone inflatable electrode balloon is shaped as an inverted triangle that unfolds when its insertion sheath is withdrawn. There are six ventral and six dorsal thin and flexible electrode plates covering the surface of the balloon, each with its own temperature sensor (Figure 3). The four cornual electrodes have pre-set temperatures at 72°C, whereas the remaining electrodes have set temperatures at 75°C. These temperatures are maintained for a 4-min treatment period with constant distension of the balloon lumen to keep the

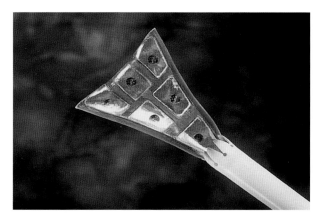

Figure 3 The Vesta System Handset Electrode Array (Valleylab, Boulder, CO, USA)

electrodes snugly against the endometrial surface. This ensures destruction to a depth of 4–5 mm into the myometrium. The cervix is dilated to 9–10 mm and the silicone balloon is inflated with 8–12 ml of air.

Preliminary results on the first 187 patients treated, at 3–24 months (mean 15 months), demonstrated 38% amenorrhea, 43% hypomenorrhea, 10% eumenorrhea and 9% no improvement. The combined amenorrhea/hypomenorrhea rate was 81%. A randomized clinical trial comparing 137 patients treated with VestaBlate™ versus 127 patients receiving resection/rollerball treatment has been completed and submitted to the FDA. The menstrual reduction was 94% versus 91% and the amenorrhea rate was 31% versus 40%, respectively[54,55]. The system is currently not in production.

HYDROTHERMABLATOR

The HydroThermAblator device (BEI Medical Systems, Hackensack, NJ, USA) was conceived by the father of endometrial ablation, Dr Milton Goldrath of Detroit[56–59]. Externally heated 0.9% normal saline is infused and circulated directly into the uterine cavity through the in-flow channel of a continuous flow hysteroscope (Figure 4). The cervix is dilated to 8 mm. The hysteroscope is introduced and the cavity is initially distended with cold saline to inspect it. Subsequently, preheated saline (at 90°C) is infused at a pressure of less than 45 mmHg for a 10-min period under hysteroscopic visualization. The cervix must be sealed tightly to prevent leakage of the circulating hot saline and it automatically shuts off flow of fluid after 10 ml is lost. This is the only device from all the global ablation techniques that allows direct visualization during the treatment cycle, which is a major safety issue. Due to the low intrauterine pressure produced by gravity alone, no flow through patent Fallopian tubes has been detected at 50 mmHg. Histological studies of the effects on the uterus of circulating hot saline prior to hysterectomy have been reported by the groups of Richart[59] and Bustos-Lopez[60].

The preliminary results on 70 treated women are as follows: 56–58% amenorrhea; 22–26% hypomenorrhea; 10–17% eumenorrhea; and 6% no improvement. The overall amenorrhea/hypomenorrhea rate at 6 and 12 months was approximately 78%[61]. A phase III randomized clinical trial comparing 181 patients treated with the HydroThermAblator with 88 patients treated with the rollerball has been completed and submitted to the FDA. At 12 months of follow-up, the amenorrhea rates were 40% versus 51% and the overall menstrual improvement was 85% versus 88%, respectively. Although its efficacy has been established, the relative safety remains to be proven. Burns to the genital tract have been encountered. Pre-thinning of the endometrium is highly recommended.

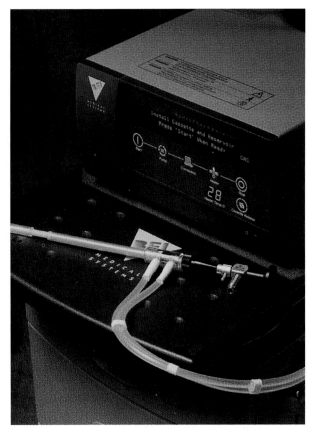

Figure 4 The HydroThermAblator System (BEI Medical Systems, Hackensack, NJ, USA)

MICROWAVE ENDOMETRIAL ABLATION

The use of microwave energy was first described by Sharp and colleagues[62]. The Microwave Endometrial Ablation (MEA™) system (Microsulis plc, Waterlooville, UK)[62-67] consists of an 8-mm diameter probe which is inserted into the uterus. Microwave power is generated by magnetron and passes along the cable to the probe at 30 W, generating energy of 1.5–9.3 kJ. The power is controlled via a foot switch operated by the surgeon (Figure 5). The temperature achieved inside the uterus is monitored continuously by thermocouples on the exterior surface of the waveguide. A computer displays temperature graphically, in real-time, and generates a hard-copy. The frequency of the microwaves is 9.2 GHz (9.2×10^9 Hz compared to the electrosurgical generator 0.5×10^6 Hz).

After appropriate analgesia (paracervical block, neuroleptic or general), the cervix is dilated to 8 mm and the microwave probe is inserted to touch the fundus. Once the probe is activated and the tip temperature reaches 95°C (within a few seconds), the probe is moved laterally to place the tip in the uterine cornua. The temperature reading falls briefly and then rises. Once 95°C is again attained, the probe is moved to place the tip in the other cornual area to repeat the procedure. The probe is then gradually withdrawn, while maintaining the

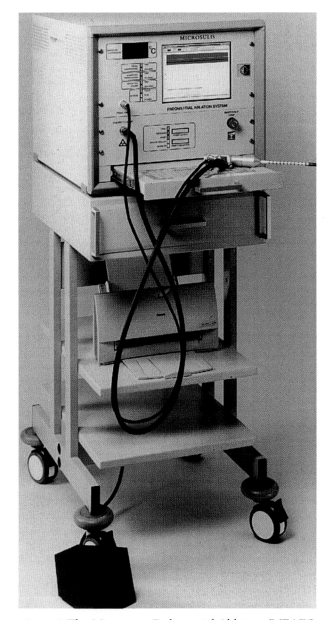

Figure 5 The Microwave Endometrial Ablation (MEA™) System (Microsulis plc, Waterlooville, UK)

probe temperature in the 80–95°C range to ensure even, complete endometrial destruction. The entire treatment is completed in 2–3 min. Pre-thinning of the endometrium is recommended.

Results after 6 months of treatment in 23 patients demonstrated 57% amenorrhea, 26% hypomenorrhea and 12% no improvement. Three patients were retreated successfully. The overall results were 83% for single treatment and 96% after retreatment[62].

This technique is safe, since the wavelength chosen provides energy which is unable to propagate further than 6 mm from the tip of the waveguide. This generates sufficient heating inside the uterine cavity and endometrial layer to ensure thorough ablation, with no risk to adjacent structures. It is currently undergoing comparative randomized clinical trials against the rollerball for FDA submission. A randomized comparative clinical trial of microwave endometrial ablation ($n = 129$) against transcervical resection of the endometrium ($n = 134$) was published recently[65]. At 12 months, 89 (77%) women in the microwave ablation group and 93 (75%) in the resection group were totally or generally satisfied with their treatment. The menstrual pattern was similar in both groups, with a combined amenorrhea/hypomenorrhea rate of 89% in both groups and satisfaction rate of 90%. Repeat resection was performed in 1% and hysterectomy in 12–13%, in both groups. The total operation time was 11 min in the microwave ablation group and 15 min in the resection group. Although the technique is short and easy to master, it is a blind procedure and the relative safety has not been established. In 1433 cases performed, in 13 centers in the UK and Canada, one small bowel burn was encountered with the microwave ablation (frequency 0.7/1000)[67]. An additional bowel injury was recently reported at the Middlesbrough Consensus Meeting in the UK[16].

CRYOENDOMETRIAL ABLATION

Cryosurgery of the endometrium using a probe to freeze the endometrium from –60°C to –100°C in six patients was first reported by Cahan and Brockunier in 1967[68]. Droegemueller and colleagues evaluated two types of cryoprobes using freon in 1970[69] (Frigitronics, Inc., Shelton, CT, USA). Ten of 16 patients with DUB developed amenorrhea during the 6–8-week interval between cryosurgery and vaginal hysterectomy. In two patients, cryosurgery was accomplished under local anesthesia[70,71].

In two subsequent studies by Pittrof and colleagues, the authors reported on 18 patients who underwent transcervical endometrial cryoablation using normal saline as a uterine distension medium[72,73]. The principle of this new technique is to distend the uterine cavity, with 3–15 ml of normal saline, and then to freeze it with nitrous oxide, an iceball forming a mold of the uterine cavity with a specially designed cryosurgical probe. The probe looks similar to a number 8 Hegar dilator. After 5 min, the ice is allowed to melt and the same procedure is repeated with the probe pointing towards the other uterine cornua. Of the 12 patients followed-up for up to 3 or more months, eight were completely satisfied with their results. There were no operative complications and 13 patients were discharged the day after their operation[72,73].

Rutherford and colleagues, in a recent pilot study involving 15 patients followed for 22 months, reported that amenorrhea was achieved in 50%. New equipment is able to freeze the endometrium down to –170°C[74]. The cervix was dilated to 8 mm and the bladder was filled with 300–400 ml of warm saline to act as a heat sink. The uterine cavity was filled with up to 10 ml of a water-soluble lubricant. An 8 mm × 27 cm conical-tip cryomed-ical freezing probe with a 4-cm freezing zone attached to a CMS 450 AccuProbe System (Cryomedical Sciences, Rockville, MD, USA) was inserted into the uterine fundus. Once freezing of the uterine cavity was begun, iceball formation was monitored using a bi-plane 7.5-MHz transrectal transducer with an ultrasound scanner. Within 3–5 min of the probe reaching –170°C, the front of the iceball was seen to be at least 50% through the myometrium. At this point, freezing was discontinued and thawing begun[74]. Fifteen patients underwent 16 procedures for DUB. Life-table calculations gave amenorrhea rates of 75.5% at 6 months and 50.3% at 22 months. One patient was retreated.

First Option™ Uterine Cryoblation Therapy™

This cryosurgical system is compressor driven and uses a new mixed gas coolant to generate temperatures of –90° to –100°C. The cryoprobe is inserted in the uterine cavity and saline is injected to bathe the cryoprobe (Figures 6 and 7). Freezing–thawing of the intrauterine iceball is monitored with transabdominal ultrasound. Endometrial cryoablation in ten women undergoing hysterectomy resulted in 9–12 mm depth of endomyometrial necrosis as determined by tetrazolium staining and electron microscopy[75–77].

Feasibility pilot studies have been performed and a multicenter randomized clinical trial comparing First Option™ (CryoGen, Inc., San Diego, CA, USA) ($n = 189$) to rollerball ($n = 86$) has been completed. At 12 months follow-up, the amenorrhea and satisfaction rates were 28% and 88% in the First Option group versus 52% and 88% in the rollerball group, respectively. Failure rates of 13% versus 9% were also reported[16]. The system was recently approved for use by the FDA.

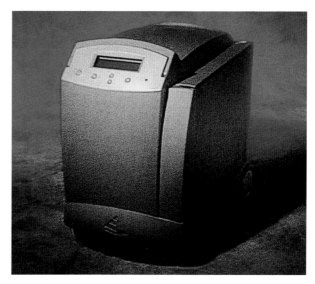

Figure 6 The First Option™ Uterine Cryoblation Therapy™ (CryoGen, Inc., San Diego, CA, USA)

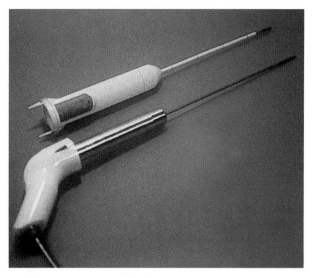

Figure 7 The First Option™ cryoprobes

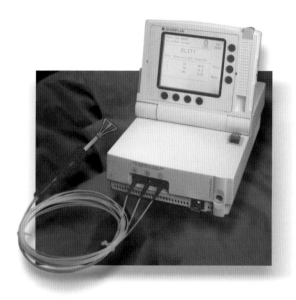

Figure 8 The Endometrial Laser Intrauterine Thermal Therapy (ELITT™) System (Gynelase™ ESC Sharplan, Needham, MA, USA)

ENDOMETRIAL LASER INTRAUTERINE THERMAL THERAPY (ELITT™)

ELITT™ (GyneLase™, ESC Sharplan, Needham, MA, USA) employs a diffuse laser light that reaches the entire uterine cavity, including inaccessible areas such as the cornua (Figure 8). It does not require direct contact with the endometrium to induce photocoagulation. The 830-nm wavelength of the diode laser light penetrates the uterine wall to a precise depth, where it is absorbed by the hemoglobin. The absorbed light is then transformed to heat, coagulating the endometrium[78–80].

This idea of the handset was conceived by Dr Jacques Donnez of Brussels and it includes three proprietary optical light diffusers that are designed to transmit laser light in all directions to effect the destruction of the endometrial tissue in the fundus and cornua, away from the cervical opening. On each side, diffusers of the handset can be manipulated individually by the operator to conform to the shape of the uterine cavity. The cervix is dilated to 7 mm, the light diffuser handpiece is inserted and deployed and the laser is activated for a 7-min, pre-programmed treatment. Therapy may not be effective in the presence of intrauterine bleeding.

Preliminary data on 75 patients followed from 6 to 24 months indicate 63–68% amenorrhea, with an additional 19–28% spotting and 0% menorrhagia[79]. In a subsequent report of the first 100 patients after 1 year of follow-up by Donnez and colleagues, the amenorrhea rate was 71%, and the rate of amenorrhea/severe hypomenorrhea rate was > 90%[80]. The ELITT procedure is an inherently safe and simple alternative, providing controlled and effective treatment of the entire endometrium. The system is presently undergoing cohort clinical trials and comparative randomized clinical trials for FDA submission and approval.

NOVASURE™ GEA GLOBAL ENDOMETRIAL ABLATION

The NovaSure™ GEA (global endometrial ablation) System (Novacept, Palo Alto, CA, USA)[16,22,23] consists of a single-use, three-dimensional bipolar ablation device and radio-frequency controller, that enables a controlled endometrial ablation in an average of 90 s, without the need for a hysteroscope or hysteroscopic skills.

Endometrial 'pretreatment' of any kind (mechanical, pharmaceutical, timing) is not required when using NovaSure GEA technology. The patient can even be treated when actively bleeding.

The NovaSure GEA ablation device (Figure 9) consists of a conformable bipolar metalized porous fabric mesh, mounted on an expandable frame. Integral to the hand-held device is the intrauterine measuring device for determining uterine cavity width (cornu-to-cornu distance). The unique geometry of the electrode controls and provides a shallower depth of myometrial desiccation in the cornual area and lower uterine segment and a deeper ablation in the mid-body of the uterus. The NovaSure GEA device can treat a uterus with a sounding length up to 12 cm and an adjustable sheath will accommodate and protect a cervix of any length, thus avoiding, or significantly reducing, the possibility of burning the endocervical canal and the subsequent stenosis and other complications related to it.

The NovaSure GEA controller (Figure 10) contains a constant power output generator, with a maximum power delivery of 180 W. Once the uterine cavity length is evaluated by sounding and the width is measured by the device, these values are key-entered into the controller and it

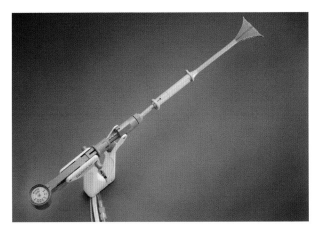

Figure 9 The NovaSure™ device (Novacept, Palo Alto, CA, USA)

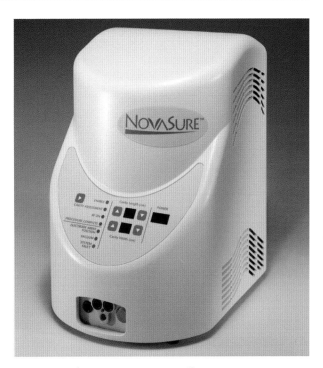

Figure 10 The NovaSure™ controller

automatically calculates the power output needed to assure an optimal confluent lesion within the uterine cavity of a given size. The depth of ablation is controlled by continuous monitoring of tissue impedance (resistance) during the procedure. The ablation of the endometrial layer is a low-impedance process, due to the high level of liquid present in the endometrial tissue. The endometrium is vaporized during the ablation and evacuated from the uterine cavity by suction. Once the myometrial layer is reached, tissue impedance (resistance) increases and quickly reaches 50 Ohms (which is equivalent to the impedance of the ablated superficial myometrium), and the NovaSure GEA System automatically terminates the ablation process. This is the key aspect of the NovaSure GEA technology. The ablation process is based not on temperature and time, but on specific, well-analyzed, physical characteristics of the tissue. This approach allows for a very well-controlled ablation process and provides consistent results.

The device is inserted transcervically into the uterine cavity; the sheath is retracted, deploying a fan-shaped bipolar electrode, which conforms to the uterine cavity. Unlike the balloon concept of other devices, where pressure distends the uterine cavity wall, a vacuum is employed to assure good electrode–tissue contact. The vacuum pump is contained within the radio-frequency controller. Paramount for the effectiveness of this technology, a vacuum is monitored and maintained within the uterine cavity throughout the endometrial ablation procedure. Constant vacuum assures an intimate apposition between the electrode and the endometrium. Constant suction also removes blood, endometrium and vaporization by-products generated during the bipolar electrosurgical process. The removal of steam during tissue vaporization maintains a controlled depth of electrosurgical effect by minimizing the otherwise irregular march of cavitational tissue penetration and destruction.

A Cavity Integrity Assessment System is an integral part of the NovaSure GEA System. This automatic safety feature was developed and implemented to assist the physician in the timely detection of uterine wall perforation, thus preventing energy delivery. It utilizes a hysteroflator-type technology. CO_2 is delivered into the uterine cavity at a safe flow rate and pressure. CO_2 pressure is monitored within the uterine cavity, the controller sensing a maintained pressure over a known period of time. Once the proper pressure is maintained, confirming good uterine wall integrity, the controller proceeds with the ablation process in an automatic or semi-automatic mode.

Over 700 patients have been treated using this novel method and technology world-wide. The NovaSure GEA System is commercially available in Europe and Canada and awaiting approval in the USA. A number of studies were conducted in order to evaluate the safety and effectiveness of the NovaSure GEA System, of which three are Grade A, randomized, controlled studies. The most important of these is the FDA multicenter clinical study, which compares the gold standard wire loop resection and roller-ball ablation to the NovaSure GEA. The treatment phase has been completed and all of the 267 patients have completed their 6-month follow-up visit. Preliminary clinical results reveal that 44% of patients in the NovaSure™ GEA arm achieved a complete cessation of bleeding (amenorrhea). The patient satisfaction rate was also very high, being 98%. Clinical data acquired from the European study suggest a similar outcome with an increase in amenorrhea rate over time and very high stability of the results. The post-ablation hysterectomy rate is approximately 1.5% (based on the analysis of all the patients treated world-wide).

Preliminary results in Europe and North America, suggest that the NovaSure GEA System can be an effective method of endometrial ablation in patients suffering from menorrhagia secondary to DUB, yielding high amenorrhea and patient satisfaction rates. Presently, the follow-up phase of the FDA-approved multicenter, randomized, controlled clinical study is near its completion.

CONCLUSIONS

(1) All these devices are easier to use than hysteroscopic endometrial ablation. However, the ease of performance and simplicity of the devices do not remove the need for adequate education and training.

(2) Sufficient outcome data on efficacy and durability have not yet been collected.

(3) The overall safety will not be determined until several hundred procedures (perhaps thousands) have been performed by each device. Most devices have not yet passed 1000 procedures. In choosing one of these devices, maximum safety should be the first criterion.

(4) If safety and outcome measures are similar, the duration of treatment and associated costs may become of importance.

(5) Since the endometrium is destroyed by all these devices, it is imperative that (pre-)malignant uterine disease be excluded.

(6) Since all procedures are performed blindly (no hysteroscopic visualization), except the hydrothermablation, it would be prudent to perform postdilatation hysteroscopy and immediately posttreatment to ensure that only the intended endometrial cavity has been treated. False passages and partial or complete uterine perforations occur at a frequency of 0.8–1.5% and may result in adjacent visceral injury.

REFERENCES

1. Bachmann GA. Hysterectomy. A critical review. *J Reprod Med* 1990;35:839–62

2. Carlson KJ, Nichols DH, Schiff I. Indications for hysterectomy. *N Engl J Med* 1993;83:792–6

3. Vilos GA, Vilos EC, King HJ. Experience with 800 hysteroscopic endometrial ablations. *J Am Assoc Gynecol Laparosc* 1996;4:33–8

4. Donnez J, Vilos GA, Gannon MJ, *et al*. Goserelin acetate (Zoladex) plus endometrial ablation for dysfunctional uterine bleeding (DUB): 3-year follow-up. *Fertil Steril* 2001;in press

5. Vilos GA. Intrauterine pregnancy following rollerball endometrial ablation. *J Soc Obstet Gynaecol Can* 1995;17:479–80

6. Brooks PG, Serden SP, Davos I. Hormonal inhibition of the endometrium for resectoscopic endometrial ablation. *Am J Obstet Gynecol* 1991;164:1601–8

7. Garry R, Khaur A, Mooney P, *et al*. A comparison of goserelin and danazol as endometrial thinning agents prior to endometrial laser ablation. *Br J Obstet Gynaecol* 1996;103:339–44

8. Vercellini P, Perino A, Consonni R, *et al*. Treatment with a gonadotrophin releasing hormone agonist before endometrial resection: a multicentre, randomised controlled trial. *Br J Obstet Gynaecol* 1996;103:562–8

9. Donnez J, Vilos GA, Gannon MJ, *et al*. Goserelin (Zoladex) plus endometrial ablation for dysfunctional uterine bleeding. A large randomized doubleblind clinical trial. *Fertil Steril* 1997;68:29–36

10. Vercellini P, Perino A, Consonni R, *et al*. Does preoperative treatment with a gonadotropin-releasing hormone agonist improve the outcome of endometrial resection? *J Am Assoc Gynecol Laparosc* 1998;5:357–60

11. Sowter MC, Singla AA, Lethaby A. Pre-operative endometrial thinning agents before hysteroscopic surgery for heavy menstrual bleeding (Cochrane Review). In *The Cochrane Library*. Oxford: Update Software, 1999: issue 3

12. Goldrath MH, Fuller TA, Segal S. Laser photocoagulation of the endometrium for the treatment of menorrhagia. *Am J Obstet Gynecol* 1981;140:14–19

13. Loffer FD. Hysteroscopic endometrial ablation with the Nd:YAG laser using a nontouch technique. *Obstet Gynecol* 1987;69:679–82

14. Overton C, Hargreaves J, Maresh M. A national survey of the complications of endometrial destruction of menstrual disorders: the MISTLETOE study. *Br J Obstet Gynaecol* 1997;104:1351–9

15. Farrell SA, Baskett TF. Endometrial ablation for dysfunctional uterine bleeding. *J Soc Obstet Gynaecol Can* 1992;14:31–41.

16. Evidence and techniques on endometrial ablation: a consensus meeting. Middlesbrough, UK. December 7–8, 2000. *Gynecol Endosc* 2001;in press

17. Martyn P. Endometrial ablation: long-term outcome. *J Soc Obstet Gynaecol Can* 2000;22:423–7

18. Vilos GA, Pispidikis JT, Botz CK. Economic evaluation of hysteroscopic endometrial ablation versus vaginal hysterectomy for menorrhagia. *Obstet Gynecol* 1996;88:241–5

19. Raders J, Vilos GA. Dispersive pad injuries associated with hysteroscopic surgery. *J Am Assoc Gynecol Laparosc* 1999;6:363–6

20. Vilos GA, Brown S, Graham G, *et al*. Genital tract electrical burns during hysteroscopic endometrial ablation: report of 13 cases in United States and Canada. *J Am Assoc Gynecol Laparosc* 2000;7:141–7

21. Vilos GA, McCulloch S, Borg P, *et al*. Intended and stray radio frequency electrical currents during resectoscopic surgery. *J Am Assoc Gynecol Laparosc* 2000;7:55–63

22. Cooper JM, Erickson ML. Global endometrial ablation technologies. *Obstet Gynecol Clin North Am* 2000;27:385–96

23. Vilos GA. Global endometrial ablation. *J Soc Obstet Gynaecol Can* 2000;22:668–75

24. Neuwirth RS, Duran M, Singer A, *et al*. The endometrial ablator: a new instrument. *Obstet Gynecol* 1994;83:792–6

25. Singer A, Almanza R, Gutierrez A, *et al*. Preliminary clinical experience with a thermal balloon endometrial ablation method to treat menorrhagia. *Obstet Gynecol* 1994;83:732–4

26. Vilos GA, Vilos EC, Pendley L. Endometrial ablation with a thermal balloon for the treatment of menorrhagia. *J Am Assoc Gynecol Laparosc* 1996;3: 383–7

27. Vilos GA, Fortin CA, Sanders B, *et al*. Clinical trial of the uterine thermal balloon for treatment of menorrhagia. *J Am Assoc Gynecol Laparosc* 1997;4:559–65

28. Amso NN, Stabinsky SA, McFaul P, *et al*. Uterine thermal balloon therapy for the treatment of menorrhagia: the first 300 patients from a multicentre study. *Br J Obstet Gynaecol* 1998;105:517–23

29. Meyer WR, Walsh BW, Grainger DA, *et al*. Thermal balloon and rollerball ablation to treat menorrhagia: a multicenter comparison. *Obstet Gynecol* 1998;92: 98–103

30. Grainger DA, Tjaden BL, Meyer WR, *et al*. Thermal balloon and rollerball ablation to treat menorrhagia: two-year results from a multicenter prospective randomized clinical trial. *J Am Assoc Gynecol Laparosc* 2000;7:175–9

31. Yackel DB. Menorrhagia treated by thermal balloon endometrial ablation. *J Soc Obstet Gynecol Can* 1999;21:1076–80

32. Lissak A, Fruchter O, Mashiach S, *et al*. Immediate versus delayed treatment of perimenopausal bleeding due to benign causes by balloon thermal ablation. *J Am Assoc Gynecol Laparosc* 1999;6:145–50

33. Aletebi FA, Vilos GA, Eskandar MA. Thermal balloon endometrial ablation to treat menorrhagia in high risk surgical candidates. *J Am Assoc Gynecol Laparosc* 1999;6:435–9

34. Vilos GA, Aletebi FA, Eskandar MA. Endometrial thermal balloon ablation with a (ThermaChoice) system to treat menorrhagia: effect of intrauterine pressure and duration of treatment. *J Am Assoc Gynecol Laparosc* 2000;7:325–9

35. Fernandez H, Capella S, Audibert F. Uterine thermal balloon therapy under local anesthesia for the treatment of menorrhagia. *Hum Reprod* 1997;12:2511–14

36. Andersen LF, Meinert L, Rygaard C, *et al*. Thermal balloon endometrial ablation: safety aspects evaluated by serosal temperature, light microscopy and electron microscopy. *Eur J Obstet Gynecol Reprod Biol* 1998;79:63–8

37. Shah AA, Stabinsky SA, Klusak T, *et al*. Measurement of serosal temperatures and depth of thermal injury generated by thermal balloon endometrial ablation in *ex vivo* and *in vivo* models. *Fertil Steril* 1998;70:692–7

38. London R, Holzman M, Rubin D, *et al*. Payer cost savings with endometrial ablation therapy. *Am J Managed Care* 1999;5:889–97

39. Vilos GA. Hot water balloon endometrial ablation. International Symposium on Diagnostic and Operative Hysteroscopy Proceedings. February 25–27, Miami, Florida. *J Am Assoc Gynecol Laparosc* 2001; in press

40. Buckshee K, Barnerjee K, Bhatla H. Uterine balloon therapy to treat menorrhagia. *Int J Gynecol Obstet* 1998;63:139–43

41. Luerti M, Garuti G. Endometrial ablation with the Uterine Balloon Therapy system. A new therapeutic option for menorrhagia. *Ital J Gynecol Obstet* 1996;8:153–6

42. Gervaise A, Fernandez H, Capella-Allouc S, *et al*. Thermal balloon ablation versus endometrial resection for the treatment of abnormal uterine bleeding. *Hum Reprod* 1999;14:2743–7

43. Friberg B, Wallsten H, Henriksson P, *et al*. A new, simple, safe and efficient device for the treatment of menorrhagia. *J Gynecol Tech* 1996;2:103–8

44. Persson BRR, Friberg B, Olsrud J, *et al*. Numerical calculations of temperature distribution resulting from intracavitary heating of the uterus. *Gynecol Endosc* 1998;7:203–9

45. Friberg B, Persson BRR, Willen R, *et al*. Endometrial destruction by hyperthermia – a possible treatment of menorrhagia. An experimental study. *Acta Obstet Gynecol Scand* 1996;75:330–5

46. Friberg B, Persson BRR, Willen R, *et al*. Endometrial destruction by thermal coagulation: evaluation of a new form of treatment for menorrhagia. *Gynecol Endosc* 1998;7:73–8

47. Hawe JA, Phillips AG, Chien PE, *et al*. Cavaterm thermal balloon ablation for the treatment of menorrhagia. *Br J Obstet Gynaecol* 1999;106:1143–4

48. Cavaterm system (online). Scandinavia (AB): Wallsten Medical; 1999 (updated 1998 Aug 08); (Cited 1999 Dec 22). (9p.). Available: http://w1.463.telia.com

49. DeGrandi P, El Din A, Kochli R, eds. Hysteroscopy, state of the art. *Contrib Gynecol Obstet* 2000;20:145–53

50. Genolet PM, Friberg B, Chardonneus E, *et al*. Endometrolyse technique au Cavaterm: resultants cliniques d'une nouvelle technique d'ablation de l'endometre. *Real Gynecol Obstet* 1996;14:28–30

51. Friberg B, Joergensen C, Ahlgren M. Endometrial thermal coagulation – degree of uterine fibrosis

predicts treatment outcome. *Gynecol Obstet Invest* 1998;45:54–7

52. Gerber S. Wirz C, Genolet PM, *et al*. Endometrolyse thermique: resultats cliniques d'une nouvelle technique d'ablation de l'endometre. *J Menopause* 1999;1:9–13

53. Gerber S, Genolet PM, De Quay N, *et al*. Endometrolyse thermique: resultats cliniques d'une nouvelle technique d'ablation de l'endometre. *Med Hyg* 1998;56:822–5

54. Soderstrom RM, Brooks PG, Corson SL, *et al*. Endometrial ablation using a distensible multielectrode balloon. *J Am Assoc Gynecol Laparosc* 1996;3:403–7

55. Corson SL, Brill AI, Brooks PG, *et al*. Interim results of the American Vesta trial of endometrial ablation. *J Am Assoc Gynecol Laparosc* 1999;6:45–9

56. Goldrath MH, Barrionuevo M, Husain M. Endometrial ablation with hysteroscopic instillation of hot saline solution. *J Am Assoc Gynecol Laparosc* 1997;4:235–40

57. Dores GB, Richart RM, Nicolau SM, *et al*. Evaluation of hydrothermablator for endometrial destruction in patients with menorrhagia. *J Am Assoc Gynecol Laparosc* 1999;6:275–8

58. Romer T, Muller J. A simple method of coagulating endometrium in patients with therapy-resistant, recurring hypermenorrhea. *J Am Assoc Gynecol Laparosc* 1999;6:265–8

59. Richart RM, Botacini das Dores G, Nicolau SM, *et al*. Histologic studies of the effects of circulating hot saline on the uterus before hysterectomy. *J Am Assoc Gynecol Laparosc* 1999;6:269–73

60. Bustos-Lopez HH, Baggish M, Valle RF, *et al*. Assessment of the safety of intrauterine instillation of heated saline for endometrial ablation. *Fertil Steril* 1998;69:155–60

61. Weisberg M, Goldrath MH, Berman J, *et al*. Hysteroscopic endometrial ablation using free heated saline for the treatment of menorrhagia. *J Am Assoc Gynecol Laparosc* 2000;7:311–16

62. Sharp NC, Cronin N, Feldberg I, *et al*. Microwave for menorrhagia: a new fast technique for endometrial ablation. *Lancet* 1995;346:1003–4

63. Hodgson DA, Feldberg IB, Sharp N, *et al*. Microwave endometrial ablation: development, clinical trials and outcomes at three years. *Br J Obstet Gynaecol* 1999;106:684–94

64. Milligan MP, Etokowo GA. Microwave endometrial ablation for menorrhagia. *J Obstet Gynecol* 1999;19:496–9

65. Cooper KG, Bain C, Parkin D. Comparison of microwave endometrial ablation and transcervical resection of the endometrium for treatment of heavy menstrual loss: a randomized trial. *Lancet* 1999;354:1859–63

66. Downes E, O'Donovan P. Microwave endometrial ablation in the management of menorrhagia: current status. *Curr Opin Obstet Gynecol* 2000;12:293–6

67. Downes E, Cooper K, O'Donovan P, *et al*. Microwave endometrial ablation is a safe technique (Abstract). *J Am Assoc Gynecol Laparosc* 2000;7:S13

68. Cahan WG, Brockunier A. Cryosurgery of the uterine cavity. *Am J Obstet Gynecol* 1967;99:138–53

69. Droegemueller W, Greer BE, Makowski EL. Preliminary observations of cryoablation of the endometrium. *Am J Obstet Gynecol* 1970;107:958–61

70. Droegemueller W, Greer B, Makowski E. Cryosurgery in patients with dysfunctional uterine bleeding. *Obstet Gynecol* 1971;38:256–8

71. Droegemueller W, Makowski E, MacSalka R. Destruction of the endometrium by cryosurgery. *Am J Obstet Gynecol* 1971;110:467–9

72. Pittrof R, Majid S, Murray A. Initial experience with transcervical cryoablation of the endometrium using saline as a uterine distension medium. *Minim Invasive Ther* 1993;2:69–73

73. Pittrof R, Majid S, Murray A. Transcervical endometrial cryoablation (ECA) for menorrhagia. *Int J Gynecol Obstet* 1994;47:135–9

74. Rutherford TJ, Zreik TG, Troiana RN, *et al*. Endometrial cryoablation, a minimally invasive procedure for abnormal uterine bleeding. (Pilot Study). *J Am Assoc Gynecol Laparosc* 1998;5:23–8

75. Dobak JD, Willems J, Howard R, *et al*. Endometrial cryoablation with ultrasound visualized in women undergoing hysterectomy. *J Am Assoc Gynecol Laparosc* 2000;7:89–93

76. Dobak JD, Willems J. Extripated uterine endometrial cryoablation with ultrasound visualization. *J Am Assoc Gynecol Laparosc* 2000;7:95–101

77. Dobak JD, Ryba E, Kovalcheck S. A new closed-loop cryosurgical device for endometrial ablation. *J Am Assoc Gynecol Laparosc* 2000;7:245–9

78. Donnez J, Polet R, Mathiew PE, *et al*. Endometrial laser interstitial hyperthermy: a potential modality for endometrial ablation. *Obstet Gynecol* 1996;87:459–64

79. Donnez J, Polet R, Squifflet, *et al*. Endometrial laser intrauterine thermo-therapy (ELITT): a revolutionary new approach to the elimination of menorrhagia. *Curr Opin Obstet Gynecol* 1999;11:363–70

80. Donnez J, Polet R, Rabinovitz R, *et al*. Endometrial laser intrauterine thermotherapy: the first series of 100 patients observed for 1 year. *Fertil Steril* 2000;74:791–6

48

Hysteroscopic myomectomy

J. Donnez, M. Nisolle, M. Smets and J. Squifflet

Laser energy has some advantages in precision of tissue destruction that are not shared by the electrical energy used in the resectoscope[1,2]. Since the most popular laser in gynecology has been the carbon dioxide (CO_2) laser, efforts have been made to adapt this for hysteroscopic use. However, several features of the CO_2 laser make it impractical for hysteroscopic use. The neodymium : yttrium–aluminum–garnet (Nd : YAG) laser, however, has three specific features, making it readily adaptable for hysteroscopic myomectomy:

(1) Its ability to transmit the beam of energy easily into the uterine cavity by means of a flexible quartz fiber;

(2) Its ability to transmit laser energy to the tissue surface through a liquid distending medium;

(3) Its ability to penetrate tissue to a controlled depth.

The depth at which tissue destruction will occur can be controlled by varying the power used[3,4]; this physical quality can be applied for myomectomy and hysteroscopic myolysis[5,6]. This report describes the different techniques of hysteroscopic myomectomy.

HYSTEROSCOPIC EQUIPMENT

The fiber used to carry the laser light consists of quartz, surrounded by a thin plastic jacket, beyond which the tip of the fiber extends for several millimeters. The fiber is gas-sterilized or wiped with alcohol or cidex prior to use.

The deflecting arm is not of particular value, but allows the fiber to be stabilized. New instruments are now available in which the telescope is inserted into two different sheaths of varying diameter: one for inflow and the other for outflow. This resembles the classic resectoscope[7] and permits the constant cleaning of the uterine cavity. This system has been called the continuous flow hysteroscope (CFH). The author provides constant uterine distension by attaching one 3000-ml plastic bag of 1.5% glycine or saline solution to the blood infusion tubing. The bag is then wrapped in a pressure infusion cuff, similar to that used to infuse blood under pressure. The tubing is connected to the hysteroscope. Since the CFH has been used, overload syndrome has not occurred and this very simple system, which does not require any sophisticated and expensive pumps, allows the surgeon to perform hysteroscopic surgery in optimal conditions.

A Sharplan 2100 apparatus (Sharplan, Tel Aviv, Israel) is used for generating the laser. A power output of 80 W is used.

THE ROLE OF PREOPERATIVE GONADOTROPIN RELEASING HORMONE AGONIST THERAPY

We treated 376 women aged between 23 and 43 years (mean 33 years) with symptomatic submucous uterine fibroids, with a biodegradable gonadotropin releasing hormone (GnRH) agonist (Zoladex implant, ICI, Cambridge, UK). The implant was injected subcutaneously at the end of the luteal phase to curtail the initial gonadotropin stimulation phase always associated with a rise in estrogen. One implant was systematically injected at weeks 0, 4 and 8. Hysteroscopic myomectomy was carried out at 8 weeks. After the initial stimulation of estrogen secretion, GnRH agonist administration produces estrogen levels in the postmenopausal range (15 ± 6 pg/ml). Luteinizing hormone and follicle stimulating hormone levels were significantly suppressed within 2 weeks of treatment. Recovery of ovarian secretion occurred an average of 4–5 weeks after the last injection[6] (Figure 1).

Using the method previously described[5,6], the reduction in area of large submucous fibroids was calculated. When more than one fibroid was present, only the largest was evaluated. In all but four patients, the fibroid area decreased by an average of 38%[8] (range 4–95%). The fibroid area was found to decrease significantly ($p < 0.01$), from the baseline area (7.2 ± 4.7 cm^2) to 4.4 ± 3.5 cm^2

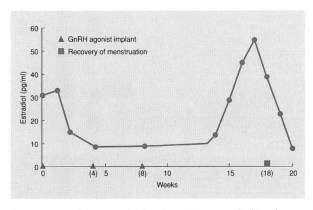

Figure 1 Hormonal levels (17β-estradiol) during gonadotropin releasing hormone agonist therapy. An implant of Zoladex was injected at weeks 0, 4 and 8

after 8 weeks of therapy. Figure 2 shows the mean fibroid area in patients with a pretreatment fibroid area < 5 cm^2 versus those with an area of > 5 cm^2 to < 10 cm^2. In all subgroups, a significant decrease ($p < 0.005$) was noted.

There was no significant difference between the different subgroups, but there was a significant difference (Figure 3) between individual myomas. About 10% of myomas did not appear to respond very well to GnRH agonist treatment.

CLASSIFICATION OF MYOMAS

According to hysterosalpingography data, submucosal fibroids were classified as:

(1) Submucosal fibroids with the greater portion inside the uterine cavity (Figure 4);

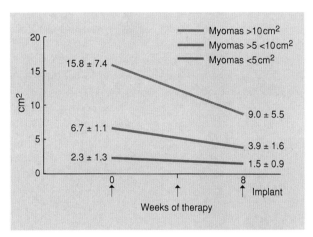

Figure 2 Decrease in fibroid area after 8 weeks of gonadotropin releasing hormone agonist therapy relative to the initial value

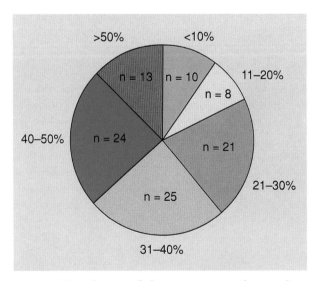

Figure 3 Distribution of the myomas according to their size decrease. Ten per cent of patients were non-responders

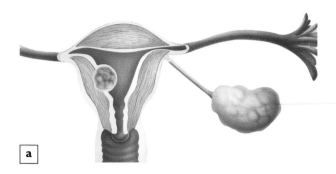

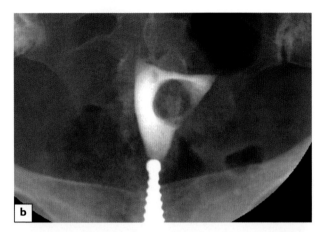

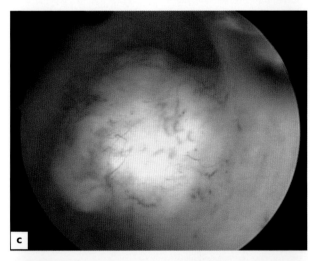

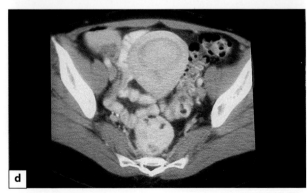

Figure 4 (a) – (d) Submucosal fibroids whose greatest diameter was inside the uterine cavity; (b) hysterography; (c) hysteroscopy; (c) computerized tomography

(2) Submucosal fibroids with the larger portion located in the myometrium (Figure 5);

(3) Multiple (> 2) submucosal fibroids (myofibromatous uterus with submucosal fibroids and intramural fibroids) diagnosed by hysterography (Figure 6) and echography.

TECHNIQUES

Submucosal fibroids with the greater portion inside the uterine cavity

All patients ($n = 233$) underwent myomectomy by hysteroscopy and Nd : YAG laser. In all but three patients,

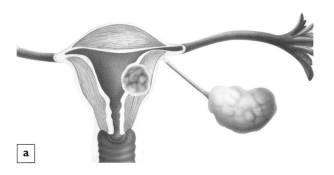

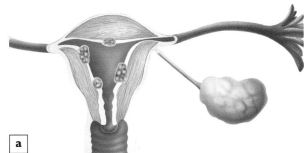

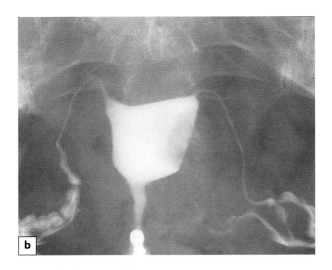

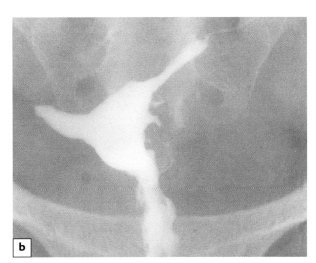

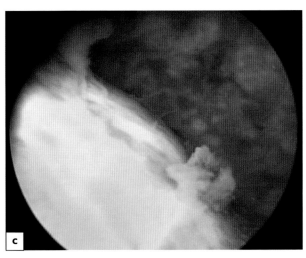

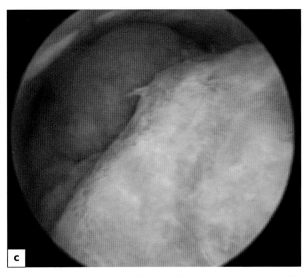

Figure 5 (a) – (c) Submucosal fibroids whose greater portion was located in the myometrium. (b) Hysterography; (c) hysteroscopy

Figure 6 (a) – (c) Multiple submucosal myomas. (b) Hysterography; (c) hysteroscopy

the operation was easily performed. The myometrium overlying the myoma was less vascular and 'shrinkage' of the uterine cavity may have accounted for the relative ease with which the myomas could be separated from the surrounding myometrium (Figures 7–9).

The myoma was left in the uterine cavity (Figure 10) unless no decrease in size was observed after GnRH agonist therapy – in this case, histological examination was required. No complications such as infection, bleeding or uterine contractions occurred. Hysteroscopy, performed

2–3 months after myomectomy, confirmed the complete disappearance of the myoma, which was probably ejected during the first menstruation after the procedure.

No hormonal therapy was given. The operating time ranged from 10 to 50 min (mean 24 ± 6 min).

Large submucosal fibroids with the greater portion located in the uterine wall

For large submucous fibroids with the greater portion not inside the uterine cavity but inside the uterine wall ($n = 78$), a two-step operative hysteroscopy was proposed[6]. After 8 weeks of preoperative GnRH agonist therapy, partial myomectomy was carried out by resecting the protruding portion of the myoma (Figure 11). The laser fiber was then directed, as perpendicularly as possible, at the remaining (intramural) fibroid portion and was introduced into the fibroid to a depth of 5–10 mm (Figure 12). During the application of laser energy, the fiber was slowly removed so that the deeper areas were coagulated. The end-point of fibroid coagulation with this technique was

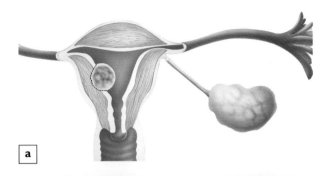

a

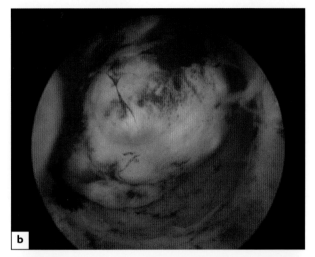

b

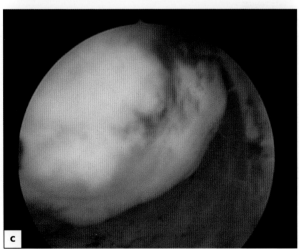

c

Figure 7 Hysteroscopy myomectomy in cases of submucosal fibroids with the greater portion inside the uterine cavity: (a) – (c) illustration of the technique

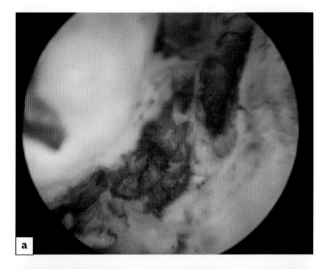

a

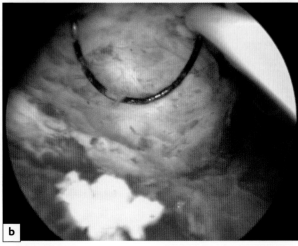

b

Figure 8 (a) Dissection of the myoma from the surrounding myometrium using the Nd : YAG laser or (b) the resectoscope

identifiable by the observation of distinct craters with brown borders on all fibroid areas. The depth of the intramural fibroid portion was already known from the results of echographic examination performed the day before surgery. The aim of this procedure was to decrease the size of the remaining myoma by decreasing its vascularity. This technique induces a necrobiosis (Figure 13) and can be called 'transhysteroscopic myolysis'[6,16].

GnRH agonist therapy was administered for another 8 weeks. At second-look hysteroscopy, the myoma was found to protrude inside the uterine cavity and appeared very white and without any apparent vessels on its surface (Figure 14). The shrinkage of the uterine cavity allowed the residual myoma portion to be easily separated from the surrounding myometrium and dissected off (Figure 15). Myomectomy was then carried out. At the end of the procedure, the myoma could be left in the uterine cavity.

In all but five patients, two-step therapy allowed successful myomectomy. In the five remaining cases, a 'third-look' hysteroscopy was necessary to achieve myomectomy. When removed, the myoma revealed areas of histological necrosis (Figure 13). In some cases, the residual myoma appeared white and necrotic (Figure 16). When performed, hysterography (Figure 17) revealed a

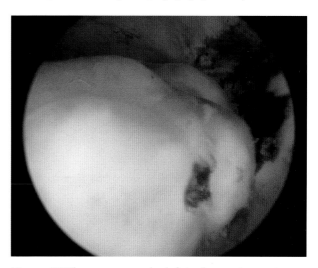

Figure 10 The myoma can be left in the uterine cavity

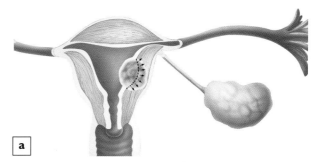

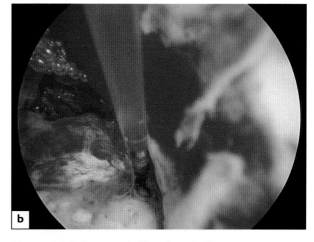

Figure 11 Submucosal fibroid with the greater portion located in the myometrium. Resection of the protruding portion of the myoma: (a) illustration; (b) hysteroscopic view

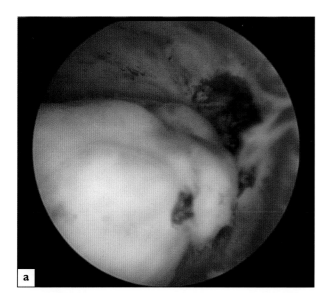

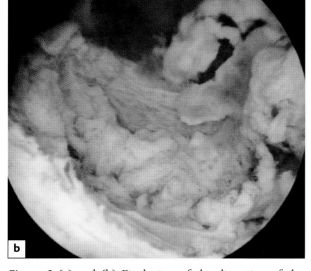

Figure 9 (a) and (b) Final view of the dissection of the myoma

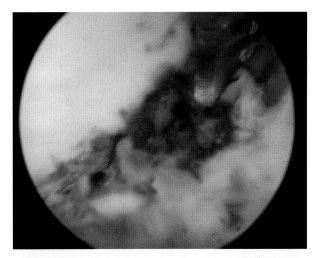

Figure 12 The laser fiber is introduced into the remaining fibroid portion to a depth of 5–10 mm and slowly removed during the application of laser energy

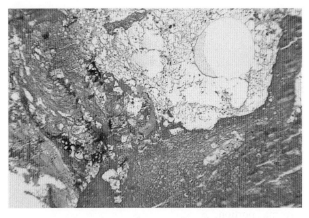

Figure 13 Myoma necrobiosis induced by the Nd : YAG laser (Gomori's trichrome, × 25). Carbonized particles phagocyted by macrophages are clearly seen. In front of them, an area of 'necrobiosis' is visible

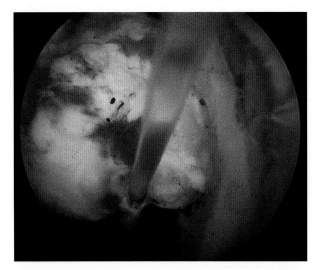

Figure 14 Eight weeks after transhysteroscopic myolysis, the intramural portion of the myoma protrudes inside the uterine cavity

normal appearance of the uterine cavity, less than 3 months after the procedure.

Fibromatous uterus

In cases of multiple submucosal fibroids, each myoma was either separated from the surrounding myometrium or totally photocoagulated (Figure 18). When only a small portion of the myoma was visible, the laser fiber was introduced into the intramural portion to a depth depending on the myoma diameter (diagnosed by echography). While firing, the fiber was slowly removed. Each myoma was systematically destroyed. At the end of surgery, endometrial ablation with the Nd : YAG laser was carried out (Figure 18) in order to induce uterine shrinkage only in women older than 35 years who did not wish to become pregnant.

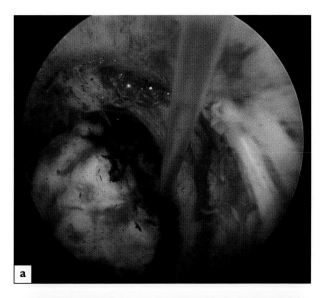

a

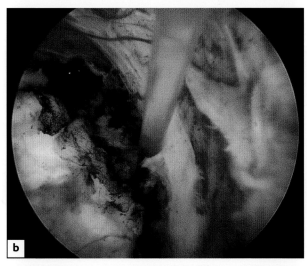

b

Figure 15 (a) and (b) Second-step hysteroscopic procedure. The residual myoma portion is easily separated from the surrounding myometrium and dissected off

RESULTS

Table 1 shows the long-term results according to the myoma classification of Donnez and Nisolle[9]. Surgery was successful in 230 of 233 patients with large submucous fibroids with the greater portion inside the uterine cavity. In three cases, a stromal tumor was diagnosed. In one of these (Figure 19), dissection of the myoma from the myometrium was impossible because the plane of dissection could not be found. Frozen histology of a biopsy revealed histological characteristics of a stromal tumor (Figure 20). Vaginal hysterectomy was then carried out. The other two cases were diagnosed by histological examination of the removed myomas, which appeared hysteroscopically as benign. The incidence of stromal tumors in apparently benign myomas is thus 1.2% (3/233). All three tumors were observed in patients who did not respond very well (< 10% decrease) to GnRH agonist therapy.

Successful myomectomy permits the restoration of normal menstrual flow. Long-term results show that recurrence of menorrhagia occurs more frequently (22%) in patients with multiple submucosal myomas than in those with single submucosal myomas[8]. Recurrence of menorraghia is provoked by the growth of myomas in other sites, as shown by hysterography and hysteroscopy.

Fertility

A first evaluation of a series of 60 women was published in 1990[6]. Twenty-four of 60 treated women wished to become pregnant and had no other infertility factors. Sixteen (66%) of them became pregnant during the first 8 months after the return of menstruation. No miscarriages

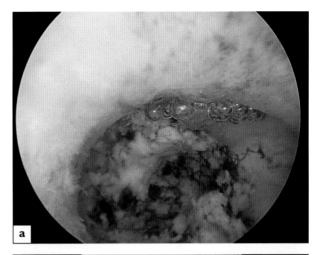

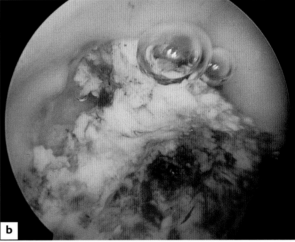

Figure 16 (a) and (b) Necrotic appearance of the residual myoma portion, 8 weeks after coagulation with the Nd : YAG laser

Table 1 Surgical procedures and long-term results according to the site of myomas

	Greater portion inside the uterine cavity	Greater portion located in the uterine wall	Multiple submucosal myomas (myomectomy and endometrial ablation)
Surgical procedures			
Total number of patients	233	78	55
Successful	230	74	51
Failed	3*	4†	4§
1-year follow-up			
Total number of patients	132	42	39
Recurrence of menorrhagia	1 (1%)	1 (2%)	8 (20%)
2-year follow-up			
Total number of patients	98	24	24
Recurrence of menorrhagia	2 (2%)	1 (4%)	6 (25%)

* Stromal tumor; † a third-look hysteroscopy allowed the removal of the myoma; § myomectomy was not totally successful (in two cases, second-look laser hysteroscopy was successfully performed. In the other two cases, vaginal hysterectomy was proposed and successfully performed)

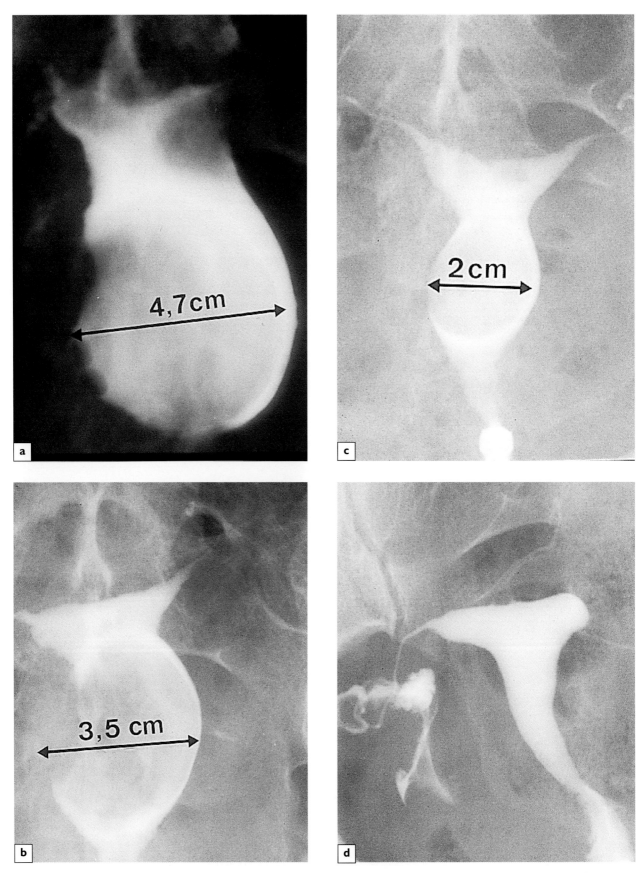

Figure 17 Hysterography (a) before gonadotropin releasing hormone (GnRH) agonist therapy; (b) after GnRH agonist therapy; (c) hysterography 8 weeks after partial myomectomy and coagulation. The residual intramural portion was found protruding again in the uterine cavity; (d) hysterography 8 weeks after the second hysteroscopic myomectomy

or premature labor occurred in these women; one Cesarean section was necessary because of fetal distress.

DISCUSSION

Because most leiomyomata return to pretreatment size within 4 months of cessation of GnRH agonist therapy, these agents cannot be used as definitive medical therapy[10–13]. Several reports have demonstrated reductions in uterine and fibroid volumes of 52–77% after 6 months of GnRH agonist therapy, as assessed by ultrasound imaging. In our study, hysterographic imaging documented an average decrease of 35% in uterine cavity size[5,14]. Another study[6] demonstrated reductions in fibroid volume

of 38% after 8 weeks of GnRH agonist therapy. The response was variable, however, ranging from 20% to 95%. There was no difference in the extent of the decrease according to the pretreatment fibroid area.

In patients with submucosal uterine fibroids, hysteroscopic myomectomy was carried out if the greater portion of the leiomyoma, as assessed by hysterography, was inside the uterine cavity. Hormonal treatment for 8 weeks before hysteroscopic myomectomy was advised since this produced a significant uterine shrinkage.

Peroperative blood loss was minimal, possibly because of the decreased vascularity of the myometrium. This was demonstrated by a significant reduction in the uterine arterial blood flow (Doppler) after treatment with a GnRH agonist[15]. In all patients (except when no decrease in the

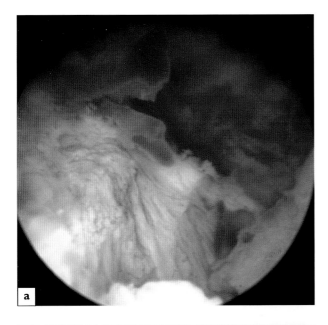

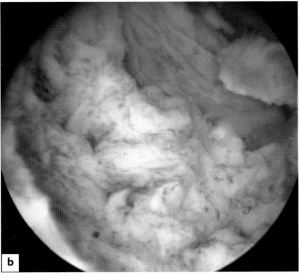

Figure 18 (a) Transhysteroscopic multiple myomectomy; (b) multiple myomectomy was associated with endometrial ablation

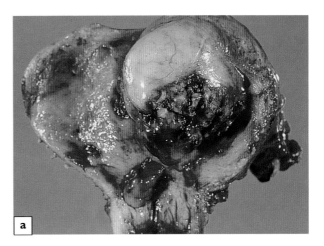

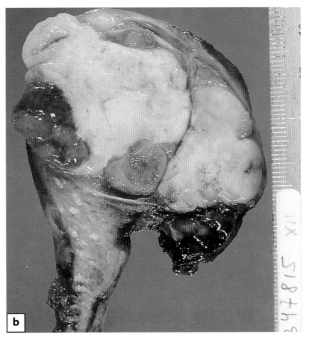

Figure 19 (a) and (b) Hysteroscopically, the intrauterine lesion appeared as benign myomas, but no plane of dissection could be found. Histology revealed a stromal tumor invading the myometrium

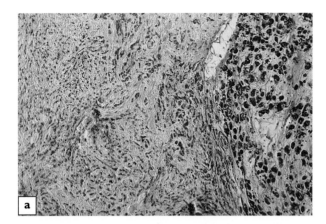

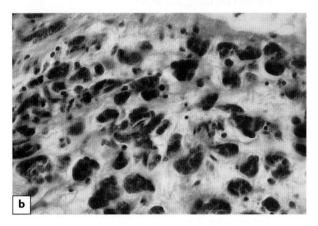

Figure 20 (a) Low-grade stromal sarcoma with areas of epithelial differentiation (on the right). In these areas, cells are considerably more atypical than those seen on the left, which resemble the stromal cells of proliferating endometrium; (b) areas of epithelial differentiation (high-power view)

myoma size was observed), the myoma was left in the uterine cavity and there were no complications. Probably, after a necrotic phase, the myoma was ejected with menstrual blood.

For very large fibroids with the greater portion not inside the uterine cavity, myomectomy was carried out in two stages. During the first surgical procedure, the protruding portion was removed and the intramural portion was devascularized by introducing the laser fiber into the myoma, to a depth of 5–10 mm, depending on the depth of the remaining intramural portion (evaluated by echography). The pelvic structures were protected from injury because the distance between the top of the fiber and the external surface of the uterus was never < 1.5 cm. There was no risk of introducing the laser fiber as much as 1 cm into the remaining portion if the diameter of the fibroid was > 3–4 cm.

A very interesting finding was that this intramural portion of the myoma became submucosal and protruded inside the uterine cavity, possibly because of the GnRH agonist-induced uterine shrinkage. In all cases, the greater

part of the remaining portion of the myoma was inside the uterine cavity, and myomectomy was easily performed by separating the myoma from the surrounding myometrium with the Nd : YAG laser.

CONCLUSION

Preoperative GnRH agonist treatment reduces tumor size and makes subsequent surgical treatment by hysteroscopy possible. In our series, even when the greater portion of the myoma was in the myometrium, a two-step hysteroscopic therapy combined with GnRH agonist therapy[6,16] represented ideal management of large submucous myomas, decreasing the need for laparotomy, which is often accompanied by increased operative blood loss and postoperative adhesion formation.

When numerous submucosal and intramural myomas were present, a higher risk of recurrence was observed than in patients with only one submucosal myoma[8]. Because of this high rate of recurrence, we prefer to perform a laparoscopic supracervical hysterectomy instead of the hysteroscopic procedure[16,17].

By preventing uterine bleeding, preoperative GnRH agonist therapy restores a normal hemoglobin concentration, and allows for the possibility of a later autologous transfusion[6]. The hormonal endometrial status is one of the factors affecting fluid absorption. Endometrial vascularization may account for liquid resorption, and this was reduced after preoperative GnRH agonist therapy. Less fluid was absorbed if the endometrium was atrophic, reducing the risk of fluid overload. This represents another major advantage of the combined medical and surgical approach to therapy.

The advantages of the preoperative use of a GnRH agonist are:

(1)   Reduction of the myoma size;

(2)   Decreased risk of fluid overload;

(3)   Restoration of normal hemoglobin concentration;

(4)   Detection of a stromal tumor.

Like Gallinat[18], we believe that, although Nd : YAG laser treatment requires experience and a thorough knowledge of the technique, it nevertheless has the lowest complication rate, when compared to the resectoscope. Nd : YAG laser treatment of large myomas must be considered the safest method in the hysteroscopic surgical treatment of large myomas.

REFERENCES

1.   Hallez JP, Netter A, Cartier R. Methodical intrauterine resection. *Am J Obstet Gynecol* 1987;156:1080

2.   Loffer FD. Laser ablation of the endometrium. *Obstet Gynecol Clin North Am* 1988;15:77

3. Goldrath MH, Fuller T, Segal S. Laser photovaporization of endometrium for the treatment of menorrhagia. *Am J Obstet Gynecol* 1981;140:14

4. Goldrath MH. Hysteroscopic laser surgery. In Baggish MH, ed. *Basic and Advanced Laser Surgery in Gynecology*. Norwalk: Appleton Century-Crofts, 1985:357

5. Donnez J, Schrurs B, Gillerot S, *et al*. Treatment of uterine fibroids with implants of gonadotropin-releasing hormone agonist: assessment by hysterography. *Fertil Steril* 1989;51:947

6. Donnez J, Gillerot S, Bourgonjon D, *et al*. Neodymium : YAG laser hysteroscopy in large submucous fibroids. *Fertil Steril* 1990;54:999

7. Neuwirth RS. Hysteroscopic management of symptomatic submucous fibroids. *Obstet Gynecol* 1983;62:509

8. Donnez J. Nd : YAG laser hysteroscopic myomectomy. In Sutton C, Diamond M, eds. *Endoscopic Surgery for Gynecologists*. London: W.B. Saunders, 1993:331

9. Donnez J, Nisolle M. Nd : YAG laser hysteroscopic surgery: endometrial ablation, partial endometrial ablation and myomectomy. *Reprod Med Rev* 1993;2:63

10. Healy DL, Fraser HM, Lawson SL. Shrinkage of a uterine fibroid after subcutaneous infusion of a LH-RH agonist. *Br Med J* 1984;209:267

11. Maheux R, Guilloteau C, Lemay A, *et al*. Luteinizing hormone-releasing hormone agonist and uterine leiomyoma: pilot study. *Am J Obstet Gynecol* 1985;152:1034

12. Andreyko JL, Blumenfeld Z, Marschall LA, *et al*. Use of an agonistic analog of gonadotropin-releasing hormone (nafarelin) to treat leiomyomas: assessment by magnetic resonance imaging. *Am J Obstet Gynecol* 1988;158:903

13. Friedman AJ, Barbieri RL, Doubilet PM, *et al*. A randomized, double-blind trial of gonadotropin releasing-hormone agonist (leuprolide) with or without medroxyprogesterone acetate in the treatment of leiomyomata uteri. *Fertil Steril* 1988;49:404

14. Donnez J, Clerckx F, Gillerot S, *et al*. Traitment des fibromes uterins per implant d'agoniste de la GnRH: evaluation per hysterographie. *Contrac Fertil Sex* 1989;17:569–73

15. Matta WHM, Stabile I, Shaw RS, *et al*. Doppler assessment of uterine blood flow changes in patients with fibroids receiving the gonadotropin-releasing hormone agonist Buserelin. *Fertil Steril* 1988;49:1083

16. Donnez J, Nisolle M. Hysteroscopic surgery. *Curr Opin Obstet Gynecol* 1992;4:439

17. Donnez J, Nisolle M. Laparoscopic supracervical (subtotal) hysterectomy (LASH). *J Gynecol Surg* 1993;9:91–4

18. Gallinat A. Hysteroscopic treatment of submucous fibroids using the Nd : YAG laser and modern electrical equipment. In Leuken RP, Gallinat A, eds. *Endoscopic Surgery in Gynecology*. Berlin: Demeter Verlag GmbH, 1993:72–88

49

Tubal sterilization

B.J. van Herendael

INTRODUCTION

Prior to the introduction of laparoscopy, hysterectomy had been the main operation to stop fertility. The great majority of patients do not want to take medication throughout their fertile lives. Laparoscopy has changed this for the better as the technique can be performed under local anesthesia. However, there are many drawbacks associated with this technique, mainly technical, but also cost.

All of these laparoscopic techniques are valid, but some are more difficult to perform than others, and there is a substantial risk for the patients with some of the techniques. The main drawback is the opening of the abdominal cavity. Even if the entry points are very small, the risk of entering large vessels, the aorta and the iliac vessels, both artery and vein, and the viscus are real and do not reflect the expertise of the operator.

Safer methods of definitive sterilization were sought. A first attempt by the World Health Organization to find a successful sterilization technique was the blind injection into the uterine cavity of caustic substances on a base of histoacrylates, quinacrine[1]. Although easy to apply, total occlusion occurred only in some 30% at a first attempt, too low a percentage to be applied in developing countries. Recanalization was a problem, even after long periods of time.

Since the advent of hysteroscopy, many hysteroscopic sterilization techniques have been tried (Table 1). Most

Table 1 Sterilization techniques by laparoscopy and hysteroscopy

Laparoscopy	
Unipolar	Palmer technique
Bipolar	the Kleppinger bipolar forceps
Endotherm coagulation	Semms technique
Tubal occluding rings	the Yoon ring
Tubal occluding clips	the Hulka Clemens clip
	the Filshie clip
Hysteroscopy	
P block	J. Brundin
Silicone plug	R.A. Erb
Hamou plug	J. Hamou
STOP device	Conceptus Inc., San Carlos, CA, USA

had to be abandoned due either to their unreliability or to their cost. Recently, major progress has been made.

In hysteroscopy[2], there were early experiments by Lindemann with unipolar coagulation of the intramural part of the tube. The main problem was recanalization, even after many years, in one case after 15 years, followed by pregnancy. The same applied to all other attempts to destroy the intramural part of the tube, even major destruction with the neodymium : yttrium–aluminum–garnet (Nd : YAG) laser[3]. The intramural part of the tube seems to have an extraordinary capacity to regenerate itself. These techniques all required general anesthesia.

As destruction techniques from outside the tube seemed to fail, many systems were created to block the tube from within. We went in search of a method which could be used in an outpatient set-up, with, or even preferably without, anesthesia.

Most attempts to obstruct the tubal lumen completely have failed. Jan Brundin[4], now the Medical Director of the Karolinska Institute in Sweden, developed a hygroscopic element, about 1.5 cm in length, with a memory of how far to swell once in contact with liquid. However, the P block was ejected in over 80% of cases.

The author has placed 20 P blocks, of which only four remained in place and not one patient had a bilateral occlusion (unpublished results).

Systems that remain in the lumen without occluding it, i.e. silicone plugs of Erb, are successful but take too long to be positioned, on average 40 min, and are too costly[5].

Therefore, we went in search of techniques that were easier to apply, that could be performed in less than 20 min, without local anesthesia. We had to develop small barrel scopes, less than 5 mm, with a working channel that accommodates 5 French instruments or a guiding wire.

The first of the fine systems, the Hamou plug, a nylon thread that anchored into the intramural area, was very effective[6] but was not passed by the Federal Drug Administration and was, therefore, abandoned. The technique for insertion is shown in Figures 1–6.

The author has inserted 30 Hamou devices. Insertion was carried out at the private office without any form of anesthesia, not even a local injection into the cervix. The Storz 'chorionoscope' (Karl Storz GmbH, Tütlingen, Germany) was used according to Perino. The outer diameter of this hysteroscope is oval and the diameter is 3.8 mm. After 11 years of follow-up, we have had two pregnancies, both due to the fact that the device was not placed correctly into the tubal ostium. The devices, however,

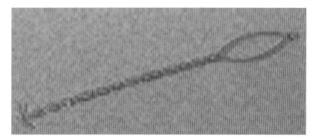

Figure 1 The original Hamou plug: a blue nylon device that was anchored into the intramural part of the tube. It had to be pushed in for at least five markers. The preformed arrow tip retained the plug in the intramural part of the tube

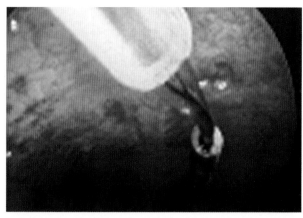

Figure 4 The guiding catheter is then withdrawn and the Hamou device is left in the tubal ostium but a large part of it resides in the uterine cavity

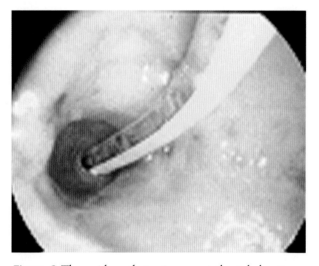

Figure 2 The guide catheter is seen at the tubal ostium, with the device inside

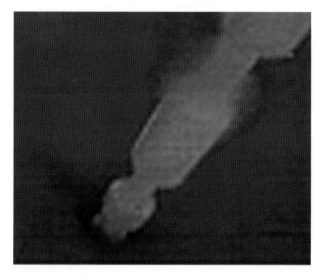

Figure 5 Correct placement of a Hamou device in the ostium of the tube

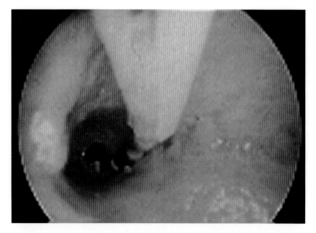

Figure 3 The device is now pushed about 2 cm into the intramural part of the tube by an occluding catheter within the first one, placed behind the device. The device is loaded into the guiding catheter from the front

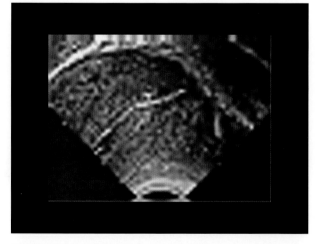

Figure 6 As the thread is made of nylon, it is easily seen with classical vaginal ultrasound as a white element in the intramural space, where normally nothing catches the eye

collect calcium crystals on the stem, as do intrauterine contraceptives devices, because more than half of their actual length remains in the cavity. The weight of these crystals causes the devices to break. The critical period seems to be 9 years. Because the devices inflict wounds to the intramural tubal epithelium, there is permanent occlusion caused by the in-growth of fibroblasts into the adhesions. For this reason, this form of intratubal device cannot be advocated as a reversible method of sterilization.

More recently, the STOP® (Conceptus Inc., San Carlos, CA, USA) system has appeared promising. Both the latter systems inflict small wounds on the tubal lumen so that a tissue reaction is gendered and its own cells, growing over the systems, obstruct the tubal lumen and occlude the tube permanently.

We use the Storz minihysteroscope (Karl Storz GmbH, Tütlingen, Germany), according to Bettocchi, and the Storz Endomat®, according to Hamou. The pump system is used with normal saline solution and the pressure does not exceed 50 mmHg when we work inside the uterus, thus avoiding cramping. The vaginoscopic technique, according to Bettocchi, is used. This means that we do not use a tenaculum to grasp the cervix. The pump is set to the maximal flow, of 400 ml/min at a pressure of 100 mmHg, and the vagina is used as a first chamber. The cervix is localized and the scope is slipped into the cervical canal. The insertion technique is shown in Figures 7–13.

Because of the small part of the device protruding into the cavity, there is no interference with the endometrium and the menstrual pattern is not altered. The average insertion time is 9 min, if the intramural part of the tube is patent and of normal anatomic configuration. Bilateral placement at first attempt is around 85%. A second attempt brings the bilateral placement up to 92%. Over 800 women with a follow-up of more than 5 years have shown only one pregnancy, due to device malfunction. The

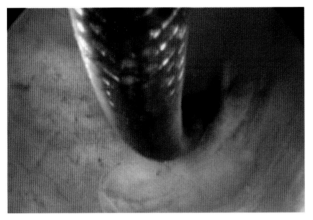

Figure 7 The STOP system: the guide wire carrying the device is inserted into the tubal ostium. Gentle pressure is used so as not to cause contractions

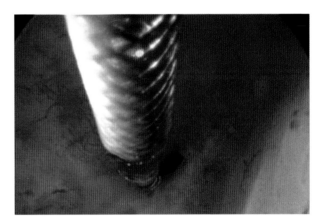

Figure 9 The STOP system: the outer catheter is removed until the wheel is blocked. At this time, the device is still not deployed and small adjustments can be made. Care is taken that the gold-colored indicator is approximately 1.5 cm from the tubal ostium

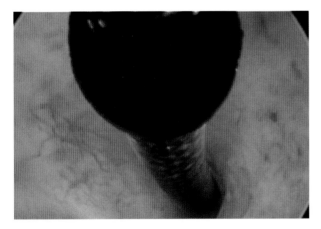

Figure 8 The STOP system: once the black 'stopper' is at the level of the tubal ostium, the wheel on the outside of the body is turned clockwise to deliver the device. The catheter is seen to come towards the end of the hysteroscope

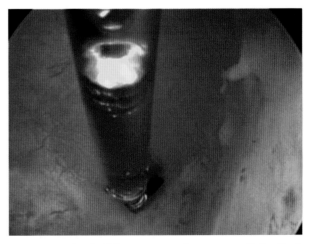

Figure 10 The STOP system: a closer view of the final stage before releasing the device so that it can be deployed in the intramural part of the tube

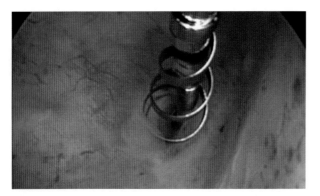

Figure 11 The STOP system: by turning the outside wheel counterclockwise, the device is now deployed so that it anchors itself in the intramural part of the tube

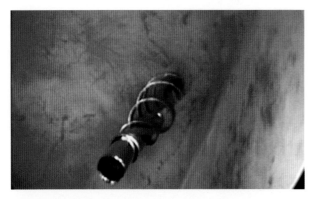

Figure 12 The STOP system: the device is now in place, the longer portion being left in the intramural part of the tube while the shorter part (approximately 1.5–2 cm) remains in the uterine cavity

fibers on the device causes a tissue reaction, which produces permanent occlusion of the intramural part of the tube.

In conclusion, we can state that a new era has begun as far as definitive contraception is concerned. Hysteroscopic placement, using thin-barrelled hysteroscopes, of small devices, causing occlusion of the intramural part of the tube, are the future of sterilization; the drawbacks are the difficulties of the hysteroscopic technique and the costs of the devices.

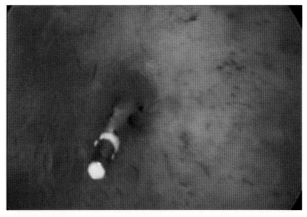

Figure 13 The STOP system: the right side of the same patient where a device had been installed exactly 1 month before. Because of an allergic reaction, the procedure had to be stopped at that time. Note the in-growths of the tissues at the tubal ostium and around the device blocking the intramural part of the tube

REFERENCES

1. Sokal DC, Zipper J, King T. Transcervical quinacrine sterilization: clinical experience. *Int J Gynecol Obstet* 1995;51(Suppl 1):S57–69
2. Sciarra JJ, Keith L. Hysteroscopic sterilization. *Obstet Gynecol Clin North Am* 1995;22:581–9
3. Donnez J, Malvaux V, Nisolle M, *et al*. Hysteroscopic sterilization. In Donnez J, Nisolle M, eds. *An Atlas of Laser Operative Laparoscopy and Hysteroscopy*. Carnforth, UK: Parthenon Publishing, 1994:337–41
4. Brundin J. Hydrogel tubal blocking device: P-block. In Zatuchni GI, Shelton JD, Goldsmith A, eds. *Female Transcervical Sterilization*. Philadelphia: Harper & Row Publishers, 1983:240
5. Ligt-Veneman NG, Tinga DJ, Kragt H, *et al*. The efficacy of intratubal silicone in the Ovabloc hysteroscopic method of sterilization. *Acta Obstet Gynecol Scand* 1999;78:824–5
6. Hamou J, Gasparri F, Scarselli GF, *et al*. Hysteroscopic reversible tubal sterilization. *Acta Eur Fertil* 1984;15:123

Complications of hysteroscopic surgery in gynecology

50

J. Donnez, P. Jadoul, F. Chantraine and M. Nisolle

INTRODUCTION

Hysteroscopic surgery has developed from a diagnostic tool into an effective surgical technique. It is now a standard investigational and therapeutic tool in gynecology which, when performed properly for the right indications in patients with no contraindications, has practically no complications. In retrospective studies, complication rates of 1–25% have been reported[1–5].

A members' survey of The American Association of Gynecologic Laparoscopists reported 17 298 operative hysteroscopies, with a complication rate of 3.8%[2]. In a recent prospective study in the Netherlands in 1997, the complication rate among 13 600 hysteroscopic procedures reached 0.28% (0.13% for diagnostic procedures and 0.95% for operative procedures)[6]. The wide variation is attributed to the varying experience of the gynecologists and to the range of pathology treated[7–9].

Although complications are infrequent, their description helps us to understand their causes and thus take steps to avoid them. There are six groups of complications of operative hystroscopy:

(1)   Traumatic complications;

(2)   Hemorrhagic complications;

(3)   Distension medium complications;

(4)   Infection;

(5)   Thermal surgery damage;

(6)   Late complications.

Less frequent complications, such as rupture of the tubes, rupture of the diaphragm leading to the patient's death, rupture of the uterine wall and trauma to pelvic vessels, have been reported. Our purpose is to describe the diagnosis, management and prevention of these complications.

TRAUMATIC COMPLICATIONS OF HYSTEROSCOPY

Traumatic complications of diagnostic hysteroscopy have been well documented. Hysteroscopic surgery, however, also involves some blind manipulation. Dilating the cervix to accommodate wide-caliber operating instruments may cause cervical laceration and/or uterine perforation, with or without hemorrhage. The frequency of these complications is unknown, and has been estimated as 1–9%[9–13].

Diagnosis

Cervical lacerations are diagnosed only if cervical bleeding occurs. Uterine perforation is suspected if the depth of passage of the sound or the dilator is greater than the apparent size of the uterus. Very rapid flow of liquid or very low distension pressure with CO_2 at the time of insertion of the hysteroscope should raise this suspicion. Diagnosis is sometimes made by visualization of the bowel. Any hemorrhage before the beginning of the surgical procedure is highly suggestive of traumatic damage.

Management

Cervical laceration is of little consequence, although sutures are occasionally required to prevent or stop cervical bleeding. Uterine perforation does not usually need surgical repair. If perforation is diagnosed before the surgical procedure, surgery must be delayed and the patient observed for 24 h. If perforation is diagnosed intraoperatively or after the surgical procedure, a diagnostic laparoscopy is recommended to ensure that no damage has been caused to adherent or adjacent structures and that there is no unsuspected laceration of the large blood vessels.

Prevention

To prevent such complications, careful placement of the tenaculum and gentle dilatation of the cervix are recommended. Advancement of the hysteroscope must always be performed under visual control, accommodating the instrument axis to the direction of the cervical canal and to the position of the uterus.

The use of laminaria tents is favored by some hysteroscopists, but avoided by others, because of the possible risk of overdilatation, resulting in loss of distension medium and intrauterine pressure, and causing poor visualization.

Some hysteroscopists prefer pharmacologic dilatation with vaginal prostaglandins. Their action is caused by softening of the cervical stroma resulting in dilatation of the canal. This is enhanced by contraction of the myometrium induced by the drug[14–16].

HEMORRHAGIC COMPLICATIONS OF HYSTEROSCOPY

Intraoperative bleeding, other than that due to cervical laceration or uterine perforation, is usually the result of inadvertent or intentional trauma to the uterine wall. The reported rate of bleeding requiring surgery or uterine tamponade ranges from 0 to 22.4%[17–20].

Hemorrhage can occur from false passages, with or without perforation, created during either the dilatation or the insertion of the hysteroscope. Bleeding can also occur after operative procedures, especially when penetration of healthy myometrium is too deep. This can occur after the use of scissors or thermal energy (laser, resectoscope).

Diagnosis

Heavy and continuous vaginal bleeding during or after surgery must be investigated, in order to determine if it is intrauterine or cervical bleeding. Management should be effected according to the origin of the hemorrhage.

Management

Intraoperatively, rapid bleeding can be controlled by coagulation, using either the tip of the laser fiber or the electrical loop. Postoperative and uncontrolled intraoperative bleeding may sometimes require intrauterine tamponade. A Foley catheter is introduced into the uterine cavity and the balloon is inflated with 15 ml of liquid. After approximately 3 h, one-half of the liquid is removed; if no bleeding recurs over the next hour, the catheter is removed and the patient is usually discharged. If active bleeding recurs, the balloon is re-inflated and left in place overnight.

Prevention

Recommendations for avoiding trauma also apply to hemorrhagic complications. In addition, the entire surgical procedure must be carried out under strict visualization of the dissection plane. If large submucosal myomas or dense intrauterine synechiae are present, performing the procedure in two parts decreases the risk of such complications. The use of intracervical vasopressin has been described to decrease the risk of bleeding[18]. This drug must be used with consideration of its systemic effects. The use of preoperative medical therapy (gonadotropin releasing hormone (GnRH) agonists, danazol, progestins) has been reported to decrease postoperative bleeding. Such therapy decreases the thickness and vascularity of the endometrium and shrinks myomas and may be helpful in preventing this type of complication[10,12,17,21,22]. A randomized double-blind study (the AZTEC study) recently proved that the use of GnRH agonists was helpful during endometrial ablation due to the significant reduction in endometrial thickness.

DISTENSION MEDIUM COMPLICATIONS

Complications specifically related to distension media occur in 0.14–4% of procedures[1,2,6] and vary with the medium used.

Carbon dioxide and air embolism

Venous gas embolism is the most feared complication when using CO_2 as a distension medium[23–26]. This risk is low when using adequate hysteroflators. Most reports of fatal CO_2 embolism during operative hysteroscopy have been the result of using inadequate or faulty insufflators[27,28]. Recently, air embolism has also been described. Air embolism can occur while using a fluid distension medium and is provoked by repeated removal and introduction of the hysteroscope, the use of pressure pumps without air detectors[29,30] and cervical trauma with subsequent dilacerated veins.

Diagnosis

Venous air embolism is marked by a sudden decrease in CO_2 pressure in the expired air. Clinical signs, such as decreased blood pressure, tachycardia, arrhythmia and increasing central venous pressure, come too late to be useful as warning signals. As soon as the end-tidal CO_2 drops in the expired air, insufflation must be stopped.

Management

The patient must be immediately ventilated with 100% oxygen[31]. If the patient is in the Trendelenburg position, this position must be maintained in order to prevent the passage of the air bubble into the pulmonary artery. If the patient is in normal decubitus, an anti-Trendelenburg position will maintain the air bubble in the right atrium. A large catheter must be inserted into the right atrium through the internal jugular vein to aspirate the gas. A transesophageal ultrasound allows vizualization of the gas embolism.

Prevention

The first rule for hysteroscopy with CO_2 is the use of adequate insufflators. The insufflation pressure must not exceed 100 mmHg. Faulty routes, especially submucosal passages, increase the risk of embolism. Cervical trauma with subsequent dilaceration of veins should be avoided to prevent air embolism. Repeated introduction of the hysteroscope must also be avoided, as must the use of CO_2 for cooling laser tips.

Fluid distension media

High-molecular-weight dextran

The major complication feared from the use of dextran 70 (Hyskon) is anaphylactic shock. The incidence of anaphylactic shock is rare at 1 in 10 000[32,33]. So-called dextran-induced anaphylactic reaction (DIAR) is not predictable and does not depend on the amount used[34]. It can be prevented by performing an intravenous injection test with a small amount of 15% dextran 2 min before using dextran 70. This distension medium also induces ascites and intravascular overload if a substantial volume is retained in the patient. Intravascular reabsorption of dextran has also been linked to non-cardiogenic pulmonary edema and to coagulation disorders[34–40].

Low-viscosity liquid complications

These fluids (mainly sorbitol, glycine and dextrose in water) are used primarily during electrosurgical intra-uterine procedures. When retained by the patient, they may cause hyponatremia and fluid overload.

Glycine solution has excellent optical and non-hemolytic properties during hysteroscopic surgery. Glycine is a non-essential amino acid which exists naturally in the body. Its normal plasma level is 120–155 μmol/l and it readily crosses the blood–brain barrier. Glycine functions as an inhibitory transmitter in the spinal cord and in the brain stem and retina. Its toxic effects on the central nervous system are also due to oxidative deamination in the liver and kidneys and to the forming of glycoxylic acid and ammonia[14].

Glycine overload results in fluid overload (hypervolemia and hyponatremia) and in neurological symptoms (Table 1). Glycine and its metabolites may be a cause of visual disturbances and encephalopathy, independent of changes in serum sodium levels and osmolarity.

In order to study the metabolism of glycine after endoscopic uterine surgery, serum concentrations of the amino acid and its metabolites were measured in seven patients with artificially induced menopause scheduled for Neodymium : yttrium–aluminum–garnet (Nd : YAG) laser endoscopic procedures in our department[41]. Fluid balance was determined by a volumetric method (comparison of in- and outflow). The mean irrigant absorption was 1128 ± 673 ml. A significant increase in glycine concentration

Table I Specific problems related to 1.5% glycine solution

Fluid overload

Electrolyte dilution

Hyperglycinemia and ammonia toxicity

during and after the procedure (up to 100 times the normal value) was correlated with a rise in serum ammonia levels (Figure 1). Recovery was uneventful in all cases. Serum sodium levels and osmolarity remained normal during and after surgery and there was no increased oxaluria.

Diagnosis

Manifestations of fluid overload and glycine intoxication are treacherous and can occur any time postoperatively. Patients present with bradycardia and hypertension followed by hypotension, nausea, vomiting, headache, visual disturbances[42], agitation, confusion and lethargy. Other important factors are the decrease in serum osmolarity and the rapid drop in the serum sodium level. If untreated, the result may be seizures, coma, cardiovascular collapse and death.

Management

The monitoring of intake and output of liquids during and after the procedure is mandatory to assess the fluid balance. A discrepancy of 1000 ml requires assessment of serum electrolytes to permit diagnosis. If a discrepancy of 1500 ml is noted during surgery, the procedure must be stopped immediately.

If the serum sodium level is normal and the patient has no particular complaint, no further treatment is necessary. In the case of decreased sodium levels and hemodilution, the patient should observe fluid restrictions and intravenous diuretics (furosemide) should be administered.

In cases of severe hyponatremia causing neurological symptoms, perfusion of hypertonic saline solution is required. If correction is too rapid, however, it may cause injury to the brain known as central pontine myelinolysis.

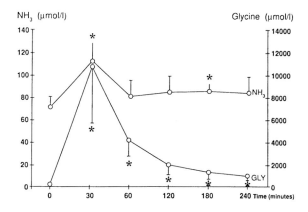

Figure I Concentrations of glycine and ammonia measured in serum of seven patients with artificially induced menopause undergoing Nd : YAG laser endoscopic procedures

Prevention

During hysteroscopy with liquid medium, monitoring of the inflow and outflow volumes is essential to prevent retention of too much distension medium by the patient. An infusion pressure of more than 150 mmHg increases the risk of fluid absorption, but intravasation of the fluid often occurs through open uterine venous channels or, in the presence of unrecognized perforation, with normal infusion pressure[43]. If uterine perforation and/or a fluid balance discrepancy of over 1500 ml is detected, the procedure must be stopped.

INFECTIOUS COMPLICATIONS

Infection is rare, with a frequency of 0.25–1%[18,44–49]. Usually, infection follows prolonged operative procedures, especially when repeated insertion and removal of the hysteroscope through the cervical canal have been necessary. It occurs about 72 h postoperatively and manifests itself with fever, vaginal discharge and pelvic pain. It can be treated successfully with broad-spectrum oral antibiotics. Hospitalization is rarely required. To prevent this complication, the use of prophylactic antibiotics is recommended. Postoperative infection can be the cause of late complications, such as synechiae and infertility.

THERMAL ENERGY COMPLICATIONS

There is little information in the gynecological literature regarding the occurrence and management of injury to viscera during hysteroscopy. Such injuries could be caused directly by the electrical current or by the thermal diffusion of energy. They often occur in the presence of uterine perforation. They can be induced by prolonged application of strong electrical or laser energy to the uterine wall, especially in the area of the tubal ostia (Figure 2).

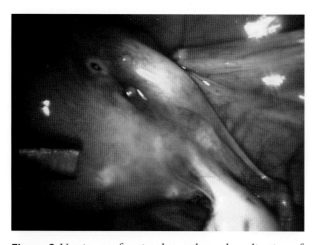

Figure 2 Uterine perforation by prolonged application of Nd : YAG laser energy during synechiae lysis by hysteroscopy

The English MISTLETOE (Minimally Invasive Surgical Techniques – Laser, Endo-Thermal Or Endo-resection) study of 10 686 endometrial resections from April 1993 to October 1994 reported a perforation rate of 0.64–2.47% with 0.07% of bowel injury[50].

This study examined the complications of endometrial resection and the influence of the surgeon's experience. It included 690 doctors performing endometrial ablation on 10 686 patients with a 6-week follow-up. Different techniques were used (loop, rollerball, laser, cryoablation, radiofrequency ablation, or the combination of loop and ball).

Perioperative morbidity and intraoperative emergency procedures are described in Table 2. Six visceral burns occurred, three with the loop associated with the rollerball and three with the loop alone. No visceral lesions occurred with the laser. There was a significant trend in the group treated by loop alone, suggesting, overall, that the more experienced the operator, the less likely the woman was to suffer immediate complications.

Diagnosis

The diagnosis is missed intraoperatively in the majority of cases. Postoperative symptoms include fever, abdominal pain, leukocytosis and signs of peritonitis. Laparoscopy is helpful in suspect cases, but this may be insufficient to evaluate the bowel fully, and laparotomy is then required[51].

Management

Guidelines described in Chapter 36 relating to vessel injuries and bowel burns with laparoscopy apply to such injuries.

Prevention

The success of prevention depends on respecting the technical conditions of surgical hysteroscopy. If uterine perforation occurs, the procedure must be delayed for the

Table 2 Immediate complications ($n = 10\,686$)

Complications	n	%
Hemorrhage	254	2.38
Perforation	158	1.48
Cardiovascular respiratory complications	53	0.5
Visceral burn	6	0.06
Total complications	474	4.44
Total emergency surgery	135	1.26

From MISTLETOE study[50]

patient's safety. In addition, the energy source must always be activated with a completely clear visualization of the tip of the laser fiber or the resectoscope loop.

LATE COMPLICATIONS

Besides the common acute complications, attention should be paid to the late complications such as uterine perforation during any subsequent pregnancy[18,52–57], incomplete resection and undesired pregnancy[58–60], post-resection infertility and post-resection pain (hematometra, synechiae, post-ablation tubal sterilization syndrome)[61–66].

Post-ablation tubal sterilization syndrome was first described by Townsend and colleagues in 1993[66]. A patient with former tubal ligation presented with lower quadrant pain following endometrial ablation. At laparoscopy, the left proximal Fallopian tube was hemorrhagic and swollen as in an ectopic pregnancy. Removal of the tube alleviated the discomfort. Over an 18-month period following this incident, six women presented with the same clinical and laparoscopic findings. Pain occurred between 6 and 10 months after endometrial ablation and at the time of an expected menstrual period. In the review by Bae and colleagues[64], six out of 71 women with a history of endometrial ablation and tubal obstruction after ligation or salpingectomy developed post-ablation tubal sterilization syndrome.

The histopathology is that of persistent endometrium in the cornual area. Because the lower uterine segment is obliterated after endometrial ablation, menstrual blood passes out into the Fallopian tube and the proximal part of the tube fills with blood, causing distension and pain. Patients describe increasing pain, cyclic in the beginning, then continuous. Ultrasonography usually fails to reveal distended Fallopian tubes but may indicate hematometra in the cornual area.

The diagnosis is made by laparoscopy. Histopathology shows hematosalpinx and microscopic findings of salpingitis and myometritis.

A bilateral salpingectomy should be performed even if symptoms are unilateral, as recurrence of symptoms on the other side after unilateral salpingectomy has been reported. Hysterectomy might be necessary because of the possibility of deep myometritis and microabscesses of the myometrium[64].

To prevent this post-ablation tubal sterilization syndrome, care should be taken to perform meticulous destruction of the uterine cornua at the time of endometrial ablation.

DISCUSSION

Operative hysteroscopy has provided new possibilities for the conservative treatment of gynecological pathologies. Although complications are not frequent, some serious problems do occur. Most of the complications described are induced by traumatic injuries. The safety of the procedure depends on the experience of the surgeon, and the increasing number of gynecologists performing operative hysteroscopy will inevitably increase the potential risk of complications. Understanding the risks inherent in the use of the instruments and media selected will minimize the chances of complications and enhance the chances of good surgical results.

REFERENCES

1. Peterson HB, Hulka JF, Phillips JM. American Association of Gynecologic Laparoscopist's 1988 membership survey on operative hysteroscopy. *J Reprod Med* 1990;35:590

2. Hulka JF, Peterson HB, Phillips JM, *et al*. Operative hysteroscopy. American Association of Gynecologic Laparoscopists 1991 membership survey. *J Reprod Med* 1993;38:572

3. Smith DC, Donohue LR, Waszak SJ. A hospital review of advanced gynecologic endoscopic procedures. *Am J Obstet Gynecol* 1994;170:1635

4. Scottish Hysteroscopy Audit Group. A Scottish audit of hysteroscopic surgery for menorrhagia: complications and follow up. *Br J Obstet Gynaecol* 1995;102:249

5. Vilos GA, Vilos EC, King JH. Experience with 800 hysteroscopic endometrial ablations. *J Am Assoc Gynecol Laparosc* 1996;4:33

6. Jansen FW, Vredevoogd CB, Van Ulzen K, *et al*. Complications of hysteroscopy: a prospective, multicenter study. *Obstet Gynecol* 2000;96:266

7. Prost AM, Liberman RF, Harlow BL, *et al*. Complications of hysteroscopic surgery: predicting patients at risk. *Obstet Gynecol* 2000;96:517

8. Cooper JM, Brady RM. Late complications of operative hysteroscopy. *Obstet Gynecol Clin N Am* 2000;27:367

9. Lindemann HJ, Mohr J. CO_2 hysteroscopy: diagnosis and treatment. *Am J Obstet Gynecol* 1976;124:129

10. Donnez J, Nisolle M. Hysteroscopic surgery. *Curr Opin Obstet Gynecol* 1992;4:439

11. Cooper JM. Hysteroscopic sterilization. *Clin Obstet Gynecol* 1992;35:282

12. Siegler AM. Risks and complications of hysteroscopy. In Van der Pas H, van Herendael B, VanLith D, Keith L, eds. *Hysteroscopy*. Lancaster: MTP Press, 1983: 75–80

13. Castaing N, Darai E, Chuong T, *et al*. Mechanical and metabolic complications of hysteroscopic surgery: report of a retrospective study of 352 procedures. *Contracept Fertil Sex* 1999;27:210

14. Van Herendael BJ. Hazards and dangers of operative hysteroscopy. In Sutton C, Diamond M, eds.

Endoscopic Surgery for Gynecologists. London: WB Saunders Company Ltd, 1993:641–8

15. Van Boven M, Pendeville PE, Singelyn FJ. Glycine and its metabolites during and after intrauterine Yag laser surgery. *Br J Anaesth* 1993;70(Suppl 1):A87

16. Preutthipan S, Herabutya Y. A randomized controlled trial of vaginal misoprostol for cervical priming before hysteroscopy. *Obstet Gynecol* 1999;94:427

17. Brooks PG, Serden SP, Davos I. Hormonal inhibition of the endometrium for resectoscope endometrial ablation. *Am J Obstet Gynecol* 1991;164:1601

18. Brooks PG. Complications of operative hysteroscopy: how safe is it? *Clin Obstet Gynecol* 1992;35:256

19. De Cherney AH, Diamond MD, Lavy G, *et al.* Endometrial ablation for intractable uterine bleeding: hysteroscopic resection. *Obstet Gynecol* 1987;70:668

20. Donnez J, Gillerot S, Bourgonjon D, *et al.* Neodymium : Yag laser hysteroscopy in large submucous fibroids. *Fertil Steril* 1990;54:999

21. Donnez J, Schrurs B, Gillerot S, *et al.* Treatment of uterine fibroids with implants of gonadotrophin releasing hormone agonist: assessment by hysterography. *Fertil Steril* 1989;51:947

22. Donnez J, Vilos G, Gannon MJ, *et al.* Gosereline Acetate (Zoladex) plus endometrial ablation for dysfunctional uterine bleeding: a large randomized, double-blind study. *Fertil Steril* 1997;68:29

23. Neis KJ, Brandner P, Lindemann HJ. Room air as the etiology of gas embolism in diagnostic CO_2 hysteroscopy. *Zentralbl Gynakol* 2000;122:222

24. Corson SL, Brooks PG, Soderstrom RM. Gynecologic endoscopic gas embolism. *Fertil Steril* 1996;65:529

25. Nishiyama T, Hanaoka K. Gas embolism during hysteroscopy. *Can J Anaesth* 1999;46:379

26. Brandner P, Neis KJ, Ehmer C. The etiology, frequency and prevention of gas embolism during hysteroscopy. *J Am Assoc Gynecol Laparosc* 1999;6:421

27. Perry PM, Baughman VL. A complication of hysteroscopy: air embolism. *Anesthesiology* 1990;73:546

28. Baggish MS, Daniell JF. Death caused by air embolism associated with neodymium : yttrium-aluminium-garnet laser surgery and artificial sapphire tips. *Am J Obstet Gynecol* 1989;161:877

29. Nachum Z, Cole S, Adia Y, *et al.* Massive air embolus, possible cause of death after operative hysteroscopy using a 32% dextrane 70 pump. *Fertil Steril* 1992;58:836

30. Overton C, Wilson-Smith E, Hunt P, *et al.* Air embolism during endoscopic resection of the endometrium: recommendations for a change in practice. *Gynaecol Endosc* 1996;5:357

31. Tur-Kaspa I. Hyperbaric oxygen therapy for air embolism complicating operative hysteroscopy. *Am J Obstet Gynecol* 1990;163:680

32. Leake JF, Murphy AA, Zacur HA. Non-cardiogenic pulmonary oedema: a complication of operative hysteroscopy. *Obstet Gynecol* 1987;48:497

33. McLucas B. Hyskon complications in hysteroscopic surgery. *Obstet Gynecol Surv* 1991;46:196

34. Witz CA, Silverberg KM, Burns WN, *et al.* Complications associated with the absorption of hysteroscopic fluid media. *Fertil Steril* 1993;60:745

35. Brandt RR, Dunn WF, Ory SJ. Dextran 70 embolization. Another cause of pulmonary hemorrhage, coagulopathy and rhabdomyolysis. *Chest* 1993;104:631

36. Jedeikin R, Olsfanger D, Kessler J. Disseminated intravascular coagulopathy and adult respiratory distress syndrome: life-threatening complications of hysteroscopy. *Am J Obstet Gynecol* 1990;162:44

37. Romero RM, Kreitzer JM, Gabrielson GV. Hyskon induced pulmonary hemorrhage. *J Clin Anaesth* 1995;7:323

38. Vercellini P, Rossi R, Pagnoni B, *et al.* Hypervolemic pulmonary edema and severe coagulopathy after intrauterine dextran instillation. *Obstet Gynecol* 1992;79:838

39. Morrison DM. Management of hysteroscopic surgery complications. *AORN J* 1999;69:194–7, 199–209, quiz 210, 213–15:21

40. Indman PD, Brooks PG, Cooper JM, *et al.* Complications of fluid overload from resectoscopic surgery. *J Am Assoc Gynecol Laparosc* 1998;5:63

41. Van Boven M, Pendeville PE, Singelyn FJ. Glycine and its metabolites during and after intrauterine Yag laser surgery. *Br J Anaesth* 1993;70(Suppl 1):A87

42. Levin H, Ben-David B. Transient blindness during hysteroscopy: a rare complication. *Anaesth Analg* 1995;81:880

43. Vulgaropulos SP, Haley LC, Hulka JF. Intrauterine pressure and fluid absorption during continuous flow hysteroscopy. *Am J Obstet Gynecol* 1992;167:386

44. Taylor PJ, Hamou JE. Hysteroscopy. *J Reprod Med* 1983;28:359

45. Mergui JL, Raossanaly K, Salat-Baroux J. Place de l'hysteroscopie opératoire en 1990. *Lett Gynécol* 1990;132:21

46. Rullo S, Boni T. Broad ligament abscess after operative hysteroscopy. *Clin Exp Obstet Gynecol* 1995;22:240

47. Amin-Hanjani S, Good JM. Pyometria after endometrial resection and ablation. *Obstet Gynecol* 1995;85:893

48. Jorgenson JC, Pelle J, Philipsen T. Fatal infection following transcervical fibroid resection. *Gynaecol Endosc* 1996;5:245

49. McCausland VM, Fields GA, McCausland AM, *et al.* Tuboovarian abscess after operative hysteroscopy. *J Reprod Med* 1993;38:198

50. Overton C, Hargreaves J, Maresh M. A national survey of the complications of endometrial destruction for menstrual disorders: the MISTLETOE study. *Br J Obstet Gynaecol* 1997;104:1351

51. Sullivan B, Kenny P, Seibel M. Hysteroscopic resection of fibroid with thermal injury to sigmoïd. *Obstet Gynecol* 1992;80:546

52. Creinin M, Chen M. Uterine defect in a twin pregnancy with a history of hysteroscopic fundal perforation. *Obstet Gynecol* 1992;79:879

53. Howe RS. Third-trimester uterine rupture following hysteroscopic uterine perforation. *Obstet Gynecol* 1993;81:827

54. Lobaugh ML, Bammel BM, Duke D, *et al.* Uterine rupture during pregnancy in a patient with history of hysteroscopic metroplasty. *Obstet Gynecol* 1994;83:838

55. Yaron Y, Shenhav M, Jaffa AJ, *et al.* Uterine rupture at 33 weeks' gestation subsequent to hysteroscopic uterine perforation. *Am J Obstet Gynecol* 1994;170:786

56. Gabriele A, Zanetta G, Pasta F, *et al.* Uterine rupture after hysteroscopic metroplasty and labor induction. A case report. *J Reprod Med* 1999;44:642

57. Tannous W, Hamou J, Henry-Suchet J, *et al.* Uterine rupture during labor following surgical hysteroscopy. *Presse Med* 1996;25:159

58. Mints M, Radestad A, Rylander E. Follow up of hysteroscopic surgery for menorrhagia. *Acta Obstet Gynecol Scand* 1998;77:435

59. Baumann R, Owerdiek W, Reck C. Schwangerschaft nach Sterilisation und Endometriumablation. *Gebürtshilfe Frauenheilkd* 1994;54:246

60. Hill DJ, Mahrer P. Pregnancy following endometrial ablation. *Gynaecol Endosc* 1992;1:47

61. Römer T, Campo R, Hucke J. Hämatometra nach hysteroskopischer Endometriumablation. *Zentralbl Gynäkol* 1995;5:278

62. Gannon MJ, Johnson N, Watters JK, *et al.* Haematometra–endometrial resection-sterilization syndrome. *Gynaecol Endosc* 1997;6:45

63. Tapper AM, Heinonen PK. Hysteroscopic endomyometrial resection for the treatment of menorrhagia – follow up of 86 cases. *Eur J Obstet Gynecol Reprod Biol* 1995;62:75

64. Bae IH, Pagedas AC, Perkins HE, *et al.* Postablation-tubal sterilization syndrome. *J Am Assoc Gynecol Laparosc* 1996;3:435

65. Webb JC, Bush MR, Wood D, *et al.* Hematosalpinx with pelvic pain after endometrial ablation confirms the postablation-tubal sterilization syndrome. *J Am Assoc Gynecol Laparosc* 1996;3:419

66. Townsend DE, McCausland V, *et al.* Post-ablation tubal sterilization syndrome. *Obstet Gynecol* 1993;3:422

A note on the medical artwork

the Editors would like to thank

Michèle Lemaire of St. Luc's University Hospital, Brussels, Belgium

for her outstanding work on the preparation of the

medical artwork in this Atlas

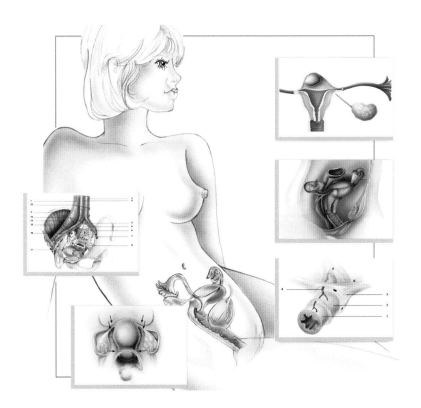

Index